T0325594

Ubiquitous Health and Medical Informatics:
The Ubiquity 2.0 Trend and Beyond

Sabah Mohammed
Lakehead University, Canada

Jinan Fiaidhi
Lakehead University, Canada

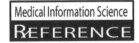

MEDICAL INFORMATION SCIENCE REFERENCE

Hershey · New York

Director of Editorial Content:	Kristin Klinger
Director of Book Publications:	Julia Mosemann
Acquisitions Editor:	Lindsay Johnston
Development Editor:	Julia Mosemann
Publishing Assistant:	Sean Woznicki
Typesetter:	Myla Harty
Production Editor:	Jamie Snavely
Cover Design:	Lisa Tosheff
Printed at:	Yurchak Printing Inc.

Published in the United States of America by
Medical Information Science Reference (an imprint of IGI Global)
701 E. Chocolate Avenue
Hershey PA 17033
Tel: 717-533-8845
Fax: 717-533-8661
E-mail: cust@igi-global.com
Web site: http://www.igi-global.com/reference

Copyright © 2010 by IGI Global. All rights reserved. No part of this publication may be reproduced, stored or distributed in any form or by any means, electronic or mechanical, including photocopying, without written permission from the publisher.

Product or company names used in this set are for identification purposes only. Inclusion of the names of the products or companies does not indicate a claim of ownership by IGI Global of the trademark or registered trademark.

Library of Congress Cataloging-in-Publication Data

Ubiquitous health and medical informatics : the ubiquity 2.0 trend and beyond
/ Sabah Mohammed and Jinan Fiaidhi, editors.
        p. ; cm.
  Includes bibliographical references and index.
  Summary: "This book is specific to the field of medical informatics and
ubiquitous health care and highlights the use of new trends based on the new
initiatives of Web 2.0"--Provided by publisher.
  ISBN 978-1-61520-777-0 (hardcover)
  1. Ubiquitous computing. 2. Medical informatics. I. Mohammed, Sabah, 1954-
II. Fiaidhi, Jinan, 1955-
  [DNLM: 1. Medical Informatics Applications. 2. Internet. 3. Telemedicine.
W 26.5 U15 2010]
  R859.7.U27U25 2010
  610.285--dc22
                        2010000388

British Cataloguing in Publication Data
A Cataloguing in Publication record for this book is available from the British Library.

All work contributed to this book is new, previously-unpublished material. The views expressed in this book are those of the authors, but not necessarily of the publisher.

Editorial Advisory Board

Sylvia Osborn, *University of Western Ontario, Canada*
Anand Ranganathan, *IBM TJ Watson Research Center, USA*
Rachid Benlamri, *Lakehead University, Canada*
Richard Khoury, *Lakehead University, Canada*
Waldemar Koczkodaj, *Laurentian University, Canada*
Robert Istepanian, *Kinsigton University, UK*

List of Reviewers

Dominic Covvey, *University of Waterloo, Canada*
Charles Jaffe, *Health Level Seven (HL7), USA*
Kim Solez, *University of Alberta, Canada*
Neil Coulson, *University of Nottingham, UK*
Soraya Kouadri Mostéfaoui, *Open University, UK*
Nilmini Wickramasinghe, *Illinois Institute of Technology, USA*
Raymond Leduc, *University of Western Ontario, Canada*
Wane Menary, *Geopac Inc., UK*
Elske Ammenwerth, *University for Health Sciences, Austria*
Mohammad Ikram, *Ajou University, Rep. of Korea*
Vivian Vimarlund, *Linköping University, Sweden*
Ritu Tiwari, *ABV-IIITM Gwalior, India*
Poh Hean Yap, *Deakin University, Australia*
Ivan Karljevski, *FON University, Republic of Macedonia*
Rachid Benlamri, *Lakehead University, Canada*
Sime Arsenovski, *European University, Republic of Macedonia*
Mikel Laurea Alava, *UPV/EHU, Spain*
Vahideh Zarea Gavgani, *Osmania University, India*
Vinod Scaria, *Institute of Genomics and Integrative Biology, India*

Table of Contents

Section 1
Background

Chapter 1

Sabah Mohammed, Lakehead University, Canada
Jinan Fiaidhi, Lakehead University, Canada

Section 2
Research Issues

Chapter 2

W. Ed Hammond, Duke University, USA

Chapter 3

Simon Y. Liu, National Library of Medicine, USA

Chapter 4

Jun Hu, University of Ottawa, Canada
Liam Peyton, University of Ottawa, Canada

Section 3
Management Issues

Section 4
Applications

Section 5
The Future

Detailed Table of Contents

Section 1
Background

Chapter 1

Sabah Mohammed, Lakehead University, Canada
Jinan Fiaidhi, Lakehead University, Canada

This chapter introduced the concept of ubiquity 2.0 trend as the roadmap for e-health improvements and differentiated it from the traditional ubiquity trend or what is called ubiquity 1.0. The ubiquity 2.0 trend is an evolving concept for achieving interoperability based on the new and emerging technologies like ubiquitous computing, Web 2.0, Web-Oriented Architectures and cloud computing. This chapter also highlights the security challenges and the emerging web-oriented identity management technologies to provide a single, common user credential that is trusted, secure, and widely supported across the Web and among various healthcare enterprises.

Section 2
Research Issues

Chapter 2

W. Ed Hammond, Duke University, USA

This chapter argues that the semantic interoperability is the key to achieving global interoperability in healthcare information technology. The benefits are tremendous, however, there are many barriers to achieving semantic interoperability. Key among these is the resolution of the many issues relating to the terminologies used in defining, describing and documenting healthcare. The terminologies conflict and overlap; the granularity is not sufficiently rich for direct clinical use; there are gaps that prevent an exhaustive set; there are major variances in cost and accessibility; and no one appears eager or willing to make the ultimate decisions required to solve the problem. This chapter defines and describes the purpose and characteristics of the major terminologies in use in healthcare today. Terminology sets are compared in purpose, form and content. Finally a proposed solution is presented based on a global master metadictionary of data elements with a rich set of attributes including names that may come from existing controlled terminologies, precise definitions to remove ambiguity in use, and complete value sets of possible values. The focus is on data elements because data elements are the basic unit of data interchange.

Chapter 3

Simon Y. Liu, National Library of Medicine, USA

This chapter suggests the open source solution as a valid solution for patient personal health records interoperability. A Personal Health Record (PHR) is a private and secure digital record that is created, managed, and owned by an individual, and contains the owner's relevant health information. The benefits of PHRs have not yet been widely realized due to several significant challenges in their adoption, including the need for privacy, security, and interoperability, and the lack of accepted standards. Although many players in the healthcare arena are beginning to offer partial solutions, none have adequately addressed the full range of challenges. The adoption of PHRs can be significantly accelerated by the development of Open Source software that enables an individual to collect, create, organize, and manage his or her own private and secure PHR, using a standardized format and controlled vocabulary.

Chapter 4

Jun Hu, University of Ottawa, Canada
Liam Peyton, University of Ottawa, Canada

This chapter argues that knowledge discovery is a critical component in improving healthcare. There are a number of issues which must be addressed before knowledge discovery can be leveraged effectively and ubiquitously in Health 2.0. Health care data is very sensitive in nature so privacy and security of personal data must be protected. Regulatory compliance must also be addressed if cooperative sharing of data is to be facilitated to ensure that relevant legislation and policies of individual health care organizations are respected. Finally, interoperability and data quality must be addressed in any framework for knowledge discovery on the Internet. In this chapter, we lay out a framework for ubiquitous knowledge discovery in Health 2.0 based on a combination of architecture and process. Emerging Internet standards and specifications for defining a Circle of Trust, in which data is shared but identity and personal information are protected, are used to define an enabling architecture for knowledge discovery. Within that context, a step-by- step process for knowledge discovery is defined and illustrated using a scenario related to analyzing the correlation between emergency room visits and adverse effects of prescription drugs. The process we define is arrived at by reviewing an existing standards-based process, CRISP-DM, and extending it to address the new context of Health 2.0.

In this chapter a social network is described, where users can formulate healthcare questions that are automatically classified under concepts of a medical ontology and assigned to experts of each topic. These questions are then answered by healthcare expert physicians. Our proposal includes a semantic classification method that provides the automatic classification of questions by means of a medical ontology, based on the tags used to annotate them, and the previously classified questions. The proposal includes an ontological model that represents the questions, the assigned tags, the answers, the physicians, and the medical concepts.

This chapter presents an overview of an integrated system for eMedicine that is implemented in the Republic of Macedonia. The system contains advanced medical information systems, various telemedicine services supported by modern telecommunication technologies, and decision support modules. The telemedicine services use wireless broadband technologies (WiMAX, 3G, Wi-Fi). A significant part of the chapter presents a web based medical expert system that performs self training using a heuristic rule induction algorithm. The data inserted by medical personnel while using the e-medicine system is subsequently used for additional learning. The system is trained using a hybrid heuristic algorithm for induction of classification rules that we developed. The SA Tabu Miner algorithm (Simulated Annealing and Tabu Search based Data Miner) is inspired by both research on heuristic optimization algorithms and rule induction data mining concepts and principles.

Chapter 7

This chapter elaborates on the potential of Web 2.0 for active and, potentially, effective learning in medicine and in health and reviews current practices and emerging advances in the field. Discussion focuses on current and emerging applications that fully exploit the potential of Web 2.0. Finally, the envisaged merit of merging with Web 3.0 technologies is also discussed.

Chapter 8

This chapter analyzes the relevant medicinal instructions such as medicinal learning objects and considers three complementary ways for the dissemination of medicinal instructions: (i) by providing keyword-based searching, (ii) by providing ontology-based searching, and (iii) by automatic integration of medicinal instructions to employers´ day-to-day work tasks. The integration can be based either on the similarity of the metadata descriptions of the tasks and learning objects, or on the ontology which specifies the relationships of the tasks and instructions. The authors argue that integration is most preferable as medicinal instructions are provided just-in-time and tailored to their specific needs.

Chapter 9

This chapter explores the essential issues of ubiquitous health information (UHI), beginning with its origins in the explosion of health information and the advent of new technologies. Challenges of UHI include privacy issues, change management, and the lack of basic infrastructure. However, benefits for patients include improvements in access to information, communication with providers, prescription renewals, medication tracking, and the ability to self-manage their conditions. Benefits at the organizational level include increased patient satisfaction, continuity of care, changes in costing models and improved standardization of care as organizations streamline processes to address this change in clinical practice.

Chapter 10

This chapter highlights the role of grid computing as the basic architecture for supporting enterprise healthcare applications through offering massive resources through collaborative framework that is offering power computing, storage devices, and services. Grid computing along with Web 2.0 technologies provides a robust model for deploying, discovering, invoking, and integrating resources in open standard format. This chapter proposes a Service Oriented Architecture (SOA) as a model for managing the mixing between Web 2.0 and grid computing technologies. SOA for Web 2.0 and Grid Computing (SOAW2G) are used throughout this chapter to offer a fabric for e-health applications.

Chapter 11

Daniel Ruiz Fernández, University of Alicante, Spain

The chapter introduces a multi-agent architecture as a framework for the implementation of healthcare decentralization. It is intended to provide the capability to implement a global distribution of healthcare, even reaching the patient's home, workplace or holiday hotel. This is a distributed architecture which is flexible to implement new functionalities and accessible from anywhere. The architecture defines different types of agents and their interactions.

Chapter 12

Mahmood Tara, Mashad University of Medical Sciences, Iran

This chapter is aimed at introducing the Semantic Web and Web Services Architectures for e-health users and professionals. In particular, the chapter focuses on the current and prospective (or practical and potential) contributions of the Semantic Web technologies in providing e-Health content and services to its potential users worldwide.

Section 3
Management Issues

Chapter 13

Christo El Morr, York University, Canada

This chapter explores the ways in which mobility within virtual communities can play an important role in facing the current and future healthcare challenges. The chapter suggests that mobile VCs (MVCs) can help patients with chronic disease to self-manage their health. The chapter shows the many advantages of this approach, particularly in terms of enhanced healthcare delivery and reduced healthcare cost, also the chapter discusses the challenges that this approach faces.

Chapter 14

Christian Stingl, Carinthia University of Applied Sciences, Austria
Daniel Slamanig, Carinthia University of Applied Sciences, Austria

This chapter provides a security analysis of Electronic Healthcare Records (EHR) systems and discuss the basic and enhanced security requirements and finally introduces levels of security to classify EHR systems.

Chapter 15

This chapter presents a privacy-based multi-agent brokering architecture that supports different privacy degrees. Unlike traditional approaches, the brokering is viewed as a set of services in which the brokering role is further classified into several sub-roles each with a specific architecture and interaction protocol that is appropriate to support a required privacy degree. To put the formulation in practice, a prototype of the proposed architecture has been implemented to support information-gathering capabilities in healthcare environments using FIPA complaint platform (JADE).

This chapter aims to critically examine the issues associated with use of Web 2.0 technologies in healthcare. The chapter concludes that Web 2.0 will enhance e-Health applications and provides an improved management from a policy perspective.

This chapter describes approaches taken and lessons learned while developing the informatics infrastructure to support interprofessional practice at with the Northern Ontario School of Medicine. Moreover, it describes how common procedures and software tools can benefit from a Web 2.0 approach, comparing commercial and open-source aspects of possible solutions.

Section 4
Applications

This chapter describes the technological challenges faced during the design and implementation of the K4Care system, an agent-based Web-accessible platform that helps medical practitioners to deliver Home Care services in an efficient way. The system incorporates a Knowledge Layer, with an explicit representation of the required medico-organizational knowledge. The administrative and care actions are performed by the coordinated operation of intelligent agents, that represent the human users of the system. Users can access the platform by means of a Web interface. Several Web 2.0 technologies have been used in order to provide a rich interaction, putting special care on connecting the Web browser with the multi-agent system in an efficient manner. An intermediate Data Abstraction Layer has been incorporated in order to allow agents to transparently retrieve the appropriate knowledge when needed. The separation of the knowledge from its actual use has allowed the development of a very dynamic, flexible and adaptable system. The platform also includes several techniques to personalize the interaction with the user both from the visual and functional points of view

This chapter provides a basic overview of care process management and active patient engagement principles. It builds upon these principles to describe in more detail the way information and communication technology can provide support for these activities. It later discusses effects on cost efficiency and quality of care. The authors specify care models suitable for ICT support, specific process support characteristics related to health care, standards and communication devices to be used to work with these environments. For practical purposes the chapter provides a description of development and implementation of such an environment to support treatment of patients with depression.

This chapter introduces a virtual reality approach for building virtual communities for health promotion using Second Life. Such approach allows health educators, researchers, and practitioners (ERPs) to engage students, participants, and patients through innovative and uniquely rewarding methods. The technology's value lies in its access to non-traditional participant pools, novel forms of social interaction, and cost-effective improvements to existing methods. These benefits are built on key Web 2.0 principles, namely social networking, community synthesis, and collaborative content generation. In light of ongoing dynamic development of virtual platforms, advancements in networking and immersion technology, and sustained consumer interest, the appeal of these environments will likely increase. Linden Lab's Second Life (SL), a widely recognized and heavily populated MUVE, illustrates the technology's broad spectrum of possibilities through the documented efforts of early adopters involved in health promotion, research, and therapy. However, ERPs must be mindful of the medium's complexities, technological and social parameters, and weaknesses before considering development within virtual worlds (in-world). As these environments operate independently of the real world in some aspects, knowledge of gathering and creating relevant in-world and real-world resources, attracting and retaining project interest, and addressing common obstacles is essential. Through an analysis of the Texas Obesity Research Center at the University of Houston's International Health Challenge in SL and the documented findings of past and existing health-related programs in SL, we seek to provide best practices to overcome these challenges and establish realistic parameters for program design and implementation.

Chapter 21

This chapter discusses the features needed to incorporate the Computer Supported Collaborative Work (CSCW) for e-health applications (e.g. dynamic creation of medical virtual teams, dynamic workflows and the automatic triggered events upon time expiration). In this respect and having in mind the new Web 2.0 characteristics, a set of new features applied to the proposed system (DITIS). Furthermore, an extensive evaluation of the system is presented, supporting the need for such enhancement.

Chapter 22

This chapter introduces a method for integrating Digital pathology and Virtual Microscopy at the format of the Electronic Healthcare Records. Digital pathology allows information sharing for diagnosis, biomedical research and education. It follows the previous efforts made in radiology and clinical laboratory. Virtual microscopy resulting in digital slides is an outreaching technology that is facilitating the shift to digital in anatomic pathology. Limiting factors in the expansion of virtual microscopy are formidable storage dimension, scanning speed, quality of image and cultural change. Anatomic pathology data and images should be an important part of the patient electronic health records as well as of clinical data warehouses, epidemiological or biomedical research databases and platforms dedicated to translational medicine Integrating anatomic pathology to the "healthcare enterprise" can only be achieved using existing and emerging medical informatics like Digital Imaging and Communications in Medicine (DICOM), Health Level Seven (HL7), and Systematized Nomenclature of Medicine-Clinical Terms (SNOMED CT), following the recommendations of Integrating the Healthcare Enterprise (IHE) Anatomic Pathology technical framework.

Chapter 23

This chapter reviews recent advances in Content-based image retrieval (CBIR) technology and discusses its expanding role in medical imaging and its particular application to mammography, provides working examples, and highlights the potential opportunities in this field for computer vision research and clinical decision making.

Chapter 24

    Ivica Dimitrovski, Ss. Cyril and Methodius University in Skopje, Macedonia
    Suzana Loskovska, Ss. Cyril and Methodius University in Skopje, Macedonia

This chapter aims to develop highly flexible web-based system for storage, organization and retrieval of medical images. The developed system besides text and metadata retrieval also supports querying by image to find visually similar images to presented query. Several algorithms and techniques were implemented in the system to support content based retrieval. For efficient and reliable search machine learning techniques were included in the system.

Chapter 25

    Alessandra Gorini, Istituto Auxologico Italiano, Italy
    Andrea Gaggioli, Istituto Auxologico Italiano, Italy
    Giuseppe Riva, Istituto Auxologico Italiano, Italy

This chapter illustrates the past and the future of different virtual reality applications for the treatment of psychological disorders. After a brief technical description of the virtual reality systems, the rationale of using virtual reality to treat different psychological disorders, as well as the advantages that the online virtual worlds offer to the promising field of the virtual therapy will be discussed. Finally, the chapter introduces "Interreality", a personalized immersive e-therapy whose main novelty is a hybrid, closed-loop empowering experience bridging the physical and virtual worlds. The main feature of interreality is a twofold link between the virtual and the real world: (a) behaviour in the physical world influences the experience in the virtual one; (b) behaviour in the virtual world influences the experience in the real one. This is achieved through: (1) 3D Shared Virtual Worlds; (2) Bio and Activity Sensors (From the Real to the Virtual World; (3) Mobile Internet Appliances (From the Virtual to the Real One).

Chapter 26

    Elizabeth M. Borycki, University of Victoria, Canada
    Andre W. Kushniruk, University of Victoria, Canada

This chapter describes an approach to applying clinical simulations to evaluate the impact of health information systems and ubiquitous computing devices on health professional work. The approach allows for an assessment of "cognitive-socio-technical fit" and the ability to modify and improve systems and devices before they are released into widespread use. The application of realistic clinical simulations is detailed, including the stages of development of such simulations (from creation of representative clinical environments to subject selection and data collection approaches). In order to ensure the success and widespread adoption of ubiquitous computing devices (UCD) it is argued that greater emphasis will need to be placed on ensuring such systems and devices have a high degree of fit with user's cognitive and work processes.

This chapter introduces the uses of technology in human resource management and how it can help improve the medical care that health professionals provide to their patients. For instance, technology can be used to maximize communication, collaboration and support between health professionals separated by distance, as well as provide immediate and up-to-date patient care information. ICT can also be used for distance training and education for those facing geographic isolation and provide a medium through which continued education can be maintained for both rural and urban health professionals. However, due to the differences in barriers of ICT use found for each group, such as computer illiteracy, geographic isolation or poor infrastructure, different steps need to be taken in order to ensure the successful implementation and use of information technologies in both urban and rural communities in developed and developing regions across the world.

Section 5
The Future

This chapter introduces an interoperability framework as a solution for the challenges facing e-health communities. The proposed interoperability framework identifies citizens, providers, policy makers and researchers. This framework is developed and related to the improvement of understanding, access, trust, discourse, and practice for the purpose of moving toward a high performing healthcare system. Web 2.0 offers great promise as an eHealth platform to synergistically catalyze significant improvements to healthcare delivery, however, caution is advised about uncritical adoption. Barriers to progress and opportunities for advancement are identified and questions for future research are posited.

Foreword

With this edited volume, IGI Global continues its tradition of publishing high quality titles that address the range of current issues in information technology utilization and management that arise in today's knowledge society. This book, edited by researchers with well-established credentials in ubiquitous systems, computer science, and medical informatics, includes contributions from a number of scholars on a wide range of topics that are relevant to the complex considerations of ubiquitous eHealth/ medical informatics. These topics touch on many issues of burning interest to the healthcare community, as the search continues for innovative ways in which healthcare quality can be improved, while at the same time realizing benefits to healthcare provider productivity and effectiveness.

It is difficult to over-emphasize the complexities involved in providing healthcare. Many of the issues to be addressed are non-technical and they interact in many ways with technical solutions, requiring careful consideration of these interactions. The reader will find in this book a good indication of the strong multidisciplinary links that result among computer and communications engineering, computer science, the health disciplines, business, and social sciences that support eHealth. When it comes to developing innovative and lasting contributions to this field, it is essential to take into account the broad scope of the underpinnings of this research.

There is a large disparity among nations in the ubiquity, depth, and expenditures, and the technology supporting healthcare, ranging from the most advanced, in Europe, to nations that still are building an appropriate infrastructure (U.S. and Canada), to developing nations such as China and India that have islands of expertise, but are far from offering ubiquitous health to their populations, to the many less developed nations. Each nation faces questions of cost, infrastructure, privacy, network infrastructure, adoption by the healthcare community, and embedded cultural beliefs in the appropriate levels of healthcare to be offered. Developing nations in particular are moving ahead rapidly with communications systems that use wireless systems to leapfrog over the fixed landline systems typical of Western nations.

We are becoming accustomed to the rapid developments in Web 2.0, the second generation of Web development and design. This has grown out of cumulative changes in how developers and end-user utilize the Web to facilitate information sharing and collaboration. Web 2.0 includes the development and evolution of Web-based communities, hosted services, and Web applications such as social networking, video-sharing, wikis (websites using wiki software for the creation and editing of interlinked Web pages using a simplified markup language to create collaborative websites, community websites, and note taking); blogs (weblogs -a type of website, containing regular commentaries, event descriptions, or other material, often allowing comments by readers); mashups (Web pages or applications that combine data or functionality from two or more external sources to create a new service, using open APIs and data sources); and folksonomies (non-hierarchical classifications generated by user-based tagging). Investments in Web 2.0 eHealth applications are becoming increasingly significant, in a way that is distinguished from previous eHealth trends. This technology has a value in its access by non-traditional participants, novel forms of social interaction, and cost-effective improvements to existing methods through social networking, community synthesis, and collaborative content generation.

Ubiquity is the property of being everywhere at once. As you will see in Chapter 1, the first generation of ubiquity, dubbed Ubiquity 1.0, is supported by the widespread adoption of XML in both syntactic and semantic communication layers, thus enhancing interoperability among heterogeneous systems. Heterogeneous systems are a characteristic of the role that eHealth plays in the healthcare system, so interoperability is essential for eHealth ubiquity. Ubiquity 2.0 derives from Web 2.0 tools and all the innovations it has generated, to enable better support that can empower both providers and consumers of healthcare. However, the specialized and innovative applications that are supported by these tools require a substantial rethinking of how they can be implemented ubiquitously. Hence the reason for this volume, which explores many of the relevant research and management issues, and demonstrates some relevant applications. The following touches briefly on the flavor of many of the works that are presented.

Interoperability is one of the most important aspects of ubiquitous solutions, since healthcare is characterized by multiple heterogeneous systems that may not support access to all the relevant information about a patient in one view within the network. Lack of interoperability in turn causes issues with continuity of care, safety, and the assessment of program delivery. An appropriate interoperability framework will lead to an improvement in understanding of the need to move towards a high performing healthcare system that can make use of some of the Web 2.0 methodologies and tools. The semantic Web, related common languages, and semantic Web services architectures that are upgrades to existing physical architectures can help provide eHealth content and services to users. Semantic interoperability that allows clinical data sharing to multiple users, with the potential for improved patient safety, better healthcare, improved outcomes, and higher quality of life may result. Before this can be achieved, there are many issues relating to terminologies that define, describe, and document healthcare. One way these can be addressed is through terminology sets with a global master meta-dictionary of data elements that have precise definitions to remove ambiguity in use.

To move towards a secure and trusted network that manages patient health record identity and ensures patient privacy is a major challenge. Ensuring patient privacy has been found to be one of the most critical factors of system success. Thus, care for the security of the health record system must always be considered, including both basic and enhanced security methods that balance privacy needs with the need for access to the system by the patient's circle of care. One way of providing the needed privacy is through a multi-agent brokering architecture that supports different degrees of privacy. Implementing new functionalities that are accessible anywhere may be supported through different types and classes of agents through a flexible distributed architecture. Experimental agent-based applications have been designed and tested to help medical practitioners deliver home care services securely and efficiently.

To ensure an affordable healthcare system, it is necessary to move towards ubiquitous patient-centered and self-managed care. This provides patient empowerment through private personal health records (PHRs) with access that is under the control of patients themselves. Development and adoption of PHRs can be accelerated by the development of open source software that uses a standardized format and controlled vocabulary. The resulting benefits for patients include improved access to information, communication with providers, medication tracking, prescription renewals, and so on. Organizational benefits include improved patient satisfaction, continuity of care, improved standardization of care, and improved costing models. However, there are many challenges before such advantages can be realized, including privacy issues, change management issues among providers and patients, and the lack of suitable support infrastructures.

Advances in interoperable systems that support access to relevant patient health records from all available sources also create opportunities for ubiquitous knowledge discovery that monitors, analyzes, and manages the health of individual patients, and potentially to enhance public health management in the face of epidemiological threats. Such knowledge discovery requires a well-crafted architecture for the patient's circle of trust that shares data while protecting identity and personal information. Knowledge discovery and management has also been used in supporting dynamic learning capabilities in telemedicine. Lifelong learning in the healthcare sector requires specialized knowledge that must be renewed frequently. The dissemination of updated medication information can be supported by keyword search, ontology-based search, and by automatic integration of instructions into regular daily tasks. An integrated system is preferable since updates are just-in-time and tailored to the specific needs of users.

Human resources management (HRM) organizations are typically responsible for employee training. As innovation continues at a rapid pace, training medical personnel can directly support the provision of superior care. Technology can maximize communication, collaboration, and support among professionals separated by distance and at the same time be used for distance training and continuing education for geographically isolated individuals. Healthcare specialists working in remote areas face many challenges that can be addressed by Computer Supported Collaborative Work (CSCW) wireless technologies that are adapted to suit medical applications. Mobile technologies can be used to develop virtual communities to help patients to self-manage chronic diseases, typically enhancing healthcare delivery at a reduced cost. Common procedures and software tools can benefit from Web 2.0, with ubiquitous remote data access for point of care decision making supported by integrating Web services, mobile devices, and multi-stream communications. Web 2.0 social networks provide a wide range of possibilities in eHealth, offering many research opportunities. These include the formulation of healthcare questions by users that can be automatically classified semantically through medical ontologies, for answers by expert physicians.

Computer architectures can support many innovations in treatment. For example, psychological disorders can be addressed through virtual online worlds that link the virtual and the real world, taking care at the same time to protect against the risks of privacy and personal safety. Care process management can describe the way information and communication can support active patient management principles, with positive effects on cost efficiency and quality of care, applied for example to an environment to support treatment of patients with depression. Clinical simulation is a tool that can be used to assess issues of information, workflow, and cognitive needs arising from proposed ubiquitous computing devices and to evaluate their impact on supporting systems and the work of health professionals.

One class of diagnostic tools involves the generation of digital images. The current trend is towards tools that generate far more high quality images (e.g. Magnetic Resonance Imaging or MRI machines) than were thought possible just a few years ago. The flood of such images has created an overwhelming load on radiologists who must read and interpret these images. The trend is towards regionalized image repositories that can be accessed, queried, and/or matched by physicians or radiologists for first or second opinions through remote high speed links, and the use of computerized detection and diagnosis of lesions (e.g. mammography), involving applications of machine learning, computer vision, and clinical decision support. Digital pathology is closely related to these technologies, through the use of virtual microscopy and digital slides. Grid computing is one solution for the massive computing power needed to support the collaborative computing environment resulting from the growing overlay of Web 2.0 technologies on healthcare architectures. At the same time, high data quality and security, computing resource availability and reliability in an open source format can be best provided by Service Oriented Architectures (SOA).

Healthcare reforms are urgently needed to address the rising costs of providing quality healthcare to aging populations. These reforms must consider how to overcome barriers linked to historical processes that have not used interoperable and collaborative information technology solutions effectively. Ubiquitous eHealth, with its Web 2.0 innovations, has great promise in catalyzing significant improvements that will help overcome the deficits in healthcare delivery.

Norm Archer
McMaster University, Canada

Norm Archer, *Ph.D. is a Professor Emeritus in the DeGroote School of Business, McMaster University, Canada, and a Special Advisor to the McMaster eBusiness Research Centre. Norm and his graduate students and colleagues are intensively involved in studies of the adoption and use of electronic health records in Canada, identity theft and fraud, and a range of eBusiness issues.*

Preface

Progress in ubiquitous computing, social networking, medical informatics and IT technologies is bringing healthcare a new generation of systems, which we term as the ubiquity 2.0 trend systems. Before embarking on a discussion of the concepts contributing to the ubiquity 2.0 trend and its effects on e-health, it is important to consider the drivers, reasons, and challenges behind such an innovative shift in healthcare. Some of challenges are common as they accompany any healthcare enhancement project such as:

- Enhancement of Quality of Care
- Providing Patient Safety
- Reducing the Delivery of Cost of Care
- Comprehensive Availability and Ubiquity
- Empowerment of e-health Providers and
- Synchronization of Content and Application Development
- Integration of e-health Segments
- Providing Context-Awareness
- Encouraging New Types of Collaborations
- Enhancing the Continuity and Coverage of Care
- Supporting Sound Research and Education

Other challenges involve the healthcare of the aging population. For example, in the United States alone, the number of people over age 65 is expected to hit 70 million by 2030, doubling from 35 million in 2000, and similar increases are expected worldwide. Moreover, many elderly people suffer from chronic diseases that require medication and clinic visits on a regular basis. The cost of the healthcare is a growing problem and challenge, too. For example, United States expenditures for healthcare make up about 16% of the US GDP (Center for Medicare and Medicaid Services, 2008), as a result of the accumulative impact of chronic degenerative diseases in the elderly and their increasing dependence on the healthcare system. Many other factors may also be added to the list of challenges, including preference of home and self care over traditional hospital care and cost advantages associated with home and self care. The ubiquitous health market is expected to attain significantly high growth in future. The next generation of networked medical devices and health management systems are envisioned to be ubiquitous networked systems for secure, reliable, privacy-preserving, cost-effective and personalized quality healthcare. This would lead not only to better healthcare delivery, but also to improving people's quality of life in general. This vision requires an innovative IT infrastructure on the Internet that encourages collaboration, flexibility and integration. The ubiquity 2.0 trend is based on such vision. An important concept in ubiquity 2.0 is that Web-based software should offer its functionality not only via the browser, but also as open Web services so that it can be mashed up in new and unintended ways. This will allow for sharing and reusing functionality and contents anywhere in a loosely-coupled and interoperable way. The ubiquity 2.0 Web services are different from traditional Web service technologies as they use simpler and more straightforward methods that *just work* and hide the protocol complexity in the application state. Essentially, the ubiquity 2.0 Web services utilize lightweight protocols like HTTP and JSON for Web service interoperability. This means that the ubiquity 2.0 supports only the REST type of Web services along with JSON (JavaScript Object Notation) instead of XML. The ubiquity 2.0 trend is also about consumer empowerment by interactively delivering what they need and thus greatly reducing their workload, time and effort spent on targeted actions performance. Moreover, the ubiquity 2.0 simplifies the highly complex processes, saves bandwidth and performs considerably faster than traditional Web applications, thus escalating customers' online interaction with the e-health websites or portals. The ubiquity 2.0 healthcare environment is about the hyper connectivity collaboration environment that involves Ubiquitous Computing (Kumar, S., Kambhatla, K., Hu, F., Lifson, M., & Xiao, Y., 2008), Web 2.0 (Karkalis, G. I., & Koutsouris, D. D., 2006), Web 3.0 (Giustini, D., 2007), Web-Oriented Architectures (Hinchcliffe, D., 2006, April 1), Cloud Computing (Wikipedia, n.d.) and Medical Informatics (Wikipedia, n.d.) technologies. Intuitively, the ubiquity 2.0 trend highlights the changes to healthcare distribution via the Internet that will significantly impact on the value exchange occurring between a health provider and consumer.

ORGANIZATION OF THE BOOK

With the obvious global need for understanding in this evolving area, this book provides a valuable insight into the various trends, innovations, and organizational challenges of contemporary ubiquitous health and medical informatics. The interest in this area was quite obvious in that we were overwhelmed with expressions of interest to submit chapters. We have managed to carefully select the most appropriate of these but, in doing so, left out many almost as deserving. All contributions underwent a double blind review process in order to ensure academic rigor. Readers can therefore be assured that only the very highest qualities of contributions were accepted for the final publication.

The book contains 28 chapters, split into five sections; the first contains one chapter dedicated to introduce the concept of ubiquity 2.0 trend. The second section is comprised of chapters that discuss some of the research issues related to the ubiquity of healthcare. The third section describes healthcare management and organizational issues. The fourth section provides a good mix of clinical and healthcare applications. The final section contains one chapter that is dedicated for introducing a future vision for e-health interoperability.

Section 1: Background

This section includes one chapter by the editors which provides a roadmap solution based on the emerging Web technologies that hold great promise for addressing the various challenges facing e-health. The roadmap is termed as the "ubiquity 2.0 trend." This chapter also highlights the security challenges and the emerging Web-oriented identity management technologies to provide a single, common user credential that is trusted, secure, and widely supported across the Web and within the healthcare enterprises.

Section 2: Research Issues

This section includes eleven chapters. William Hammond begins this section by examining the issue of standardizing medical vocabularies. The next chapter by Simon Liu discusses the issue of using the open source approach for personal healthcare records. Chapter 4 is by Jun Hu and Liam Peyton and provides a framework of knowledge discovery for Health 2.0 collaborative and ubiquitous environments. Chapter 5 is by Fracisco Echart et. al., where they provide a semantic model to address health queries to professionals in a healthcare social networking environment. Chapter 6 is by Ivan Chorbev and Boban Joksimoski, where they provide a vision for producing an integrated e-medical system. Chapter 7 by Eleni Kaldoudi et. al. introduces Web 2.0 based collaborative approaches for health and medical learning. Chapter 8 is by Juha Puustjärvi and Leena Puustjärvi, which provides a research vision on integrating medical learning objects for lifelong learning. Chapter 9 is by David Wiljer, Sara Urowitz and Erin Jones, where they provide a vision on treating personal health information for the age of ubiquitous health. Chapter 10 is by Wail Omar, who introduced an ontological approach for dealing with a Web 2.0 Service-Oriented healthcare system. Chapter 11 is by Daniel Ruiz Fernández, who provides an agent-based architecture for modeling ubiquitous healthcare systems. Finally, chapter 12 is by Mahmood Tara, who examined the paradigm of Semantic Web and its suitability providing ubiquitous contents and services.

Section 3: Management Issues

This section contains five chapters. In chapter 13, Christo El-Morr introduces his mobile virtual communities' model for the management of ubiquitous health. The next chapter is by Christian Stingl and Daniel Slamanig, where they introduced a privacy enhancing technology as a solution for sharing electronic healthcare records. The following chapter is by AbdulMutalib Masaud Wahaishi and Hamada Ghenniwa, where they introduced a Multi-agent Brokering Architecture for Privacy enforcement of Ubiquitous Healthcare Systems. Chapter 16 is by Benjamin Hughes, who evaluated the impact of Web 2.0 on managing e-health systems. The final chapter of this section is by David Topps, who provided a vision on managing academic family health teams.

Section 4: Applications

This section contains ten chapters providing very interesting healthcare application. The first chapter of this section is by David Isern et. al., where they provided the K4Care agent-based Web-accessible platform that helps medical practitioners to deliver Home Care services. Chapter 19 chapter introduces a case study for treating depression for integrated care management. The following chapter is by Sameer Siddiqi and Rebecca E. Lee, where they employed virtual reality via Second Life to build virtual communities for health promotion. The following chapter is by Dimosthenis Georgiadis et. al., where they analyzed the virtual communities in the wireless e-health environment. The next chapter is by Marcial Rojo, who provided a digital pathology virtual microscopy for Integration in eHealth records. Chapter 23 is by Issam El Naqa, Liyang Wei and Yongyi Yang, where they introduced content-based image retrieval for searching for digital mammography repository. The next chapter is by Ivica Dimitrovski and Suzana Loskovska, where they used content image retrieval for features evaluation and classifications of medical images. The following chapter is by Alessandra Gorini, Andrea Gaggioli and Giuseppe Riva, where they experimented with virtual reality as a method for psychological interventions. Chapter 26 is by Elizabeth M. Borycki and Andre W. Kushniruk, where they examined the use of clinical simulations and their impacts on ubiquitous health. The last chapter in this section is by Stefane Kabene and Candace Gibson, where they examined the use of technology and human resource management in the future of e-health.

Section 5: The Future

This section contains one chapter by Donald W. M. Juzwishin, who introduced a future vision for a challenging framework to enable e-health interoperability.

REFERENCES

Centers for Medicare and Medicaid Services (2008, January). *National Health Expenditure Projections 2007-2017, National Health Expenditures (NHE)*. Retrieved from http://www.cms.hhs.gov/National-HealthExpendData/Downloads/proj2007.pdf

Kumar, S., Kambhatla, K., Hu, F., Lifson, M., & Xiao, Y. (2008). Ubiquitous Computing for Remote Cardiac Patient Monitoring: A Survey. *Int J Telemed Appl., 2008*; 2008. Retrieved from http://www.pubmedcentral.nih.gov/articlerender.fcgi?artid=2442250

Karkalis, G. I., & Koutsouris, D. D. (2006). *E-health and the Web 2.0*. Paper presented at the ITAB 2006 Int. Conference, Ioannina - Epirus, Greece, October 26-28, 2006.

Giustini, D. (2007). Web 3.0 and medicine: Make way for the semantic web. *BMJ*, 335, 1273-1274.

Hinchcliffe, D. (2006, April 1). The SOA with reach: Web-Oriented Architecture. ZDNet Blog. Retrieved from http://blogs.zdnet.com/Hinchcliffe/?p=27

Wikipedia (n.d.). Cloud Computing. Retrieved from http://en.wikipedia.org/wiki/Cloud_computing

Wikipedia (n.d.). Health Informatics. Retrieved from http://en.wikipedia.org/wiki/Health_informatics

Acknowledgment

This book has been an interesting, emotional, and intellectual journey for both of us. Many people helped during the process of writing and editing this book; it is impossible to keep track of them all. To all that we have forgotten to list, please don't hold it against us! First and foremost, we need to thank Dr. Maurice Benson, the chair of Computer Science at Lakehead University, for his kind encouragement and support. We would also like to thank IGI Global for their forms of assistance. The editors extend a special thanks to many external reviewers whose thoughtful comments improved this book and whose enthusiasm for the book was very welcome. The list of external reviewers includes: Dr. Dominic Covvey (Director of Waterloo Institute for Health Informatics Research, University of Waterloo, Canada), Dr. Charles Jaffe (CEO of Health Level Seven (HL7), USA), Dr. Kim Solez (Director of Experimental Pathology as well as Director of NKF cyberNephrology, University of Alberta, Canada), Dr. Neil Coulson (Institute of Work Health & Organisations, University of Nottingham, UK), Dr. Soraya Kouadri Mostéfaoui (Open University, UK), Dr. Nilmini Wickramasinghe (Director Center for the Management of Medical Technology, Illinois Institute of Technology, USA), Raymond Leduc (University of Western Ontario, Canada), Dr. Wane Menary (Director of Geopac Inc., UK), Dr. Elske Ammenwerth (Director of the Institute for Health Information Systems, University for Health Sciences, Austria), Mohammad Ikram (Muhammad Ikram, Information Communication & Security Lab - Ajou University, Rep. of Korea), Dr. Vivian Vimarlund (Dept. of Computer and Information Science, Linköping University, Sweden), Dr. Ritu Tiwari (Dept. of Info. & Comm. Technology, ABV-IIITM Gwalior, INDIA), Poh Hean Yap (Deakin University, Australia), Dr. Ivan Karljevski (FON University, Republic of Macedonia), Dr. Rachid Benlamri (Lakehead University, Canada), Dr. Sime Arsenovski (Faculty of Informatics, European University - Republic of Macedonia), Dr. Mikel Laurea Alava (Facultad de Informatica, UPV/EHU, Spain), Vahideh Zarea Gavgani (Osmania University, India) and Dr. Vinod Scaria (Institute of Genomics and Integrative Biology, India). Finally, the editors would like to thank the authors of this book for acting as internal reviewers.

Sabah Mohammed
Jinan Fiaidhi
Editors

Section 1
Background

Chapter 1
Identifying the Emerging e–Health Technologies:
To Ubiquity 2.0 and Beyond

Sabah Mohammed
Lakehead University, Canada

Jinan Fiaidhi
Lakehead University, Canada

ABSTRACT

Achieving improvements and optimum healthcare delivery has become a bipartisan top priority for several governments and institutions. The ability to meet this goal depends on the exchange of information within and across healthcare communities. The real challenge for any healthcare initiative is at the application level, where patient data may be stored on hundreds of different clinical systems such as lab, radiology, or pharmacy systems, and various clinical applications such as electronic medical record (EHRs), that use different protocols and schemas. In an attempt to overcome these challenges, many organizations have used enterprise-oriented integration platforms to transform and translate information so that disparate systems could exchange information internally and externally. However, the development and ongoing maintenance of such healthcare systems has become extremely expensive due to the growing complexity of healthcare organizations as they acquire more systems to meet clinical and business needs. As a result, healthcare communities continue to face the same challenge: how to achieve a level of interoperability for accessing all relevant information about a patient from a single point, which is universally becoming the Web, as well as to ensure accuracy, security, and privacy of all the relevant data. This chapter provides a roadmap solution based on the emerging web technologies that hold great promise for addressing these challenges. The roadmap is termed as the "ubiquity 2.0 trend." This chapter also highlights the security challenges and the emerging web-oriented identity management technologies to provide a single, common user credential that is trusted, secure, and widely supported across the Web and within the healthcare enterprises.

DOI: 10.4018/978-1-61520-777-0.ch001

Copyright © 2010, IGI Global. Copying or distributing in print or electronic forms without written permission of IGI Global is prohibited.

THE XMALIZATION TECHNOLOGIES: THE ROADMAP OF UBIQUITY 1.0

During the last decade, a number of health initiatives have been undertaken to address various issues related to the e-health quality of service. In spite of the technical improvements, the current healthcare systems often lack adequate integration among the key actors, and commonly fail to consider variety of social aspects. Actually, there is a misconception that e-Health is just about the usage of the Information and Communications Technologies (ICT). Dealing with e-health applications, requires measures and technologies beyond the mere qualified communication networks infrastructure. The challenge will be to make the e-health technology as invisible and as possible to attract widespread use. This means, it will need to be ubiquitous (i.e. present in every place) and widely accepted. For that to true, there will need to be social as well as technological changes. Thus, ubiquitous healthcare technologies become an emerging and challenging paradigm that is gradually reshaping the old disease-centered model, where treatment decisions are made almost exclusively by physicians based on clinical experience, into a patient-centered model where patients are active participants in the decision making process about their own health. Although the Internet has played a drastic role in this movement by giving people access to an extreme amount of health information and providing access to variety of e-health services, it fails short to present an effective media of participation and collaboration. With the other emerging unprecedented technological innovations (e.g. Wireless communication, Sensors Technology), many aspects of the e-health and health care systems are in need of serious modernization and fundamental shift. These current e-health systems are ripe with inefficiencies, inequities, and errors. If we study the changing trend in the demographic and health profiles of the population, we can anticipate the challenges that we need to face over the next 20 years in the management of chronic and multiple diseases in an aging population. At present, about 80% of ill health, disability-caused, and premature deaths are due to chronic diseases (Vitacca, Mazzù and Scalvini; 2009). Due to people's concern for a healthy life, there is a rising need for e-health systems available anytime, anywhere; this causes a paradigm shift from reactive care to preventive care, and thus enhancing our quality of life.

In general, e-health is a highly fragmented and heterogeneous enterprise, with complex processes and few standards for either the processes themselves or the data they generate. Obstacles in the path of e-health are numerous and include legal, ethical, economic, social, medical, organizational, and cultural aspects as well as the fact that a further market downturn may choke development resources. However, the lack of ubiquity and interoperability in systems and services, such as electronic health records, patient summaries, and emergency data sets, has been identified as a major obstacle to the widespread take-up of the e-health applications in the world. The full benefits of e-health services and tools will not reach patients unless a high level of ubiquity and interoperability is integrated at the heart of their design and deployment. Fortunately, Internet-based integration frameworks have helped solve similar problems in other industries and paradigms (e.g. eBusiness), and there is good reason to believe that they will be equally effective in healthcare. The optimism stems from a belief that healthcare faces integration challenges similar to those in other domains:

- Sharing data and information among heterogeneous systems that were never designed to interoperate;
- Automating and integrating ad hoc paper-based processes within and across organizations;
- Managing identities and authorizations across trust boundaries; and

- Minimizing the need for custom systems integration, so that small organizations can afford to participate.

The probability that e-Business can revolutionize health care delivery depends on the development activities and the collaborative works in a comprehensive environment where information exchanged between healthcare users and/or patients is simple, fast and reliable. Consequently, this environment requires great deal of standardization and harmonization. This status can be obtained by means of a common effort of industries and public institutions to define and to harmonize standards like HL7, Cen/TC 251 and DICOM in order to improve the ubiquity and/ or interoperability between healthcare systems. The world Health Organization (WHO) takes this issue very seriously (WHO; 2006): " *If used consistently, the standardization and harmonization process enhances accuracy, efficiency, reliability and comparability of health information at local, regional, national and international levels.*" By standard harmonization and utilization of approved standards, the various information systems and software applications will have the ability to work together and hence achieving the ultimate goal of having a ubiquitous healthcare.

One of the problems facing e-health ubiquity and interoperability is the fact that data is invariably stored in ASCII plain text format. This format does not reflect the underlying structure of the data. Consequently, e-health software tools need to unearth this structure for ubiquity and interoperability purposes. For this purpose, efforts are being made around the world to explore the possibility of adopting XML format to represent the structure of the data for e-health systems. The popularity and press surrounding the release of XML has created widespread interest in standards within particular e-health communities that focus on representing content. The dream is that these standards will enable consumers and e-health systems to more accurately search information on the Web within these communities. We generally identify this trend as the ***ubiquity 1.0*** where XMLization is the main catalyst for e-health ubiquity and interoperability. Figure 1 illustrates the first wave of e-health ubiquity.

The ubiquity 1.0 trend can be categorized in two major layers: The *Syntactic XMLization layer* and the *Semantic XMLization layer*. Syntactic XMLization defines the messaging layer and involves the ability of two or more systems to exchange information. Syntactic XMLization involves several sub-layers: The network and

Figure 1. The e-health ubiquity 1.0 XMLization trend

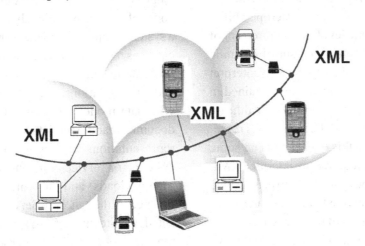

transport layer (such as the Internet), the application protocol layer (such as HTTP or email), the messaging protocol and message format layer (such as ebXML messaging or SOAP), and the sequencing of the messages. Syntactic XMLization guarantees the message to be delivered but does not guarantee that the content of the message will be machine processable at the receiving end. To guarantee message content interoperability, the message content should conform to an agreed semantic. Semantic XMLization is the ability for information shared by systems to be understood at the level of formally defined domain concepts. Around the world, considerable gains have been achieved already, through standardization based on syntactic XMLization. The requirements of semantic XMLization far exceed those of syntactic XMLization, requiring a stable reference information model, vocabulary bindings to controlled terminologies, formally defined data types and structures, a mechanism for defining and constraining clinical statements and documents, a common repository of consensus-based reusable clinical concepts, and an agreed interchange format. Currently the only viable candidates for this role are HL7 version 3 (with or without CDA), openEHR and CEN 13606. Yet, it is not realistic to expect all the healthcare institutes to conform to a single standard. Furthermore, different versions of the same standard (such as HL7 Version 2 and Version 3) do not interoperate. Therefore, there is a need to address the ubiquity and interoperability problem at the semantic level. At the forefront of the semantic XMLization is the issue of semantic translation; that is, the ability to properly interpret the elements, attributes, and values contained in an XML file. In many cases, specific healthcare domains have standardized the way data is represented in XML. When this does not occur, some type of mediation is required to interpret XML formatted data that does not adhere to pre-defined semantics. Although this mediation and interpretation process is at the heart of the ``schema-wars'', which are currently raging at forums such as www.

w3c.org, www.oasis-open.org, www.rosettanet. org, www.schema.net, etc.; this fundamental aspect of XML is not yet widely recognized or solved. Such mediation is actually needed before data exchange can be established between applications where a model of the domain of interest has to be built, since it is necessary to clarify what kind data is sent from the first application to the second. This model is usually described in terms of objects and relations. From the domain model a DTD or an XML Schema is constructed. Since the DTD or the XML Schema is just a grammar, then there exist multiple possibilities to encode a given element. To achieve semantic XMLization, one needs to have constrained the specifications of XML Schemas/DTD so that a single translation mechanism can be used to transform any XML instances compliant with Ontology-based Naming and Design Rules into standard RDF or OWL structures. In this way, ontologies can be used to integrate, interoperate and mediate information exchange. However, building such mediators is an extremely complicated process even for different versions of the same healthcare system. For example, the semantic mediation between HL7 Version 2 and HL7 Version 3 messages requires two phases of complicated translations: *Message Ontology Mapping Phase*; and *Message Instance Mapping Phase* (see Figure 2):

Nevertheless, the semantic XMLization challenge is much more complex than just those basic codes of schema mapping. It is about the ability of a system to operate on data from other systems as easily as it operates on its own data. This involves both static and dynamic data representations and interpretations. Static representations deal with data models of such constructs as clinical documents and genetic testing results. Dynamic representations deal with interactions among systems (or services carrying static data as message payloads) and the workflows that must be fulfilled. Although, Web Services and Service Oriented Architectures (SOA) provide such dynamic representations enabling interoperability between

Figure 2. Transcoding Hl7 version 2.3 to HL7 version 3

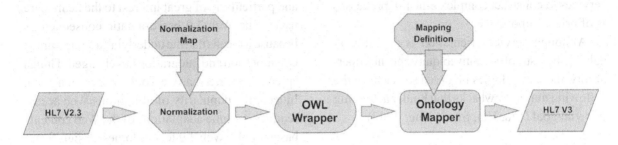

software components that can communicate between different companies and can reside on different infrastructures, they utilize heavyweight Semantic Web tools, policies and techniques (e.g. SOAP, WSDL, UDDI). However, current Web service technology is evolving towards a simpler approach to define Web service APIs that challenge the assumptions made by existing heavyweight Web services. RESTful Web services, for example, introduce a new kind of abstraction which does not require the message-oriented paradigm of the Web service description language (WSDL) and its SOAP messaging protocol (Pautasso, Zimmermann, and Leymann; 2008). REST API's haven't been around for very long, so REST is definitely the trendy way to create a web service, if creating web services could ever be trendy. The main advantages of REST web services are:

- Lightweight - not a lot of extra XML coding
- Human Readable Results
- Easy to build - no toolkits required

Compared to the traditional web services (or so called SOAP (Simple Object Access Protocol) Based Web Services), one can identify the following disadvantages:

- Heavyweight- requires lots of extra XML coding

- Very difficult to build, requires lots of development tools
- Rigid – uses type checking,

However, choosing REST or SOAP web service is not a simple decision based who is lightweight or not. For instance, Google's AdWords web service is hard to consume, it uses SOAP headers and a number of other things that make it kind of difficult. On the converse, Amazon's REST web service can sometimes be tricky to parse because it can be highly nested, and the result schema can vary quite a bit based on what you search for. Indeed, people seem to argue from the perspective that the success or failure of a given approach (REST or SOAP) can be boiled down to something entirely technical, when in reality success or failure is often determined almost completely by non-technical forces, such as *market effects* or social effects. Yes, the e-health scenarios demand systems that can be built upon notions of service-orientation. As most of the services in this domain, have to be flexibly adapted to meet exceptional or unforeseen situations. However, e-health scenarios are also very sensitive with regard to privacy issues. Therefore, an adequate security and access right management is essential as well. One of the most important benefits of using Web services is to build new business processes, services and values through compositing existing services quickly and reliably. Hence, the flexibility and simplicity of composing web services to construct complex e-health processes is of prime importance.

Although service orientation is one step in solving the issue of e-health ubiquity and interoperability, the technologies involved suffer from the following major drawbacks that hinder achieving this vial goal (Liu, Hui, Sun, Liang; 2007):

1. Service oriented technologies involve relatively strong requirements overhead about developer's skill and supporting infrastructure. The developers usually need to spend major effort to master many of such technologies, e.g. BPEL, WSDL, as well as tools, e.g. design-time IDE tools, and runtime middleware servers (BPEL server). Most of these tools demand for major investment on hardware and software infrastructure;
2. Secondly, these technologies cannot support service composition's customization on the fly.
3. The service-oriented technologies cannot well support the composition of legacy or existing web applications, which don't or can't provide web service interfaces.

These issues have become the barriers for faster and wider adoption of service orientation in e-health. However, the emergence of web 2.0 related technologies [e.g. AJAX (Asynchronous JavaScript and XML), Wiki, mashup] provide opportunities for overcoming these drawbacks. Mashup, for example, allows consumers to draw upon content retrieved from external data sources (web services, data store, web application) to create entirely new and innovative services. In our opinion, mashup essentially introduces a much simpler, more cost-effective, self-served approach for service composition that significantly reduces the complexity and barriers of the traditional Web service composition. Obviously, mashup is an extremely "consumer-centric" and lightweight service composition technology, which would be

more applicable to all consumers all over internet and particularly of great interest to the healthcare users. The Web 2.0 has dramatic consequences because it means that the underlying architecture of collaboration and integration has changed. Things spread far greater than we would've ever imagined. Indeed, the popularity of ubiquitous Web access requires runtime adaptations of the Web contents based on the Web 2.0 technologies. A significant trend in these content adaptation services is the growing amount of personalization required by users. Personalized services and developing Rich Internet Applications (RIA) are and will be a key feature for the success of the ubiquitous Web. We term this new trend of ubiquity as **Ubiquity 2.0**. This chapter is dedicated to introduce the ubiquity 2.0 trend and its implications on the future e-health applications.

THE WEB-ORIENTED TECHNOLOGIES: THE UBIQUITY 2.0 TREND

Before embarking on a discussion of the standards and possible directions for ubiquity 2.0 and its effects on e-health, it is important to consider the reason for undertaking such works. Internationally, the key Health IT enhancement drivers are (Tan; 2005,Eng; 2001):

*   **Enhancement of Quality of Care:** as the previous attempts are marked with inconsistencies between the management of similar patients.
*   **Providing Patient Safety**: as significant diagnostic and therapeutic error rates are observed in all jurisdictions based on the previous IT systems.
*   **Reducing the Delivery of Cost of Care**: there is an international trend of increasing healthcare costs due to the ageing population, increasing burden of chronic disease, increasingly expensive care options, and

wastage of resources through inappropriate, unnecessary or duplicated interventions.

- **Comprehensive Availability and Ubiquity:** as most of the e-health services are available at urban areas.
- **Empowerment of e-health Providers and Consumers**: Most of the e-health services are confined to the provider's servers with very little empowerment on the consumer side.
- **Synchronization of Content and Application Development:** Development efforts of e-health services are typically uncoordinated and essentially independent.
- **Integration of e-health Segments**: There is a need to integrate the various features and functions of e-health tools, including health information and support, transaction processing, electronic health records, clinical and public health information systems, compliance and disease management programs, and behavior change and health promotion
- **Providing Context-Awareness:** There is a need for e-health services that are aware of the patients' presence and context, and are sensitive, adaptive, and responsive to their needs, habits, gestures and emotions.
- **Encourage New Types of Collaborations**: e-health needs to provide many new collaborative relationships (e.g. provider to provider, virtual teams)
- **Enhancing the Continuity and Coverage of Care**: Patients are increasingly seen by an array of providers in a wide variety of organizations and places, raising concerns about fragmentation of care. Healthcare needs to have wider coverage too (e.g. pervasive, mobile, RFID-Based).
- **Support Sound Research and Education**: There is an increasing level of demand from various healthcare sections (e.g. pharmaceutical industry, genomic research) to have e-health research data available and

accessible based on standard format for research and education purposes.

By leveraging these IT drivers and technologies we can provide better e-health services in underserved areas, networked health systems and patients can gain access to seamless, coordinated, and continuing care. This vision requires an innovative IT infrastructure on the Internet that encourages collaboration, flexibility and integration. The ubiquity 2.0 trend is the backbone that can take this abstract vision to the concrete reality. Based on the ubiquity 2.0 trend, we can leverage web as the design-time and runtime tool for service composition, to significantly reduce overhead to composite service consumers. We can perform On-the-fly customization and deployment to make the service composition more responsive for consumer's requirement changes and certainly, we can reuse and remix the existing applications and data to be accessed through the web. The Ubiquity 2.0 trend is also about consumer empowerment through interactively delivering what they need and thus greatly reducing their workload, time and effort spent on targeted actions performance. Moreover, the ubiquity 2.0 simplifies the highly complex processes, saves bandwidth and performs considerably faster than traditional Web applications, thus escalating customers' online interaction with the e-health websites or portals. Intuitively, the ubiquity 2.0 trend highlights the changes to healthcare distribution via the Internet that will significantly impact the value exchange occurring between a health provider and consumer. It is now timely to consider the impact of ubiquity 2.0 on healthcare brought about by the new technological and market forces. For this purpose, let us zoom more into the notion and elements of the ubiquity 2.0 trend. Figure 3 illustrates the main features of the ubiquity 2.0 trend.

An important concept in ubiquity 2.0 is that Web-based software should offer its functionality not only via the browser, but also as open Web services so that it can be mashed up in new and

Figure 3. The main contributors to the ubiquity 2.0 trend

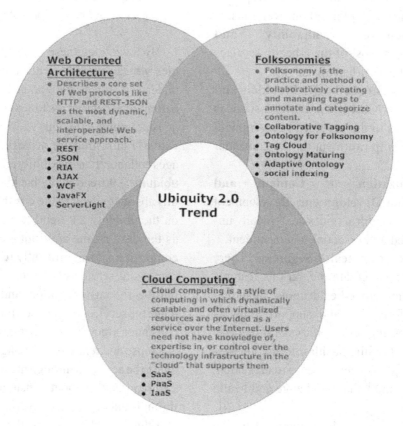

unintended ways. This takes software from being a mere isolated application and turns it into a true collaborative platform by sharing the application's pieces as Web services that allows functionality and data to be useful to others. Mashup allows business users to move — when appropriate — from their current so-called "end-user development tools", such as Microsoft Excel, that are highly isolated and poorly integrated to much more deeply integrated models that are more Web-based and hence more open, collaborative, reusable, ubiquitous, shareable, and in general make better use of existing sources of content and functionality. Although the ubiquity 2.0 mashup concept is based on Web services that resemble the notion of the traditional Web services which in turn makes it possible to share and reuse functionality and contents anywhere inside an organization

in a loosely-coupled and interoperable way, the ubiquity 2.0 web services uses simpler and more straightforward methods that *just work*, and hide the protocol complexity in the application state. Essentially, the ubiquity 2.0 Web services utilize lightweight protocols like HTTP and JSON for Web services interoperability. This means that the ubiquity 2.0 supports only the REST type of Web services along with JSON (JavaScript Object Notation) instead of XML. Compared to the traditional Web services, interoperability is achieved via XML and SOAP. There are many reasons why Web services interoperability is better with REST-JSON than XML-SOAP: (1) JSON is a lot simpler than XML+XML Schema and is more isomorphic with the relational data stores most services use for persistence; (2) Browsers can consume large amounts of JSON much more efficiently than they can consume large amounts of XML and the gap is widening because the latest versions of the browsers are now providing native, safe support for encoding and decoding JSON; (3) REST interfaces are much easier to design and implement than SOAP interfaces; for example: Verbs are already defined, exception semantics are already defined, caching semantics are already defined, versioning semantics are already defined, authentication and access control are already defined. All you really need to focus on are modeling resources using JSON, modeling URL hierarchies, modeling search patterns and modeling batching for performance improvements; and (4) One of the obvious JSON advantages over XML is that it can be directly evaluated in JavaScript and for the AJAX-world we live in, it is not a small thing. Interestingly, some researchers coin the REST based Web services architectures as "Web Oriented Architecture (WOA)" in contrast to the traditional "Service Oriented architectures (SOA)" (Hinchcliffe; 2008). Certainly, the gap will continue to widen between WOA and SOA as the open web stack matures and things like Open ID, Oauth, Flex/AIR, JavaFX, uniPaaS and Silverlight become more widely spread.

Another important factor contributing to the ubiquity 2.0 trend is the notion of collaborative tagging or folksonomy. Applications based on this concept are gaining in popularity across the web as it has emerged as a popular way to organize ideas on social networks. These tools have made information more accessible on consumer sites such as del.icio.us and Flickr. Now, e-health is starting to take notice. What are some of the best practices for implementing social tagging and folksonomies in the Healthcare Enterprise? For example, how do you manage and merge folksonomies and existing taxonomies? Do folksonomies and taxonomies even belong in the e-health environment? Folksonomy, a term that combines the people or "folks-y" approach to building a taxonomy. Folksonomy can be defined as a type of distributed classification system. It is usually

created by a group of individuals, typically the resource users. Users add tags to online items, such as images, videos, bookmarks, and text. These tags are then shared and can sometimes be refined" (Guy, and Tonkin; 2006). In other words, folksonomy is a naturally created classification system which arises as a result of user-based tagging. Although there is an ongoing debate over the issue of how useful folksonomy is compared to the traditional notion of taxonomy or ontology, it is obvious that folksonomies play an important part in cataloging information by adding metadata and using tags to organize digital collections, categorize the content of others and build bottom-up classification systems. Folksonomies is all about another dimension of user empowerment as no longer do the experts or the centralized ontologies have the monopoly (Beth; 2008). The major criticism against using folksonomies is the lack of hierarchy. The lack of hierarchy *leads to low search precision and poor resource navigation and retrieval* (Laura; 2006). Contrary to folksonomies, controlled vocabulary is characterized by rigid structures and slow responsiveness to new terminology. But its systematic organization, hierarchy and careful formulation of terms and relationships would be complementary to the disadvantage of folksonomies. Thus building ontologies from a combination of both folksonomies and controlled vocabulary became a hot research issue and a promising solution to the advance search engines for information that are categorized by tagging (Lin, Davis, and Zhou; 2009), (Echarte, Astrain, Córdoba, and Villadangos; 2008), (kim, Scerri, Breslin, Decker, and Kim; 2008).

The third and last factor contributing to the ubiquity 2.0 trend is the notion of *cloud computing* which is the natural advancement or bi-product related to the flexibility offered by the Web 2.0 trend (e.g. RIA, and Folksonomies). Cloud computing is a "paradigm in which information is permanently stored in servers on the Internet and cached temporarily on clients (Hewitt; 2009)." The cloud is merely a metaphor for the Internet, and thus, unlike traditional application architectures that rely on the infrastructure and services provided and controlled within an enterprise, cloud computing uses the Internet and its emerging set of technologies and services to satisfy the computing needs of individual users and organizations (Hutchinson, Ward, Castilon; 2009). Instead of relying on the traditional enterprise architectures with controlled, internal resources, the cloud computing enterprise can look outward, accessing and integrating applications and services that others have created and controled. The cloud computing enterprise relies on the Internet for satisfying the computing needs of the users. Cloud computing services usually provide common business applications online that are accessed from a web browser, while the software and data are stored on the servers. Cloud services - computation services, storage services, networking services, whatever is needed - are delivered and made available in a simplified way - "on demand" regardless of where the user is or the type of device they are using (Jones; 2008). It enables both rapid innovation and support of core business functions based on technologies that are termed as SaaS (Software as Service), dSaaS (Data Storage as Service), PaaS (Platform as Service) and IaaS (Infrastructure as Service) (Youseff, Butrico, and Silva;2008), (Lin, Dasmalchi, and Zhu; 2008), (Mika, and Tummarello;2008), (Kaliski; 2008). Currently there are many venders who offer such services: (Google Apps, Microsoft "Software+Service"—SaaS), (Nirvanix SND, Amazon S3—dSaaS), (IBM IT Factory, Google AppEngine—PaaS) and (Amazon EC2, IBM BlueCloud—IaaS). Any cloud computing architecture can have a wide variety of reusable components, including portals, mashup servers, RSS feeds, database servers, mapping servers, gadgets, user interface components, and legacy Web servers. Architects can integrate these elements to form an edge application in which multiple services and components are overlaid or "mashed" together (Hutchinson, Ward, and Castilon; 2009).

THE REALAM OF E-HEALTH BASED ON UBIQUITY 2.0 TREND

For community and public health, the ubiquity 2.0 trend offers the opportunity to create a common working backbone for all healthcare users and stakeholders to improve interoperation and collaborations. There are many studies that anticipated the need for such trend in creating an effective e-health paradigm (Breton; 2005), (Kamel, and Wheeler; 2007),(McLean, Richards and Wardman; 2007). Moreover, there are numerous applications that have implemented many elements of the ubiquity 2.0 trend technologies in e-health. Table 1 list some of these applications:

However in today's ubiquity 2.0 environment, hyper connectivity and new and complex technologies require a shift from individualized proprietary Enterprise applications such as those listed in Table 1 to a more open and dependent world of web-oriented architecture and cloud computing. The future vision of the e-health architecture needs to set out plans to incrementally shape the information technology to support the delivery of improved healthcare. The architecture vision must be based on a mix of bottom-up and top-down implementation strategies. Unlike the traditional e-health application architecture which is relatively of static structure, the ubiquity 2.0 e-health architecture is a dynamic collection of moving parts, with no clear concept of a baseline; it's far more dependent on relationships and interactions between organizations as well as healthcare users. In this architecture, applications can reuse several different components—the servers can exist on the Internet or within the enterprise. Combining these components lets organizations build new, powerful applications, thereby delivering greater business value faster and at a lower cost. Figure 4 provides a general vision for the ubiquity 2.0 e-health architecture. The lowest level of this architecture is the ubiquity 2.0 hub, which represent an IaaS service. This means the ability of leasing services and data with specific quality-of-service

Table 1. Notable medical applications based on some notions of ubiquity 2.0 trend.

e-Health Application	Purpose	Examples-URL
Blogs	Provides a community entry for discussions about clinical cases, images and special clinical, medical and health interest topics	**Oldlarmed** http://odlarmed.com/ **Healthcare Blog** www.thehealthcareblog.com/
Wikis	Server software that allows users to freely create and edit web page content using any web browser.	**Ask Dr Wiki** http://askdrwiki.com **Medical Portal** http://en.wikipedia.org/wiki/Portal:Medicine
Podcats/Vodcasts	Allows audio and video downloads from websites to MP3 and MP4 players (including iPods) based on RSS feeds and an aggregator.	**Medical Podcasts** www.medicinenet.com **Cleveland Clinic** http://my.clevelandclinic.org
Social Bookmarking and Folksonomies	A method for Internet users to store, organize, search, and manage bookmarks of web pages on the Internet with the help of metadata, typically in the form of tags that collectively and/or collaboratively become a folksonomy.	**Hub Med** www.hubmed.org **CiteMD** http://citemd.com/
Mashup Servers	The server based ability to easily create useful new applications from existing services and Web applications. By combining data from multiple sources across the Web, and from within the enterprise, mashups can help distill important health information for people who would otherwise need to gather and distill it manually.	**WSO2** http://wso2.com/ **Kapow** http://kapowtech.com/
Microformat Based Applications	A web-based approach to that seeks to re-use existing XHTML and HTML tags to convey metadata and other attributes. This approach allows information intended for end-users (such as contact information, calendar events) to also be automatically processed by software.	**XFN** http://microformats.org **relTag** http://microformats.org
Social Networking	Providing social networking enterprise for linking people with the same interest.	**MDjunction** www.mdjunction.com/ **TiroMed** www.tiromed.com/
Search Engines	Medical search engines use peer-reviewed sources and sites selected by experts providing the most relevant and reliable medical information of the best quality.	**Healthline** http://www.healthline.com/ MedHunt http://www.hon.ch/MedHunt/

constraints that has the ability to execute an arbitrary operating system and software. An example of such hub is the Microsoft "Connected Health and Human Services Hub" (El Maliki, and Seigneur; 2007). The other levels of the ubiquity 2.0 architecture include one or more PaaS services. Each PaaS can be represented as Portal service such as Liferay (Hamlin; 2005), which allow applications from a variety of different mashups, widgets, and iframes to be included in different user panels. Portals also let users build applications through simple customizations in which the user specifies a URL for a panel or pane. Web 2.0 users can customize their own interfaces, reusing the components they need without programming. This new deployment model gives end users more control over their applications. The upper level of the ubiquity 2.0 architecture includes many

Figure 4. Essential ubiquity 2.0 elements for constructing e-health systems

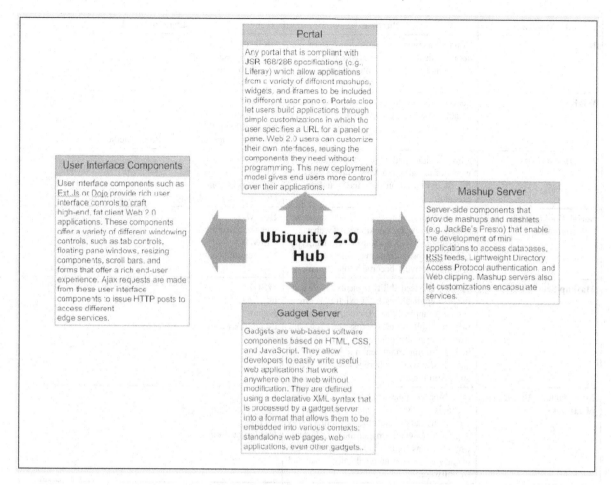

services that are dynamic in nature, operate in a SaaS form. These services can be in the form of services used by a local application or a remote application observed through a Web browser. Remotely executing applications commonly rely on an application server to expose needed services. An *application server (e.g. Red Hat JBoss, Apatche Geronimo)* is a software framework that exposes APIs for software services (such as transaction management or database access). Among the most important SaaS services are the followings:

- **The UI SaaS:** To provide rich user interface controls to craft high-end fat client application.

- **The Gadget SaaS:** Allows developers to easily write useful web applications that work anywhere on the web without modification.
- **The Mashup SaaS:** To provide mashup and customization services that enable the development of mini applications.

Certainly, the ubiquity 2.0 architecture, coupled with increased standardization, convergence and ambient computing, will enable improvements in the availability of clinical and non-clinical information to clinicians and managers, and support the service to manage the patient empowerment.

BEYOND THE UBIQUITY 2.0 TREND: THE SECURITY CONCERN

As always, working in a new environment presents new and different challenges for developers as well as users. Concern about security is one of the greatest hurdles to implementing the notions of ubiquity 2.0 trend for the e-health paradigm. Privacy and security problems are compounded by the use of remote, distributed services operated by third parties. E-health institutions employing these emerging technologies must take a comprehensive approach to security across on-site and cloud infrastructure, and learn how to assess and manage it. This encompasses protection, access *and* management, all built around user identity and integrated with a highly secure, interoperable platform for a broad set of partner solutions. Identity is a core part of any security strategy, because it allows for more contextual protection and access to information and resources. Identity is important to identify the user for different purposes including personalization, authorization, communication, content publishing and maintaining public identity across different e-health providers. In general, the identity management systems are elaborated to deal with the following core facets (El Maliki, and Seigneur; 2007):

- **Management:** The amount of digital identities per person will increase, so the users need convenient support to manage these identities and the corresponding authentication.
- **Reachability**: The management of reachability allows users to handle their contacts to prevent misuse of their address (spam) or unsolicited phone calls
- **Authenticity:** Ensuring authenticity with authentication, integrity and non-repudiation mechanisms can prevent identity theft.
- **Anonymity and pseudonymity:** providing anonymity prevents tracking or identifying the users of a service.

- **Organization of personal data management**: A quick method to create, modify or delete work accounts is needed, especially in big organizations

The roadmap of identity management started with Enterprise Identity Management but later been developed into more general management that is currently known as User-Centric Identity Management (Hansen; 2008). On one hand, enterprise identity management provides centralized security and authentication that is closed to third parties. On the other hand, the user centric identity management is based on decentralized authentication but it allows users to keep at least some control over their personal data. With the advancement in user-centric and URI-based identity systems over the past few years for accessing open applications and services on the web, it has become clear that a single specification will not be the solution to all security problems. Rather, like the other layers of the Internet, developing small, interoperable specifications that are independently implementable and useful will ultimately lead to market adoption of these technologies. Currently, there are wave of specifications, tools and techniques that are termed "identity 2.0" (Hamlin; 2005) to deal with sharing applications and services on the web and outside the boundary of the enterprise. Identity 2.0 is the anticipated revolution of identity verification on the internet using emerging user-centric technologies such as OpenID (http:// *openid.net/), Open SSO (*https://opensso.dev.java.net*), Open SAML* (http://OpenLiberty), *Live ID (*www.passport.net/*) and OAuth (http://oauth.net)*. Identity 2.0 stems from the Web 2.0 initiative of the World Wide Web transition. Its emphasis is a simple and open method of identity transactions similar to those in the physical world, such as a driver's license. The goal is to centralize security around users instead of organizations. Figure 5 illustrates the two main themes of identity management.

While OpenID seems to have the upper hand in terms of market share and competent execu-

Figure 5. Enterprise versus web identity management

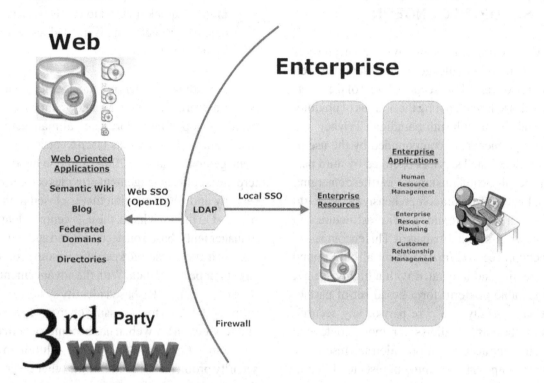

tion, it's still too early to declare a winner in the Web identity sweepstakes. OpenID is an open, decentralized standard for user authentication and access control, allowing users to log onto many services with the same digital identity. As such, it replaces the common login process that uses a login-name and a password, by allowing a user to log in once and gain access to the resources of multiple software systems (Eldon; 2009). Figure 6 illustrates how OpenID protocol works (Ho; 2009).

Open ID gives you one login for multiple sites. Each time you need to log into a WebSite - a site using Open ID - you will be redirected to your Open ID site where you login, and then back to the WebSite. However, Open identity like OpenID does push users into considering their Terms of Service of their provider much more carefully, since they're making a long-term strategic decision with whom they'll will invest with their Web identity, and whether they offer a good home for

what may be their last new Web account ever. According to (Clancy; 2008), there are some important questions the users of open identity should carefully ask and analyze. The following provides a list of such questions:

- What are the sign-on, access and authentication policies?
- Who handles penetration testing, and how is it done?
- What encryption policies will protect data as it is transferred, or when it is being stored?
- Is there a single-tenant hosting option separated from that of other customers?
- Who manages the application on the back end, and what policies are in place to thwart insider breaches?
- What is the backup and recovery plan?
- How well does the provider's security policy match my company's

Figure 6. OpenID protocol

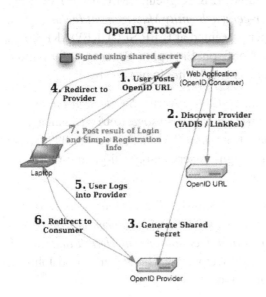

However, if you want to ease your mind regarding security in the identity 2.0 environment, then you need to ask if the provider is SAS 70 Type II certified. This certification is highly comprehensive, includes regular audits to retain certification and covers just about everything you can think of regarding operating a business in the cloud. SAS 70 is a widely recognized auditing standard developed by the American Institute of Certified Public Accountants (AICPA) (www.sas70.com). The SAS 70 Type II certification ensures comprehensive change management documentation (including at the application level), backup and recovery requirements, disaster recovery requirements, physical level security requirements of the data center including access and mirrored data centers.

CONCLUSION

The interaction between medicine and technology has a rich history. Healthcare professionals and policy makers have always been resourceful in finding ways to utilize technology to enhance the provision of clinical care. However, the prolifera-

tion of computers and the Internet has vastly expanded the possibilities. The Internet, in particular, has ushered in the new field of e-Health as a model for global or ubiquitous healthcare. E-Health is currently facing increasing pressure to improve the quality of care delivered to patients through effective prevention and post-operative care. This comes at a time when there is a need to curtail growth in healthcare spending fuelled by ageing populations, increasing rates of chronic diseases, rising expectations from health consumers, fractured systems of healthcare delivery (e.g. limited information-sharing capabilities) and the decline in health workforce. Once ubiquitous healthcare services are in place, e-health will always be 'on'; working anytime and anywhere. The key goals of such an e-health vision must be to enhance the efficiency and effectiveness of the healthcare system by making services more accessible, affordable, and accountable. Open source and open standard solutions are thus needed for interoperability and integration of the various services offered by different institutions and enterprises. During the last few years, we have seen a gradual shift from the traditional healthcare delivery systems to more ubiquitous forms of healthcare. The evolution involves ubiquitous healthcare concepts, infrastructure, technologies, applications, interfaces, and strategies all of which contribute to the paradigm shift from tethered to ubiquitous wellness. This chapter focused on the e-health evolution based on the emerging internet technologies. The chapter identified two types of e-health emerging ubiquity streams. An earlier ubiquity stream that is based on XMLization, which termed *"The Ubiquity 1.0 Trend"* and a more recent ubiquity trend that is based on rich internet applications, which are termed *"The ubiquity 2.0 Trend."* The ubiquity 2.0 vision promises far greater advantages in producing highly interactive and portable applications compared to the earlier vision of ubiquity 1.0. However, the realization of ubiquity 2.0 healthcare services on the Web requires that these services should meet reliable and high quality of service

(QoS) constraints. This chapter shed some light on the security issue related to providing ubiquity 2.0 services on the Web. The chapter identified an emerging technological solution for the security of the ubiquity 2.0 Web services based on Open Web Identity Management. However, the use of the ubiquity 2.0 emerging technologies in eHealth field is still in its infancy and must address numerous challenges. Feasibility and efficacy trials, particularly related to healthcare Internet interventions (e.g. prevention and post-operative care) and sharing electronic healthcare records over the Web, need to be conducted to fully trust the ubiquity 2.0 trend.

REFERENCES

Beth, D. S. (2008). Folksonomy and Health Information Access: How can Social Bookmarking Assist Seekers of Online Medical Information? *Journal of Hospital Librarianship, 8*(1), 119–126. doi:10.1080/15323260801943570

Bicer, V., Laleci, G. B., Dogac, A., & Kabak, Y. (2005, September). Artemis Message Exchange Framework: Semantic Interoperability of Exchanged Messages in the Healthcare Domain. *SIGMOD Record, 34*(3), 71–76. doi:10.1145/1084805.1084819

Clancy, H. (2008, May). 7 Security Questions to Ask Your SaaS Provider. *Information Security Magazine*. Retrieved January 25, 2009, from http://searchsecurity.techtarget.com/magazineFeature/0,296894,sid14_gci1313252,00.html

Echarte, F., Astrain, J. J., Córdoba, A., & Villadangos, J. (2008). Self-adaptation of Ontologies to Folksonomies in Semantic Web. In *Proceedings of World Academy of Science* (*Vol. 33*). Engineering and Technology.

El Maliki, T., & Seigneur, J. M. (2007). *A Survey of User-centric Identity Management Technologies*. Paper presented at IEEE SECUREWARE 2007, Int. Conf. on Emerging Security Information, Systems and Technologies.

Eldon, E. (2009, April). *Single sign-on service OpenID getting more usage*. Retrieved January 25, 2009, from http://venturebeat.com/2009/04/14/single-sign-on-service-openid-getting-more-usage/

Eng, T. R. (2001). *The eHealth Landscape: A Terrain Map of Emerging Information and Communication Technologies in Health and Health Care*. Princeton, NJ: The Robert Wood Johnson Foundation.

Guy, M., & Tonkin, E. (2006, January). Folksonomies Tidying up Tags? *D-Lib Magazine, 12*(1). doi:10.1045/january2006-guy

Hamlin, K. (2005). *Identity 2.0 Gathering: Getting to the Promised Land*. Retrieved January 25, 2009, from http://www.oreillynet.com/pub/a/policy/2005/10/07/identity-workshop.html

Hansen, M. A. (2008). User-controlled identity management: the key to the future of privacy? *International Journal of Intellectual Property Management, 2*(4), 325–344.

Hewitt, C. (2009). Perfect Disruption: The Paradigm Shift from Mental Agents to ORGs. *IEEE Internet Computing, 13*(1), 90–93. doi:10.1109/MIC.2009.15

Hinchcliffe, D. (2008). *What Is WOA? It's The Future of Service-Oriented Architecture (SOA)*. Retrieved March 22, 2009, from http://hinchcliffe.org/archive/2008/02/27/16617.aspx

Ho, D. (2009, January). *Tutorial: OpenID authentication with SSO (PHP)*. Retrieved April 3, 2009, from http://www.mti.epita.fr/blogs/serveur/2009/01/12/tutorial-authentification-sso-avec-openid-en-php/

Hutchinson, C., Ward, J., & Castilon, K. (2009). Navigating the Next-Generation Application Architecture. *IT Professional*, *11*(2), 18–22. doi:10.1109/MITP.2009.33

Jones, M. T. (2008). Cloud computing with Linux Cloud computing platforms and applications. *IBM Research Journal*. Retrieved April 25, 2009, from http://www.ibm.com/developerworks/library/l-cloud-computing/index.html

Kaliski, B. (2008, October). *Multi-tenant Cloud Computing: From Cruise Liners to Container Ships*. Paper presented at the Trusted Infrastructure Technologies Conference, APTC '08. Third Asia-Pacific, 4 – 4.

Kamel, B. M. N., & Wheeler, S. (2007). The emerging Web 2.0 social software: an enabling suite of sociable technologies in health and healthcare education. *Health Information and Libraries Journal*, *24*(1), 2–23. doi:10.1111/j.1471-1842.2007.00701.x

Kim, H. L., Scerri, S., Breslin, J. G., Decker, S., & Kim, H. G. (2008). The state of the art in tag ontologies: a semantic model for tagging and folksonomies. In *Proceedings of the 2008 International Conference on Dublin Core and Metadata Applications, Berlin, Germany* (pp. 128-137).

Laura, G. M. (2006, June). Social bookmarking, folksonomies, and Web 2.0 tools. *Searcher,* *14*(6), 26-38. Retrieved March 22, 2009, from http://www.accessmylibrary.com/coms2/summary_0286-16124325_ITM

Lin, G., Dasmalchi, G., & Zhu, J. (2008, September). *Cloud Computing and IT as a Service: Opportunities and Challenges*. Paper presented at ICWS '08. IEEE International Conference on Web Services, 5 – 5.

Lin, H., Davis, J., & Zhou, Y. (2009). *An Integrated Approach to Extracting Ontological Structures from Folksonomies*. Presented at 6th Annual European Semantic Web Conference (ESWC2009)

Liu, X., Hui, Y., Sun, W., & Liang, H. (2007). Towards Service Composition Based on Mashup. *IEEE Congress on Services (SERVICES 2007)*.

McLean, R., Richards, B. H., & Wardman, J. I. (2007). The effect of Web 2.0 on the future of medical practice and education: Darwikinian evolution or folksonomic revolution? *The Medical Journal of Australia*, *187*(3), 174–177.

Mika, P., & Tummarello, G. (2008). Web Semantics in the Clouds. *Intelligent Systems. IEEE*, *23*(5), 82–87. doi:10.1109/MIS.2008.94

Pautasso, C., Zimmermann, O., & Leymann, F. (2008). RESTful Web Services vs. "Big" Web Services: Making the Right Architectural Decision. WWW 2008 / Refereed Track: Web Engineering - Web Service Deployment Beijing, China

Solomonides, T. (Eds.). (2005). *From Grid to Healthgrid: Prospects and Requirements*. IOS Press.

Tan, J. (Ed.). (2005, April). E-Health Care Information Systems: An Introduction for Students and Professionals.

Vitacca, M., Mazzù, M., & Scalvini, S. (2009). Socio-technical and organizational challenges to wider e-Health implementation. *Chronic Respiratory Disease*, *6*, 91–97. doi:10.1177/1479972309102805

WHO. (2006, May). *WHO eHealth: standardized terminology*. EXECUTIVE BOARD EB118/8, 118th Session 25, Provisional agenda item 8.4. Retrieved January 13, 2009, from http://apps.who.int/gb/ebwha/pdf_files/EB118/B118_8-en.pdf

Youseff, L., Butrico, M., & Da Silva, D. (2008, Nov. 12-16). Toward a Unified Ontology of Cloud Computing. *Grid Computing Environments Workshop, 2008. GCE, 08*, 1–10.

Section 2
Research Issues

Chapter 2
Semantic Interoperability:
Issue of Standardizing Medical Vocabularies

W. Ed Hammond
Duke University, USA

ABSTRACT

Semantic interoperability is the key to achieving global interoperability in healthcare information technology. The benefits are tremendous – the sharing of clinical data for multiple uses including patient care, research, reimbursement, audit and analyses, education, health surveillance, and many other uses. Patient safety, higher quality healthcare, more effective and efficient healthcare, increased outcomes, and potentially improved performance, higher quality of life and longer lifetimes are potential results. Decision support and the immediate linking of knowledge to the care process become easier. Semantic interoperability is a worthy goal. There are many barriers to achieving semantic interoperability. Key among these is the resolution of the many issues relating to the terminologies used in defining, describing and documenting health care. Each of these controlled terminologies has a reason for being and a following. The terminologies conflict and overlap; the granularity is not sufficiently rich for direct clinical use; there are gaps that prevent an exhaustive set; there are major variances in cost and accessibility; and no one appears eager or willing to make the ultimate decisions required to solve the problem. This chapter defines and describes the purpose and characteristics of the major terminologies in use in healthcare today. Terminology sets are compared in purpose, form and content. Finally, a proposed solution is presented based on a global master metadictionary of data elements with a rich set of attributes including names that may come from existing controlled terminologies, precise definitions to remove ambiguity in use, and complete value sets of possible values. The focus is on data elements because data elements are the basic unit of data interchange.

DOI: 10.4018/978-1-61520-777-0.ch002

Copyright © 2010, IGI Global. Copying or distributing in print or electronic forms without written permission of IGI Global is prohibited.

INTRODUCTION

The most widely used word today in health informatics is "interoperability", and the most frequently used adjective with that word is "semantic". Interoperability's importance results from the current model for the effective use of Health Information Technology (HIT) that requires the aggregation and sharing of health-related data and knowledge. Semantic interoperability requires the ability of both humans and computers to read and understand shared data as it is received (in the sense of knowing what the data represents and how it is to be used). If the sender and receiver know each other, a business agreement as to what data will be exchanged and in what format provides a working solution. The more severe problem, and the one we are trying to solve, requires semantic interoperability among previously unknown exchange partners.

We have been aware of the need for semantic interoperability for over five decades. Even within the same setting, healthcare professionals used different terms to express themselves, and the real meaning is left to the imagination of the receiver. Many medical errors are a direct result of ambiguous or misinterpreted terminologies. Patient care, clinical trials, performance and quality evaluation, and the like depended on an interpretation of the terms used. In some cases, life and death decisions were made on the basis of unclear data. Different groups solved the problem in local settings by developing their own vocabularies. That process worked until the need arose to communicate with an external group. The result was several hundred sets of similar but different, redundant and competing medical vocabularies. Now, as each nation tries to build a national linked network sharing health data, the solution seems costly and overwhelming. A global harmonized solution challenges what is possible.

This chapter addresses what is required to meet this need and where we are along that pathway. Major controlled vocabularies are introduced, including some of their characteristics and what they represent, and what role they might play in the future. Further, the chapter will discuss both an ideal solution and a workable, though less desirable, solution. The solution moves the focus from vocabulary to data elements.

BACKGROUND

The need for communication and the ability to communicate among humans is perhaps one of the most important human characteristics that define who and what we are. Without the ability to communicate among like creatures, we would be unable to share experiences and knowledge. The Biblical Book of Genesis makes this point very well. The opening sentence in Chapter 11 states: "Now the whole world had one language and a common speech." The story goes on to relate that the men of the community decided to build a tower, the Tower of Babel, to reach heaven. God saw this work and said "If as one people speaking the same language have begun to do this, then nothing they plan to do will be impossible for them." God then confused the language of the people, and they were unable to complete the building. Today's world of health care uses a confused language and, as a result, we cannot build the best healthcare system.

The evolution of the many different sets of controlled vocabularies is further confounded by the labels attached: vocabulary, terminology, nomenclature, classification, taxonomy, and more recently, ontologies. Are the products of these differently named sets the same or different? Clearly the intent and purposes of each are slightly different. On the other hand, the terms that appear are similar. These terms are defined and discussed below.

Vocabulary

Vocabulary is perhaps the most frequently used, everyday term to describe the words we use in defining and documenting the health care process.

Simply defined, a vocabulary is a set of words used to express concepts or thoughts. We frequently use the words "controlled vocabulary" to mean that some group has placed some constraints, organization and control on the set of words and manages content and provides maintenance. A controlled vocabulary includes an organized list of words and phrases that identify concepts and content. An example of a controlled vocabulary is LOINC ® (Logical Observation Identifiers Names and Codes).

Terminology

Terminology, perhaps, is a little more formal than vocabulary but largely is considered to be a synonym of vocabulary. A terminology is a structured collection of specialized terms, assigned to or used for a particular purpose and is a symbolic representation of conceptual information. Terminology presents a finite, enumerated set of terms intended to convey information unambiguously. de Keizer (2000) does an excellent job of defining terminology and providing an overview of terminological systems.

Nomenclature

Nomenclature refers to a system of names or terms used in a particular science or art. The set of names of anatomical structures or organs of the body are usually referred to as a nomenclature. An Englishman, William Farr, in 1939, stated "The nomenclature is of much importance in [public health] as weights and measures in the physical sciences and should be settled without delay." An example of a nomenclature is SNOMED ® (Systematized Nomenclature of Medicine). SNOMED® provides for an internationally recognized set of terminologies for diseases, pathology, clinical indications, body parts, treatments and surgical operations.

Classification

Classification is the grouping of objects into classes according to some common relationships or attributes. An example of a classification system is the World Health Organization's ICD – n (International Classification of Disease). Examples of classes include such groups as diagnoses, drugs, allergies, findings, anatomies, etc.

Taxonomy

Taxonomy is defined as the practice and science of classification. Taxonomies are typically arranged in a tree or hierarchical structure with parent-child relationships.

Ontology

Ontologies deal with questions concerning what entities exist or can be said to exist, how such entities should be grouped, related within a hierarchy and subdivided according to similarities and differences. An ontology is a formal representation of a set of concepts within a domain and the relationships between those concepts. An ontology provides a vocabulary that can be used to model a domain. Examples of ontologies include the Gene Ontology and the Web Ontology Language (OWL). An OWL ontology may include descriptions of classes, properties and their instances. Protégé is a free, open-source ontology editor and knowledge-based framework that can be represented in an OWL-based ontology.

As should be evident from the definitions, these words are related and overlap in use. Each word is used for a specific purpose, but those purposes have less and less distinction as the purposes merge. For the most part, in the remaining sections of this chapter, vocabulary or terminology will be used interchangeably to identify the area we are discussing.

BASIC FEATURES OF A TERMINOLOGY

The different controlled vocabulary sets use different models – some no apparent model at all, different code schemes, and different attributes. The major requirement of any vocabulary is completeness with the ability to convey meaning or concept unambiguously, regardless of the context in which it is used. A data element is the fundamental unit of data interchange and, in its simplest form, is called an atomic element. Vocabulary components start as atomic elements, but the components must represent concepts not words. From these atomic data elements, phrases are built by adding atomic concepts together. There are two approaches to building the phrases. The first is a pre-compositional approach in which atomic data elements are added together, prior to use, in a meaningful way to name only possible conditions. Such an approach does not ensure completeness and creates a large number of terms. The second approach is post-compositional in which the atomic terms are put together dynamically as used. The challenge to the value of this approach is that it may lead to ambiguity or more than one way to define the same concepts. A compromise solution is the construction of a template that defines composition and constrains compositional extensibility.

J. Cimino (Cimino, 1998) defined the characteristics most desired in a vocabulary model. Each vocabulary term is associated with a concept identified by a non-semantic concept identifier, e.g., a numeric identifier. Codes that have meaning, such as M for male and F for female, quickly lose significance as the value set increases in number. The code should include a check digit, particularly if the code is input manually. The check digit serves to recognize data entry errors such as reversal of digits. The code should also not attempt to imply a hierarchical relationship among the concepts. The primary reason is that the relationships are polyhierarchial and relation-ships are best represented with link attributes. With automatic capture of data, check digits have less importance. A number of groups propose using an object identifier (OID) across all of health care to identify all objects used in health care. The OID consists of a node in a hierarchically-assigned namespace, formally defined using the International Telecommunication Union's ASN.1 standard. The root of the arc (the first digit) identifies one of three paths: 0 = ITU-T, 1 = ISO, and 2 = joint-ISO-ITU-T. Health Level Seven (HL7), a standards-developing organization in the area of electronic health care data exchange, is an assigning authority at the 2.16.840.1.113883 node [joint-iso-itu-t (2).country (16).us (840). organization (1).hl7 (113883)]. HL7 maintains its own OID registry, and as of January 1, 2008 it contained almost 3,000 nodes, most of them under the HL7 root.

One of the problems with many of the existing controlled vocabularies is that, in an attempt to be complete, include codes such as "Not Elsewhere Classified" (NEC) or "Not Otherwise Specified" (NOS). The classic example that illustrates the problem with the use of those terms is the vocabulary that included a code for Hepatitis A, a code for Hepatitis B, and a code for non-A-non-B. When Hepatitis C was given its own code later, one could not assume that non-A –non-B was actually Hepatitis C.

One of the benefits of using structured data with coded terms is to drive decision support algorithms. This feature requires a fine granularity in the atomic terms available. The groupings and awkward phrasing of several of the terminology sets are inadequate to serve this function.

Classes of Data

The definition of a term includes the unique concept identifier, the preferred name, a unique unambiguous definition, data type, units, class, value sets, synonyms, short name, and potentially other attributes. The general classes include:

- Demographic
- Signs and symptoms
- Anatomy
- Physical findings
- Diagnostic procedures
- Organisms
- Chief complaint
- Diagnoses
- Medications
- Immunizations
- Allergies
- Adverse events
- Therapeutic
- Genomic
- Billing and insurance
- Administrative
- Other

Different sets of controlled terminology address different classes. The consequence is that no single controlled terminology provides a complete set of concepts. In many cases, a controlled vocabulary does not include atomic terms for the value set. For example, the method of transportation for a patient encounter is a frequently collected term. Few systems include this value set or even the root term. In addition, other identifiers are required to completely express coded events. These other identifiers include persons, providers, places, health plans, etc.

CONTROLLED TERMINOLOGIES

International Classification of Disease

The International Classification of Disease (ICD) is one of the oldest lasting controlled terminologies. Developed and owned by the World Health Organization, it was first published in 1900. It is designed for the classification of morbidity and data for statistical purposes, for the purpose of indexing medical records by disease and op-

erations. The current version is the 10th revision (ICD-10) which is used by most of the world. The United States currently uses ICD-9-Clinical Modification (CM), but is committed to changing to ICD-10 with a compliance date of October 1, 2013. The main reason the U.S. is one of the last countries to update to ICD-10 is the resistance of the payers to the change. Estimates for the cost of the change ranged from 5 billion dollars to 15 billion dollars. The U.S. will also use a local replacement of CM procedural codes known as Procedure Coding System (PCS).

ICD-9-CM is used in the U.S. for professional billing. That requirement seems unlikely to change, so it is most likely that ICD-9/ICD-10 will exist for an indefinite period of time. ICD-10/9 is the most frequently used controlled terminology globally and that trend also is likely to continue. ICD-9 and 10 are not clinically pure coding systems. Expressions used in the concept names are not clinically used terms. It also includes "NEC" codes and uses pre-coordinated terms.

ICD-11 is currently under development with a completion data of 2015. Dr. Chris Chute of the Mayo Clinic is the chief editor.

There are supplements to the ICD coding system, including the Diagnostic and Statistical Manual of Mental Disorders (DSM IV), published by the American Psychiatric Association. This coding system standardizes diagnoses in psychiatry and mental health disorders. DSM IV includes diagnostic definitional criteria. DSM uses a multi-axial approach to coding to accommodate the linkage of mental health problems to other disease states. The five axes are clinical syndromes, development disorders and personality disorders, physical conditions, severity of psychosocial stresses, and highest level of functioning. It uses a coding scheme consistent with ICD. These codes are important because most disease and other factors in life have an impact on mental health. Future electronic health records will include mental health coding; most diseases, even in primary care, will have a mental health

Table 1. Example of ICD 9 codes

018.0 Acute military tuberculosis
018.8 Other specified miliary tuberculosis
018.9 Miliary tuberculosis, unspecified
780.01 Coma
V10.9 Unspecified personal history of malignant neoplasm
E828 Accident involving animal being ridden

Table 2. Examples of CPT codes

99201 New Patient office visit
99211 Established Patient office visit
11100 Biopsy of skin
19316 Reduction mammaplasty
30100 Biopsy, intranasal
39501 Repair, laceration of diaphragm
93042 Rhythm ECG

involvement. DSM has changed little over time and has a licensing fee.

Current Procedural Terminology (CPT)

Current Procedural Terminology, owned by the American Medical Association, is medical nomenclature used to report medical procedures and services for purposes of reimbursement. The use of CPT coding is required by the Centers for Medicare & Medicaid Services (CMS). CPT is licensed by American Medical Association (AMA). Table 2 shows examples of CPT codes.

Healthcare Common Procedure Coding System (HCPCS)

The HCPCS Level II Code Set is a comprehensive classification system that classifies similar products that are medical into categories for the purpose of efficient claims processing. HCPCS is divided into two subsystems: Level I is the CPT code set described above; Level II is used primarily to identify products, supplies and services not included in the CPT codes. Examples of products coded in HCPCS, Level 2 include ambulance services, durable medical equipment, prosthetics, orthotics, and supplies used outside a physician's office. Table 3 shows example HCPCS coding.

Diagnosis Related Groups (DRGs)

DRGs were created in the early 1980s by Fetter and Thompson at Yale University with support from Health Care Financing Administration

(now CMS) with an original purpose of classifying patients into groups relating to the resources they consumed. DRGs are based on ICD-9-CM diseases and procedures codes and use some rather complex coding algorithms. DRGs are known as groupers in that the DRG groups a set of codes that are expected to have similar hospital resource use and are used by the Centers for Medicare and Medicaid Services (CMS) as the basis for a prospective payment system. DRGS are assigned by a grouper program based on ICD 9-CM, procedures, age, sex, and the presence of complications or comorbidities. Current version is Version 2.6. Table 4 shows examples of DRG codes.

Logical Observation Identifiers Names and Codes (LOINC®)

LOINC® development was led by Dr. Clem McDonald at the Regenstrief Institute and was developed primarily for identifying medical laboratory observations (Huff, 1998), (McDonald, 2003). The current version of LOINC® is v2.2. LOINC® is available at no cost.

Actually there are two sections of LOINC®: the laboratory section, which is the most widely used; and the clinical portion that has more limited

Table 3. Examples of HCPCS coding

A0040 Ambulance Service, air, helicopter service, transport
A0999 Unlisted ambulance service
A4200 Gauze pads, medicated or nonmedicated, each
A4367 Ostomy belt
B9999 NOC for parenteral supplies
E1139 Standard wheelchair, fixed full length arms, swing away detachable elevating leg rests

Table 4. Examples of DRG codes

75 Respiratory disease with major chest operating room procedure, no major complication or comorbidity
76 Respiratory disease with major chest operating room procedure, minor complication or comorbidity
77 Respiratory disease with other respiratory system operating procedure, no complication or comorbidity
79 Respiratory infection with minor complication, age greater than 17
80 Respiratory infection with no minor complication, age greater than 17
89 Simple Pneumonia with minor complication, age greater than 17
90 Simple Pneumonia with no minor complication, age greater than 17
475 Respiratory disease with ventilator support
538 Respiratory disease with major chest operating room procedure and major complication or comorbidity
539 Respiratory disease, other respiratory system operating procedure and major complication or comorbidity
540 Respiratory infection with major complication or comorbidity
631 Respiratory infection with secondary diagnosis of bronchopulmonary dysplasia
740 Respiratory infection with secondary diagnosis of cystic fibrosis
770 Respiratory infection with minor complication, age not greater than 17
771 Respiratory infection with no minor complication, age not greater than 17
772 Simple Pneumonia with minor complication, age not greater than 17
773 Simple Pneumonia with no minor complication, age not greater than 17
798 Respiratory infection with primary diagnosis of tuberculosis

use. Lab LOINC® is used dominantly in the U.S. for laboratory test names. It includes chemistry, hematology, serology, microbiology (including parasitology and virology), and toxicology; drugs and cell counts for blood smears and cerebrospinal fluids; and antibiotic susceptibilities. Clinical LOINC® includes vital signs, hemodynamics, intake/output, ECG, obstetric ultrasound, cardio echo, urologic imaging, pulmonary ventilator management, survey instruments, and other categories of data. LOINC® also includes codes and definitions for clinical documents.

LOINC® codes meet very well the criteria for the desiderata for controlled vocabularies. The codes are numeric, permanently unique, and have no meaning or implied hierarchical linkages. A LOINC® code has a format of NNNNN-C, where C is the check digit. LOINC® codes are defined by six definitional axes:

- **Component name**: what is measured, evaluated, or observed
- **Property**: characteristic of what is measured (length, mass, volume, etc.)
- **Timing**: interval of time over which the observation or measurement is made
- **System**: context or specimen type on which observation is made

- **Type of scale**: quantitative, ordinal, nominal, or narrative
- **Type of method**: procedure used to make measurement or observation

LOINC® continues to evolve with new codes including terminology for genomes. The current LOINC® database contains over 51,000 terms. The international use of LOINC® is growing rapidly. LOINC® has been translated into German, Spanish, Portuguese, and Simplified Chinese. The Regenstrief Institute provides a Windows-based mapping utility called the Regenstrief LOINC ®Mapping Assistant (RELMA) to facilitate searches through the LOINC® database and to assist efforts to map local codes to LOINC® codes. REMLA is also free for use. Table 5 below illustrates examples of LOINC®.

National Drug Codes (NDC)

Drug products are identified and reported using a unique, three-segment number called the National Drug Code (NDC) and are controlled by the Food and Drug Administration (FDA). Product names are generally supplied by the manufacturer or "labeler". Labelers get a 4 or 5 digit code that is assigned by the FDA. The product code is 3 or 4

Table 5. Examples of LOINC® coding

```
4764-5 | GLUCOSE^3H POST 100 G GLUCOSE PO | SCNC | PT | SER/PLAS | QN|
1530-5 | GLUCOSE^3H POST 100 G GLUCOSE PO | MCNC | PT | SER/PLAS | QN |
5955-0 | COAGULATION THROMBIN INDUCED | TIME | PT | PPP^CONTROL | QN | TILT TUBE
12189-7 | CREATINE KINASE.MB/CREATINE KINASE.TOTAL | CFR | PT | SER/PLAS | QN | CALCULATION
13969-1 | CREATINE KINASE.MB | MCNC | PT | SER/PLAS | QN |
```

digits assigned and the package code has 2 digits assigned by the labeler. The NDC is limited to 10 digits. The drug database includes the product name, the NDC code, dosage form, routes of administration, active ingredients, strength, unit, package size and type, major drug class, and the FDA approved application number.

RxNorm

RxNorm is a standardized nomenclature for clinical drugs and is produced by the National Library of Medicine (NLM). The name of the clinical drug combines its ingredients, strengths, and form. Form is the physical form in which the drug is administered. RxNorm is intended to cover all prescription medications in the United States. The clinical drug name includes the active ingredients, strengths, and dose form. If any of the components change, then it has a different RxNorm entry. RxNorm is not efficient for data entry. For example, searching for ampicillin will yield a pick list of over 60 items.

RxNorm is contained with the NLM Unified Medical Language System (UMLS) and is available at no cost. Although RxNorm has yet to come into wide-spread use, it appears to be positioned as the prescription drug naming scheme of choice in the United States. RxNorm has little international use.

RxTerms

RxTerms is a drug interface terminology derived from RxNorm for prescription writing or medication history. RxTerms solves the data entry problems of RxNorm by separating drug name + strength + dose form + route into separate selectable components. RxTerms includes synonyms, abbreviations, and "tall man" lettering recommended by the FDA to avoid medication errors. It also includes both Brand names and generic names. RxTerms does not include drugs that are unavailable. It is available at no user cost, but it is largely U.S. specific.

VA National Drug File Reference Terminology (NDF-RT)

The NDF-RT is produced by the U.S. Department of Veterans Affairs and is used for describing drug characteristics including ingredients, chemical structure, dose form, physiologic effect, mechanism of action, pharmacokinetics, and related diseases (Brown, 2004).

International Health Terminology Standards Development Organization (IHTSDO)

IHTSDO was formed in 2007 with nine charter members: Australia, Canada, Denmark, Lithuania, The Netherlands, Sweden, United Kingdom, and the United States. Members of IHTSDO can be either an agency of a national body or an endorsed body. IHTSDO owns and administers rights to SNOMED-CT® and other health terminologies and related standards. The purpose of IHTSDO is to develop, maintain, promote and enable the uptake and correct use of SNOMED-CT® around the world. The organization is based in Denmark, and is supported by dues and fees charged to its members.

Systematized Nomenclature of Medicine (SNOMED®)

SNOMED® has its roots in the Systematized Nomenclature of Diseases and Organisms (SNDO) started in 1928 by the NY Academy of Medicine. From this beginning, next came the Systematized Nomenclature of Pathology (SNOP), in 1965, under the efforts of the College of American Pathology (CAP). An expanded version with a name change occurred in 1979 when the Systematized Nomenclature of Medicine (SNOMED 2®) evolved, defined around seven axes. SNOMED 2® was the most widely developed terminology used in pathology worldwide. This SNOMED® had several evolutions and became an international standard in 1993, renamed SNOMED 3®. In 1999, SNOMED - RT® (Reference Terminology) made its appearance, and in 2002, the current version, SNOMED-CT® (Clinical Terminology), made its appearance. SNOMED-CT® is the result of a merger of SNOMED®, primarily a code set for pathology, with the Reed Clinical Terms System from the United Kingdom. Reed codes had evolved since 1984, and the version merged with SNOMED® was Clinical Terms, Version 3. Reed codes were used mostly in primary care by the National Health Service. Dr. Roger Côté of the Université de Sherbrooke played a major role in the development of SNOMED (Rothwell, 1996). ® His persistence, loyalty to the concept, leadership and work have contributed over the years to SNOMED's becoming the world's premier controlled terminology.

The core components of SNOMED-CT® include concept codes, descriptions, and relationships. It constitutes a semantic network with definitions (Spackman, 1998). A concept is a basic unit of meaning and is designated by a unique code, a unique name and a description, including a preferred term and synonyms. Codes are a string of digits with length 6-18 digits; there is one code per meaning. Codes are organized in a directed acyclic graph (i.e., a hierarchy). SNOMED® codes can be used in a post-coordinated fashion. SNOMED-CT® includes 19 higher level hierarchies; each of which has sub-hierarchies. The relationships are link concepts either within a hierarchy or across hierarchies.

The SNOMED® axes are:

- Findings and disorders [F]
- Procedures [P]
- Body structures (anatomy) [T]
- Morphology [M]
- Organisms [L]
- Substances [L]
- Physical Agents [A]
- Events
- Observations
- Occupations
- Social context
- General
- Other

SNOMED-CT® has 344,000 concepts, 450,000 medical descriptions, and 700,000 concept interrelations. It has been cross mapped to ICD9-CM, ICD10 and LOINC. SNOMED® continues to grow, with several other controlled vocabularies being integrated into SNOMED®. The same context, however, can be coded different ways in SNOMED®, making complete retrievals of data a challenge.

Under the guidance of IHTSDO, SNOMED® is rapidly becoming the dominant controlled terminology in the world. SNOMED-CT® is available without charge in those countries holding membership in IHTSDO. IHTSDO recently announced a sliding scale for "buy-in", opening access to SNOMED® to more countries, particularly the developing world. There are still issues with SNOMED® and its underlying model.

International Classification for Primary Care (ICPC)

ICPC is a classification system for primary care encounters (WONCA, 1998). It includes reason for encounters (chief complaint), problems managed, primary care interventions, and data created during the encounter. The coding scheme is based on body system, and the same disease is coded differently, depending on the body system involved. ICPC contains 17 groupings, including such categories as Digestive, Blood, Eye, Ear, Respiratory, Pregnancy, social problems, etc. It is based on ICD. ICPC focuses on the patient perspective and includes coding for fear of disease, request for preventive services, and request for treatment.

The 17 groupings are:

- A General and unspecified
- B Blood, blood forming organs, lymphatics, spleen
- D Digestive
- F Eye
- H Ear
- K Circulatory
- L Musculoskeletal
- N Neurological
- P Psychological
- R Respiratory
- S Skin
- T Endocrine, metabolic, nutritional
- U Urology
- W Pregnancy, childbirth, family planning
- X Female genital system, breast
- Y Male genital system
- Z Social Problems

ICPC was first published in 1987 by the Oxford University press. ICPC is being developed by the World Organization of National Colleges, Academies, and Academic Associations (WONCA) International Classification Committee. ICPC continues to evolve with periodic releases. The current version is tagged ICPC-2 with a release date. It has been translated into 19 languages, and it is included in the UMLS. It is used primarily in Europe and Australia for individual family practices and group practices. It is useful for statistically defining family practices and the nature of patient encounters. For some reason, ICPC has never caught on in the U.S. Table 6 shows a sampling of ICPC codes.

MEDCIN®

MEDCIN® is a proprietary medical vocabulary developed by Medicomp Systems. It includes over 250,000 clinical data elements and includes terms for symptoms, medical history, physical examination, tests, diagnoses and treatments. The vocabulary, itself, is available at no cost. Medicomp has developed additional tools and knowledge-based linkages available at a cost. Medicomp is probably one of the best controlled vocabularies for coding history and physical exam data. MEDCIN® is used by the U.S. Department of Defense. Medicomp was founded in 1978.

Medical Dictionary for Regulatory Activities (MedDRA)

MedDRA is an international terminology used by regulatory authorities and regulated biopharmaceutical industry. It includes the adverse event classification dictionary endorsed by the International Conference on Harmonization of

Table 6. Examples of ICPC codes

R05 cough
A03 Fever
A25 Fear of death, dying
A26 Fear of cancer, NOS
Z01 Poverty/financial problems
R01 Pain, respiratory system
K01 Heart pain
L04 Chest symptom/complaint
A11 Chest pain NOS

Table 7. Examples of MedDRA

10017789 Gastric hemorrhage (LLT)
10017788 Gastric haemorrhage (LLT)
10017947 Gastrointestinal disorders (SOC)

Technical Requirements for Registration of Pharmaceuticals for Human Use (ICH). It is mandated for use in Europe and Japan and is also used in the United States. MedDRA is managed by the Maintenance and Support Services Organization that reports to the International Federation of Pharmaceutical Manufacturers and Associations (IFPMA). MedDRA is free for regulators and has a revenue-based cost for industry. It is updated twice a year. The MedDRA Dictionary is organized into High-Level Group Terms, High-Level Terms, Preferred Terms, and Lower-Level Terms. The MedDRA codes are unique 8-digit numbers, starting with 10000001. As terms are added, the codes are assigned sequentially. Examples of MedDRA codes are shown below. Note different codes for different spellings of the same concept.\

Medical Subject Headings (MeSH)

MeSH is the NLM's controlled vocabulary thesaurus whose purpose is the indexing, cataloging, and searching biomedical and health-related documents and literature. MeSH terms are used to tag medical abstracts with concept-based informa-

Table 8. Examples of MeSH codes

D011014: Pneumonia
D018410: Pneumonia, bacterial
D007877: Legionnaires' disease
D011018: Pneumonia, pneumococcal
D011019: Pneumonia, mycoplasma
D009175: mycoplasma Infections
D011002: Pleuropneumonia, contagious
D011022: Pneumonia, Rickettsial
D011023: Pneumonia, Staphylococcal
D001996: Bronchopneumonia
D011024: Pneumonia, Viral

tion. MeSH terms are arranged in a hierarchical structure to permit searching a various levels. The 2009 MeSH contains 25,186 descriptors and over 160,000 entry terms, words that map to specific MeSH descriptors. The MeSH thesaurus is used for indexing over 5200 biomedical journals worldwide. MeSH is available free from the NLM. Examples of MeSH terms are shown in Table 8. Note the hierarchical structure.

Health Level Seven Tables

HL7 tables were defined for controlled terminologies for terms required for messages that did not exist in other controlled vocabularies or were so universal that they were inconsistently defined in many controlled terminologies (Bakken, 2000). Examples of HL7 tables include administrative gender, marital status, race, religion, patient type, billing status, admission source, admission type, relationship, etc. HL7 has defined over 500 of these tables. An example of an HL7 for admission type is shown in Table 9.

Gene Ontology

Gene Ontology (GO) is a controlled ontology (The Gene Ontology Consortium, 2000) that defines terms representing gene and gene product attributes in any organism. The ontology covers three domains: cellular component – the parts of

Table 9. Example of a HL7 code set for admission type

#	Value	Description
1	A	Accident
2	E	Emergency
3	L	Labor and Delivery
4	R	Routine
5	N	Newborn (Birth in this facility)
6	U	Urgent
7	C	Elective

Table 10. Examples of gene ontology

```
id: GO:0000023
name: maltose metabolic process
namespace: biological_process
def: "The chemical reactions and pathways involving the
disaccharide maltose (4-O-alpha-D-glucopyranosyl-D-
glucopyranose), an intermediate in the catabolism of glycogen
and starch." [GOC:jl, ISBN:0198506732 "Oxford Dictionary
of Biochemistry and Molecular Biology"]
subset: gosubset_prok
exact_synonym: "malt sugar metabolic process" []
exact_synonym: "malt sugar metabolism" []
exact_synonym: "maltose metabolism" []
is_a: GO:0005984 ! disaccharide metabolic process
```

Table 11. Example of GO annotation

```
Gene product: Actin, alpha cardiac muscle 1,
UniProtKB:P68032
GO term: heart contraction ; GO:0060047 (biological process)
Evidence code: Inferred from Mutant Phenotype (IMP)
Reference: PMID:17611253
Assigned by: UniProtKB, June 06, 2008
```

a cell or its extracellular environment; molecular function – the elemental activities of a gene product at the molecular level; and biological process – operations or sets of molecular events with a defined beginning and end, pertinent to the functioning of integrated living cell units (cells, tissues, organs, and organisms). Each term has a term name, a unique alphanumeric identifier, a definition with cited sources, and a namespace indicating the domain to which it belongs. Terms may also have synonyms. The GO ontology is structured as a directed acyclic graph, and each term has defined relationships to one or more terms in the same domain or to other domains. A typical entry is shown below. The GO Ontology has 16,148 biological process; 2315 cellular component, and 8513 molecular function terms. GO is available for no charge.

Another component of the GO is the annotation of genes and gene products, using terms from the GO. The annotation includes the gene product identifier, the relevant GO term and the reference (journal article use to make the annotation, and evidence code denoting the type of evidence upon which the annotation is based, and the date and time of the annotation. The Table 11 shows an example of a GO annotation.

Nursing Terminologies

There are a number of nursing terminologies in use today (Ozbolt, 2000), (Hardiker, 2000), Coenen, 2001). Each has a slightly different purpose, but the overlap in content. Basically, the nursing terminologies address these concepts:

- Diagnoses/judgments
  - *Example*: "ineffective individual coping" [NANDA]
- Interventions
  - *Example*: "care giving/parenting – teach" [Omaha]
- Outcomes
  - *Example*: "family functioning' [NOC]
- Goals
  - *Example*: "patient moods will stabilize" [PCDS]

These nursing terminologies are identified below:

North American Nursing Diagnosis Association (NANDA)

NANDA is an international nursing association that has defined nursing diagnoses classification terminology to describe clinical judgments nurses make in providing nursing care. These diagnoses are the basis for selection of nursing outcomes and interventions. NANDA concepts are available in multiple languages.

Clinical Care Classification System (CCC)

The CCC System, developed by Dr. Virginia Saba (Saba, 1989) and colleagues at Georgetown University, was developed to provide a method for predicting home care resource needs and measure patient outcomes. The CCC is a structured clinical vocabulary and provides a standardized, coded, nursing terminology that identifies the discrete data elements of nursing practice. It provides a unique framework for capturing the 'essence of care' in all healthcare settings. The CCC is thee first national nursing terminology standard accepted for the encounter message component in clinical data for chief complaint and nurses/triage notes for the EHR. The CCC was accepted as a named standard within the Healthcare Information Technology Standards Panel (HITSP) Interoperability Specification for EHRs, Biosurveillance and Community Empowerment in 2006.

The CCC consists of two interrelated terminologies: Nursing Diagnoses & Components and Nursing Interventions & Actions. They are classified by 21 care components that represent the physiological, psychological, functional and health behavioral patterns of care. The Clinical Care Classifications include 182 nursing diagnoses, 792 nursing interventions, and 546 nursing outcomes. The CCC uses a five character alphanumeric coding structure based on ICD 10.

Patient Care Data Set (PCDS)

The Patient Care Data Set was developed by Dr. Judith Ozbolt, beginning in 1992. PCDS is a data dictionary of elements to be used in clinical information systems. The elements are defined at an atomic level and can be pre-coordinated to describe clinical activities. The vocabulary set is multiaxial and is organized into 22 components related to nursing activities. Each component contains three axes: Problems, Goals, and Orders. Version 4.0 (1998) contained 363 patient problems, 1357 patient care orders, and 311 patient care goals.

Omaha System

The Omaha System is a comprehensive documentation system for multidisciplinary healthcare practitioners during an inpatient stay. The system is based on three components: Problem Classification Scheme (assessment), Intervention Scheme (service delivery), and Problem Rating Scale for Outcomes (evaluation). The Omaha System is designed to be used with individuals, families and communities in all settings. It supports quality improvement by linking clinical data to demographic, financial, administrative, and staffing data. It presents a framework for integrating and sharing data since its beginning in the early 1970s. The Omaha System is used in home care, public health, school health practice settings, nurse-managed center staff, and hospital-based and managed care case managers. Its users include occupational health nurses, parish nurses, acute care and rehabilitation hospital/long term care staff, educators and students, and researchers.

AORN Perioperative Nursing Data Set (PNDS)

PNDS is a standardized terminology that facilitates the documentation of the care provided by perioperative nurses. It covers the perioperative patient experience from pre-admission until discharge. It assists in the measurement and evaluation of patient care outcomes. It helps informing decisions about the relationship of staffing to patient outcomes. PNDS is the only nursing terminology that is developed by a specialty organization.

International Classification of Nursing Practice

The ICNP provides a structured classification vocabulary that enables comparison of nursing data.

Its purpose is to provide a common vocabulary through which nurses can communicate among and between nurses. ICNP also describes nursing care of people in a variety of settings and permits comparison of nursing data across populations and settings.

The three primary elements of ICNP are:

- **Nursing diagnoses**: the focus of nursing
- **Nursing interventions**: actions nurses perform
- **Nursing outcomes**: results of nurses' actions that impact outcomes

Nursing Interventions Classification (NIC)

NIC is the first comprehensive classification of treatments performed by nurses. It is used for both nurse-initiated and physician-initiated nursing treatments. Over 400 interventions have been identified. Each intervention includes a label, a definition, and a set of activities a nurse does to carry out the intervention. Examples of interventions include acid-base management, airway suctioning, pressure ulcer care, anxiety reduction, home maintenance assistance, hyperglycemia management, ostomy care, fall prevention, illness prevention, health promotion, and family support. A taxonomic structure has been introduced to the system, and a feedback and review system implemented to validate the interventions. NIC extends across numerous specialties.

Nursing Outcomes Classification (NOC)

NOC is a classification system which describes patient outcomes as a consequence of nursing intervention. NIC is closely related to NOC. NOC contains 330 outcomes; each has a definition, a list of indicators that can be used to evaluate patient status in relation to patient outcome, place to identify source of data, a five-point Likert scale to indicate patient status, and a short list of references used in the description of outcome. Outcomes are rated from 1 to 5, with descriptive meanings of extremely compromised, substantially compromised, moderately compromised, mildly compromised, and not compromised. This scale provides quantifiable data about patient outcomes can be used to analyze the impact of various interventions on groups of patients. This feature is most important in doing risk assessment. The outcomes are grouped into 31 classes and 7 domains. The seven domains are: Functional Health, Physiologic Health, Psychosocial Health, Health Knowledge & Behavior, Perceived Health, and Community Health. Each outcome is assigned a code.

Table 12. Comparison of content of nursing terminologies

	Diagnoses	Interventions	Outcomes	Goals
NANDA	X			
NIC		X		
NOC			X	
CCC	X	X	X	
PCDS	X	X		X
Omaha	X	X	X	
AORN	X	X	X	
ICNP	X	X	X	X

Nursing Terminologies Summary

The American Nursing Association has endorsed NANDA, Omaha, CCC, NIC, NOC, PCDS, and PNDS. Several of the above nursing terminology sets have been mapped into SNOMED-CT, including NANDA, NIC, NOC, the Omaha System and CCC. In some cases, the mapping is only approximate. However, the advantage of mapping the various nursing languages into SNOMED is that fewer different controlled terminology sets that have to be accommodated.

Unified Medical Language System

The Unified Medical Language System (UMLS) is a compendium of many controlled vocabularies in biomedicine and health (Lindberg, 1993). UMLS was designed and is maintained by the National Library of Medicine. It provides a mapping structure among these controlled vocabularies, permitting some degree of translation, among the vocabulary systems.

UMLS consists of three knowledge sources:

- **The Metathesaurus**: a multi-purpose, multi-lingual vocabulary database that contains information about biomedical and health-related concepts including names, codes, and relationships. The Metathesaurus contains the sources of all the included vocabularies with the mappings. The purpose of the Metathesaurus, which is organized by concepts, is to link alternate names of the same concepts together (mapping) and to identify meaningful relationships between different concepts.
- **The Semantic Network**: a set of semantic types that provide a consistent categorization of concepts represented in the Metathesaurus and a useful set of meaningful relationships (Semantic Relations) that exist between Semantic Types. Major groupings include anatomic structures, biologic function, chemicals, events, organisms, physical objects, and other concepts. The primary link is the *"isa"* link that establishes a hierarchy of semantic types. There are also non-hierarchical links: *physically related to, spatially related to, temporally related to, functionally related to, and conceptually related to.*
- **The Specialist Lexicon**: a general English lexicon that includes both commonly occurring words as well as biomedical terms. An entry includes the syntactic, morphological and orthographic information. The primary purpose of the Specialists Lexicon is to support Natural Language Processing (NLP). The Specialist Lexicon includes spelling variants of a word in different parts of speech. The Specialist Lexicon includes most frequently used words from *Dorland's Illustrated Medical Dictionary, The American Heritage Word Frequency Book,* and *Longman's Dictionary of Contemporary English.* The Lexicon contains approximately 20,000 entries.

DATA ELEMENTS

The distinction between what a data element is and what a terminology is may differ only in the perspective of the viewer. Data represent the ability to measure and understand characteristics of health and health care, effects of interventions and treatments, outcomes, and quality of life. Data becomes the source from which knowledge can be extracted. Reusability of data requires a common understanding of every data element. One of the first activities among groups sharing data is the creation of a minimum data set. Sharing of data requires a common set of data elements with a common understanding of their meaning. Unfortunately, this process most frequently occurs, each time, without using existing materials.

This section presents an approach to the semantic interoperability from the perspective of defining a set of data elements with vocabulary being the name attribute of a data element. A number of groups are taking this approach, and some of them will be discussed below. Most of the work uses ISO 11179, Specification and Standardization of Data Elements. The section closes with a discussion of how a Master Set of Data Elements might be generated and shared internationally to provide true semantic interoperability.

ISO 11179 – INFORMATION TECHNOLOGY – SPECIFICATION AND STANDARDIZATION OF DATA ELEMENTS

ISO 11179 is a standard dating from 1999 that has been used globally to create metadata registries of data elements. The standard was created by Subcommittee SC 32 of the Joint Technical Committee ISO/IEC JTC 1.

The standard consists of six parts:

- **Part 1**: Framework for the specification and standardization of data elements
- **Part 2**: Classification for data elements
- **Part 3**: Basic attributes of data elements
- **Part 4**: Rules and guidelines for the formulation of data definitions
- **Part 5**: Naming and identification principles for data elements
- **Part 6**: Registration of data elements

ISO 11179 emphasizes such data element characteristics as identifiers, definitions, representation, and classification categories. A data element is defined as having three parts:

- The **object class**: a set of things, abstractions or ideas in the real world whose meaning, properties and behavior follow defined rules;

- **Property:** a feature common to all members of an object class;
- **Representation**: description of how the data are represented – the attributes, including data types, units, and value domain.

The value domain is the set of permissible (or valid) values for a data element. Value domains may be enumerated or non-enumerated. Values may be numeric, coded, or textual.

ISO 11179 has been used to create metadata registries in other areas than health care, for example, the U.S. Census.

United States Health Information Knowledgebase (USHIK)

USHIK is a metadata registry, begun in 1998, for healthcare data and contains content contributed by several Standards Developing Organizations and other healthcare organizations. USHIK uses methodology based on ISO 11179 and is sponsored by the Agency for Health Research and Quality (AHRQ). The registry contains over twelve thousand data elements. USHIK contains high level Information Models to permit the grouping of data elements. Data elements are linked to model views and are linked to other data elements. The Healthcare Information Technology Standards Panel (HITSP) uses USHIK to compare standards for demographic data, to perform gap analysis among selected standards, and to support feedback to SDOs for requirements of existing standards to meet specific use cases.

Clinical Data Interchange Standards Consortium (CDISC)

The CDISC Terminology Initiative's objective is to define and support the terminology needs of the CDISC models across the clinical trial continuum. That initiative led to the development of controlled terminology for the Study Data Tabulation Model (SDTM) Implementation Guide. The philosophy behind SDTM was to evaluate and use existing terminology when available and, working with the developer and owner of existing terminology, to expand existing terminology to meet CDISC needs. SDTM is harmonized across CDSIC models and with pre-existing vocabulary initiatives.

The Clinical Data Acquisition Standards Harmonization (CDASH) Standard describes recommended (minimal) data collection sets for 16 domains, including demographic, adverse events, and other safety domains that are common to all therapeutic areas and types of clinical research. CDASH is focused on the development of consensus-based content standards, (specifically: element name, definition, and metadata) for a basic set of global data collection fields based on the CDISC SDTM model.

National Cancer Institute (NCI)

The National Cancer Institute has created a national cancer Data Standards Repository (caDSR) and a core terminology set, the Enterprise Vocabulary Services (EVS), to support core semantics of the cancer community. The controlled vocabulary set includes external terminologies such as LOINC, MedDRA, VANDF-RT, HL7 and others. The NCI also has developed unique content where needed and incorporates other data sources including GO, Swissprot, drug formularies, and trial protocols. The EVS also links to UMLS and NCI has created a NCI Thesaurus that is a filtered UMLS Metathesaurus extended with additional required vocabularies. The NCI Metathesaurus contains over 1,100,000 concepts and over 2,200,000 terms and phrases with definitions. Over 55 controlled vocabularies are incorporated into the Metathesaurus.

The common data elements repository includes structured data reporting elements that are precisely defined. The caDSR uses ISO 11179 methodology. NCI supports the following collaborations:

- **FDA**: terminology for drugs, devices and clinical trial initiatives
- **VA**: drugs, clinical trials semantics
- **CDC**: cancer incidence and prevention
- **Cancer Centers**: clinical trials, experimental organism terminology, open terminology servers
- **CDISC/HL7**: clinical research data standards
- Others

A number of tools are available from NCI as part of the application support. Those tools include:

- **Common Data Element (CDE) Browser**: supports browsing, searching and exporting CDEs across contexts
- **CDE Curation Tool**: supports creating and editing data elements concepts, value domains, and data elements
- **Form Builder**: organizes CDEs in forms for Case Report Forms and other forms
- **UML Model Browser**: supports browsing and searching UML models loaded into caDSR
- **caDSR Sentinel Tool**: allows users to create and manage Alert Definitions for the caDSR Databases
- **SIW**: a Java Web Start application that assists users in adding consistent metadata to their UML model by matching their concepts with similar items from the NCI Thesaurus.

Cancer Biomedical Informatics Grid (caBIG)®

The cancer Biomedical Informatics Grid is an organization that brings together data, research tools, scientists, and organizations in order accelerate the discovery of new approaches for the detection, diagnosis, treatment and prevention of cancer. caBIG® uses NCI's caDSR and EVS as well as the full set of tools available from NCI to achieve its goals. caBIG® is federated, open development, open access and open source.

One activity of caBIG® is focused on vocabularies and common data elements - the VCDE Workspace. This Workspace is responsible for developing standards for the representation of ontologies and vocabularies used throughout the caBIG® system, as well as assessments of existing systems proposed for use within the caBIG®. Twenty CDEs have been defined and accepted by the group.

caBIG® recognizes four levels of compatibility in defining interoperability in a federated environment (https://cabig.nci.nih.gov/guidelines_documentation/). These levels are used to rate both syntactic and semantic interoperability and are applied to interface integration; vocabularies, terminologies, and ontologies; data elements; and information models. The levels range in the degree of interoperability provided.

- **Legacy**: implies no interoperability; free text or uncontrolled narrative
- **Bronze**: products created outside the caBIG program but compliant with the caBIG compatibility certification program. Items may be interoperable to some extent.
- **Silver**: products have undergone a compatibility review within the caBIG. Items are largely interoperable.
- **Gold**: products totally structured and defined and includes all attributes; fully interoperable.

ISSUES AND PROPOSED SOLUTIONS

The question of which terminology to use is ambiguous and confusing. Most institutions avoid the problem by using a local terminology. Even large enterprise systems, such as the Veterans Admin-istration, have left the choice up to the individual sites. These choices prevent semantic interoperability even within a single institution, and computer understanding of shared data among a larger audience is essentially impossible. Proprietary controlled vocabularies represent large revenues for the owners, and typically these owners have great influence over the use of their vocabularies in specific applications. For example, will the Centers for Medicare and Medicaid (CMS) ever be willing to change from the use of ICD vocabularies? Even the transition from ICD-9 to ICD-10 has been a bitter fight. Would the American Medical Association permit CPT codes to be replaced? SNOMED-CT has made considerable strides in world-wide use of SNOMED-CT through its new governance organization IHTSDO. The United Kingdom has invested considerable money into SNOMED and has legislated the use of SNOMED-CT in the United Kingdom. MedDRA has the strong support of the International Conference on Harmonization and the European Medicines Agency (EMEA) and is unlikely to change.

The survivability of most of the controlled vocabularies is very high. So what might be a solution? One approach is commonly used today – the mapping among the various vocabulary sets. That approach loses information and is prone to errors. If two vocabularies could be mapped without the loss of information, then why have two sets. Maintenance of mapping rules and synchronization of mapping data sets are very difficult and expensive.

Another approach is to define the use of a particular vocabulary for a particular purpose. For example specify LOINC® for laboratory test names and SNOMED-CT® for the value set. This approach is a step forward, but leaves a number of remaining vocabularies out of the solution, and each of these vocabularies will have a following and a community of users. For example, ICPC is extremely popular in many countries outside the US, and that condition is unlikely to change.

There also is the question of granularity. All existing controlled vocabularies have some underlying purposes that meet someone's needs. Most, if not all, vocabulary sets include some grouping, whether for reimbursement, reporting, comorbidities or other relationships. The granularity of terms varies, but most have a coarser granularity. There are few vocabulary sets defined from a pure clinical view point. If a terminology set is to be at the level of clinical expression, and used to drive clinical algorithms and clinical decision making, the granularity has to be five. Terms must be defined at an atomic level, and structures built from those basic terms. The argument is that there is a difference in what is required for clinical purposes and what is required by the variety of reporting purposes. The reuse of data also requires a finer granularity than exists today in controlled vocabularies.

Finally, there is the issue of what will vendors support. Although there is some freedom in what HIT vendors support, most vendors are now moving toward a preferred vocabulary. Further, those sets are often constrained and may not match the desires of the purchaser. Vendors suggest that there is not business case for a particular vocabulary and are reluctant to change.

If a particular user wishes to use, for example, a grouper or classifying terminology, that user could do a one-of translation for a clinical terminology set, rather than requiring every user to do the required mapping locally. For example if CMS wished to continue to use DRG and ICD codes sets, claims could be submitted using a rich clinical terminology, and CMS could do the mapping.

Health Level Seven, along with other organizations, has started an effort to bring together all medical societies plus government groups, such as NIH, CDC, CMS, FDA, FHA, VA, DOD plus terminology-related groups. The proposal is based on creating a global master set of data elements, where each data element has a set of defined and required attributes. Each data element would have a primary steward that would be the ultimate authority for the definition and attributes of the data element. The work would be done primarily within each medical society, using a common process. For overlaps and disagreements, a Clinical Information Interchange Council (CIIC) has been created to bring the groups together to agree on common attributes. If disagreements cannot be resolved, two data elements will be defined with clear distinctions between the data elements. The final decision of the characteristics of a data element will lie with experts identified by the stewarding group. There would, however, be feedback from the stewardship community and then from the outside world. Work would include the global community. Figure 1 shows the proposed process.

The data elements would be defined at an atomic level. Higher level structures would also be created using templates, archetypes, clinical statements and other structuring architecture. These structured data elements would each be assigned a unique code and include a set of attributes. One challenge of this approach is to engage the international community together in the defining and vetting process.

The many required languages would be accommodated through a language attribute. Content experts would be hired to translate concepts, not words, for each required languages. Cultural requirements and the accommodating of both eastern and western medicine terminology must be addressed. The master data element set would be mirrored in multiple datasets stored around the world. Updates would be in real time. Access to and use of the data elements repository would be at no cost to users. Obviously, a cost would be involved in creating and maintaining this repository; likely candidates would be the World Health Organization, the United Nations, or a group of the economically-leading countries of the world.

Figure 1. Proposed process for creating and maintaining data elements

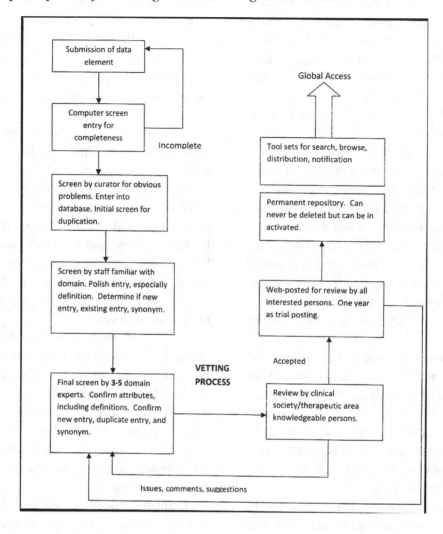

Characteristics of the Master Data Element Repository

Semantic interoperability requires more than just the use of common names and terms. It requires a rich set of attributes for both definition and maintenance. The section below discusses many of the defined attributes and the role they play is achieving semantic interoperability.

Definition

A major goal for creating the master set of data elements would be to remove all ambiguity

for each data element used. The first and most important requirement would be the definition attribute. A literature review, in 1994, identified 67 different definitions of unstable angina in use (Jones, 1994). One of the challenges in accepting and acting on data from other sources is the uncertainty of the meaning of the word used. The value of the master data element set is the dedication to unique and unambiguous definition of each term with the understanding of what a term means when it is used. The definitions can go a step further: definitions can include criteria required for use of the term. For example, the definition of acute myocardial infarction could include what must be present to make that diagnoses. If those conditions are presented in computer-readable terms, using other data elements with specific values, the diagnoses could be validated. If one of the logical components is missing, the system can prompt for the value. This approach would not only avoid ambiguity in use but would also validate the use. Similarly, data integrity could be strengthened by including constraint specifications. Certain diseases can only occur in males and others in females. Finally, definitions should include, when appropriate, how the measurement should be made. For example, the measurement of Length of Stay is the Discharge Date minus the Admit Date; Height should be measured with shoes removed and top of head level with floor.

Coding

Codes should be unique and likely numeric and may include a check digit. One recommendation for codes is to use the ISO Object Identifiers to guarantee uniqueness of codes. Once assigned, a code is never reused. Data elements may be deprecated, however, and future input of that term would be restricted. An example may occur, if, in the defining of a data element, agreement cannot be reached, so two data elements are defined. Later evaluation of use determines that the two terms are in fact the same. One term would be deprecated, but would remain in the database so existing data would still be identifiable.

Name

The preferred name should be the term the clinical experts use when referring to the data element. It is the long name and does not contain any abbreviations or acronyms. At least in a transition period, these terms may be mapped to a term in an existing controlled vocabulary set. This approach would preserve the intellectual property value on existing vocabulary sets and permit groups to migrate from existing terminologies to the preferred names.

Short Name

The short name is the display name and is used when display space is limited. It is derived from the preferred name and may contain acronyms and abbreviations.

Synonyms

One of the biggest problems in the use of today's terminologies is the confusion between preferred names and synonyms. Synonym tables should be rich and include name variants, abbreviations, and alternate spellings. Synonyms permit compliance with preferred names but with more freedom in input. Meeting definitional requirements still, however, remains a challenge.

Units

Units must be specified for each data element, including no units. A standardized set of units should be used, most likely, scientific units.

Data Type

Data Type is one of a set of distinct values that has defined properties and format. Examples include numeric, integer, date-time, string, Boolean, etc. Data type may also be specified as coded with the source code set specified. The data type must be specified. The data type is likely to be a primitive data type and should be chosen from the ISO 21090 – Health Informatics - Harmonized Data Types for Information Exchange. Data types may also be complex, representing structures of data such as addresses or names.

Value Set

The value set represents the set of permissible values. Elements in the value set are frequently coded items that are also data elements. They may be numeric or textual. Value sets should include the permissible set of null flavors such as unavailable, unknown, not applicable, etc. Null flavor is the term used when the actual value is not available. For example, the null flavor for gender might be unavailable (not asked) or unknown (anatomically ambiguous). A value set for numeric might include a maximum and a minimum. A value set for a text string might include length.

Classes

Classes define the type of data element. Examples include demographic, administrative, reimbursement, diagnosis, procedures, studies (laboratory tests, radiology, diagnostic test), therapy (prescription drug, allergy (drug, animal, environment), blood product, immunization), adverse event, findings and history, physical exam, supplies, scheduling/appointments, protocols, providers, health plans, facilities, and others.

Classifications

Classifications identify class and subclasses into which the data element falls. Examples include antihistamine, beta blocker, antibiotic, respiratory disease, cardiac disease, heart murmur, etc. More than one classification may exist. Classifications may be hierarchical, and the permissible sets may vary with the category of data.

Citation

The citation identifies the authoritive source from which the definition and other attributes for the data element is taken.

Relational Links

Links to other data elements show relationships between data elements. These links may be hierarchical showing general to specific; showing parent/children relationships; showing equivalence; showing opposites; showing causes, or showing

manifestations. Flags may be included showing high level concepts, down to leaf level concepts. A data element may contain several links, appropriately identified.

Language

This set of attributes contains the name equivalent in all languages. It is likely that initial efforts will be limited to the most frequently used languages, but over time, all languages used for health care should be included.

Purpose

A new attribute is proposed that identifies the purpose of the data element. For example, why is gender included in an EHR? Obviously, gender is used to constrain the use of certain data elements, e.g., normal limits are gender dependent and certain diagnostic tests are gender-dependent. Other purposes would include key to certain diagnoses; show effect of treatment; show severity of disease, etc.

Administrative Attributes

There are a number of administrative attributes include with each data element. These attributes include:

- Steward of the data element
- Submitting organization
- Registration or certification authority
- Status (active/inactive/deprecated)
- Version (refined definition, added purposes are examples)
- Date of entry or last update

Use of Master Data Element Repository

All data elements used in any application must be taken from the master set of data elements, respecting their definitions and all their attributes. No site will use every data element but will derive the set it does use from the master set. Minimum data sets, defined as business sets, would be derived from the master set. Every site would have a web-accessible database containing the data elements it collects. Given proper authority, another site, needing to share or exchange data, would know what data was available. The content of disease registries would be defined from this master set. Health Plans and reimbursement requirements would be defined from the master data element set. Data exchanged between sites of care, for example a hospital and a nursing home, would be defined from the master set. Decision support, clinical guidelines, and evidence based care plans would be defined from the common repository. The real advantage would be that, through the use of the common set of data elements, knowledge could be shared globally and be immediately implementable. Audit reports, infectious disease reports, health surveillance, and geo-analysis could be accomplished in any setting, region or country and compared with other regions or countries. Rule-driven data sharing becomes routine.

The ease of use of the master data element registry would depend on the set of tools available. The tool sets available from the NCI are examples of the kind of tools required but need to be extended.

Application systems could be designed so that, as a site adds to the set of data elements collected, data entry screens automatically added those elements. A bit of imagination will extend what might be accomplished if such a registry exists. Tools and processes must be defined to permit the migration from the chaos of current vocabularies to the standards set.

The cost of setting up and maintaining the common data element registry would be minimal. Redundant activities will be virtually eliminated. As the data elements are identified and defined by experts, acceptance should be relatively quick and easy.

CONCLUSION

Mapping is the current way of dealing with terminology issues. However, if two code sets are not identical, then there will always be a loss of information. If code sets are identical, we only need one set. Mapping additionally challenges synchronization of databases and requires additional resources for maintenance and upkeep.

The vocabulary dilemma has existed for at least four decades with little progress. Current solutions leave much to be desired, and they are expensive. No one appears to be willing to step forward and force a solution. Vocabularies are a big business, and the market pressures to keep existing sets are strong. As long as the problem exists, semantic interoperability at national levels will not exist. It is possible that agreements at regional levels ease the problem, but it doesn't go away. Every region has a boundary, and patients cross that boundary. If the approach suggested in this chapter is successful, the potential of what can be achieved will be huge. The rewards will be overwhelming, and the money saved will be orders of magnitude more than the cost of making those decisions. The question is who will step forward.

ACKNOWLEDGMENT

I would like to acknowledge the use of examples, presentations, conversations and other education from many of my colleagues including Drs. Clem McDonald, Stanley Huff, James Cimino, Chris Chute, Judy Ozbolt, Virginia Saba, and Suzanne Bakken. I also express appreciation to the reviewers for their most constructive comments and suggestions in reviewing this chapter.

REFERENCES

Bakken, S., Campbell, K. E., Cimino, J. J., Huff, S. M., & Hammond, W. E. (2000). Toward Vocabulary Domain Specifications for Health Level 7–Coded Data Elements. *Journal of the American Medical Informatics Association, 7,* 333–342.

Brown, S. H., Elkin, P. L., Rosenbloom, S. T., Husser, C., Bauer, B. A., & Lincoln, M. J. (2004). VA National Drug File Reference Terminology: A Cross-Institutional Content Coverage Study. *Medinfo, 2004,* 477–481.

Cimino, J. J. (1998). Desiderata for Controlled Medical Vocabularies in the Twenty-First Century. *Methods of Information in Medicine, 37,* 394–403.

Coenen, A., Marin, H. F., Park, A., & Bakken, S. (2001). Collaborative Efforts for Representing Nursing Concepts in Computer-based Systems: International Perspectives. *Journal of the American Medical Informatics Association, 8,* 202–211.

de Keizer, N. F., Abu-Hanna, A., & Zwetsloot-Schonk, J. H. M. (2000). Understanding Terminological Systems I: Terminology and Typology. *Methods of Information in Medicine, 39,* 16–21.

Hardiker, N. R., Hoy, D., & Casey, A. (2000). Standards for Nursing Terminology. *Journal of the American Medical Informatics Association, 7,* 523–538.

Huff, S. M., Rocha, R. A., McDonald, C. J., DeMoor, J. E., & Fiers, T. (1998). Development of the logical observation identifier names and codes (LOINC) vocabulary. *Journal of the American Medical Informatics Association, 5,* 276–292.

Lindberg, D., Humphreys, B., & McCray, A. (1993). The Unified Medical Language System. *Methods of Information in Medicine, 34,* 281–291.

McDonald, C. J., Huff, S. M., Suico, J. G., Hill, G., Leavelle, D., & Aller, R. (2003). LOINC, a Universal Standard for Identifying Laboratory Observations: A 5-Year Update. *Clinical Chemistry, 49*(4), 624–633. doi:10.1373/49.4.624

Ozbolt, J. (2000). Terminology Standards for Nursing: Collaboration at the Summit. *Journal of the American Medical Informatics Association, 7*(6), 517–522.

Rothwell, D., & Côté, R. (1996). Managing Information with SNOMED: Understanding the Model. *SCAMC,* 80-83.

Saba, V. K. (1989). *Nursing Information Systems. Classification systems for describing nursing practice: working papers* (pp. 55–61). American Nurses Association.

Spackman, K., & Campbell, K. (1998). Compositional concept using SNOMED: towards further convergence of clinical terminologies. *J Am Med Inform Assoc Annual Symposium*; 740-744.

The Gene Ontology Consortium. (2000). Gene Ontology: tool for the unification of biology. *Nature Genetics, 25,* 25–29. doi:10.1038/75556

WONCA International Classification Committee. (1998). *ICPC-2, International Classification of Primary Care* (2nd ed.). Oxford University Press.

Chapter 3
Personal Health Records:
Status–Quo and Future Perspectives

Simon Y. Liu
National Library of Medicine, USA

ABSTRACT

Consumers, industry, and government have recently focused attention on the potential of personal health records to empower patients in the health care process, improve patient-provider relationships, facilitate patient access to health information, and improve the quality of health care. A Personal Health Record (PHR) is a private and secure digital record that is created, managed, and owned by an individual, and contains the owner's relevant health information. The benefits of PHRs have not yet been widely realized due to several significant challenges in their adoption, including the need for privacy, security, and interoperability, and the lack of accepted standards. Although many players in the healthcare arena are beginning to offer partial solutions, none have adequately addressed the full range of challenges. The adoption of PHRs can be significantly accelerated by the development of Open Source software that enables an individual to collect, create, organize, and manage his or her own private and secure PHR, using a standardized format and controlled vocabulary.

INTRODUCTION

Healthcare today is facing many critical challenges. One of the biggest is the lack of electronic health information. Studies suggested that over 80% of the doctors in the US manage healthcare information on paper. In other words, individual health information is housed independently by doctors or care providers. Therefore, access to individual's health information is difficult, especially in the event of an emergency. The concept of the *electronic* personal health record (PHR) has been suggested as a significantly improved method for collecting and using personal health information.

Recent surveys suggest that the general public wants PHRs. The Markle Foundation commissioned a survey of 1,003 Americans in November 2006, examining public opinion toward PHRs

DOI: 10.4018/978-1-61520-777-0.ch003

Copyright © 2010, IGI Global. Copying or distributing in print or electronic forms without written permission of IGI Global is prohibited.

(Markle Foundation, 2006a; Markle Foundation, 2006b).The survey found that 79% of the public believes that PHRs would provide major benefits to individuals in managing their health and 46.5% of the public expressed an interest in having a PHR. Eighty-four percent said it would be important to have electronic copies of health records if changing doctors or moving to another city. Similar percentages said they wanted access to their medical information to ensure that it is accurate, and to check for errors. However, most of those surveyed were very concerned about the potential that their personal health information might be misused or accessed without their authorization. Nearly 57% of the public express concern over the privacy and security of their data and more than 90% felt that their expressed consent should be required for each use of their information. Three quarters of those surveyed said the government has a role in establishing privacy and confidentiality protections for electronic personal health information.

PHR Benefits

There are many benefits to PHRs. In general, PHRs allow a greater patient access to a wide variety of health information, best medical practices, and health knowledge. Instead of several paper files locked away in various doctors' offices, all of an individual's medical records are in one place and fully accessible by that individual. A number of authors have recently described the benefits of PHRs and PHR systems (Endsley, S., Kibbe, D.C., Linares, A., & Coloafi, K., 2006; Tang, P.C., Ash, J.S., Bates, D.W., Overhage, J.M., & Sands, D.Z., 2006; U.S. Department of Health and Human Services, 2006). The key benefits include:

- **Improved quality of care**: PHRs can provide the opportunity for automated analysis of an individual's health profile, and identify potential improvements to healthcare based on an analysis of drug-drug interactions, current best medical practices, identification of gaps in the current medical care plan, and identification of medical errors. Patients with chronic illnesses will be able to track their diseases in conjunction with their providers, promoting earlier interventions when they encounter a deviation or problem.

- **Reduced healthcare cost**: In a recent study titled *The Value of Personal Health Records* (The Center for Information Technology Leadership, n.d.), the Center for Information Technology Leadership at Partners Healthcare System stated that adopting interoperable PHRs could save the United States more than $19 billion annually after expenses. The financial estimate is based on making the PHRs available to 80% of the population in a 10-year rollout period. The initial start-up costs are $3.7 billion and the annual maintenance costs are $1.9 billion. Primary sources of cost savings include sharing test results and medication lists, monitoring chronic disease conditions, visit support, automated medication renewals, electronic appointment scheduling, and administration of pre-visit questionnaires.

- **Better provider and patient relationship**: PHRs improve communication between patients and clinicians, allow documentation of interactions with patients and convey timely explanations of test results. PHR-mediated electronic communication between patients and caregivers can free clinicians from the limitations of telephone and face-to-face communication or improve the efficiency of such personal contacts (Tang, P., Ash, J., Bates, D., Overage, M., Sands, D., 2006).

- **Empower patient control**: A PHR provides continuity in healthcare records as an individual obtains medical services from multiple healthcare providers in different locations over time. A PHR enables individuals to be better informed about their healthcare, and empowers them to ensure that their records are complete and accurate.

- **Improved health information access**: One of the most important PHR benefits is greater patient access to a wide array of credible health information, data, and knowledge. A PHR system can enable personalized links to relevant health information sources, and assembly of health information that is customized to the needs of the individual.

Despite significant interest in PHRs and benefits of PHRs, less than 7 million U.S. adults actually use them, according to Manhattan Research's Cybercitizen Health v8.0 study (Manhattan Research, n.d.). Although there was recent buzz about offerings from companies such as Google, Microsoft, IBM, Intel, Manhattan Research says average consumers face barriers to adoption. Primary barriers include the difficult of data collection, the lack of portability and interoperability, the concern about privacy and security, and others. The full potential of PHRs will not be realized until they are widely adopted. An Open Source approach will promote and accelerate the adoption rate.

Interoperability refers to the technical capacity for the exchange of health information between different healthcare information systems. If PHRs cannot exchange data with other health care systems, they will become "information islands" that contain subsets of data. To facilitate interoperability, PHRs must support open communications, messaging, and content encoding standards as other health information systems. For example, Integrating the Healthcare Enterprise (IHE, www. ihe.net) is a global initiative that creates the framework for passing vital health information seamlessly across multiple healthcare enterprises. IHE brings together healthcare information technology stakeholders to implement standards for communicating patient information efficiently throughout and among healthcare enterprises by developing a framework for interoperability.

BACKGROUND

In 2001, the National Committee on Vital & Health Statistics (NCVHS) issued the "A Strategy for Building the National Health Information Infrastructure (NHII)" (The National Committee on Vital and Health Statistics, n.d.). In this report it mentions the *personal health dimension* supporting individuals in managing their own wellness and healthcare decision-making. It specifically mentions a personal health record (PHR) that is maintained and controlled by the individual or family. In 2004, President Bush announced that all citizens would have access to electronic medical records in 10 years. To this end, there is increasing interest in the consumer's role in his or her own health care and health care management. The PHR is an adjunct tool related to the provider based electronic medical record. The U.S. Secretary of Health and Human Services, the National Coordinator for Health Information Technology, and the Administrator of the Centers for Medicare and Medicaid Services (CMS) have all identified PHRs as a top priority. In 2005, American Health Information Management Association (AHIMA) formed an electronic health information management workgroup to examine the role of the PHR in relation to the electronic health record (EHR). In 2006, NCVHS released a comprehensive report and recommendations on "Personal Health Records and Personal Health Record Systems" that further promoted the needs and benefits of PHRs (U.S. Department of Health and Human Services, 2006).

Several organizations have recently initiated efforts to promote PHRs. As a free public service, the American Health Information Management Association (AHIMA) has created a Web site called "myPHR – Personal Health Record – A guide to understanding and managing your personal health information" (American Health Information Management Association, n.d.) Other health information technology organizations, such as the Healthcare Information and Management Systems Society (HIMSS) (Healthcare Information Management and Systems Society, n.d.) are creating committees and projects to develop strategies for increasing the adoption of PHRs.

Medical organizations are also beginning to support the adoption of PHRs. The American Academy of Family Physicians (AAFP) Center for Health Information Technology (CHIT) and the American Academy of Pediatrics (AAP) Council for Clinical Information Technology (COCIT) are participating in the development of standards related to PHRs (AIIM, 2006) and organizing information about standards-compatible products (American Academy of Family Physicians, n.d.).

PHR Defined

Currently, this is no standard or generally-accepted definition of "personal health record" in industry or government. The term PHR is variably used to describe either a data file or a software application, using either personal computer or Internet technologies, and with data ownership either by the individual or by somebody else. The wide range of PHR definitions was noted by Endsley, et al (2006) who described the following alternatives:

- A provider-owned and provider-maintained digital summary of clinically relevant health information made available to patients.
- A patient-owned software program that lets individuals enter, organize, and retrieve their own health information.
- A portable, interoperable digital file in which selected, clinically relevant

health data can be managed, secured, and transferred.

In 2002, Kim and Johnson defined PHRs as a simple data repository that stores core health information from both providers and patients and allows this information to be reviewed or sent to outside users (Tang, P., Ash, J., Bates, D., Overage, M., Sands, D., 2006). In 2005, the International Organization for Standardization (ISO) defined key features of the PHR as that it is under the control of the subject of care and that the information it contains is at least partly entered by the subject (consumer, patient) (International Organization for Standardization, n.d.). In 2006, Tang *et al.* envisioned PHRs as both the personal data and tools that allow patients to manage their health more independently, such as remote monitoring for chronic disease management and related content to support patient decision making about their care. The common thread throughout all of these definitions is the emphasis on increased patients' involvement in their care.

The Markle Foundation defined PHRs in their recent report, "A Common Framework for Networked Personal Health Information," (Markle Foundation, 2006c) by identifying the attributes of an ideal PHR as follows:

- Each person controls his or her own PHR.
- PHRs contain information from one's entire lifetime.
- PHRs contain information from all health care providers.
- PHRs are accessible from any place at any time.
- PHRs are private and secure.
- PHRs are transparent. Individuals can see who entered each piece of data, where it was transferred from, and who has viewed it.
- PHRs permit easy exchange of information across health care systems.

The U.S. Department of Health and Human Services (HHS) report "Personal Health Records and Personal Health Record Systems"(U.S. Department of Health and Human Services, n.d.) proposes that the term "personal health *record*" be used to refer to a collection of information about an individual's health and health care, stored in electronic format. The report uses the term "PHR *system*" to refer to the addition of computerized tools that help an individual understand and manage the information contained in a PHR. The report describes a PHR and PHR system as intended for use by consumers, patients, or their care givers, in contrast with an electronic health record (EHR) system, which is intended for use by healthcare providers.

The definition of PHR in this article is based on the HHS report, and amplified with key ideas from the Markle work and AHIMA (Pickard, B., 2007): *A PHR is a collection of information about an individual's health and health care, described using controlled medical vocabulary, stored in a private and secure digital file that is owned and controlled by the individual. The file is portable, and has access rights determined by the individual. The PHR is ideally interoperable with EHRs and other health information systems.*

PHR Design Attributes

AHIMA (American Health Information Management Association, n.d.) and others (Tang, P.C., Ash, J.S., Bates, D.W., Overhage, J.M., & Sands, D.Z., 2006) have categorized PHR systems on the basis of data storage location and the degree of integration with EHR systems. The Markle report (Markle Foundation, 2006) describes six dimensions for classifying the PHRs in the market today. The HHS report (U.S. Department of Health and Human Services, 2006) defines an initial framework of seven attributes for characterizing PHRs and PHR systems. The list of attributes below synthesizes ideas from these several sources, and can serve as a checklist of PHR design alternatives:

- **User population**: Many PHRs are intended to be used by the general public. Others are designed for selected populations, such as members of an insurance plan, patients of a healthcare provider, or employees of a company.

- **Scope and nature of content**: Some PHRs contain only personal information, such as information about providers and insurers, personally-generated medical history, and personal health journals. Other PHRs contain clinical information, including lab reports, diagnostic images, and physician notes. Some PHRs have components that are disease or condition-specific.

- **Source of information**: Data in PHRs may come from the individual, a caregiver, a healthcare provider, an insurer, a medical device, or all of the above. Data originated from the individual is usually entered manually, while data from a healthcare provider or insurer may be transferred from an EHR system.

- **Integration and interoperability**: Some PHRs are tightly integrated ("tethered") to an EHR system, such that the PHR is essentially a patient view into a provider EHR. Other PHRs are interconnected (or interoperable) with provider and insurer health information systems, so that data from those systems can be imported into the PHR. Other PHRs are standalone – not connected to other information systems.

- **Storage location (data portability and accessibility)**: The PHR data may be stored in a variety of locations, including a Web-based data base, a provider's EHR, the individual's personal computer, or a portable storage device such as a USB flash drive, smart card, portable music player, or cell phone. Hybrid approaches are also possible, in which the PHR is stored in more than one location: e.g., on a secure Web server and also on a portable storage device.

- **Access to the data (privacy and security):** With some PHRs, the party controlling access to the data is the sponsor; in others it is the individual. With some PHRs, the individual can permit healthcare providers and others to access all or a subset of the data. Other PHRs make part of the data easily accessible to emergency care providers.
- **Custodian of the PHR data (sponsor):** PHR systems can be differentiated by the entity that sponsors the system, and is therefore the custodian of the PHR data. Alternatives include the individual, an insurance plan, a healthcare provider, a pharmacy service, an employer, a healthcare information service, an affinity group, or some other organization.
- **Business model:** The business model defines the value offered to the sponsor of the PHR system. A PHR system may provide direct revenue from software sales, service fees, or advertising; or indirect value in terms of loyalty and marketing, increased healthcare delivery efficiency, or improved healthcare information and outcomes provided to users.
- **Features and functions:** PHR systems may offer a wide variety of additional functions, including scheduling appointments, reminders for reordering prescriptions, health information retrieval, and healthcare decision support tools such as medication interaction alerts.

PHR Evolution

As PHR systems become more widely used, they will increase in capability and level of interoperability with other health information systems. Dunbrack (2007) has suggested a five-stage maturity model for PHR systems that describes their evolution from basic health records to fully interoperable PHRs:

- **Basic PHRs:** Records are paper-based, or constructed manually using standard word processor or spreadsheet software.
- **Standalone PHRs:** Personal computer or Web-based software with templates that guide the manual entry of personal health information.
- **Sponsored PHRs:** Web-based PHR systems sponsored by employers, providers, or insurers, with some population of data from sponsor's health information systems.
- **Portal PHRs:** PHR is integrated with portal functions, including health information access and health decision aids.
- **Interoperable PHRs:** Interoperable data sharing with electronic health records (EHRs).

The HL7 Personal Health Record System Functional Model defines the level of PHR functionality as follows: (Health Level Seven, Inc., n.d.)

- **Basic:** Provides technology foundation for PHR growth. Consists of users populated health information. Provides complementary decision support tools.
- **Personalized:** Information and decision support tailored to the unique needs and preferences of users. Applies EHR populated-related standards of care. May include external data such as claims-derived data, lab results.
- **Connected:** Supports integration with EHR and care management capabilities and platforms. Serves as platform for advanced communication tools and tracking. Applies EHR clinical setting and provider specialty standards.
- **Interoperable:** Is interoperable with EHRs/PHRs based on industry standards. Applies EHR interoperability standards.

PHR Models

Based on the framework discussed above, several PHR models emerge in the industry. The following models are classified primarily on the storage location.

- **PC Based**: These are standalone PC applications owned by individual consumers. PHR applications and data are stored on user owned PCs. They allow users to collect and record their own health information. These applications are installed on the user's computer and rely primarily or entirely on self-reported information. The data can be printed out for presentation to a physician.

- **Device Based**: These are standalone applications owned by individual consumers. PHR applications and data are stored on portable devices such as a USB flash drive or a smart card. The PHR application can be run on any available computer, allowing data to be viewed or updated at the site of care. The portable device itself is usually encrypted and requires authentication to access the patient's data. Like PC based PHRs, portable PHRs rely primarily or entirely on self-reported information.

- **Web Based**: These are Internet based applications provided by sponsors. PHR applications and data are run and stored at the sponsor sites. Sponsors could include payers, employers, health information services providers, or internet service companies. They provide an application interface which allows users to enter their own health information. Web based PHRs offered by payers (usually insurance plans and employers) may also incorporate information from insurance claims, reducing the patient's data entry effort. Web based PHRs offered by internet service companies such as Microsoft and Google also provide tools to collect health information from various sources.

- **Portal Based**: These are tethered PHRs provided by sponsors. PHR applications and data are run and stored at the sponsor sites. Many hospitals and clinics have rolled out patient portals attached to their internal Electronic Medical Record (EMR) system. Users can log in and are given a view into the data stored within the hospital's EMR systems. The portal based "PHR" is not, by the definitions above, a Personal Health Record at all, since the data is not owned by the patient unless it is exported. This PHR model requires minimal effort from the patient, but is limited in its ability to integrate data from different providers.

- **Health Bank Based**: These are Health Record Bank offered by companies or agents who are moderating a PHR on behalf of the owner of the PHR. PHR applications and data are run and stored at the provider sites. PHR applications aggregate data from multiple providers in a centralized, patient controlled data repository. The health record bank is responsible for making the record available to authorized users, and for giving the patient a mechanism to identify who may access what parts of their record, and under what circumstances. As standards develop, the health bank may or may not provide a direct user interface for manipulating the PHR data. Instead, the health bank provides the data in a standard form via a standard interface to third party software which presents the information in a user-appropriate manner (to a physician via an EHR, to a patient with translations of clinical terms, etc.).

PHR Stakeholders

PHRs are sponsored by a variety of stakeholders. A number of healthcare providers, health insurers, employers, and healthcare information services have recently offered PHR systems or announced plans for such tools. However, none of these efforts adequately address the full range privacy and security concerns, portability needs, and interoperability requirements. The adoption of these PHR systems will likely be limited by these deficiencies. The value proposition varies among different stakeholders.

Healthcare Providers

A number of U.S. healthcare providers offer PHR-like systems to their patients, such as the Cleveland Clinic's *MyChart* PHR, Kaiser Permanente's *My Health Record* PHR, the U.S. Veterans Affairs *MyHealtheVet*, and the Kettering Health Network's *DaytonHealthKonnect*. Many of these systems are integrated (tethered) with provider EHR systems, and enable patients to view portions of their electronic medical records. Kaiser Permanente began offering its *My Health Record* PHR in 2005, and reports that 1.3 million members have signed up, representing 25% of the membership age 13 and up (Reese, S., 2007). Kaiser Permanente, the University of Pittsburg Medical Center, Humana, and others are participating with the Centers for Medicare and Medicaid Services (CMS) in a new PHR pilot to help Medicare beneficiaries better manage their health (America's Health Insurance Plans, 2006). The pilot identify PHR features that are most attractive to Medicare beneficiaries, and the best methods to encourage adoption and ongoing usage of PHRs.

Health Insurers

Aetna announced in October 2006 a new Web-based PHR system for members that will provide online access to personal information, detailed health history, personalized alerts, and integrated information to help members make informed decisions about their health care. The Blue Cross Blue Shield Association (BCBSA) and America's Health Insurance Plans (AHIP) announced (McGee, M.K., 2006; America's Health Insurance Plans, 2006) in December 2006 the creation of a "health plan-based" PHR model and a portability standard for PHR data. The PHR model defines the core data elements that all insurers should provide in their PHR tools. The portability standard will allow consumers to move their data when then change insurers. Individual insurance companies can add their own features to their PHR offering, for example providing electronic reminders to get medications refilled.

Employers

In 2006, a consortium of employers announced (Omnimedix Institute, 2008) the formation of the Dossia Founders Group (http://www.dossia. org), which is developing the Dossia Network. The network is a Web-based framework that U.S. employees and dependents of the consortium members can use to maintain lifelong PHRs. Members of the consortium include Wal-Mart, BP America, Intel Corporation, Pitney Bowes, Applied Materials, and Cardinal Health. Users could create and update their PHRs on a secure web site. Data could also be obtained from selected pharmacies, labs, insurers, physician and hospital EHR systems, and automatically added to the PHRs. Verizon Communications, Inc. announced (Verizon Communications, Inc., 2007) in 2007 a new *Electronic PHR* tool. The Web-based system provides employees secure 24/7 access to personal medical and prescription history, and a snapshot of personal health status that can be shared with healthcare providers.

Healthcare Information Services

In 2007, Microsoft (http://www.microsoft.com) launched HealthVault, a platform that enabled consumers to collect, store, and share their personal health information. Data feeds into HealthVault coming from payers, pharmacy benefit managers, providers, commercial laboratories, and personal health devices.

In 2008, Google (http://www.google.com) launched Google Health for consumers to create a PHR with data feeds from various sources.

WebMD (http://www.webmd.com) provided consumers a free *WebMD Personal Health Record*. A *Master Assessment* tool is also offered to provide personal health action guidance, based on data recorded in the PHR. LifeSensor (https://www.lifesensor.com/us/us/us-hn/consumers/lifesensor-phr.html) offered a Web-based personal health record allowing users to store, manage, and view their medical histories. LifeSensor PHR also included emergency records such as the existence of an advance directive, an organ donor card, or information on x-rays.

OPEN SOURCE PHRS

Fundamentally, Open Source is about creating a collaborative environment for problem solving. As healthcare technology standards evolve and healthcare IT systems adopt standards-based software technologies that enable greater interoperability, the opportunities for PHR collaboration will only grow. The compelling economics of Open Source and its collaborative development model will improve the affordability of PHR systems that is crucial to improving the quality of personal health.

PHR Adoption Challenges

Despite their many benefits, PHRs are not yet widely used. Adoption is being constrained by several key challenges that must be addressed.

Privacy and Security

Some individuals are reluctant to use PHRs because they fear their personal data will be used for unauthorized purposes, or will be accessed by unauthorized persons. With employer- and insurer-offered PHR systems, individuals are concerned that their data might be misused to limit their job prospects, or to reduce their life or health insurance coverage. The president of AHIMA recently told a House Subcommittee on information policy that current laws and the Health Insurance Portability and Accountability Act (HIPAA) privacy rule provide only weak privacy protections for PHRs (American Health Information Management Association, 2007; Pickard, B., 2007). The HHS report (U.S. Department of Health and Human Services, 2006) notes: "The privacy considerations of PHR systems are complex, but addressing them adequately is essential if PHR systems are to become widely accepted and used. Consumers want to be able to control access to their personal health information." Individuals are also uncertain about the security of Web-based data. The HHS report cautions that "widespread adoption of PHRs is not likely to happen until consumers are confident that they have adequate security protections."

Interoperability

Only the most committed individuals will manually enter all the data needed to maintain their PHRs. Most PHR users will demand that data be automatically populated from provider or insurer information systems, but most current PHR systems don't do this. PHRs tethered to a single provider's EHR don't receive data from other providers. Insurer-provided PHRs can receive information from insurance claims about physician visits, lab tests performed, and medications purchased, but details of physician notes, lab results, and medication instructions are available only from the healthcare provider. Interoperability is the term used to describe the capability to exchange data between PHRs, EHRs, and other health information systems. The HHS report (U.S. Department of Health and Human Services, 2006) notes: "The full potential of PHR systems will not be realized until they are capable of widespread exchange of information with EHRs and other sources of personal and other health data." Data content and exchange standards will be essential to achieving interoperability.

Portability

Individuals will have to invest some time and effort to create their PHRs. Unfortunately, with current employer-based, provider-based, or insurer-based PHR systems, they will have to redo much of this work when a change in employer, healthcare provider or insurer forces them to move to a new PHR system. PHRs will not widely be adopted until they are portable – the data can be easily moved from one PHR system to another.

Standards

Further limiting the adoption of PHRs is the lack of standards for PHR content, and for PHR data interchange and portability. A *PHR content standard* should specify the data elements included in a PHR, and the format and vocabulary used for each data element. For example, a defined set of terms should be specified for medical conditions, e.g., from SNOMED CT. A *PHR data interchange and portability standard* should specify the format of a digital file used to transport a PHR between PHR systems, or to store a PHR on a portable storage device.

Several health information interoperability standards exist, or are being developed, that may play roles in defining future PHR standards:

- **CCR**: The Continuity of Care Record (CCR) standard (ASTM International, 2005), published by ASTM International in December 2005, defines a core data set of the most relevant administrative, demographic, and clinical information facts about a patient's healthcare, covering one of more healthcare encounters. The

standard enables a healthcare provider to aggregate pertinent data about a patient and forward it to another provider when the patient is transferred. The standard suggests that fields be coded with terms from controlled vocabularies such as SNOMED CT, LOINC, and RxNorm, but specific terms are not specified. Although this XML-based standard is designed primarily for data exchange between healthcare providers, the standard notes that it can be used as the basis for a PHR.

- **CDA**: The Clinical Document Architecture (CDA) Release 2.0 standard (Health Level Seven, n.d.) developed by Health Level Seven (HL7) and approved as an ANSI standard in May 2005, provides an exchange model for clinical documents such as discharge summaries and progress notes.

- **CCD**: The Continuity of Care Document (CCD) standard (Health Level Seven, n.d.) developed by HL7 and ASTM and approved in February 2007, integrates the CCR and CDA standards to provide a harmonized format for the exchange of clinical information, including patient demographics, medications, and allergies.

- **PDF/H**: The Portable Document Format (PDF) Healthcare Best Practices Guide (AIIM, 2006; AIIM, n.d.) is being developed by AIIM, with the participation of several medical groups, including the American Academy of Family Physicians (AAFP) and the American Academy of Pediatrics (AAP). The Guide will describe a standard way to use a PDF file as a portable, secure, and universal healthcare data exchange container for PHR and EHR data. PDF is an attractive choice because of its ability to contain text, graphics, and images – and its widespread use in business and government. The Guide will describe how standard CCR, CDA, and CCD data can be contained, along with medical images.

Accelerating PHR Adoption through Open Source

Open Source is a software development model and philosophy characterized by freely redistributable source code. Unlike the traditionally closely guarded trade secret of proprietary software companies, Open Source software encourages the free sharing of software blueprints. This sharing empowers a robust ecosystem of contributors who collaborate in advancing the development of software. The collaborative ecosystem enables all users of the software to amortize their development costs and share knowledge across a larger install base than that of traditional proprietary software. Customers, partners, and competitors alike can all contribute and benefit from participating in the community. As a result, no single software vendor is capable of dominating a truly successful Open Source project.

The adoption of PHRs can be significantly accelerated by the creation of an Open Source PHR software tool that adequately addresses the privacy and security, interoperability, and portability needs described above. The Open Source software development paradigm has been used successfully in many computer systems and application areas to develop robust products that earn user confidence. Open Source projects frequently harness the innovation of highly motivated developer communities to produce products that excel in satisfying user's needs.

McDonald et al.(2003) review the history of Open Source software, and describe its growing role in medical informatics applications. The authors make the case that the expanded development of Open Source medical informatics applications will benefit both commercial medical system developers and medical informatics researchers. The authors conclude that a traditional, "closed source," or proprietary PHR tool will not achieve the accelerated adoption rate possible with Open Source software. Open Source PHR software has the following clear advantages:

- **No vested interests**: The Open Source PHR software will be free of the vested interests that individuals may associate with PHR tools sponsored by insurers, healthcare providers, and employers. Individuals will be free of concerns that vested interests may misuse their personal health data. In addition, since the intellectual property of Open Source software belongs to the community, no one organization can have a monopoly on the software, and vendors must continuously compete on service and support.

- **Better security and privacy**: User concerns about the security and privacy of their personal health data will be mitigated by the fact that experienced developers will examine the Open Source code, verify that privacy and security provisions are adequate, and publicly share their assessments. Similar to the practice of peer review in academic circles, the open publication of all source code, coupled with a community of reviewers, testers, and users, drives security and privacy in Open Source software.

- **Improved interoperability**: An Open Source PHR is more likely to be built to open standards, so interoperable with other open standards systems.

- **Free**: An Open Source PHR tool will be available at no cost. Users can easily download the software, try it out, and begin to use it without making any purchases.

- **High quality and innovative**: With a motivated and broad-based developer community, the software will evolve into a PHR tool that is recognized for its reliability, functionality, ease of use, and innovative features.

- **Past success**: Over the past two decades, open source software, such as the Linux operating system, the Apache web server, the Firefox web browser, the JBoss application server, and the MySQL database management system, have come to represent significant portions of their respective markets. In each case, the same confluence of factors— expansion of Internet connectivity and email, clearly defined technical problems that demanded robust solutions, frustration with proprietary solutions—led to the rapid adoption of open source software into the mainstream.

Open Source PHR software also has the following two major disadvantages:

- **No guarantee development**: It is not possible to know if a project will ever reach a usable stage, and even if it reaches it, it may die later if there is not enough interest. This disadvantage could be overcome once a self sustained Open Source PHR ecosystem is established.
- **Uncertain support**: Unlike propriety software supported by vendors, Open Source software users could face challenges in getting needed technical support in a timely manner. This disadvantage can be addressed by actively participate in the Open Source PHR community to tap into virtually limitless resources.

Open Source PHR System Architecture

Although several PHR system architectures exist in the industry, most PHR systems work like a hub and spoke model as illustrated in Figure 1. Under this architecture, a patient-controlled PHR works at the center and is connected to different stakeholders who exchange data and interact with patients. Stakeholders include individuals, family members, healthcare providers, hospitals, pharmacies, labs, payers/insures, health information exchange organizations, and health information databases. Ideally, the PHR should include as much relevant data as possible over the individual's lifetime, from multiple sources. The more comprehensive the data contained in a PHR are, the more useful the data will be to patients and care providers. In addition, the bigger the hub (i.e., the more functions the PHR has) is, the more spokes it has (i.e., the more connected it is to other sources of health information), and the thicker the spokes are (i.e., the more complete the sources of health information are), the more valuable the PHR will become.[35]

Open Source PHR Contents

A wide variety of health and health care information might be included in a PHR. Broader than a medical record, the PHR should contain any information relevant to an individual's health. The following types of information have been included in existing PHR tools, or have been suggested for future PHR tools:

- Patient administrative information
- Patient identification, patient support providers and contacts.
- Living wills, advance directives, or medical power of attorney.
- Organ donor authorization.
- Patient health information
- **Current health status**: Problems, medications, allergies and adverse drug reactions, recent procedures, plan of care, vital signs, medical equipment used, implants, current exercise, nutrition and diet, functional status.
- **Medical history**: Surgeries and other procedures, physician encounters, medications, written orders, hospitalizations, immunizations and vaccinations, family medical history, social history

Figure 1. PHR system architecture

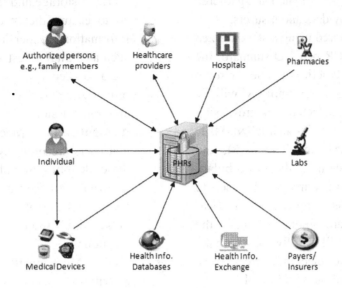

- **Results:** Laboratory test results, diagnostic medical images
- **Personal health monitoring data**: Personal measurements of BP, weight, and other personal health observations and notes
- Healthcare provider information
- Payer information
- Medical insurance information, claims and payments data
- Personal genetic information
- Inherited traits, personal genome data

Open Source PHR Functionalities

Although detailed requirements and design are yet to be agreed upon by the industry, the high-level capabilities of the Open Source PHR software have been defined. Requirements and architecture working groups that include experts in healthcare, medical informatics, medical vocabulary, and information technology will create detailed functional, user interface, data interface, and security specifications.

Data Creation, Collection, and Aggregation

The Open Source PHR software will enable an individual to create and update their own PHR. The architecture working group will determine if the software will run locally on a user's personal computer, or on a Web server accessed via a Web browser over a secure network connection. If the PHR software is Web-based, it may be hosted by any organization that chooses to provide this PHR service for a user community, e.g., an employer, a healthcare provider, a school, a professional society, a credit union, a church, or a special-interest association.

The Open Source PHR software will enable individuals to receive healthcare data from their healthcare and insurance providers and add it to their PHR, and to share selected data from their PHR with their doctors. The software will import data that is received in standard formats from EHR systems at physicians, hospitals, and other healthcare providers. It will also import data received in standard formats from online personal health records systems operated by insurance providers and pharmacies. In this way, an individual can update their PHR with data created and gathered by their healthcare providers and insurers.

The PHR will be stored using a standardized format, such as the CCR or CCD standard, the PDF Healthcare Best Practices Guide, or some future standard. Medical terminology will be used as specified by the selected standards, using controlled medical vocabularies such as SNOMED CT, LOINC, RxNORM, and ICD-9-CM, and reflecting best practices in medical vocabulary usage. Lists of standard terms will be used to indicate medical problems, procedures, medications, immunizations, and other data items in the PHR. The Open Source PHR software will make it easy for individuals to select the correct terms, even if they are not familiar with formal medical terminology. For example, some individuals will recognize the term "heart attack," but not the medical term "myocardial infarction." Research in the area of consumer health vocabulary will be applied to this effort (Zeng, Q.T., & Tse, T., 2006).

Security & Privacy

The PHR contains health information that is owned and controlled by an individual. The individual controls what information is included in their PHR, and controls what portion of their PHR can be shared, and with whom. Information in a PHR cannot be accessed or used by anyone without the explicit knowledge and permission of the owner. Fundamental security and privacy functionalities include:

- **Administration**: Tools to manage user identity and access. This includes tools for granting, managing, and auditing user access privileges for family caregivers, health and human service providers, and other trusted individuals.
- **Authorization**: Mechanisms to ensure that users can only access what they are authorized. Proper data encryption (National Institute of Standards and Technology,

2001) in storage and transmission is needed to ensure the confidentiality of PHR information. Proper integrity mechanisms such as digital digest and backup schemes are also needed to protect PHR from improper alteration or·destruction in storage and transmission.

- **Authentication**: Mechanisms to ensure that users are properly identified and that these identities are validated to access authorized PHR information. Two or three factor authentication schemes and public-key infrastructure (PKI) are possible solutions.
- **Audit**: Mechanisms to ensure that the activities associated with user access are logged for monitoring and investigative purposes.

Accessibility

A segment of the PHR will be designated for access by emergency care providers, and is stored without password protection or encryption. This segment of the PHR may contain data about drug allergies and other important information that emergency healthcare providers should have in the event that an individual cannot speak for himself. Emergency healthcare providers may access this segment of the PHR from a portable storage device, or from a Web site.

The Open Source PHR software will also extract owner-specified portions of a PHR to be shared with a healthcare provider. The extracted file can be printed or stored in a computer file using a standard format that can be read by a healthcare provider's EHR system.

Transportability

The PHR file is portable, and can be moved to wherever it is needed. The owner can move his or her PHR file to any computer that hosts the Open Source PHR software, provided that the owner has access rights. The owner can also take the PHR file to a physician's office, hospital, or other healthcare facility by storing the file on a portable storage device such as a USB flash drive, cell phone, or digital music player. The encrypted PHR file can be sent as an email attachment, for example to a physician or to a family member. The owner controls where the PHR is transported and stored.

Personal Health Management

The Open Source PHR software will enable individuals to easily access personalized health information from Web-based health information resources, according to the contents of their PHR. The National Library of Medicine (www.nlm.nih. gov) health information sources such as Medline-Plus, NIHSeniorHealth, DailyMed, ClinicalTrials, and PubMed can be automatically searched for information relevant to the individual's medical conditions, based on data stored in the individual's PHR. The use of controlled medical vocabularies in the PHR will enable accurate linkages to these health information resources.

The software will generate PHR summary reports and statistics that will help individuals manage their personal health. The software will also be extensible with plug-in modules that provide a range of personal health management functions, such as appointment scheduling, reminders, and specialized disease tracking and management.

Clinical Decision Support

The Open Source PHR software will be used as a core, around which more advanced software modules will be configured to analyze the PHR data and provide improved healthcare opportunities to the PHR owner. Many of these advanced software modules will provide clinical decision support functions. For example, the PHR can be analyzed to detect adverse drug-to-drug interactions in the individual's current medication regi-

men. Medical errors can be reduced by analyzing the PHR data to determine if the medication and care plan fall within general guidelines for the medical problems identified. Gaps in medical care can be identified by analyzing the PHR data to determine if the individual's medical status indicates medical conditions that should be treated, but are not listed in the care plan. And the PHR can be analyzed to determine if current best medical practices would suggest alternative treatment plants to be considered.

FUTURE RESEARCH DIRECTIONS

Patients, providers, payers, employers, and others have increasing interest in using personal health records (PHRs) to improve healthcare costs, quality, and efficiency. PHR related research has increased in the past few years. Kaelber et al. suggested that past PHR research focused primarily in the following seven areas: (Kaelber, D.C., Jha, A.K., Johnston, D., Middleton, B., & Bates D.W., 2008)

- PHR adoption and attitudes
- PHR function description
- PHR function evaluation
- PHR position statement/editorials
- PHR privacy and security
- PHR architecture
- Others

Despite increasing interest and activity, PHR definitions, standards, architectures, value and propositions are not universally agreed upon and PHR adoption rate is low. Targeted research investment in PHRs appears inadequate. Additional PHR research is need in the following areas.

- **PHR standards & interoperability**: One of the greatest technology issues barring improvements in the U.S. healthcare environment is the absence of data, integration, formatting, and presentation standards. For example, a PHR content standard is needed to specify the data elements included in a PHR, and the format and vocabulary used for each data element. Consumers change health plans and providers with some frequency. Research is needed to mature the standard and to enable interoperability and to improve portability.

- **PHR functions**: Better delineation of PHR functions and of their impact on healthcare costs, quality, and efficiency is needed (Kaelber, D.C., Jha, A.K., Johnston, D., Middleton, B., & Bates D.W., 2008). Primary research for PHR functions falls into four general categories:
- Information collection functions that help patients to enter their own health information and to retrieve their information from external sources
- Information sharing functions that support patients to engage in one-way sharing of their health information with others
- Information exchange functions that enable patients to engage in two-way data exchange with others
- Health Management functions that enable patients to better manage their own health/healthcare
- **PHR privacy and security**: Patients' greatest concern about nearly every type of electronic healthcare applications, including PHRs, is security and privacy (Kaelber, D.C., Jha, A.K., Johnston, D., Middleton, B., & Bates D.W., 2008; Tang, P., Ash, J., Bates, D., Overage, M., Sands, D., 2006). Several important issues regarding PHR privacy and security need better evaluation. The first involves who controls sharing and accessing of the information in a PHR. This is critical when many organizations and individuals are sharing data within the PHR. A second concern is how to optimally design PHR systems in order

to allow patients to maximize the security of their PHR. PHR issues around control over sharing and access to PHR data present even more complex issues, especially considering a patient controlled PHR and patient proxies. All of these issues around PHR privacy and security present opportunities for research.

- **Sustainable PHR ecosystem**: Efforts are needed to research effective ways of developing a sustainable PHR ecosystem. This includes ways to build a motivated community of Open Source PHR developers, vendors, partners, and users. Developers develop PHR tools. Vendors and partners contribute to tool development, distribute packaged executable tool through its own brand, and generate revenue. Users are the ultimate consumers of PHR technology. Better understanding and addressing adoption barriers among patients and healthcare providers represents an important research area to achieving widespread implementation and use of PHRs.

CONCLUSION

Considerable interest has been focused recently on the definition, potential benefits, and barriers to adoption of PHRs. Health care information technology organizations and medical associations are leading their memberships to a fuller understanding of the field, and are promoting the development of relevant standards. A variety of insurers, health care information services, employers, and software companies are beginning to provide PHR tools and services. However, several key challenges to the widespread adoption of PHRs have not been fully addressed, including privacy and security, interoperability, portability, and controlled medical vocabulary.

The adoption of PHRs will be significantly accelerated with the development of an Open Source

PHR software that is personal, private, secure, portable, based on emerging industry content and format standards, and uses controlled medical vocabularies. Individuals will use this software to collect, create, organize, and mange their own PHRs, and software development organizations will use this software as the basis for enhanced tools and services.

REFERENCES

Aetna, Inc. (2006, October 3). *Aetna introduces powerful, interactive personal health record.* Press release. Retrieved December 11, 2008, from http://www.aetna.com/news/2006/pr_20061003.htm.

AIIM. (2006, October 20). *Industry leaders join forces to advance portable healthcare document practices; new Best Practices Guide addresses exchange of healthcare information.* Press release. Retrieved November 8, 2008, from http://www.aiim.org/article-pr.asp?ID=32097.

AIIM. (n.d.). *PDF Healthcare Committee Web site.* Retrieved December 5, 2008, from http://www.aiim.org/standards.asp?ID=31832.

America's Health Insurance Plans. (2006, June 20). *Health plans participate in CMS PHR pilot to help Medicare beneficiaries better manage their health.* Press release. June 20, 2006. Retrieved December 11, 2008, from http://www.ahip.org/content/pressrelease.aspx?docid=20043.

America's Health Insurance Plans. (2006, December 13). *Industry leaders announce personal health record model; collaborate with consumers to speed adoption.* Press release. Retrieved December 14, 2008, from http://www.ahip.org/content/pressrelease.aspx?docid=18328.

American Academy of Family Physicians. (n.d.). *ASTM Continuity of Care Record (CCR) Web site.* Retrieved November 8, 2008, from http://www.centerforhit.org/x201.xml.

American Health Information Management Association. (2007, June 19). *AHIMA calls on Congress to expand and standardize personal health information privacy protections.* Press release. Retrieved February 7, 2009, from http://www.ahima.org/press/press_releases/07.0619.asp.

American Health Information Management Association. (n.d.). *myPHR Web site.* Retrieved October 13, 2008, from http://www.myphr.com.

ASTM International. (2005). Designation [*Standard specification for continuity of care record*] [*CCR*]. E (Norwalk, Conn.), •••, 2369–05.

Dunbrack, L.A. (2007, April). The PHR maturity model: the road to interoperability. *Health Industry Insights.* #HI206237.

Endsley, S., Kibbe, D. C., Linares, A., & Coloafi, K. (2006). An introduction to personal health records. *Family Practice Management, 13*(5), 57–62.

Fogel, K. (2005). *Producing open source software: how to run a successful free software project.* Retrieved January 7, 2009, from http://producingoss.com

Freudenheim, M. (2007, April 16). AOL Founder hopes to build new giant among a bevy of health care Web sites. *New York Times.*

Health Level Seven. (n.d.). *HL7 receives ANSI approval of three version 3 specifications including CDA, release 2.* Press release. May 5, 2005. Retrieved December 11, 2008, from http://www.hl7.org/documentcenter/public/pressreleases/20050505.pdf.

Health Level Seven. (n.d.). HL7 Continuity of Care Document, a healthcare IT interoperability standard, is approved by balloting process and endorsed by healthcare IT standards panel. Press release. February 12, 2007. Retrieved December 11, 2008, from http://www.hl7.org/documentcenter/public/pressreleases/20070212.pdf.

Health Level Seven. (n.d.). *The Clinical Document Architecture (CDA) Release 2.0*. Retrieved November 2, 2008, from http://www.hl7.org.

Health Level Seven, Inc. (n.d.). *Personal Health Record System Functional Model*. Retrieved April 17, 2009, from http://www.hl7.org/ehr/.

Healthcare Information Management and Systems Society. (n.d.). *Personal Health Record Web site*. Retrieved July 3, 2008, from http://www.himss.org/ASP/topics_phr.asp.

International Organization for Standardization. (n.d.). *ISO/TR 20514:2005 Health informatics — Electronic health record — Definition, scope, and context*. Retrieved January 17, 2009, from http://www.iso.org/iso/iso_catalogue/catalogue_tc/catalogue_detail.htm?csnumber=39525.

Kaelber, D. C., Jha, A. K., Johnston, D., Middleton, B., & Bates, D. W. (2008). A research agenda for personal health records (PHRs). *Journal of the American Medical Informatics Association, 15*(6), 729–736. doi:10.1197/jamia.M2547

Mamlin, B. W., Biondich, P. G., Wolfe, B. A., Fraser, H., Jazayeri, D., Allen, C., et al. (2006). Cooking up an open source EMR for developing countries: OpenMRS – a recipe for successful collaboration. *AMIA 2006 Symposium Proceedings* (pp. 529-533).

Manhattan Research. (n.d.). *Cybercitizen Health v8.0*. Retrieved January 7, 2009, from http://www.manhattanresearch.com/products/Strategic_Advisory/CCH/default.aspx.

Markle Foundation. (2006a, November). Survey finds Americans want electronic personal health information to improve own health care. News release. Retrieved July 3, 2008, from http://www.markle.org/downloadable_assets/research_doc_120706.pdf.

Markle Foundation. (2006b, December). Americans see access to their medical information as a way to improve quality, reduce health care costs. News release. Retrieved October 13, 2008, from http://www.markle.org/downloadable_assets/news_release_120706.pdf.

Markle Foundation. (2006c, December). *Connecting Americans to Their Health Care: A Common Framework for Networked Personal Health Information*. Retrieved November 8, 2008, from http://www.connectingforhealth.org/common-framework/docs/P9_NetworkedPHRs.pdf.

McDonald, C. J., Schadow, G., Barnes, M., Dexter, P., Overhage, J. M., Mamlin, B., & McCoy, J. M. (2003). Open source software in medical informatics – why, how and what. *International Journal of Medical Informatics, 69*, 175–184. doi:10.1016/S1386-5056(02)00104-1

McGee, M. K. (2006, December 13). Insurers push patients toward e-health records. *InformationWeek*. Retrieved December 19, 2008, from http://www.informationweek.com/story/showArticle.jhtml?articleID=196603941.

National Institute of Standards and Technology. (2001, November 26). *Federal Information Processing Standards (FIPS) Publication 197, Advanced Encryption Standard (AES)*.

National Library of Medicine. (n.d.). *Unified Medical Language System Web site*. Retrieved January 11, 2009, from http://www.nlm.nih.gov/research/umls/umlsmain.html.

National Library of Medicine Board of Regents. (2006, September). Charting a Course for the 21st Century: NLM's [from http://www.nlm.nih.gov/pubs/plan/lrpdocs.html.]. *Long Range Planning*, ▪▪▪, 2006–2016. Retrieved November 5, 2008.

Omnimedix Institute. (2008, December 11). *Major U.S. employers join to provide lifelong personal health records for employees; independent system will give individuals access to complete medical information whenever and wherever they need it.* Press release. December 6, 2006. Retrieved December 11, 2008, from http://www.omnimedix.org/pr_2006.12.06.html.

Pickard, B. (2007, June 19). *Hearing on protecting patient privacy in healthcare information systems.* U.S. House of Representatives Committee on Oversight and Government Reform, Subcommittee on Information Policy, Census and National Archives (Testimony of the President of the American Health Information Management Association (AHIMA)). Retrieved November 8, 2008, from http://ahima.org/dc/CommentsTestimony.asp.

Reese, S. (2007, June 1). The value of PHRs depends on the quality of data inputs. *Managed Healthcare Executive.* Retrieved December 14, 2008, from http://www.managedhealthcareexecutive.com.

Tang, P. C., Ash, J. S., Bates, D. W., Overhage, J. M., & Sands, D. Z. (2006). Personal health records: definitions, benefits, and strategies for overcoming barriers to adoption. *Journal of the American Medical Informatics Association, 13*(2), 121–126. doi:10.1197/jamia.M2025

The Center for Information Technology Leadership. (n.d.). *The Value of Personal Health Records.* Retrieved January 7, 2009, from http://www.citl.org/_pdf/CITL_PHR_Report.pdf

The National Committee on Vital and Health Statistics. (n.d.). *A Strategy for Building the National Health Information Infrastructure (NHII).* Retrieved January 21, 2009, from http://aspe.hhs.gov/sp/NHII/Documents/NHIIReport2001/default.htm.

U.S. Department of Health and Human Services. (2006, February). Personal Health Records and Personal Health Record Systems: A Report and Recommendations from the National Committee on Vital and Health Statistics. *National Cancer Institute, National Institutes of Health, and National Center for Health Statistics, Centers for Disease Control and Prevention.* Retrieved July 3, 2008, from http://www.ncvhs.hhs.gov/0602nhiirpt.pdf.

Verizon Communications, Inc. (2007, May 9). *Verizon CEO announces implementation of new online personal health records program for company employees.* Press release. May 9, 2007. Retrieved December 19, 2008, from http://newscenter.verizon.com/press-releases/verizon/2007/verizon-ceo-announces.html.

WorldVistA Web site. (n.d.). Retrieved December 11, 2008, from http://www.worldvista.org

Zeng, Q. T., & Tse, T. (2006). Exploring and developing consumer health vocabularies. *Journal of the American Medical Informatics Association, 13*(1), 24–29. doi:10.1197/jamia.M1761

ADDITIONAL READING

Ball, M. J., Costin, M. Y., & Lehmann, C. (2008). The personal health record: consumers banking on their health. *Studies in Health Technology and Informatics, 134,* 35–46.

Bodily, N. J., Carlston, D. A., & Rocha, R. A. (2007). Personal health records: key features within existing applications. *AMIA Annual Symposium Proceedings* (p. 875).

Botts, N. E., & Horan, T. A. (2007). Electronic personal health records and systems to improve care for vulnerable populations. *AMIA Annual Symposium Proceedings* (p. 880).

Detmer, D., Bloomrosen, M., Raymond, B., & Tang, P. (2008). Integrated personal health records: transformative tools for consumer-centric care. *BMC Medical Informatics and Decision Making, 8*(45).

Dimick, C. (2008). The great PHRontier. Private business stakes a claim in personal health records. *Journal of American Health Information Management Association, 79*(6), 25–28.

Foxhall, K. (2007). Now it's personal. Personal health records may be next on deck for the certification process. *Healthcare Informatics, 24*(3), 30.

Grossman, J. M., Zayas-Cabán, T., & Kemper, N. (2009). Information gap: can health insurer personal health records meet patients' and physicians' needs? [Millwood]. *Health Affairs, 28*(2), 377–389. doi:10.1377/hlthaff.28.2.377

Halamka, J. D., Mandl, K. D., & Tang, P. C. (2008). Early experiences with personal health records. *Journal of the American Medical Informatics Association, 15*(1), 1–7. doi:10.1197/jamia.M2562

Hudson, D. L., & Cohen, M. E. (2008). Temporal trend analysis in personal health records. *Conference Proceedings IEEE Engineering in Medicine and Biology Society* (pp. 3811-4).

Johnston, D., Kaelber, D., Pan, E. C., Bu, D., Shah, S., Hook, J. M., & Middleton, B. (2007). A framework and approach for assessing the value of personal health records (PHRs). *AMIA Annual Symposium Proceedings* (pp. 374-8).

Kaelber, D., & Pan, E. C. (2008). The value of personal health record (PHR) systems. *AMIA Annual Symposium Proceedings* (pp. 343-7).

Kahn, J. S., Aulakh, V., & Bosworth, A. (2009). What it takes: characteristics of the ideal personal health record. [Millwood]. *Health Affairs, 28*(2), 369–376. doi:10.1377/hlthaff.28.2.369

Keselman, A., Slaughter, L., Smith, C. A., Kim, H., Divita, G., Browne, A., et al. (2007). Towards consumer-friendly PHRs: patients' experience with reviewing their health records. *AMIA Annual Symposium Proceedings* (pp. 399-403).

Lafky, D. B., & Horan, T. A. Health Status and Prospective PHR Use. *AMIA Annual Symposium Proceedings* (p. 1016).

Morales Rodriguez, M., Casper, G., & Brennan, P. F. (•••). Patient-centered design. The potential of user-centered design in personal health records. *Journal of American Health Information Management Association, 78*(4), 44–46.

Neupert, P., & Mundie, C. (2009). Personal health management systems: applying the full power of software to improve the quality and efficiency of care. [Millwood]. *Health Affairs, 28*(2), 390–392. doi:10.1377/hlthaff.28.2.390

Pagliari, C., Detmer, D., & Singleton, P. (2007). Potential of electronic personal health records. *BMJ (Clinical Research Ed.), 335*(7615), 330–333. doi:10.1136/bmj.39279.482963.AD

Raisinghani, M. S., & Young, E. (•••). Personal health records: key adoption issues and implications for management. *International Journal of Electronic Healthcare, 4*(1), 67–77. doi:10.1504/IJEH.2008.018921

Reti, S. R., Feldman, H. J., & Safran, C. (2009). Governance for personal health records. *Journal of the American Medical Informatics Association, 16*(1), 14–17. doi:10.1197/jamia.M2854

Shah, S. S., Kaelber, D. C., Vincent, A., Pan, E., Johnston, D., & Middleton, B. (2008). A Cost Model for Personal Health Records (PHRs). *AMIA Annual Symposium Proceedings* (pp. 657-61).

Tang, P. C., & Lee, T. H. (2009). Your doctor's office or the Internet? Two paths to personal health records. *The New England Journal of Medicine, 360*(13), 1276–1278. doi:10.1056/NEJMp0810264

Terry, K. (2008). Will PHRs rule the waves or roll out with the tide? *Hospitals & Health Networks, 82*(8),36-9, 1.

Van Deursen, T., Koster, P., & Petković, M. (2008). Reliable personal health records. *Studies in Health Technology and Informatics, 136*, 484–489.

Vincent, A., Kaelber, D. C., Pan, E., Shah, S. S., Johnston, D., & Middleton, B. (2008). A Patient-Centric Taxonomy for Personal Health Records (PHRs). *AMIA Annual Symposium Proceedings* (pp. 763-7).

Zayas-Cabán, T., & Valdez, R. (2007). Do patients understand how PHRs work? *AMIA Annual Symposium Proceedings* (p. 1169).

KEY TERMS AND DEFINITIONS

Personal Health Record: A Personal Health Record (PHR) is a collection of information about an individual's health and health care, described using controlled medical vocabulary, stored in a private and secure digital file that is owned and controlled by the individual. The file is portable, and has access rights determined by the individual.

PHR System: A PHR System is computerized tools that help an individual understand and manage the information contained in a PHR.

Electronic Health Record: An Electronic Health Record (HER) is an aggregation of patient-centric health data that originates in the patient record systems of multiple independent healthcare organizations for the purpose of facilitating care across multiple organizations.

Electronic Health Record System: An EHR system is a combination of information systems that perform the functions of an EHR. An EHR system is intended for use by healthcare providers.

Controlled Medical Vocabulary: A controlled medical vocabulary is a mechanism used to standardize health information for purposes of capturing, storing, exchanging, searching, and analyzing data.

Interoperability: Interoperability is the technical capacity for the exchange of health information between different healthcare information systems.

Open Source: Open Source is a software development model and philosophy characterized by freely redistributable source code to empower a robust ecosystem of contributors who collaborate in advancing the development of software.

Chapter 4
A Framework for Privacy Assurance and Ubiquitous Knowledge Discovery in Health 2.0 Data Mashups

Jun Hu
University of Ottawa, Canada

Liam Peyton
University of Ottawa, Canada

ABSTRACT

Knowledge discovery is a critical component in improving health care. Health 2.0 leverages Web 2.0 technologies to integrate and share data from a wide variety of sources on the Internet. There are a number of issues which must be addressed before knowledge discovery can be leveraged effectively and ubiquitously in Health 2.0. Health care data is very sensitive in nature so privacy and security of personal data must be protected. Regulatory compliance must also be addressed if cooperative sharing of data is to be facilitated to ensure that relevant legislation and policies of individual health care organizations are respected. Finally, interoperability and data quality must be addressed in any framework for knowledge discovery on the Internet. In this chapter, we lay out a framework for ubiquitous knowledge discovery in Health 2.0 based on a combination of architecture and process. Emerging Internet standards and specifications for defining a Circle of Trust, in which data is shared but identity and personal information protected, are used to define an enabling architecture for knowledge discovery. Within that context, a step-by-step process for knowledge discovery is defined and illustrated using a scenario related to analyzing the correlation between emergency room visits and adverse effects of prescription drugs. The process we define is arrived at by reviewing an existing standards-based process, CRISP-DM, and extending it to address the new context of Health 2.0.

DOI: 10.4018/978-1-61520-777-0.ch004

Copyright © 2010, IGI Global. Copying or distributing in print or electronic forms without written permission of IGI Global is prohibited.

INTRODUCTION

Knowledge discovery is a critical component in improving health care. Web 2.0 technologies provide us an increasing ability to integrate and share data from a wide variety of sources on the Internet. Health 2.0 leverages those technologies to create on-line communities within which patients, caregivers, medical professionals, and other health stakeholders can collaborate and share data. In particular, both Google Google Health, 2009) and Microsoft Healthvault (HealthVault, 2009) are proposing services to maintain personal electronic health records on behalf of consumers, and share them as needed with physicians, clinics, and other health care providers. Consolidating all health care records across a broad spectrum of health care providers, provides a potentially very valuable source of information about health, disease and health care especially with respect to detecting trends in the spread of disease (SARS, Swine Flu) as well as measuring the efficacy of prescription drugs and the number of side effects. But to leverage that collective source of information, a framework for knowledge discovery is needed which defines a managed process for collecting, analyzing and publishing data relevant to healthcare decisions based on large, statistically significant data patterns within a Health 2.0 data architecture. Such a framework can promote a continuous process of evidence-based medicine and performance management to ensure that health care services are meeting the needs and objectives of the communities which use them.

There are a number of issues which must be addressed before knowledge discovery can be leveraged effectively and ubiquitously in Health 2.0. Trust is of paramount concern. Health care data is very sensitive in nature so privacy and security of personal data must be protected. Normally, in a single enterprise, data can be collected from multiple data sources within a single organization into a single data warehouse in a controlled fashion to build a model of the overall enterprise that can support knowledge discovery through analysis and data mining. In a Health 2.0 environment, though, different organizations each have their own independent sources of data that could be published, shared and linked over the Internet to support knowledge discovery.

Interoperability and data quality are also major issues. Typically, each organization stores its data in a different format, according to different standards, or in an ad hoc manner. Most family doctors still maintain paper records and write notes in natural language. In order to effectively process data in a consistent automated fashion, mechanisms must be put in place to standardize the data that is collected and linked. One of the biggest challenges is finding a mechanism for reliably identifying patients from different data sources, while still protecting privacy.

More importantly business agreements and regulatory oversight must be in place amongst the different organizations in order to collect and analyze data in this manner to ensure that the relevant legislation and policies of individual health care organizations are respected. As well, patient consent forms and access controls to ensure compliance with privacy laws (HIPAA, 1996; PIPEDA, 2000; PHIPA 2004) must be in place. Special care must be given, if public access is granted to data and knowledge discovery within a Health 2.0 network. Decisions based on health care data are complex and life affecting, so continuous monitoring to ensure validity, reliability and compliance of a Health 2.0 framework must be as ubiquitous as the data sharing it supports.

In this chapter, we lay out a framework for ubiquitous knowledge discovery in Health 2.0 based on a combination of architecture and process. First, we provide a summary and background of relevant technologies and trends in Health 2.0, paying attention to how privacy is protected via federated identity management. Then we introduce our framework. Emerging Internet standards and specifications for creating a Circle of Trust are used to define an enabling architecture for knowledge discovery, in which data is shared but identity and personal information protected. Within that context, a step-by-step process for knowledge discovery is defined and illustrated using a scenario related to analyzing the correlation between emergency room visits, clinic symptoms and adverse effects of prescription drugs. The process we define is arrived at by reviewing an existing standards-based process, CRISP-DM (Shearer, 2000; CRISP-DM, 2009), and extending it to address the new context of Health 2.0.

BACKGROUND

In this section, we introduce some of the key concepts and technologies that form a basis for our proposed framework.

Master Patient Index

A Master Patient Index is a database that contains a unique identifier for each patient which can be used to lookup, access and link health records (paper or electronic) for a patient from a variety of sources (each of which may have their own way independent mechanism for identifying patients). This concept has been quite common in healthcare both with paper and electronic health records. Many countries have created initiatives to build a national Master Patient Index (Tan, 1995; Neame & Olson, 1996; Walker, 1998) in support of integrated health services. Linking a Master Patient Index with electronic delivery of data would be desirable to construct a distributed electronic health record. This has been done within the context of a single organization, by for example creating an enterprise Master Patient Index that links records for a single institution like a hospital (Adragna, 1998). For Health 2.0, there are a number of technical and policy-based issues that must be resolved to enable to deliver health records across organizations over the Internet, but doing so would make possible sophisticated and

timely data integration to give a complete medical picture for a patient even in dynamic emergency response situations (Shapiro et al, 2006).

One of the issues in leveraging a Master Patient Index for knowledge discovery is to ensure privacy protection when sharing and analyzing data. One approach to this has been to anonymize data records by removing patient identities or encrypting them (de-identifying). (Li and Shaw, 2005) presented an attribute analysis framework to de-identify personal health information for data mining. (El Emam et al, 2006) has analyzed algorithms for "re-identifying" individuals based on combining "de-identified" data from distributed sources in order to evaluate just how well the practice of de-identification protects privacy. A comparison of different approaches to managing patient identities and linking patient records across different organizations is given in (Hu & Peyton, 2009) including a discussion of the Liberty Alliance Circle of Trust specifications and standards used in this paper.

Federated Identity Management

A Circle of Trust is a key concept for protecting personal data that is shared between organizations over the Internet. An architecture to support this has been developed by the Liberty Alliance project (Landau, 2003; Cahill et al, 2008). Liberty Alliance was established in 2001 as a consortium of technology enterprises to create an open standard and set of specifications for federated identity management. A Circle of Trust is a business to business network in which an individual's identity and personal information is protected by a designated Identity Provider, while still allowing cooperating organizations within the Circle of Trust to access and share the individuals personal information over the Internet in a systematic manner that ensures the individual's permission is obtained and their identity protected. The cooperating organizations have trust relationships and operational agreements established amongst them.

There are a number of tools and services available for federated identity management. OpenID (Recordon & Reed, 2006) is a free single-sign on solution originating with open source community efforts that simplifies and consolidates logins for internet users. Currently it falls short of the standards proposed by Liberty Alliance, but is improving with each release. Microsoft's Windows Live ID (Live, 2006) replaced its earlier Passport Service which was criticized for its proprietary approach wherein Microsoft was the sole authority that acts as the Identity provider. The Liberty Alliance consortium was formed in part as a response to Microsoft. Sun has an implementation based on Liberty Alliance called OpenSSO (OpenSSO, 2009).

Anonymous and pseudonymous identities are two ways of protecting identity (Koch & Möslein, 2005). With anonymous identity, the identity is unknown and one cannot refer to an identity beyond the single session in which it is used. With pseudonymous identity, one can link events across sessions to an identity created for a specific organization, without knowing the actual identity. Pseudonyms are central to how identity is protected in a Circle of Trust. The Identity Provider provides a given user with a different pseudonym for each organization it interacts with, while hiding the user's real identity and protecting their personal information. Access to personal information and sharing of data between organizations is managed and controlled by the Identity Provider. The pseudonym is a key with allows each organization to recognize the user they are interacting with and access only the data they are permitted to see. (Peyton et al, 2007) explored audit trail mechanisms for ensuring privacy compliance for e-Health in a Circle of Trust.

Data Mining and Methodology

The CRoss-Industry Standard Process for Data Mining, CRISP-DM (Shearer, 2000; CRISP-DM, 2009) was created by the European Union to define an industry- and tool-neutral data mining process. CRISP-DM organizes the data mining process into six phases: business understanding, data understanding, data preparation, modeling, evaluation, and deployment. These phases provide a road map to follow while carrying out any data mining project. However, CRISP-DM assumes that a single organization is pursuing the data mining project, based on data collected within a single organization, and that the results of the data mining project are used by a single organization. It assumes a relatively straight forward and static data architecture. Privacy issues are also not addressed in a systematic fashion because of the assumption of a straight forward data architecture within a single organization. (Peyton & Hu, 2007) made a preliminary assessment of these gaps in CRISP-DM.

Several research communities however have made contributions to address privacy preserving data mining, especially in the context of a distributed data architecture. One approach is based on statistical methods. In this approach, the data is altered before delivering it to the data mining tool so that real values are obscured (Agrawal, 2001; Evfimievski et al., 2002). The second approach is based on cryptographic protocols that encrypt the data in a systematic fashion that still enables linking and processing. The distributed sites cooperate to learn the global data mining results without revealing the data at their individual sites (Vaidya & Vaidya, 2004).

Health 2.0 Technologies

Health 2.0 is a broad label that refers to the transformation of our health care systems based on leveraging emerging Web 2.0 technologies, principles and practices (O'Reilly, 2004) for building applications and services around the unique features of the Internet. A good analysis of this technology driven transformation is provided in (Goldstein et al, 2007), while (Porter & Teisberg, 2006) looks at the business drivers for such a transformation, and (Coffield & DeLoss, 2008) reviews the legal and privacy challenges faced by the technology.

Web 2.0 encompasses a broad spectrum of technologies, including Rich Internet Applications that allow users to participate in and add value to the content of the application. It also pre-supposes ubiquitous connectivity in which data and rich content is available instantly as it happens, anywhere and anytime from a plethora of mobile devices. Scalability and processing power is presumed infinite and readability available as a hosted service. The focus of our paper however is mainly related to Web 2.0 technologies for open interoperability and data integration in a Service Oriented Architecture (SOA) using RSS, REST, SOAP and other Internet protocols to support the concept of a data mashup.

Data mashups are based on integrating data from web pages or a set of services or data feeds published by a Web site. We will refer to such Web sites, throughout this paper as Data Providers. The web pages, sevices and data feeds enable a data mashup Web site (referred to throughout this paper as a Mashup Provider) to generate integrated content and reports by take information from the various sites, and mix features from multiple sources, as well as continuously querying over Web services (Tatemura et al., 2006). Currently, Data mashups are largely defined in an ad hoc fashion, in that each individual mashup filters, interprets and links data from Data Providers in a manner specific to its use. There are some systems and tools (Aboulnaga & El Gebaly, 2007; Sarma et al, 2008) that take a more reusable model-based approach to representing and integrating data across Data Providers. Due to the volumes and real-time nature of the data feeds, support for mining of data streams as well as data sets is important (Han & Kamber 2006) including the ability to monitor such data streams for patterns (Baron et al 2003).

Health 2.0 applications, services and tools are emerging along five themes: social networking, participation, apomediation, collaboration and openness (Eysenbach, 2008). Google Health (Google Health, 2009) and Microsoft Healthvault (HealthVault, 2009) are two major initiatives for Health 2.0 services. Both have search as their business model, and build a platform for other smaller services to tap into. Google Health allows users to build online health profiles, download medical records, get personalized health advice and share information with doctors and others. Microsoft Healthvault is designed as a health organizer to enable users to collect, store and share their health information only with those granted permission. In Canada, Telus Health Space (Telus Health, 2009) is tapping Microsoft HealthVault Web portal to enable Canadians to manage their own health records.

Data Integration Standards and Tools

There are a number of standards that attempt to facilitate sharing of data in the eHealth industry. Health Level Seven (HL7, 2009) is an ANSI-accredited Standard Developing Organization (SDOs) which provides standards for interoperability among all healthcare stakeholders. The Clinical Document Architecture (HL7 CDA, 2009) is a XML-based HL7 standard for the representation and machine processing of clinical documents for the purpose of exchange. It provides an exchange model in a way which makes the documents both human readable and machine processable. The European Committee for Standardization (CEN) develops CEN 13606 (CEN 13606, 2006), an electronic health record (EHR) extract standard using the openEHR archetype methodology (OpenEHR, 2009). In (Patrick et al, 2007), an approach to encoding doctors notes using SNOMED defined codes is described.

In general, though, even if organizations use the same standard to encode data and use the same standard to define interfaces to those data, there is no guarantee that there will be interoperability. For interoperability, there has to be a standardized common data model that all organizations agree to, and they have to follow the same methodology for encoding and linking between their data sources. Communication of data between organizations is also an issue. HL7 and web services provide a standard interface for accessing data on an as needed basis. But it is not designed for handling large amounts of data. Often ETL tools are used to extract, transform and load data into standardized data sets that can be published or communicated in bulk.

HEALTH 2.0 KNOWLEDGE DISCOVERY FRAMEWORK

Our approach to defining our Health 2.0 knowledge discovery framework (shown in Figure 2) is to start with the CRISP-DM process that has been defined by the European Union for data mining in general (shown in Figure 1), and extend it to address the new realities of Health 2.0.

CRISP-DM defines six steps or phases in a data mining project, starting with "Business Understanding" and ending with "Deployment" which center on the collection and analysis of a dataset and the building of a data mining model used to interpret the data that can be deployed

to address a business issue for an organization. The data mining project is typically a standalone project not tightly integrated into the organization's online systems. As such, it can be viewed as a process of

- Data Understanding to see what data to extract from existing data sources within the organization in order to address a need based on Business Understanding
- Data Preparation to create a standalone dataset that can be used as a basis for data mining Modeling
- Evaluation of the model to ensure it meets the need based on Business Understanding
- Deployment into business operations

In our proposed framework, this process is revisited in the context of a Health 2.0 Data Sharing Architecture that allows for the continuous integration of data from multiple organizations across the Internet. To emphasize this change in context from mining a standalone dataset we use the term "knowledge discovery" instead of data mining to emphasize that it is fully integrated into the ongoing publishing and sharing of data on the Internet, as another mechanism for contributing new content. In particular, the data mining or

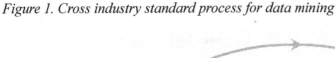

Figure 1. Cross industry standard process for data mining

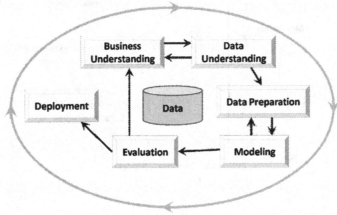

knowledge discovery model is packaged as a data mashup that is itself published as a data source on the Internet that can be used by others.

In order to address the special requirements of Health 2.0, three new phases are added to the process model for a knowledge discovery project and three existing phases are modified. Due to the dynamic nature of Data Providers and the data they publish, a Monitoring phase is added to ensure the ongoing quality of published data mashups, and verify regulatory compliance in terms of who is accessing what data. Two new phases are also added for Privacy-Preserving Data Publishing and Data Integration in order to handle the sharing of data across organizational boundaries. Each Data Provider has to carefully control and package the data they publish in a way that protects or anonymized identities, while the knowledge discovery framework must flexibly and accurately integrate, link and combine data from several Data Providers. The Data Preparation, Modeling and Deployment phases are shown in grey to indicate

that while the phases still exists in our framework, they have evolved and been modified from their original conception in CRISP-DM.

The rest of the paper will elaborate on the details of our framework, including the Health 2.0 Data Sharing Architecture, in the context of an e-Health knowledge discovery scenario.

E-HEALTH KNOWLEDGE DISCOVERY SCENARIO

The main components and participants of our e-Health knowledge discovery scenario are shown in Figure 3. The scenario takes place within the context of a Liberty Alliance Circle of Trust that creates an e-Health B2B network of online services related to an emergency room in a hospital (eHospital), a clinic (eClinic) and a pharmacy (ePharmacy). In particular, each one is a Data Provider that can contribute date to our knowledge discovery process. The Circle of Trust is the foundation for

Figure 2. Health 2.0 knowledge discovery framework

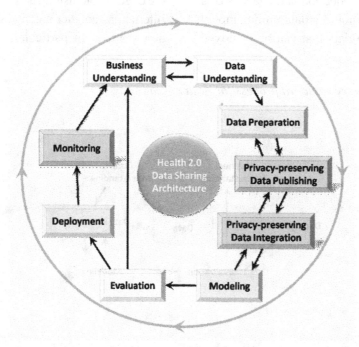

our Health 2.0 data sharing architecture. It includes an Identity Provider which is used to protect and manage identity for both Patients and Health Care Workers. Patients and Health Care Workers will log in to the Identity provider, but after that their interaction with the different services is based on special security tokens or pseudonyms that protect their true identity. In addition, patient's privacy is protected since data published by a Data Provider can only be accessed based on the consent of the patient and applicable privacy regulations. The Identity provider controls access to their data records, and it "pseudonymizes" the data. Each Data Provider has its own pseudonym for each patient so that it can only recognize its own data. A Mashup Provider is able to integrate and link data from the different Data Providers, in collaboration with the Identity Provider which resolves the Pseudonyms based on its Master Patient Index, and generates a new set of pseudonyms for the Mashup Provider. The Mashup Provider has registered knowledge discovery processes that are registered and carefully reviewed. These discover processes model the data from Data Providers in order to generate data mashups and reports that are used by analysts to improve and manage the performance, health trends and quality of care in the network and ensure compliance. Some of these may also be made available for public use.

We know define the scenario for our example knowledge discovery process as follows. Variations on this scenario have been used as a basis for analysis in (Hu et al, 2008; Hu & Peyton, 2009):

1) A patient U1 goes to eClinic to see his family doctor. The pseudonym for the patient at eClinic is "C1". The doctor may observe symptoms like high blood pressure, nausea, headache etc. and record the fact. If such symptoms are observed, the doctor may take no action, or they might prescribe a drug ("Drug A", "Drug B", etc.)

2) If a drug is prescribed, the patient then goes to ePharmacy to fill a prescription, for example "Drug A". The pseudonym for the patient at ePharmacy is "P1". A pharmacist records the fact that a prescription has been fulfilled.

3) If, sometime later, the patient arrives at the Emergency Room (eHospital) with a severe condition like a "Cardiac Arrest" or "Stroke". This will be recorded for the patient at eHospital where the pseudonym for the patient is "H1".

In this scenario, it raises the question as to whether there is any relationship between the symptoms observed at eClinic, the prescription dispensed at ePharmacy and the resulting severe condition treated at eHospital. In a traditional health setting, such a question could only be addressed by setting up an approved clinical trial at a great cost in terms of time, human resources and expense. In a Health 2.0 setting, it would be advantageous if medical analysts could collect data on all patients from eHospital, ePharmacy, and eClinic on a continuous basis in order to discover if there are any patterns that might cor-

Figure 3. Liberty alliance e-health scenario for knowledge discovery

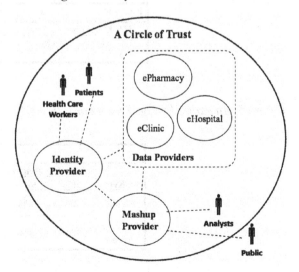

relate Emergency Room visits to symptoms or prescriptions.

Figure 4 shows a "Consolidated Data Set" created by the Mashup Provider that could be used for knowledge discovery. Each column of data comes from a different service: eHospital has data on emergency room events, ePharmacy has data on prescriptions, and eClinic has data on symptoms. Note, also that this dataset has a pseudonym specific to the Mashup Provider and the data set. It uniquely identifies each row in the dataset, but it is an identifier that is meaningless outside that purpose. Neither eHospital, nor eClinic, nor ePharmacy would recognize or be able to use the pseudonym. Only the Identity Provider, responsible for enforcing privacy regulations and access control is able to correlate using the Master Patient Index. Note that in order to create this consolidated data set across many clinics, pharmacies and hospitals, one needs a consistent mechanism for identity resolution and standardization of the format and possible values for Events, Prescriptions, Doses and Symptoms within a Circle of Trust.

Statistics based on the consolidated data set from Figure 4, might result in the performance management report shown in Figure 5. (Note that the report shown is fabricated for illustration purposes.) From this report we can see that it looks like there might be an increased risk of Cardiac Arrest for those who took Drug A when having Chest Pain symptoms (48% versus 1% in all other cases), and an increased risk of Stroke for those who had Chest Pain but did not take any medication (19% versus 1 or 2% in all other cases).

HEALTH 2.0 DATA SHARING ARCHITECTURE

The architecture we propose to use to support Health 2.0 data sharing is shown in Figure 6. It complies with the Liberty Alliance Circle of Trust specifications but extends it in a few key areas. It is a Service Oriented Architecture in which all the Data Providers, the Identity Provider and the Mashup Provider implement web services based on the Liberty Alliance Web Service Framework (Cahill et al, 2008). Generically, in terms of the Liberty Alliance specifications, all of the "providers" in the figure are Service Providers. The Identity Provider is a special type of provider

Figure 4. Consolidated dataset used for knowledge discovery

Pseudonym	Event	Prescription	Dose	Symptom
U1 M	Cardiac Arrest	Drug A	20/day	Chest Pain
U2 M	Stroke	Drug B	50/day	Vision Loss
U3 M	None	Drug C	10/day	Migraine

Figure 5. An example report from consolidated dataset

	Chest Pain				
	Drug A	Drug B	Drug C	No Drug	Total
No Event	50%	98%	98%	80%	80%
Stroke	2%	1%	1%	19%	10%
Cardiac Arrest	48%	1%	1%	1%	10%

identified in the Liberty Alliance specifications, but Data Providers and the Mashup Provider are a new type of provider that we have defined specifically for supporting data publishing and integration in support of knowledge discovery for Health 2.0. While all the providers coordinate and communicate via the standard web service interface, they also support specific API calls related to data collection and integration that enable the delivery of data feeds. As specified by Liberty Alliance, all sharing of data is brokered by the Identity provider which enforces privacy policies and provides "Pseudonym translation". Each of the providers is described in more detail below

Data Provider is a data source owned by some organization in the Circle of Trust that publishes data for use by other organizations in the Circle of Trust. The Data Provider is responsible for the integrity and quality of the data it provides. Typically, wholesale access to its data is not provided, rather it must carefully define the data sets that can be requested or the restricted types of queries that it can process. It enforces access to data within its own organization and ensures that any data sets or queries it publishes are consistent with its organizational policy. However, consent

Figure 6. Architecture for ubiquitous knowledge discovery in health 2.0

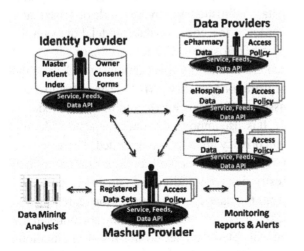

for sharing the data is managed by the Identity Provider on a patient by patient basis. As well, access to the data sets and queries are managed by the Mashup Provider and not the Data Provider. The Data Provider publishes its data by registering it with the Mashup Provider.

Identity Provider provides federated identity management. It provides single sign on for patients and health care workers. It is the only place where identification information is stored (other than pseudonyms). It also stores, tracks and manage the consent provided by patients for allowing the use and sharing of their personal information which includes both identity information and information maintained by any of the Data Providers in the Circle of Trust. Where possible, signed consent forms are put in place which give permission for the Mashup Provider to collect, integrate and analyze the information in the Health 2.0 Circle of Trust for the purposes of knowledge discovery to improve the health care services provided.

Encryption technology is used to create a Master Patient Index of pseudonyms for each person for each data provider and provide federated trust relationships with a high level of granularity, allowing the participated organization to expose only a subset of their data; and enable real-time mapping of attributes. When the Mashup Provider makes requests or queries which result in data sets from the Data Provider, the Identity Provider is responsible for mapping and transforming the Pseudonym attributes from the Data Provider into a recognizable set meaningful to the Mashup Provider. All data sharing is brokered by a the Identity Provider and Mashup Provider working together so that identity (managed by the Identity Provider) is kept separate from data (managed by the Mashup Provider).

Mashup Provider makes requests or queries for data sets from the Data Providers and it links and integrates those data sets to make consolidated data sets that can be used for knowledge discovery in order to create data mashups and reports. This can be done on a continuous basis and can include monitoring of the resulting data streams to detect patterns and raise alerts. Requests can only be made for registered data sets for which all necessary business and legal approvals are obtained. The Mashup Provider maintains a registry which controls who can have access to what data sets, data mashups or reports and is responsible for regulatory compliance. In addition, the Mashup Provider must monitor the network in terms of what Data Providers are available, any changes in the type or quality of data returned and respond adaptively to unexpected disruptions. Performance metrics can be tracked.

Note that for the purposes of this chapter, we have assumed that the communication channels between the components in figure 6 are secure, and that each of the components is well-behaved, and not malicious. In practice, a complete threat analysis of the architecture would be needed as well as appropriate scalability reviews. The focus of this chapter is strictly on addressing legal and functional requirements of the data sharing architecture and process for knowledge discovery.

KNOWLEDGE DISCOVERY PROCESS FOR HEALTH 2.0

In the context of our data sharing architecture, we can now step through the knowledge discovery process outlined in Figure 2, for our example e-Health scenario (Figure 3). This analysis builds upon and extends the preliminary gap analysis of CRISP-DM that was presented in (Hu & Peyton, 2007).

Business Understanding

The first phase focuses on understanding the business requirements for knowledge discovery, and the definition of a suitable, possibly continuous, knowledge discovery process. In addition, to identifying a business need to link emergency room events to prescriptions and symptoms seen in a clinic, there are two main requirements specific to Health 2.0 that must be addressed from a business point of view. Namely, establishing the business relationships and agreements that allow data to be collected from different organizations and ensuring that appropriate patient consent and privacy safeguards are in place. In our e-Health scenario, data from each of eClinic, ePharmacy and eHospital may be relevant to understanding how emergency events might be related to symptoms at a medical clinic and drugs that were prescribed for those symptoms. To allow knowledge discovery process to take place, there must be business agreements in place from the three Data Providers, and the organization must have reviewed and explicitly given permission for the data to be published. Ideally, in our situation, the patients would have signed a consent form for their health data to be shared within the Circle of Trust for knowledge discovery purposes. Note that in our scenario, all data has been de-identified. And in the final report that is the output of our knowledge discovery, we are only using aggregated data.

Data Understanding

The data understanding phase involves understanding what data must be collected from which data sources at what organizations as well as understanding what attributes can be used to link and integrate the data. It is important, that if data is published within the Circle of Trust that it conforms to a common data model. For example, each of eHospital, eClinic and ePharmacy should represent time in a consistent fashion. Part of the registration process with the Mashup Provider can assure conformance to a common data model.

It is also important to understand how identity and privacy are to be safeguarded. There may be patient-defined as well as organization-defined restrictions on individual attributes collected from the data sources. In addition, care must be taken to ensure that the resulting attributes in the consolidated data set do not result in situations where patients become potentially identifiable or sensitive data can be inferred. For example, if geographic attributes like postal code are combined with other attributes, then it might be possible to deduce the identity of a patient without needing to resolve pseudonyms with the Identity Provider (El Emam et al, 2006). As another example, consider if the resulting consolidated data set contained only one patient with a cardiac arrest at a rural hospital over a one week period. It would be very easy for many people in that rural community to infer the actual identity of that patient.

Data Preparation

In CRISP-DM, the goal of the data preparation phase was to produce standalone datasets as a basis for a single organization data mining model. Tasks included selecting data, cleaning data, constructing data, integrating data, and formatting data. In a Circle of Trust, the goal of the data preparation phase is to prepare data so it can be published to make it accessible by other organizations. There are four main requirements specific to Health 2.0 in this phase. The first is data standardization that requires exchange of database schema information and collection of relevant meta-data information, typically coordinated with the Mashup Provider. The second is normalization and data cleaning that address distributed management of data scaling, handling missing data and other data cleaning issues. The last is de-personalization that protects the patient's privacy which is partially achieved by the Master Patient Index system of pseudonyms, but which may also involved filtering or obfuscating other attributes.

In our e-Health scenario, the attributes from each of eClinic, ePharmacy and eHospital will have to be identified, selected, cleaned and formatted. For example, symptoms in eClinic, drug names and dose in ePharmacy and events in emergency room are selected to be shared. The personal information is removed from the shared dataset. Each of eClinic, ePharmacy and

eHospital is then ready to publish its data and metadata information to allow other organizations to subscribe to it.

Privacy-Preserving Data Publishing

After data is prepared in the previous phase, it is published so that it can be used in a knowledge discovery process. The four main requirements specific to Health 2.0 that must be addressed in this phase are patient consent for sharing, standardization of publishing, security of the data, and protection of privacy.

In our e-Health scenario, eClinic, ePharmacy, eHospital publish their data by registering with the Mashup Provider. All requests to access the published data are brokered by a collaboration between the Mashup Provider and Identity Provider. The Mashup Provider ensures that the datasets conform to the common data model (i.e. a consistent handling of Events, Prescriptions, Doses, Symptoms, and Dates) and that proper organizational authorization has been given to use the data sets in the knowledge discovery process. The Identity Provider holds the patient consent forms that permit the sharing of data. However, it is the right of the patient to refuse to allow their data to be shared for such purposes. When the Mashup Provider requests a data set on behalf of an analyst or other authorized user, the pseudonyms are mapped from the Data Provider to the Mashup Provider, and any patient records for which consent is not granted are filtered out. (The details of this mechanism are explained in more detail in the next paragraph on data integration and shown in Figure 7). The use of encryption, SSL and Liberty Alliance specification provides security and additional privacy protection.

Privacy-Preserving Data Integration

The Privacy-preserving Data Integration is a new phase, which we introduce to address integrating data sets from several Data Providers, which may

Figure 7. Correlate data using a master patient index

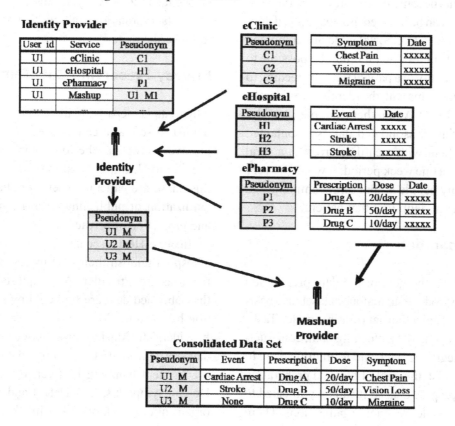

be arriving continuously and asynchronously, and link them via pseudonyms without compromising identity. The Mashup Provider, through its interaction with the Identity Provider requests the data sets it desires from each Data Provider. The data sets however are returned in two pieces. The pseudonym attributes for each row are returned via the Identity Provider which transforms them into pseudonyms meaningful to the Mashup Provider for that request using the Master Patient Index. The rest of the attributes are returned to the Mashup Provider directly by the Data Provider. It is important that the Master Patient Index is kept separate from the actual data otherwise one would be able to link all health data in the network to the real identities.

Figure 7 shows the situation for our scenario. The Mashup Provider requests Symptom, Prescription and Event data sets from each of eClinic,

ePharmacy, and eHospital. However, it is the Identity Provider that receives the distinctive pseudonym data sets from each Data Provider ("Ci", "Pi", "Hi") and transforms them into the pseudonyms understood by the Mashup Provider ("Ui_M"). The Mashup Provider receives three such data sets from the Identity Provider, corresponding to each of the data sets returned by the Data Providers. All six data sets may arrive at different times, and in fact may be arriving continuously on a scheduled basis or as events occur. The Mashup Provider must correlate records for its target consolidated data set as they arrive. Note that if patients have not given consent then the Identity Provider will return NULL instead of a meaningful pseudonym, and the Mashup Provider will drop the records from the integration.

Modeling

In the modeling phase, depending on the specific knowledge discovery task, various techniques are selected and applied, and their parameters are calibrated to optimal values. This phase considers various models and chooses the best one based on their predictive performance. There are two main issues specific to Health 2.0. The consolidated data set may result in potentially identifiable records based on the attributes, so they may need to be filtered or obfuscated as appropriate just like in the data preparation phase for individual Data Providers. The second is that the modeling techniques are not only traditional data mining algorithms, but also include statistical techniques, OLAP data models, text mining and event or data stream mining to handle processing of large quantities of data arriving on a continuous basis.

Statistical Techniques

Statistical techniques can sometimes be just as effective as data mining algorithms for discovering new knowledge, especially detecting patterns in streaming event data and building predictive models. Markov chain analysis is particularly relevant for continuous streams of event data. A thorough treatment of discrete event analysis for health care is given in (Jun et al, 1999). Statistics can help greatly to answer several important questions about data: what is the pattern? Which patterns are significant? What is a high level summary of the data and its trends?

OLAP Data Model

An On-Line Analytic Processing (OLAP) (Thomsen, 2002) data model creates a multi-dimensional view of the data that is optimized for reporting and analysis, in particular for aggregating data. It can be maintained in memory by the Mashup Provider, or persisted to the file system. Although Data Mining techniques can operate on any kind of unprocessed or even unstructured information, they can also be applied to the data views and summaries generated by OLAP to provide more in-depth and often more multidimensional knowledge. Like data mining, OLAP could be considered as an analytic technique. (Ledbetter and Morgen, 2001) give a thorough treatment of knowledge discovery for health care based on leveraging an OLAP models assembled from electronic patient records.

Text Mining Methods

Text mining is a technique to extract useful information from unstructured text and convert to attributes. Much web content such as web pages, news article and email in unstructured, but even information stored in a Data Provider database may be unstructured. For example, the amount of the prescription might be a text field in which different doctors and pharmacists write equivalent amounts differently. Data Providers may publish unstructured data, or the Mashup Provider may have decided to include general Internet sources for data that is only available as text.

Data Streams

In most real-time applications, event data is usually represented as a continuous data stream often associate with, for example, RFID tags. Continuous collecting and querying streaming event data enables organizations to monitor, analyze and act for decision-making. In streaming data mining, where data stream may arrive asynchronously at a rapid rate, answer may be computed with incomplete information and hence may in error. Therefore it is not practically feasible to store continuous data streams in a traditional data model, as they are not designed for rapid and continuous storage of data. Rather the data model must include the notion of time, while the query should support continuous queries and evaluated over unbounded data sets. A good treatment of both traditional data mining, and stream based data mining is given in (Han & Kamber 2006)

Evaluation

Evaluation is the process of determining if the discovered knowledge has meaning in the targeted business scenario, and also to determine if there still exist some important business issues that need to be further considered. It is important to more thoroughly evaluate the model and review the steps executed to mine the data to be certain it properly achieves the business objectives before proceeding to deployment. Evaluation criteria that can be used to measure success include quality of model (accuracy, reliability, and timeliness), cost (how much data over what time period must be processed), security and privacy. While security and privacy are largely handled within our Circle of Trust-based architecture, care must be taken with respect to potentially identifying attributes, and with respect to which users will have access, and what risks are associated with their possession of the data. In our e-Health scenario, the following should be verified:

1. The knowledge discovery process generates data that is available in a timely fashion, and accurate. And there is evidence that the data is being used in a useful manner.
2. Data is collected and integrated with reasonable performance and is scalable.
3. Consent has been obtained from patients for their data, and the use of that data in the knowledge discovery process, and the knowledge created is consistent with that consent.
4. Business agreements are in place between the relevant organizations that cover both data collection from Data Providers and access to the results generated by the knowledge discovery process.
5. The knowledge discovery services and registered users of the consolidated data

sets have the required access rights at each Data Provider for the data required.
6. The consolidated data sets created by the knowledge discovery process will not compromise privacy by making it possible for identities or sensitive data to be inferred.
7. The knowledge generated by the knowledge discovery process should be statistically sound, and all potential business and legal implications should be carefully examined.

Deployment

Once the knowledge discovery process has been evaluated and cleared for deployment, the results of the knowledge discovery process are published by the Mashup Provider and registered in its dataset registry. Both the consolidated data set and the performance management report from our scenario are potentially publishable in this fashion. The Mashup Provider is itself a Data Provider and the results of one knowledge discovery process can be a data source that is used by another knowledge discovery process. All the usual constraints and process that apply to a Data Provider during the privacy-preserving data publishing phase, apply to the Mashup Provider when it deploys its knowledge discovery process and publishes the results.

Monitoring

Due to the dynamic nature of Health 2.0 environment, and the need for regulatory compliance, a new phase, "Monitoring", is added in our knowledge discovery process. Both the data sets published by Data Providers and the results published by the Mashup Provider must be monitored on an ongoing basis to ensure the quality and consistency of the data, as well as the availability and reliability of the Data Provider. An audit trail of data collected and accessed must also be maintained to monitor regulatory compliance.

Choosing an effective monitoring mechanism is vital for completing a successful knowledge discovery project. (Baron et al, 2003) focus on the monitoring of patterns and the detection of interesting changes. (Peyton et al, 2007) proposes an audit trial service for verifying compliance with privacy regulations in a Circle of Trust for eHealth.

ESSENTIAL ELEMENTS OF HEALTH 2.0 KNOWLEDGE DISCOVERY

Table 1 shows the essential elements of Health 2.0 knowledge discovery that are supported by our framework in comparison with the traditional approach to data mining as defined by CRISP-DM. In many ways these mirror the essential elements of Health 2.0 itself. Our framework supports B2B networks over the Internet on a continuous, ubiquitous basis so any organization is potentially a source of data, knowledge discovery collaborator and/or consumer of data. Whereas the traditional

model is Intranet or Standalone oriented, planned and deployed by a single organization.

Our framework leverages Liberty Alliance Circle of Trust standards for security, privacy and federated identity management and Web 2.0 technologies for data sharing and data integration to flexibly support continuous, automatic knowledge discovery that is grounded in explicitly secured patient consent and organizational agreement. In the traditional approach this is largely irrelevant as the entire process takes place within a single organization and is commissioned on a case by case basis. Finally, the dynamic nature of Health 2.0, and the sheer volumes of continuous data possible require continuous monitoring and new modeling techniques for knowledge discovery.

FUTURE RESEARCH DIRECTIONS

The architecture and process underlying our proposed framework require further study in a number

Table 1. Essential elements of health 2.0 knowledge discovery

	Health 2.0 Knowledge Discovery	**CRISP-DM Process Model**
Platform	B2B network, Internet	Intranet, Standalone
Availability	Continuous and Ubiquitous	Planned
Data	Multiple sources on the Internet from different organizations	Single organization
Authorization	Permission-based, Automatic	Commission-based
Trust model	Circle of Trust	Single organization
Privacy protection	Business agreement, Patient consent form, Regulatory compliance, Federated identity management, Master Patient Index	Single organization privacy policies. Patient consent.
Data sharing	Web 2.0 technologies, Web Services, Data feeds	Enterprise Data Model
Data integration	Web 2.0 technologies, Mashups Dynamical and flexible configuration Efficient, lower cost development	ETL Static integration per project. High cost development
Modeling techniques	Statistics, Data mining algorithms, OLAP model Text mining, Streaming Event Data	Statistics, Data mining algorithms OLAP model
Monitoring	Real-time, dynamic, continuous	N/A
Security	Liberty Alliance security specifications	Single Organization security.

of areas. Privacy-preserving data sharing, privacy-preserving data integration and monitoring are new phases introduced to ubiquitous knowledge discovery in Health 2.0. Each phase itself is a complex process that can be further investigated. The protocol, algorithms, standards, and tasks for each phase are all good opportunities for future research. In particular, there are still many organizational challenges to be faced in setting up and leveraging the technologies we have described here. Many are not yet commonly used.

Data mashup technology makes it easy to draw on multiple data sources to create new applications but there are also risks and challenges in terms of quality, reliability, security, and scalability that need to be addressed and managed. This is still an active area of research. The ability to process massive amounts of streaming data into an OLAP data model and event-based data mining are also active areas of research. Many mashup platforms leverage the pipes integration pattern to create business logic. This approach is simplicity for modeling the flows, but better support is needed for enforcing a common data model, and integrating access controls. How to support flexible integration of data sources inside and outside the Circle of Trust requires more work, as does how to determine what data and knowledge discovery results can be safely published to a Data Provider, Circle of Trust or the Internet public as a whole. The latter must take into account, how that data is retained, stored, or combined once released.

More importantly, careful analysis of electronic personal health record services like Google Health and Microsoft Health Vault is required with possible regulation by governments to ensure that patient privacy and publishing of health data is properly controlled. Currently, governments have not fully understood the implications and potential benefits of Health 2.0. This regulation and standardization is essential, not only to protect consumers, but also to make possible the potential benefits of Health 2.0 for improving quality of care.

CONCLUSION

Health 2.0 presents both opportunities and challenges, as we have shown through our analysis of the proposed framework and the example e-Health knowledge discovery scenario. The major contribution of this work has been to highlight the need for a well-defined, open, standards-base architecture for data sharing in a Health 2.0 context, and to articulate the major phases of a continuous knowledge discovery process to give guidance to organizations. A balance must be struck between the exciting possibilities of the new technology, and the care that must be taken in ensuring the quality, security and regulatory compliance of the health services the framework would support and improve. In particular, this chapter:

1. Identified the requirements of each phase of ubiquitous knowledge discovery in Health 2.0 based on the CRISP-DM model in the context of a Circle of Trust.
2. Proposed additional phases in a knowledge discovery process, privacy-preserving data sharing, privacy-preserving data integration, and monitoring, to address the requirements of trust, privacy and quality of data and results in a B2B network.
3. Defined a trusted architecture that enables ubiquitous knowledge discovery in Health 2.0.

REFERENCES

Aboulnaga, A., & El Gebaly, K. (2007). µBE: automatic source selection and schema mediation for Internet scale data integration. In *Proceedings of IEEE International Conference on Data Engineering* (pp.186-195). Istanbul, Turkey: IEEE.

Adragna, L. (1998). Implementing the enterprise master patient index. *Journal of American Health Information Management Association, 69*(9), 46–52.

Agrawal, D., & Aggarwal, C. (2001). On the design and quantification of privacy preserving data mining algorithms. In *Proceedings of the Twentieth ACM SIGACT-SIGMOD-SIGART Symposium on Principles of Database Systems* (pp. 247–255). Santa Barbara, California, USA: ACM.

Baron, S., Spiliopoulou, M., & Günther, O. (2003). *Efficient monitoring of patterns in data mining environments. Advances in Databases and Information Systems* (pp. 253–265). Berlin, Heidelberg: Springer.

Cahill, C., Canales, C., Le Van Gong, H., Madsen, P., Maler, E., & Whitehead, G. (2008). Liberty Alliance Web Services Framework: A Technical Overview. Liberty Alliance Project, New Jersey. Retrieved May 1, 2009, from http://www.project-liberty.org/liberty/resource_center/papers

CEN 13606. (2006). HealthInformatics – Electronic Health Record communication, Part1: Reference Model. European Standard. Retrieved May 1, 2009, from http://www.chime.ucl.ac.uk/resources/CEN/ EN13606-1/N06-02_prEN13606-1_20060209.pdf

Coffield, R. L., & DeLoss, G. E. (2008). The Rise of the Personal Health Record: Panacea or Pitfall for Health Information. *American Health Lawyers Association - Health Lawyers News, 12*(10). Retrieved May 1, 2009, from http://www.fsbwv.com/pdf/The_Rise_of_the_PHR_AHLA.pdf

CRISP-DM. (2009). Cross Industry Standard Process for Data Mining. Retrieved May 1, 2009, from http://www.crisp-dm.org/Process/index.htm

El Emam, K., Jabbouri, S., Sams, S., Drouet, Y., & Power, M. (2006). Evaluating common de-identification heuristics for personal health information. *Journal of Medical Internet Research, 8*(4), e28. doi:10.2196/jmir.8.4.e28

Evfimievski, A., Srikant, R., Agrawal, R., & Gehrke, J. (2002, July). Privacy preserving mining of association rules. In *Proceedings of The Eighth ACM SIGKDD International Conference on Knowledge Discovery and Data Mining* (pp. 217–228). Edmonton, Alberta, Canada.

Eysenbach, G. (2008). Medicine 2.0: Social Networking, Collaboration, Participation, Apomediation, and Openness. *Journal of Medical Internet Research, 10*(3), e22. doi:10.2196/jmir.1030

Goldstein, D., Groen, P. J., Ponkshe, S., & Wine, M. (2007). *Medical Informatics 20/20: Quality and Electronic Health Records Through Collaboration, Open Solutions, and Innovation.* Sudbury, MA: Jones & Bartlett Publishers.

Google Health. (2009). *Google Health.* Retrieved May 1, 2009, from https://www.google.com/health

HL7. (2009). *Health Level Seven.* Retrieved May 1, 2009, from http://www.hl7.org

HL7 CDA. (2009). *Clinical Document Architecture* (CDA). Retrieved May 1, 2009, from http://xml.coverpages.org/healthcare.html #cda

Han, J., & Kamber, M. (2006). *Data Mining: Concepts and Techniques* (2nd ed.). Morgan Kaufmann Publishers.

HealthVault. (2009). *Microsoft HealthVault.* Retrieved May 1, 2009, from http://www.healthvault.com

HIPAA. (1996). *Health Insurance Portability and Accountability Act.* United States Congress, United States. Retrieved May 1, 2009, from http://aspe.hhs.gov/admnsimp/pl104191.htm

Hu, J., & Peyton, L. (2009). Integrating Identity Management with Federated Healthcare Data Models. In *Proceedings of the 4th International MCeTech Conference on eTechnologies* (pp. 100-112). Ottawa, Canada. LNBIP 26, Springer.

Hu, J., Peyton, L., Turner, C., & Bishay, H. (2008). A Model of Trusted Data Collection for Knowledge Discovery in B2B Networks. In *Proceedings of the 3rd International MCETECH Conference on e-Technologies* (pp. 60-69). Montreal, Canada.

Jun, J. B., Jacobson, S. H., & Swisher, J. R. (1999). Application of discrete-event simulation in health care clinics: A Survey. *The Journal of the Operational Research Society, 50*(2), 109–123.

Koch, M., & Möslein, K. M. (2005). Identity Management for Ecommerce and Collaborative Applications. *International Journal of Electronic Commerce, 9*(3), 11–29.

Landau, S. (Ed.). (2003). Liberty ID-WSF and Privacy Overview, version 1.0, Liberty Alliance Project. Retrieved May 1, 2009, from http://www.projectliberty.org/liberty/resource_center/papers

Ledbetter, C. S., & Morgan, M. W. (2001). Toward Best Practice: Leveraging the Electronic Patient Record as a Clinical Data Warehouse. *Journal of Healthcare Information Management, 15*(2). Retrieved May 1, 2009, from http://www.himss.org/content/files/jhim/15-2/him15205.pdf

Li, J., & Shaw, M. (2004). Protection of Health Information in Data Mining. *International Journal of Healthcare Technology and Management, 6*(2), 210–222. doi:10.1504/IJHTM.2004.004977

Live. (2006). *Introduction to Windows Live ID, Windows Live Development Center.* Retrieved May 1, 2009, from http://msdn.microsoft.com/en-us/library/bb288408.aspx

Neame, R. L., & Olson, M. (1996). Measures implemented to protect personal privacy for an on-line national patient index: a case study. *Topics in Health Information Management, 17*(2), 18–25.

O'Reilly, T. (2005). *What is Web 2.0: design patterns and business models for the next generation of Software.* Retrieved May 1, 2009, from http://www.oreillynet.com/pub/a/oreilly/tim/news/2005/09/30/ what-is-web-20.html

OpenEHR. (2009). *The openEHR Foundation.* Retrieved May 1, 2009, from http://www.openehr.org/shared-resources/getting_started/openehr_primer.html

OpenSSO. (2009). *Sun OpenSSO.* Retrieved May 1, 2009, from http://www.sun.com/software/products/ opensso_enterprise/index.xml

Patrick, J., Wang, Y., & Budd, P. (2007). An automated system for conversion of clinical notes into snomed clinical terminology. In *Proceedings of the fifth Australasian symposium on ACSW frontiers* (pp. 219–226). Darlinghurst, Australia: Australian Computer Society, Inc.

Peyton, L., & Hu, J. (2007). Knowledge Discovery in a Circle of Trust. In Zanasi, A., Brebbia, C., & Ebecken, N. (Eds.), *Data Mining VIII: Data, Text and Web Mining and their Business Applications* (pp. 235–244). Billerica, MA, USA: WIT Press.

Peyton, L., Hu, J., Doshi, C., & Seguin, P. (2007). Addressing privacy in a federated identity management network for e-health. In *Proceedings of Eighth World Congress on the Management of eBusiness,* Toronto.

PHIPA. (2004). *Personal Health Information Protection Act.* Government of Ontario, Canada. Retrieved May 1, 2009, from http://www.e-laws.gov.on.ca/html/statutes/english/elaws_statutes_04p03_e.htm

PIPEDA. (2000). *The Personal Information Protection and Electronic Documents Act.* Department of Justice, Canada. Retrieved May 1, 2009, from http://laws.justice.gc.ca/en/P-8.6/text.html

Porter, M. E., & Teisberg, E. O. (2006). *Redefining health care.* Boston: Harvard Business School Press.

Recordon, D., & Reed, D. (2006), OpenID 2.0: a platform for user-centric identity management. In *Proceedings of the Second ACM Workshop on Digital Identity Management* (pp. 11-16). Alexandria, Virginia, USA. DIM '06. ACM, New York, NY, 11-16.

Retrieved May 1, 2009, from http://doi.ieeecomputersociety.org/10.1109/MCETECH.2008.22

Sarma, A., Dong, X., & Halevy, A. (2008, June). Bootstrapping pay-as-you-go data integration systems. In *Proceedings of ACM SIGMOD International Conference on Management of Data.*

Shapiro, J. S., Kannry, J., Lipton, M., Goldberg, E., Conocenti, P., & Stuard, S. (2006, October). Approaches to Patient Health Information Exchange and Their Impact on Emergency Medicine. *Annals of Emergency Medicine, 48*(4), 426–432. doi:10.1016/j.annemergmed.2006.03.032

Shearer, C. (2000). The CRISP-DM model: the new blueprint for data mining. *Journal of Data Warehousing, 5*(4), 13–22.

Tan, L. T. (1995). National patient master index in Singapore. *International Journal of Bio-Medical Computing, 40*(2), 89–93. doi:10.1016/0020-7101(95)01130-7

Tatemura, J., Sawires, A., Po, O., Chen, S., Candun, K., Agrawal, D., & Goveas, M. (2007). Mashup feeds: continuous queries over Web services. In *Proceedings of ACM SIGMOD International Conference on the Management of Data* (pp. 1128-1130). Beijing, China.

Telus Health. (2009). Telus Health Solutions. Retrieved May 1, 2009, http://telushealth.com

Thomsen, E. (2002). *OLAP Solutions: Building Multidimensional Information Systems.* New York: John Wiley & Sons, Inc.

Vaidya, J., & Clifton, C. (2004). *Privacy-preserving data mining: why, how, and what for?* IEEE Security & Privacy.

Walker, A. (1999). South Australia: best practice guidelines for patient master index maintenance. *Health Information Management, 29*(1), 43–45.

Chapter 5
A Semantic Model to Address Health Questions to Professionals in Healthcare Social Networks

Francisco Echarte
Universidad Pública de Navarra, Spain

José Javier Astrain
Universidad Pública de Navarra, Spain

Alberto Córdoba
Universidad Pública de Navarra, Spain

Jesús Villadangos
Universidad Pública de Navarra, Spain

ABSTRACT

Internet social networks offer a wide variety of possibilities, including communication between users, sharing information, and the creation of virtual communities on many different subjects. One of these subjects is healthcare, where different social networks are now appearing and covering different objectives. In this chapter, a social network is described, where users can formulate healthcare questions that are automatically classified under concepts of a medical ontology and assigned to experts of each topic. These questions are then answered by healthcare expert physicians. This chapter includes a semantic classifying method that provides the automatic classification of questions by means of a medical ontology, based on the tags used to annotate them, and the previously classified questions. The chapter includes an ontological model that represents the questions, the assigned tags, the answers, the physicians, and the medical concepts.

DOI: 10.4018/978-1-61520-777-0.ch005

Copyright © 2010, IGI Global. Copying or distributing in print or electronic forms without written permission of IGI Global is prohibited.

INTRODUCTION

Nowadays, we assist to the emergence of different social networks based on some of the features offered by Web 2.0 technologies. Users of social networks are the main actors in this kind of webs: creating new content that are accessible to other users of the Web, interacting with other users, creating relationships, and defining, in a great extent, the evolution of theses networks.

Healthcare social networks (HSNs) provide new social and commercial possibilities. They provide new communication and interaction channels among patients and physicians, they provide new healthcare services, and offer new business trends.

There exist many ways to apply social networks to the healthcare field:

i)   Patients sharing their own treatment experiences with other patients (PatientsLikeMe[1]).

ii)   Physicians retrieving knowledge by reading medical literature and interacting with peers (Sermo[2], PeerClip[3], Within3[4]).

iii) Medical students, residents improving their knowledge (knowledge discovery and collective wisdom) (SocialMD[5])

iv)   Online support groups (MDJunction[6]);

v)   Rating physicians (RateMDs[7]).

vi)   Physicians and patients sharing experience both together (WegoHealth[8]). HSNs concern patients (iMedix[9]), physicians (Sermo, PeerClip, Within, SocialMD, Ozmosis[10]), students (SocialMD, Tiromed[11], DOctorsHangout[12]) and nurses (Nursing World[13], Nurselinkup[14]).

From the **physician** point of view, healthcare information is hierarchical and formally well classified by means of **ontologies**. Healthcare terminologies like SNOMED[15], openGalen[16], MeSH[17], UMLS[18] or ICD[19] are used in healthcare environments for different purposes as clinical history encoding, statistical analysis of medical activities and procedures, etc. These terminologies are often lengthy and complicated to use even for healthcare professionals, and of course very complex and often unintelligible to be used by common users of social networks without healthcare knowledge. In this sense, **folksonomies** (Vander Val, 2007) provide an easier way to create, browse and search information since they are less restrictive and rigid than the medical terminologies.

One of the more interesting features of this kind of social networks is that users can address questions concerning their health directly to medical specialists, and also to patients with similar pathologies (a way to share experiences). The main problem is the difficulty addressed to **question** classification. Users classify healthcare questions easily by means of **tags**, but this produces fuzziness in the classification. The classification of tags using folksonomies is less strict than that obtained with other more formal methods like **ontologies**. Therefore, there not exists any kind of general classification criteria. Users tag their questions following their own medical knowledge (often limited). This makes navigation among the questions difficult, since other users (i.e. medical specialists) must browse and search the questions using the limited capabilities of folksonomies.

Our contribution concerns the semantic model used to solve the addressed problem of automatic assignation of health questions from patients to physician professionals in HSNs. Our proposal includes the generation of a **folksonomy** from the user's questions and the assigned tags, and the modelling of this folksonomy using some existing ontological models. We model the folksonomy using Social Semantic Cloud of Tags (SCOT[20]) and we extend the SCOT's model using: i) Semantically-Interlinked Online Communities (SIOC[21]), in order to represent the different elements of the HSN and its behaviour; and ii) Simple Knowledge Organisation System (SKOS[22]), in order to define the ontology containing the set of necessary healthcare topics used in the clas-

Figure 1. Healthcare social network proposal

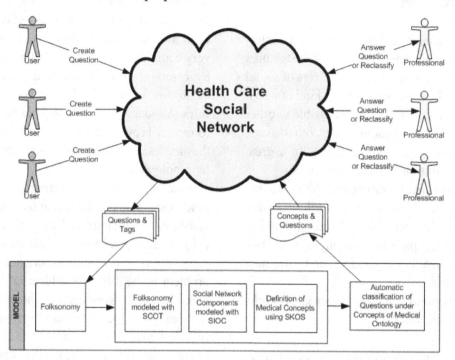

sification of the questions. These topics are either created explicitly, either incorporated from any pre-existing healthcare ontology. We perform an automatic classification of the questions under the concepts of the ontology using similarity measure techniques. The system provides the questions (classified by specialities) to the physicians, in order to assign each question to the more appropriated expert. Physicians answer the questions and all the information (both questions and answers) remain accessible in the web. If necessary, physicians can reassign the questions to new topic groups, or to any pre-existing one. Figure 1 illustrates the HSN here proposed.

Let assume a **healthcare social network** where questions are addressed to experts (physicians) instead of other community members (common users). Once a user creates a question with its associated tags, this question is automatically addressed to the right person to answer the question. This assignation requires an ontology containing all the topics, terms and concepts organized

in an ontology. The creation of a new question then implies the acquisition of its tags and the calculus of the distances (or similarities) with the questions previously classified in the ontology. Once classified, the question is answered by the expert in charge of this ontology subject. When a healthcare expert finds a misclassification of a given question, he can assign it directly to the correct subject. Since new questions are compared with previously existing ones, the classification performed by the expert ensures better future classification results. The contribution of this work is the proposal of a semantic and automatic classification system. This system classifies annotated resources of a folksonomy using the tags assigned and the previously classified resources. We use SCOT to model the folksonomy in an ontology and we extend this model with SIOC and SKOS. We use SIOC to model the healthcare social network and SKOS to model the concept and terms of the classification system.

BACKGROUND

Social networks can be considered as social structures of nodes and links. Individuals and/or organizations actors are the nodes of the social network that are linked by one or more specific types of interdependency. The resulting structures are often very complex, making difficult the information generation and the navigation among this information. Folksonomies can be considered a social classification method by collaborative tagging where users create and manage tags to annotate and categorize content. In contrast to classical subject indexing where metadata is generated only by experts, folksonomies do not follow a controlled and well known vocabulary and are not restricted to expert users.

In order to be effective, social networks require easy and intuitive methods to allow users generating and browsing information. Although ontologies are formal methods to organize and classify information commonly used, they are often inaccessible for non expert users. Once defined an ontology for a given knowledge domain, the system is rigid and static, and its evolution is difficult and implies large efforts in time and resources. Folksonomies are: i) user-generated, ii) a useful low-cost alternative to more formal systems, iii) collaborative, they allow the distribution of work tasks.

Folksonomies are based on the free allocation of tags to resources. There are two main approaches to the use of folksonomies: users can freely assign tags to resources, known as broad folksonomy, as del.icio.us[23]; and users can only assign tags to their own resources (created by them), known as narrow folksonomy, as flickr[24]. As result of the collaboration among users, either resources or tags can be interpreted semantically.

However, the simplicity and flexibility observed by users becomes a problem when dealing with resources classification. The users' ability to freely create and assign tags, causes the appearance of synonyms, polysemy, syntactic variations, syntactic errors, different granularity tags, tags that do not contribute to enrich the information system, etc. (Golder, 2005; Guy, 2006). Tags are located in a flat space without any a priori relationship among them. Tag browsing, tag navigation and tag classification become the main difficulties associated to folksonomies.

Tom Gruber defines ontologies as "a formal and explicit specification of a shared conceptualization" (Gruber, 1993) in contrast with the flexibility of folksonomies. The explicit definition refers to the need of enumerating all the concepts and elements in the formal domain and using a formalized language in its representation. In the same way, shared conceptualization refers to the need of including in the representation the users' point of view. Ontologies are structured knowledge containers where concepts, instances, and their attributes and relationships are modelled.

Ontologies provide a formal specification of a set of concepts that can be used by different agents in order to interact with a common language since they model a domain in a rigorous manner. What make ontologies appealing is their formalism, the knowledge sharing, and the possibility to reason and draw conclusions. Ontologies are widely used in applications ranging from knowledge management and natural language processing to Health Sciences and are the principles of the Semantic Web (Berners-Lee, 2001). However, ontologies also have their own drawbacks, mainly related to the difficulty of design and use. They do not easily apply to collaborative environments such as Web 2.0 and social networks, mainly due to its complexity and difficulty of use, maintenance and evolution.

RELATED WORK

Let consider a social network like iMedix where users can find and share healthcare information. iMedix is a free website that helps people to find and share health information. Members of the iMedix community share their experiences and rank medical content in order to make health information organized and accessible to everyone.

iMedix' users have different options, common to other social networks, to create contents and communities. Users can be members of different communities, in which users share interests in some health subjects and also establish friendship relations with other members. The most important feature of this HSN is that users can create questions about health topics and other users can answer them, and that users can assign positive or negative ratings to these answers. Medical knowledge can be enriched with personal experiences of other patients.

In this HSN, users collaborate among themselves sharing their own experiences and assessing different healthcare content. iMedix offers users the ability of asking medical questions that can be answered by other community members. These questions could be also automatically addressed to medical experts with the aid of adequate classification systems.

In order to formulate their healthcare questions, users demand a simple, intuitive and flexible information classification mechanism. The use of medical ontologies is suitable for the collective of physicians, but common users (patients) are not familiarized with such terminologies. Ontologies allow a precise classification of questions but they require higher effort than other techniques like folksonomies. Folksonomies deal better than ontologies with imprecise, incomplete or incorrect information classification. Furthermore, while ontologies deal with static knowledge representations, folksonomies deal with dynamic knowledge representation. The occurrence of a new topic in a question can imply its misclassification when considering ontologies. However, in the case of a folksonomy, users can assign a new label to the question automatically becoming as a part of the classification system. While users' domain (patient) fits better with folksonomies, physicians' domain fits better with ontologies.

Users create new questions using forms as illustrated in Figure 2. This form asks for a title question, its summary and a more detailed description of the question. iMedix allows users to annotate the questions using tags. This allows users to classify on an intuitive and easy way avoiding the use of more complex solutions based on common healthcare terminologies. In order to reduce the tag variability, the number of erroneous tags, the number of misspellings, and in general, the noise in the folksonomy, as the user writes down in the tag field, a list of proposed tags is provided. This tag list includes tags previously used by this user or by the rest of users, and therefore defined in the folksonomy, that fit the written pattern. It would also be possible to feed the folksonomy initially with a set of terms obtained from a pre-existing terminology, obtaining an initial set of tags that becomes the basis for the introduction of tags by users.

Questions introduced by users are immediately available in the HSN, so any user can see it (Figure 3). iMedix do not provide medical experts to answer the questions. These questions are answered by the HSN users, and other users can assign their positive or negative ratings to these answers.

When a user wants to answer a question, he fills the answer form as depicted on Figure 4.

Then, the answer is automatically associated to the question, and presented just below it, so other users can read it and provide their positive or negative rating. As Figure 5 shows, a disclaimer is used just below the question and before the answers. This disclaimer informs users that the answers are written by patients, so these answers should never be construed as medical advice or substitute for professional care.

Many works in the literature deal with the resolution of some of the well-known problems of folksonomies, reducing the existing gap between ontologies and folksonomies. Folksonomy tags co-ocurrence is analyzed in (Hassan-Montero, 2006) which focuses in the effort of improving the

Figure 2. New question creation form

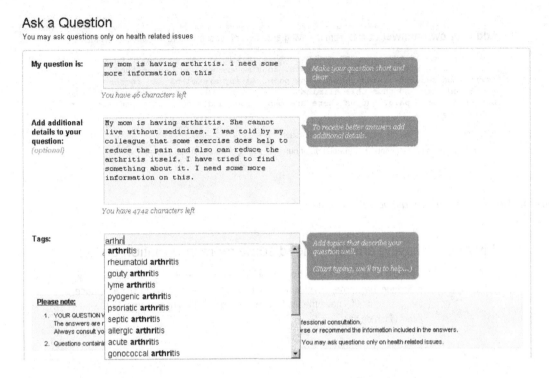

Figure 3. A question of a user using the tag "Arthritis"

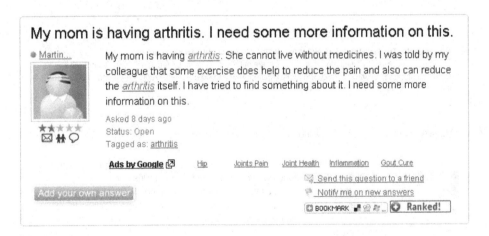

quality of tag clouds for browsing and searching. Tag clustering is addressed in (Heymann, 2006; Zhou, 2007), the problem of exploring hierarchical semantics from social annotations is annalyzed in (Heymann, 2006); and (Zhou, 2007) deals with the conversion of a large corpus of tags into a navigable hierarchical taxonomy using a graph of similarities. The problem of syntactic variations is explored in (Echarte, 2008; Echarte, 2009). Other works as (Passant, 2007; Echarte, 2007; Kim, 2008) relate folksonomies with formal information classification systems as ontologies and person-

Figure 4. Form used by other users to answer a previously created question

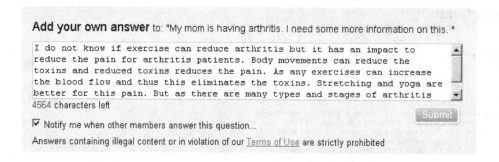

Figure 5. A question with its associated answers

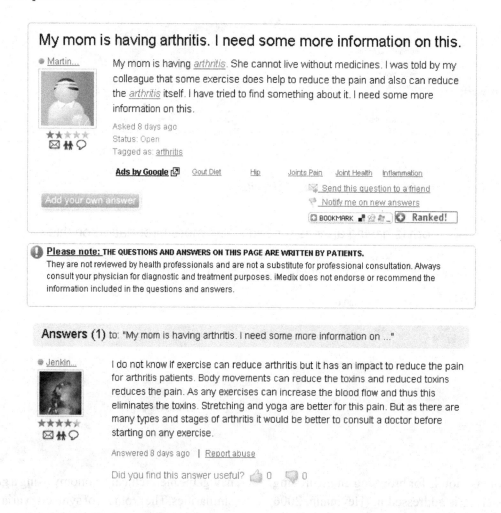

alized recommendations (Xu, 2006; Shepitsen, 2008). In (Specia, 2007) Specia and Motta create clusters of semantically related tags and makes a semantic enrichment of the folksonomy using external ontologies, and (Catutto, 2008) makes a sistematic characterization of different similarity measures in folksonomies, by a semantic grounding provided by Wordnet[25].

SEMANTIC MODEL AND METHOD TO ADDRESS QUESTIONS TO PROFESSIONALS

Semantic Model Description

This section describes an ontology based semantic model which describes the behaviour of the social network, and the classification system based on a set of concepts and terms represented by a pre-existing medical ontology.

We propose the use of OWL (Dean, 2004; Smith, 2004) in order to represent the knowledge of this semantic model. Ontologies can be defined in different ways due to the existence of different languages to represent them. Therefore, it is very important to use mature standards to define them. From this point of view, OWL is the best option. Proposed by the Wide Web Consortium (W3C), it is one of the main elements of the Semantic Web, a project initiated by T. Berners-Lee to include semantic in the Web (Berners-Lee, 2001). OWL is supported by different technologies (XML, XML Schema, RDF (Graham, 2004), RDF Schema (Brickley, 2004), and all together provides a way to define a structure for documents and the explicit semantic relationship between different resources. All these technologies are open standards, tested and accepted.

The semantic model must consider the different components of the social network: physicians and users; the questions formulated by users with the tags assigned and the answers provided by the experts; and finally, the set of topics where questions are classified. In order to define this model, we use some pre-existing ontologies like SIOC, SCOT and SKOS. SIOC allows describing the components of an online community. Its classes allow representing users, user groups, forums, comments, and any kind of user gener-

ated content. This ontology is used to represent the components of the proposed HSN: physicians, users, questions and answers. SCOT describes a given folksonomy. It is based on a set of users, a set of resources and a set of tags. It also describes the set of tags assigned by users to resources. This ontology has a set of classes and properties that allow representing some of the relationships among tags as synonyms, syntactic variations, different granularity levels, and so on. We use this ontology in order to represent the folksonomy generated by users. We populate this ontology when user creates questions and they assign tags. SKOS allows describing classification systems based on taxonomies, thesauruses, etc. Its classes and properties allow defining concepts and relationships among them. We use this ontology to define a main concept. This concept allows classifying the questions proposed by users.

Ontology Components

We define a new ontology in order to represent the semantic model of the healthcare social network here described. This new ontology takes into account both classes and properties of previously defined ontologies. Figure 6 shows these components: white ellipses represent the different classes; grey ellipses describe the classes that use foreign ontologies; and arrows represent the relationship among classes. Class *Question* is a subclass of *sioc:Item* and it is associated to the classes' *scot:Tag*, *HealthConcepts* and *Answer*.

Folksonomy components can be described as follows:

- **ProfessionalGroup**: it gathers the physicians of the social network. This class inherits from *sioc:UserGroup* which represents groups of users with similar interests in the community.
- **PatientGroup**: it gathers the users of the social network that not have assigned a physician role, that is, the patients. As

Figure 6. Ontology representing the healthcare social network

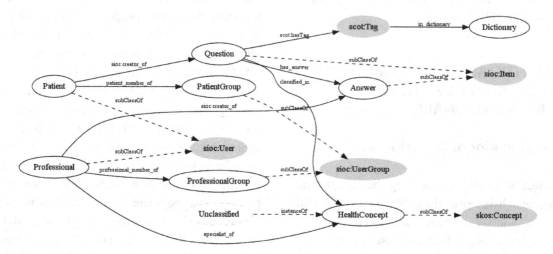

occurred with physicians, this class also inherits from *sioc:UserGroup*.

- **Professional**: it represents a medical professional, a physician. This class inherits from *sioc: User* and provides the community user account. This class is associated to the different elements that a physician can create. In this case, it is related with the answers of the questions proposed by the users.

- **Patient**: it represents a user (patient) in the social network. Inherited from *sioc:User,* this class is associated with the elements that can create a patient (questions for physicians).

- **Question**: it represents the question asked by a user. It inherits from *sioc:Item* that allows representing whatever element that users of the community could create. It provides a set of properties that represent the content of the question.

- **Tag**: it represents the **tags** assigned by patients to questions. It uses the class *scot:Tag* to represent the free text strings used to annotate the question. Narrow folksonomies restrict the annotation of questions to their creators, while broad folksonomies allow

annotating questions to both creators and rest of users. This model does not make any assumption between the uses of narrow or broad folksonomies. iMedix is based in a narrow folksonomy.

- **Dictionary**: folksonomies allow users to create tags following their own criteria, producing that the number of tags in the folksonomy increases very fast. Some works (Golder, 2005; Michlmayr, 2005) consider that annotations follow a power law distribution that produces resources trend to concentrate the majority of annotations in a reduced set of tags that define their semantics. So, this class contains a set of tags with a high degree of semantic relevance in the folksonomy. These tags are used to represent annotated **questions** as well as the classification **concepts**. Tags relevance is evaluated using some criteria like a minimum number of annotations, a minimum number of annotated questions, or a minimum number of users using them. The **dictionary** is built using a set of tags with a high degree of semantics. These tags are used to: i) encode a question; ii) encode each concept of the classification system, and iii) measure the degree of similarity of these concepts with the question.

- **Answer**: it represents the answer provided by a physician expert to a question created by some user of the community. It uses the class *sioc:Item*.

- **HealthConcept**: it represents the different concepts of the medical classifications system, under which questions are automatically classified. The classification structure in which questions are classified (i.e. a taxonomy) is created using the *skos:Concept* class. *HealthConcept* class allows to create a new classification structure or to reuse a pre-existent ontology. The class contains a special instance named *Unclassified* that is used to classify all the questions which cannot be classified under any other concept. For example, in order to avoid exceeding a minimum threshold. Each physician is associated al least with one (or more) of these concepts, representing that they have an expertise degree in the field and are in charge of answering the questions associated. Table 1 summarizes some

relevant properties of the ontology. These properties relate the elements of the classes defined in the ontology depicted in Figure 6.

Automatic Classification of Questions

This section describes a method that classifies automatically the questions created by users (*Question*) of the healthcare social network, on a set of classification concepts (*HealthConcept*). The method needs as seed a set of questions previously classified.

As Figure 7 depicts, given a new question, the method compares it with the existing classification concepts in order to classify the question under the most adequate classification concept. In order to perform this comparison, the question and the classification concepts are encoded taking into account the dictionary tags.

For a given question, the encoding process provides a tuple with n elements, where n is the number of tags included in the dictionary. This process provides a value for each element of the tuple

Table 1. Relevant properties of the ontology.

Property	Domain / Range	Description
specialist_of	Domain: Professional Range: HealthConcept	This relationship relates physicians with their expertise topics. This property has an inverse called *has_specialist*.
profesional_member_of	Domain: Professional Range: ProfessionalGroup	This relationship relates a given physician with a group of physicians. This property has an inverse called *has_professional_member*.
patient_member_of	Domain: Patient Range: PatientGroup	This relationship relates social network user with a group of patients (other users of the network). This property has an inverse called *has_patient_member*.
has_answer	Domain: Question Range: Answer	This relationship relates a given question with the answer provided by an expert. This property has an inverse called *answer_of*.
in_dictionary	Domain: scot:Tag Range: Dictionary	This relationship relates a tag with a dictionary. Although this dictionary uses to be unique, there can be more than one according to different criteria.
classified_in	Domain: Question Range: HealthConcetp	This relationship relates a given question its representative topic. After the classification of a question, the question is associated to a certain topic in order to be assigned to the more indicated expert. This property has an inverse called *has_classified*.

where $value_i$ is the number of annotations referred to the *i-th* tag of the dictionary. For example, for a dictionary *D={cat, dog, hot-dog, door}*, and a question *Q={dogs}*, the tuple provided could be (0, 12, 2, 0), indicating that twelve annotations refer to tag *dog*, and two to tag *hot-dog*. So, a question is represented by the number of its annotations that are associated to each tag of the dictionary. In the same way, classification concepts are represented as the addition of the encoded representations of the questions classified under them. Using these encoded representations, the method compares a question and the classification concepts obtaining a similarity measure and the concept with the higher similarity value. When the similarity

measure is greater than a certain threshold, the question is classified under the classification concept and otherwise the question is classified under a generic *Unclassified* concept. Once the question has been classified under a classification concept, the question becomes accessible for the professionals associated to this concept. Professionals can answer or reclassify this question under any other classification concept if they consider that the question does not fit the automatically provided classification concept. Performing this reclassification, professionals help to improve the classification process. Questions classified under *Unclassified* concept could be checked later if they receive more annotations, or they could be

Figure 7. Ontology representing the healthcare social network

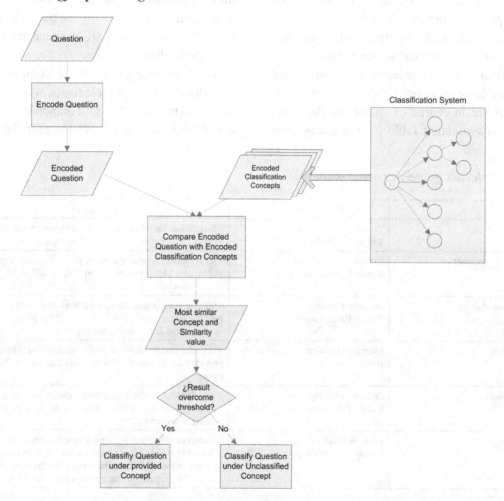

used to guide the evolution of the classification system using clustering techniques over them in order to detect the convenience of creating new classification concepts, merging two existing concepts or splitting an existing one.

Different alternatives can be used to provide an initial set of preclassified questions. For example, the creation of an ontology representing a classification system based in medical specialities creating a classification concept for each speciality. These classification concepts can be initially represented using terms obtained from a medical terminology given more weight to the terms that better represent each concept. Then, the dictionary would be initialized with these medical terms and could also be used to provide tagging suggestions to users. Another alternative is the execution of an initial classification of existing questions using clustering techniques. Each obtained cluster would represent a classification concept, and the elements of the cluster would represent the questions classified under it. The clustering method could be applied iteratively to the clusters in order to get finer classification concepts.

The size of the initial set affects the whole classification algorithm, since the larger this dictionary is, the higher computational cost the method has (the number of similarity measures to compute increases as the dimension of the dictionary does). A wide dictionary minimizes the need of using clustering techniques to reduce the number of resources classified under the concept *Unclassified*. As classification process reaches stability (new questions are almost always classified under existing classification concepts), the dictionary grows and the need of concept clustering decreases.

Social networks described in previous section can be defined like a 9-tuple $HN:= (U,P,Q,T,D, A,C,Y,f_a)$, where U represents the set of users in the community, P the set of physicians, Q the set of questions, T the set of tags associated to the questions, D a subset of T, A the set of answers created by the physicians, and C the set of clas-

sification concepts. Y represents a ternary relation among a user, a question and the set of tags assigned by the user to the question, $Y \in U \times T \times R$. Function f_a represents the automatic classifier that determines, for a given question, the most suited concept of the classification system using the questions previously classified. The subset of tags D represents the dictionary described in the semantic model section. It is built using those tags used by users that meet a certain condition, like a minimum number of annotations.

Given the described tuple, we can define a bipartite graph that relates the dictionary tags used by users and the concepts of the classification system created under *HealthConcept*, that are distinct that *Unclassified*. Lets define a graph $G=(V,E)$, where $V=\{D,C\}$ and where $\forall d_1, d_2 \in D, c_1, c_2 \in C, \neg \exists e \in E \mid e = (d_1, d_2) \vee e = (c_1, c_2)$. Two graph nodes c_i y d_i are connected by an edge if it exists at least one question previously classified on the concept represented by c_i and if the question has assigned the dictionary tag d_i. The weight of the edge is determined by the number of resources classified on the concept which have assigned the tag.

Using the relations described by this graph among concepts of the classification system and tags, we can encode any *HealthConcept* concept of the classification system like a weights vector $v_c \in R^D$. Where each vector position is associated with a dictionary tag d' and which value is determined by the number of relations between the concept and the tag; that is the edge weight that links the node c and the node d'.

Moreover, we can also encode any question using the tags assigned by the user, like a weights vector $v_q \in R^D$, where each position corresponds to the number of times that a tag has assigned to the question.

We can use both encodings to encode the concepts of the classifying system and the questions created by users, like vectors belonging to R^D. This allows measuring the similarity between a vector that represents a question and the vectors that represent the classifications concepts. We can use the cosine similarity measure, as usual in Information Retrieval (Salton, 1989).

$$Similarity(v_q, v_c) := \cos(v_q, v_c) = \frac{v_q \bullet v_c}{\left|v_q\right|\left|v_c\right|} \quad (1)$$

The cosine similarity measures the angle between the two encoded vectors providing values in the interval [0, 1]. It provides a value of 1 if both vectors point at the same direction and 0 if they are orthogonal. If we avoid the use of a dictionary, the described encodings could be done using the whole set of tags T. However, this would produce very sparse vectors affecting to the performance of the classification.

Therefore, to automatically obtain the most adequate classification concept for a given question, we need to obtain the concept with the higher similarity degree with this question. The angle of the vectors is desired to be as small as possible. Once the most suitable concept has been found, the similarity value could be rate to check if it overcomes a predefined threshold. In those cases where the similarity value does not overcome the

Figure 8. Classification algorithm

```
(1) Input: Question
(2) Vq = encode(Question)
(3) Max_similarity = 0;
(4) Max_concept  = Unclassified;
(5) For each HealthConcept hc ≠ Unclassified do
(6)    Vc = encode(hc)
(7)    Similarity = cosine(Vq, Vc)
(8)    if (similarity > max_similarity ) then
(9)       max_similarity = similarity;
(10)      if (threshold()) then
(11)         max_concept = hc
(12)      end if
(13)   end if
(14) end do
```

threshold value, the questions could be assigned to the *Unclassified* concept, and then an expert must reclassify the question. Figure 8 shows the described algorithm.

The classification system provides the questions classified on the concepts and then physicians can access to their associated concepts (topics) and answer the new questions. Physicians, as experts on the topic of each concept, are able to reclassify manually a question that could be misclassified. Performing this reclassification, experts help to improve the automatic classification of future questions.

Experimental Results

In order to evaluate the proposed automatic classification method, two elements are required: i) a folksonomy, and ii) an ontology with some resources of the folksonomy previously classified under the ontology concepts. As far as we know those requirements cannot be satisfied regarding to Healthcare, so we have obtained this information from del.icio.us as a folksonomy in order to evaluate the method. del.icio.us offers a bookmark service to users to keep their favourites web pages using tags to classify them. A combined view of all the bookmarks aggregated by users is also provided, allowing information browsing and searching. As ontology we have considered the information offered by DMOZ project[26], which consists of several millions of web pages classified under a hierarchical structure defined by an ontology.

The selection of DMOZ and del.icio.us is due to the fact that both systems work with web pages as resources and a high number of resources are defined in both systems. In order to carry out the experiments, we have obtained some resources defined in both DMOZ and del.icio.us. Then, for a given resource (web page in this case) we compare the classification concept suggested by the automatic classification method using the tags of del.icio.us with the classification concept of the web page in DMOZ.

The information of DMOZ has been downloaded from the DMOZ web site in RDF format and has been loaded in a triple store. Once loaded the DMOZ information, an initial selection of resources has been made in order to evaluate the classification method. As del.icio.us contains mainly information about computers subjects, only resources classified in DMOZ under the Top/Computers category have been considered. A total of 22 categories with depth level of 3 (i.e. Top/Computers/Programming Languages/Java) have been selected grouping under them the resources classified under deeper categories, getting a total amount of 21,489 initial resources.

With the aid of a page scraper program, we have captured the information of these resources from the html web pages in del.icio.us. This program checks, for each one of the initially 21,489 selected resources, if the page exists in del.icio.us and if it does, the program obtains all the annotations associated to this resource. After carrying out this process, 10,201 resources have been obtained, with an average number of 437.02 annotations and with an average number of different tags by resource of 54.48. The remaining 11,288 resources were not defined in del.icio.us.

Due to the reduced number of annotations, resources with less than 10 annotations (3,138) have been dropped from the 10,201 resources obtained from del.icio.us. The remaining 7,063 resources have been used to build two evaluation data sets. These resources have 4,812,592 annotations and 121,901 different tags associated. The two datasets consist of: testset1 with the 80% (5,648) of the resources and testset2 with the remaining 20% (1,415) resources. The testset1 resources have been used as pre-classified resources under the selected 22 categories, and have been used to get the representation vector of each concept. On the other hand, testset2 has been used to evaluate the automatic classification method, comparing its resources vectors with the concept vectors.

It is necessary to define some minimum criteria that tags must fulfil in order to be considered in the encoded representation of resources and concepts as vectors. The number of resources annotated by each tag and the number of annotations associated to each tag have been calculated. We have obtained experimentally that a minimum number of 20 annotations and 20 annotated resources (3,074 tags) allows representing almost all the resources in the experiment (7,062 out of the existing 7,063). Using these minimum values, the dictionary consists on 3,074 tags, a 2.52% of the folksonomy tags (121,901).

Experimental results show that our approach allows, in a great extent, the automatic classification of the folksonomy resources. Table 2 shows a summary of these experimental results. It shows the results obtained applying the automatic classification method to the 1,415 resources of *testset2*, without using a threshold in the first row and using a threshold in the last row. As can be shown, the method provides a correct classification rate of 77.81% without using any threshold increasing to 93.15% when using a threshold based on the distance between the maximum similarity value and the closest one.

Extensions to the Method

The proposed model can be extended to other similar systems in with other physicians as experts on each concept. This kind of systems require the use of any kind of rating in order to measure the authority degree of the physicians in their associated concepts. This authority degree could be based in the ratings provided by other specialist on his answers.

Let $A(p,c)$ be the authority degree for a given physician on a concept. The goodness measure of an answer could be the sum of the authority scores of all physicians who have rated the answer, multiplied by the rating value.

Table 2. Relevant properties of the ontology.

	Correct	Incorrect	Unclassified
Without threshold	1,101 (77.81%)	314 (22.19%)	0
Using threshold	802 (93.15%)	59 (6.85%)	554 (39.15%)

$$S(a) = \sum_{p \in professional\_rate(a)} A(p,c) * rate(p)$$

In this formula, *professional_rate(a)* denotes the set of physicians who have rated a given answer a, *A(p,c)* denotes the authority degree of each professional on the topic associated to the question, and *rate(p)* denotes the ratings given by them.

A simple way to measure the authority degree of a physician on a concept is to determine this value according to the average quality of his previous answers.

$$A(p,c) = \frac{\sum_{a \subset answer(p,c)} S(a)}{|answer(p,c)|}$$

In this equation, *answer(p,c)* denotes the set of answers supplied by physician *p*, on questions associated to the concept *c*. The equation measures the average quality of a given professional in a given topic.

In order to illustrate the behaviour of the proposal, we present as a case of study iMedix.

A CASE STUDY

This case is based in a real health care social network, iMedix (see Figure 9), and shows how this HSN could be extended using the proposed semantic model. As indicated in the introduction section, iMedix is a free website that helps you to find and share health information. Members of the iMedix community share their experiences and rank medical content in order to make health information organized and accessible to everyone.

The proposed semantic model and the automatic classification of questions could be applied to this web in order to classify the questions under some medical concepts associated to medical professionals. This approach could be used to create new business opportunities in HSNs. For example, users could have the option of requesting a professional answer and be charged for that, or professionals could answer the questions and users could pay for having access to these answers, or professionals could be paid a percentage of the advertisements shown beside his answers, even taking into account the answers ratings.

In this example, each component of iMedix, like tags, questions and answers, could be modelled as instances of the described classes in the semantic model proposed in the previous section. Some of these instances can be adapted in order to allow users to answer the questions or include their own personal experiences, or to allow the users or even the professionals' ratings, as occurs with Question and Answer respectively.

Figure 10 shows an example with the ontology instances representing a user, a question associated to this user, and a tag used to classify this question in the folksonomy. iMedix uses a narrow folksonomy, so only the creator of the questions can assign tags to the questions. This behaviour could be extended to a broad folksonomy, so any user could annotate whatever question.

In order to complete the proposed semantic model, we have to add the professionals and the classification concepts. We are going to use an example set of classification concepts based in some medical specialities and we are going to

Figure 9. Home page of the iMedix social network

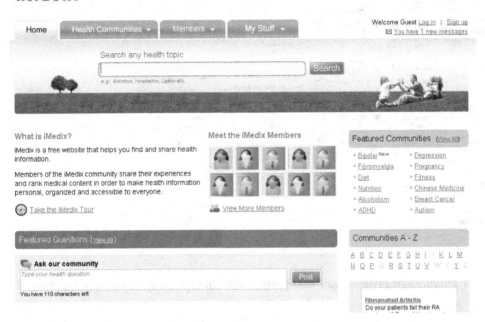

Figure 10. Ontology model instances representing a user, question and tag

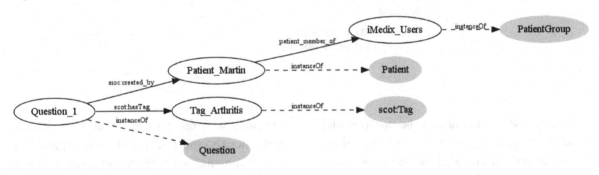

define some professionals associated to them, indicating they are specialists in those specialities. Figure 11 shows a subset of this system with some specialities modelled in the classification system and with some professionals defined associated to the specialities.

Then, we have the HSN modelled with the semantic model proposed, including these new components, like *Professionals* and *Classification Concepts*. A professional could log in the social network and get a list with his specialities (Figure 12), and with the new questions created by users and automatically classified under them.

From this page a professional could access some pending questions. He could have several options, like not answering it marking it as answered (so the question does not appear as pending), reclassify it under another speciality in the classification system if he considers that the automatic classification has made an introduced any error, or he could answer it (Figure 13).

Figure 11. Ontology instances representing a set of specialities and professionals associated to them

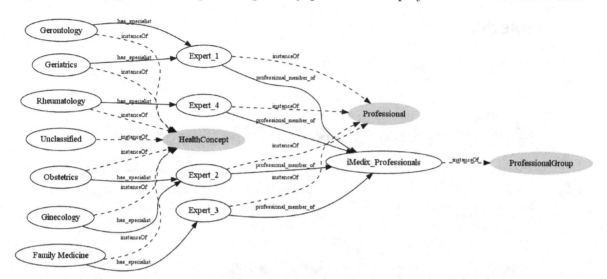

Figure 12. A template of professional main page, with his specialities and the number of new questions

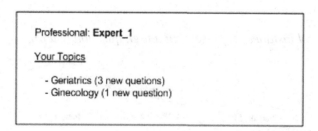

Finally, users could access the question and could see (depending on the business model selected) the answer provided by the professional, and even could rate it, according to the clearness or utility of the answer.

CONCLUSION

The popularity of Social Networks increases each day as more and more projects appear in the web arena. Social Networks offer new opportunities in the Healthcare field, creating new communications and interaction channels among patients, professionals, etc. One of the opportunities offered by HSNs is the possibility of discussing health questions with other users, or even healthcare professionals, and information and experiences sharing among them. In this chapter we have proposed a method that allows the automatically classification of questions asked by users under the concepts of an ontology, in order to be answered by healthcare experts on the subject. This method allows users to use an easy and intuitive classification method like folksonomies creating a bridge between these folksonomies and more formal and complex classification systems like the ontologies used by the professionals.

In this chapter we have proposed an automatic method that classifies by means of an ontology the annotated questions of a folksonomy in a HSN. This fact allows physicians to focus their

Figure 13. Answer form for a professional

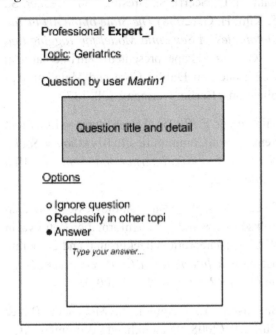

efforts on answering the questions, reducing the time spent in the classification and assignment of the questions.

We have used a semantic model to represent the different elements and relationships existing in the HSN. We have also performed an evaluation of the proposed method using two existing web applications like DMOZ and del.icio.us. This evaluation shows that our approach allows, in a great extent, the automatic classification of the folksonomy resources. Experimental results provide a correct classification rate of 78% without using any threshold. This rate increases to 93% when using a threshold based on the distance between the maximum similarity value and the closest one.

The semantic model described can be expanded by defining the degree of authority of each physician in its field (or fields), based on an assessment that other users do according to the as provided by him. This feature makes not necessary to distinguish between common users and experts (physicians) in a field, since the degree of expertise and specialization would be determined by the authority of the users on each medical concept of the ontology.

The method can also be used to maintain and guide the evolution of ontologies.

ACKNOWLEDGMENT

Research supported by the Spanish Research Council under research grants TIN2006-14738-C02-02 and TIN2008-03687.

REFERENCES

Berners-Lee, T., Hendler, J., & Lassila, O. (2001). *The Semantic Web*. Scientific American.

Brickley D., & Guha, R.V. (2004, February). *RDF Vocabulary Description Language 1.0: RDF Schema*. W3C Recommendation.

Cattuto, C., Benz, D., Hotho, A., & Stumme, G. (2008). Semantic Grounding of Tag Relatedness in Social Bookmarking Systems. In A.P. Sheth, S. Staab, M. Dean, M. Paolucci, D. Maynard, T. Finin, K. Thirunarayan (Eds), *International Semantic Web Conference (ISWC 2008)* (LNCS 5319, pp. 615-631). Springer Verlag.

Dean, M., & Schreiber, G. (2004). *OWL Web Ontology Language Reference*. W3C Recommendation.

Echarte, F., & Astrain, J. J. Córdoba, & A., Villadangos, J. (2008). Pattern Matching Techniques to Identify Syntactic Variations of Tags in Folksonomies. In M.D. Lytras (Ed.), *First World Summit on the Knowledge Society: Emerging Technologies and Information Systems for the Knowledge Society* (WSKS 2008) (LNAI 5288, pp. 557–564). Springer Verlag.

Echarte, F., Astrain, J. J., Córdoba, A., & Villadangos, J. (2007). Ontology of Folksonomy: A New Modeling Method. In S. Handschuh, N. Collier, T. Groza, R. Dieng-Kuntz, M. Sintek, A. de Waard (Eds.), Semantic Authoring, Annotation and Knowledge Markup Workshop (SAAKM2007), CEUR-WS Vol. 289. SITE Central Europe: RWTH Aachen University.

Echarte, F., Astrain, J. J., Córdoba, A., & Villadangos, J. (2009). Improving Folksonomies Quality by Syntactic Tag Variations Grouping. In S.Y. Shin, S. Ossowski (Eds.), *24th Annual ACM Symposium on Applied Computing* (pp. 1226-1230). New York: ACM.

Golder, S. A., & Huberman, B. A. (2005). The Structure of Collaborative Tagging Systems. *Journal of Information Science, 32*(2), 198–208. doi:10.1177/0165551506062337

Graham K., & Jeremy J.C. (2004, February). *Resource Description Framework (RDF): Concepts and Abstract Syntax*. W3C Recommendation.

Gruber, T. (1993). A Translation Approach to Portable Ontology Specifications. *Knowledge Acquisition, 5*(2), 199–220. doi:10.1006/knac.1993.1008

Guy, M., & Tonkin, E. (2006). Folksonomies - Tidying up Tags? *D-Lib Magazine, 12*(1). doi:10.1045/january2006-guy

Hassan-Montero, Y., & Herrero-Solana, V. (2006). Improving tag-clouds as visual information retrieval interfaces. In V.P. Guerrero-Bote (Ed.) *International Conference on Multidisciplinary Information Sciences and Technologies* (InSciT2006).

Heymann, P., & García-Molina, H. H. (2006). *Collaborative Creation of Communal Hierarchical, Taxonomies in Social Tagging Systems* (Tech. Rep. No. 2006-10). Stanford InfoLab.

Kim, H. L., Scerri, S., Breslin, J. G., Decker, S., & Kim, H. G. (2008) *The State of the Art in Tag Ontologies: A Semantic Model for Tagging and Folksonomies*. Paper presented at 8th International Conference on Dublin Core and Metadata Applications, Berlin, Germany 128–137.

Michlmayr, E. (2005). A Case Study on Emergent Semantics in Communities. In *Workshop on Social Network Analysis, International Semantic Web Conference*.

Passant, A. (2007). Using Ontologies to Strengthen Folksonomies and Enrich Information Retrieval in Weblogs: Theoretical background and corporate use-case. In *International Conference on Weblogs and Social Media* (ICWSM 2007).

Shepitsen, A., Gemmel, J., Mobasher, B., & Burke, R. (2008). Personalized Recommendation in Social Tagging Systems Using Hierarchical Clustering. In J.A. Konstan (Ed.), *2nd ACM Conference on Recommender Systems* (pp. 259–266). New York: ACM.

Smith, M.K., Welty, C., & McGuinness, D.L. (2004, February). *OWL Web Ontology Language Guide*. W3C Recommendation.

Specia, L., & Motta, E. (2007) Integrating Folksonomies with the Semantic Web. In *European Semantic Web Conference* (ESWC 2007), *The Semantic Web: Research and Applications* (LNCS 4519, pp. 624-639). Springer Verlag.

Vander Wal, T. (2007). *Folksonomy*. Retrieved February 2, 2007, from http://vanderwal.net/folksonomy.html.

Xu, Z., Fu, Y., Mao, J., & Su, D. (2006). Towards the Semantic Web: Collaborative Tag Suggestions. In *Workshop on Collaborative Web tagging* (WWW2006).

Zhou, M., Bao, S., Wu, X., & Yu, Y. (2007). An Unsupervised Model for Exploring Hierarchical Semantics from Social Annotations. In K. Aberer, K.S. Choi, N. Noy, D. Allemang, K.I. Lee, L.J.B. Nixon, J. Golbeck, P. Mika, D. Maynard, G. Schreiber, & P. Cudré-Mauroux (Eds.) *International Semantic Web Conference* (ISWC 2007) (LNCS 4825, pp. 673-686). Springer Verlag.

ENDNOTES

[1]   PatientslikeMe, http://www.patientslikeme.com

[2]   Sermo, http://www.sermo.com

[3]   PeerClip, http://www.peerclip.com

[4]   Within3, http://www.within3.com

[5]   SocialMD, http://www.socialmd.com

[6]   MDJunction, http://www.mdjunction.com

[7]   RateMDs, http://ratemds.com

[8]   WegoHealth, http://wegohealth.com

[9]   iMedix, http://www.imedix.com/

[10]   Ozmosis, http://www.ozmosis.com

[11]   Tiromed, http://www.tiromed.com

[12]   DOctorsHangout, http://doctorshangout.com

[13]   Nursing World, http://www.nursingworld.com

[14]   Nurselinkup, http://www.nurselinkup.com

[15]   SystematizedNomenclature of Medicine -- Clinical Terms, SNOMED, http://www.ihtsdo.org/snomed-ct/

[16]   openGalen, http://www.opengalen.org/

[17]   MeSH, U.S. National Library of Medicine, http://www.ncbi.nlm.nih.gov/sites/entrez?db=mesh

[18]   Unified Medical Language System (UMLS), http://www.nlm.nih.gov/research/umls/

[19]   International Classification of Diseases (ICD), http://www.cdc.gov/nchs/icd9.htm

[20]   SCOT, Let's share tags!, http://scot-project.org

[21]   SIOC, http://sioc-project.org

[22]   SKOS, http://www.w3.org/2004/02/skos/

[23]   del.icio.us, http://delicious.com/

[24]   Flickr, http://www.flickr.com/

[25]   Wordnet, http://wordnet.princeton.edu/

[26]   DMOZ open directory project, http://www.dmoz.org/s

Chapter 6
An Integrated System for E-Medicine (E-Health, Telemedicine and Medical Expert Systems)

Ivan Chorbev
Ss. Cyril and Methodius University, Republic of Macedonia

Boban Joksimoski
European University, Republic of Macedonia

ABSTRACT

This chapter presents an overview of an integrated system for eMedicine that the authors propose and implement in the Republic of Macedonia. The system contains advanced medical information systems, various telemedicine services supported by modern telecommunication technologies, and decision support modules. The authors describe their telemedicine services that use wireless broadband technologies (WiMAX, 3G, Wi-Fi). A significant part of the chapter presents a web based medical expert system that performs self training using a heuristic rule induction algorithm. The data inserted by medical personnel while using the e-medicine system is subsequently used for additional learning. The system is trained using a hybrid heuristic algorithm for induction of classification rules that we developed. The SA Tabu Miner algorithm (Simulated Annealing and Tabu Search based Data Miner) is inspired by both research on heuristic optimization algorithms and rule induction data mining concepts and principles.

INTRODUCTION

E-medicine can be viewed as a symbiosis between medicine, informatics and telecommunication technologies. Basically, e-medicine incorporates the use of computer technologies, multimedia systems and global networking in the provision of medical services. It is an area of great scientific and research interest, followed by fast implementation of novel commercial functionalities. A common simple definition describes e-medicine as the use of multimedia technologies like text, pictures, speech and/or video for performing medical activities.

The goal of our research is to define a prototype of an integrated system for e-medicine that enables

DOI: 10.4018/978-1-61520-777-0.ch006

Copyright © 2010, IGI Global. Copying or distributing in print or electronic forms without written permission of IGI Global is prohibited.

application of information and communication technologies over a wide spectrum of functionalities in the health sector including medical personnel, diagnostics, therapy, managers, medical insurance and patients. Additionally we aim at incorporating artificial intelligence in various modules of the system making it a useful partner to all entities using the system. We present algorithms for building medical decision support and expert systems as part of the e-medicine system.

The chapter is organized as follows. The first section gives a short overview of e-medicine, telemedicine and medical expert systems. The second part explains in detail our model of a system for e-medicine, its main modules, the used technologies and the implemented functionalities. The third section gives as overview of the medical expert subsystem we implemented, along with the SA Tabu Miner rule induction algorithm for classification that we developed for that purpose.

BACKGROUND

E-medicine (sometimes referred to as e-medicine or eHealth) is a rather new term for describing the medical care that is supported by modern electronic processes and modern telecommunications. It is sometimes used to describe the use of computers in health institutions, for providing medical services via Internet or simply a new name for telemedicine. In fact, it is used to describe a wide spectrum of services that are part of the medical practice supported by the aid of information technology. The provided services include:

- The use of Electronic Medical Records (EHR) for easy storing, retrieving and sharing data between medical personnel (doctors, pharmacists, therapists etc).
- Telemedicine, as a way to provide medical services remotely and as a way for providing teleconsultations and assistance to other doctors

- Public Health Informatics, where the population and/or patients could get informed about relevant medical information.
- Management of medical information and medical knowledge, using the data in data mining research
- Mobile e-medicine, a field that includes the use of mobile devices for various purposes including real-time monitoring of patients, diagnosis, gathering and providing data for the doctors and mobile telemedicine

Medical Information Systems

Information systems have been developing rapidly through the past decades, and we have now means of managing and organizing large quantities of data, methods of validating the data, and ways of processing the data for retrieving valuable information as well as learning from the data. However, for practical implementations, there are a lot of requirements that should be satisfied in order to make a healthcare information system usable. A lot of the tasks are concerned with gathering and manipulation of data provided by patients, doctors and insurance companies. The medical information is critical, and should be accessible, up to date and coherent at all times. Also, the data must be secure, confidential and protected from unauthorized access. Security of medical data is regulated by various requirements, like HIPAA and European Commission's Directive, and all systems should strictly implement them.

The evolution of Healthcare Information Systems has gone through different phases (Vogel & Perreault, 2006). The first phase was marked by development of specific applications that would help healthcare workers in a specific area (like patient registration or laboratory results). Access to data was mostly at department level, and there was the problem of transferring data between departments in a hospital. To overcome the inoperability between different systems, an approach was taken to interconnect them. The second phase was the development of appropriate interface engines to make interconnection possible. The goal is to make data accessible wherever it is required. Progress is still made in interconnecting different countries or regions and it has been regarded as a challenging task.

Telemedicine

Initially telemedicine was defined by Bird (1971) as "the practice of medicine without the usual physician-patient confrontation …via an interactive audio-video communications system" (p.67). Telemedicine basically provides options for neutralizing the geographical distance between the users. It is useful to spare the ill patients from the discomfort and expenses of traveling. Saving the medical personnel from travelling to remote areas leaves more time for the medical problems. The transfer of data from site to site ensures better judgment and informed decisions. Application areas of telemedicine expand to almost all the fields of medicine (Zielinski & Duplaga, 2006). Applications of telemedicine include: Consultation, Diagnostic Consultation, Monitoring, Education, Disaster management (Olariu et al., 2004), Virtual Microscopy (Fontelo et al., 2005), Homecare, Diagnosis, Treatment and Therapy (Psychology). Along the development of telemedicine, new terms like eHealth have emerged. According to (Maheu, 2001), "E-health refers to all forms of electronic healthcare delivered over the Internet, ranging from informational, educational, and commercial "products" to direct services offered by professionals, nonprofessionals, businesses or consumer themselves" (p. 3).

The history of telemedicine shows evident correlation with the developments in communication technology and IT software development. Researches categorize the telemedicine history into three eras based on the technological development (Bashshur et al., 2000; Tulu & Chatterjee, 2005). All the definitions during the first era of telemedicine focused on medical care as the only function of telemedicine. The first era can be named as telecommunications era of the 1970s (Bashshur et al., 2000). Applications in this era were dependent on broadcast and television technologies. Telemedicine was not integrated with any other clinical data. It was based on transmission of a TV and audio signal both ways, and lacked the ability to connect other devices and transmit data automatically. Hence, the use was limited to basic teleconsultations and low quality video communication with patients.

The second era of telemedicine evolved with the digitalization in telecommunications (Bashshur et al., 2000). The transmission of data was supported by various communication mediums ranging from telephone lines to Integrated Service Digital Network (ISDN) lines. However, the high costs attached to the communication mediums that can provide higher bandwidth became an important bottleneck for telemedicine. This era overcame a lot of the problems in the first era, like patient feedbacks, data transfer, but was not applicable for general use, mostly because the expensive services needed (ISDN, satellite communication).

The third era has been named "Internet era", where the main burden for interconnecting is transferred to the Internet network, as a robust system that is accessible, already deployed, relatively cheap and constantly growing. Also, the technologies to access the Internet are constantly evolving for better performance and higher speeds. Regardless of the technology used to access the network, previous services still function without modifications, even faster and more capable (Bashshur et al., 2000). The development of mobile wireless Internet access, by using 3G wireless networks and high-speed WiMAX provides new ways of implementing telemedicine services.

Other telemedicine projects are based on alternative ways of establishing communication, like satellite-based telemedicine (Healthware project - http://healthware.alcasat.net/), and although this provides effective large scale connectivity, its deployment and maintenance is difficult and thus its services are expensive. The wireless networks are ultimately the best cost-effective solution for fast deployment and large area covering, and WiMAX as the leading technology for fast, broadband Internet access.

Expert Systems

Expert Systems belong to the broader class of Decision Support Systems, and are viewed as consultants to human decision makers. The use of expert systems in medical problems has always been a topic of interest, and an integrated system for e-medicine must include a decision support system in order to gain the advantages that artificial intelligence can offer. Some of the reasons why decision support systems are necessary include the following challenges that the medical personnel is facing:

- Classification – deciding who is treated first, and who is sent back
- Treatment - the decisions for treatment must be informed and expert consulted
- The physicians' knowledge in a particular area might be outdated, and the time for reading new publications is always limited
- Physicians go into diagnostic habits
- The physician might be inexperienced with diagnosing or treating particular rare diseases
- The treatment might be too expensive and the doctor is hesitating to prescribe
- Time constraints to make a decision
- The doctor might be unaware of the existence of some new drugs or their side effects

Medical expert systems have been an area of research and implementation since the 1970s. A major part of the research in Artificial Intelligence was focused on expert systems. Various programming languages like LISP and Prolog were introduced for the purpose of declarative programming and knowledge representation, later to be used for development of expert systems. Famous medical expert systems include Mycin®, designed to identify bacteria causing severe infections and to recommend antibiotics, CADUCEUS®, embracing all internal medicine, also Spacecraft Health Inference Engine (SHINE)®, STD Wizard® etc.

There are two fundamental approaches for knowledge base construction for the expert system: knowledge acquisition from a human expert, and empirical induction of knowledge from collections of training samples. In our research we choose the later. We used an algorithm for rule induction that we developed to create a medical expert system.

MODEL OF AN INTEGRATED SYSTEM FOR E-MEDICINE

Services in E-Medicine are growing rapidly with the development of the underlying telecommunication and computer technologies. The developed applications quickly get replaced by newer services that use the bandwidth and accessibility of the newest communication technologies. Still, by analyzing the incoming technologies and anticipated commercial needs, the medical services, architectures and design of the e-medicine systems of the future can be predicted to some extent.

The system must be based on reliable communication technologies. Cable and optical networks will always be faster, more secure and reliable than wireless technologies, hence ensuring their infrastructural function as backbones. Wireless networks have the drawbacks of providing less resource in terms of data traffic and bandwidth, but add the very significant mobility to the users. Speeds in wireless networks are constantly growing, and with standards like WiMAX of 4G mobile telephony, the implementation of cheaper and faster e-medical services is ensured.

Integrating different multiplatform services is the crucial phase of the development of an integrated system for e-medicine. IT Systems in general are in constant development, and as such should have modular design. Older modules should be replaced with newer without interfering with the overall functioning of the system. The Healthcare Information System should be designed to provide complete and reliable storage of electronic records, implementing the concerns of privacy, confidentiality and security. Furthermore, the use of unique electronic identifications in form of chip cards, proximity cards or RFID can help improve patient care by identifying and getting medical records from patients that can't communicate (unconscious patients).

The diagram of an integrated system is shown on Figure 1. Users of the system can use various devices to access parts of the system. With the implementation of encrypted communication with XML web services, the modules do not depend on the telecommunication technology or the devise used for access (Notebook, PDA, mobile phone or other terminal). Because of modularity, newer services can be deployed when devices that sup-

port that service will be available. Of course, the new devices should support older services that are still in use.

The integrated and coherent patient data, through wireless network, are accessible to personnel in hospitals, ambulance vehicles, in a medical campus and even in homes. Data that can be transmitted can be in form of text, patient records, video streaming, audio recordings, real-time data from sensors etc. The services can also be used for management purposes, like allocation of human resources, checking supplies of medical equipment, making appointments, control of patients etc.

Implementing an E-Medicine System in a Developing IT Society

In the Republic of Macedonia there is no integrated health information and communication system. There are only individual multiplatform systems at some of the hospitals, usually based on Microsoft SQL Server databases supporting various Windows forms or recently web applications. The analysis of the current solutions show

Figure 1. Diagram of a modular e-health system

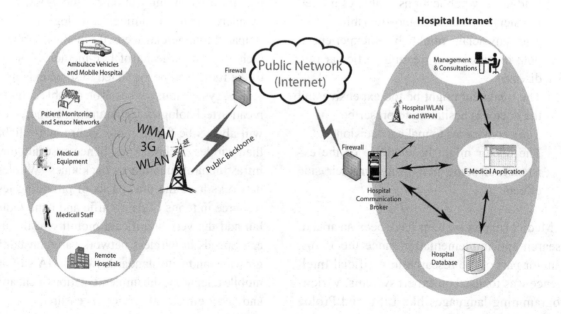

significant differences among hospitals, but the overall conclusion is serious lack of Information and Communication Technology (ICT) and nonexistence of integrated hospital information systems, with small number of exceptions. Also, it is evident that information systems that operate in some facilities are challenging to integrate and extremely difficult to enable information exchange.

While researchers in developed countries can have different goals, our objectives locally had to be scalable, ranging from establishment of basic telemedicine services up to advanced up to date functionalities. The main concepts that our system was based on included creation of necessary basic Medical Information Systems (MISs) where hospitals had none, interfaces for various MISs, using modern telecommunication technologies for creating an integrated MIS and provision of advanced medical services at remote locations and other telemedicine applications. (Chorbev & Mihajlov, 2008)

There are many prerequisites for the integrated e-medicine system to be implemented. Organizational prerequisites include cooperation and communication between actors in the complex organizational structures. Human resources need to be trained to a level of understanding and familiarity with ICT. Legal prerequisites include regulating patient related information.

The Republic of Macedonia already integrates Diagnosis Related Groups (DRG) into patient's medical data, but the records have so far been distributed among various hospitals. In developed integrated medical information systems there are numerous standardized records of patient data. With some initial organized data we already started research with diseases that are endemic for the region. By using data mining techniques, we developed modules that serve as diagnosis consultants. We used already available data in form of blood tests from 70000 patients in the Ohrid Orthopedic hospital. This data serves as training data input in our research where our rule induction

algorithm SA TABU Miner (Chorbev et al., 2009) is used for generating classification rules.

Other aspects of artificial intelligence, like combinatorial optimization, can also be integrated in the system. Using optimization tools to obtain optimal drug amounts in treatment can reduce the burden on the state health insurance fund. The limited number of existing surgery teams and equipment, kidney dialysis sets, MRI devices can be scheduled for use with combinatorial optimization, achieving maximal utilization according to specific patient needs and urgency. However, scattered results in research must be integrated in an e-medicine system for the benefits to be readily available. The modularity will enable every new diagnostic tool to be quickly integrated and delivered to physicians and patients.

All developed modules of the integrated MIS need to be readily available to both patients and physicians throughout the country. By designing the system as a web and PDA application, available through statewide wireless network and secured with adequate authentication and encryption methods, it is expected that it will increase severely the quality of medical service.

Wireless Infrastructure

In order to implement our telemedicine system we used the backbone network of a fast growing privately owned data communication provider. The backbone network consists of some fiber optic connections in the city limits of Skopje and among some major cities and mostly 802.16 (WiMAX) base stations throughout the country. The optic fiber connections are used for provision of fast bandwidth services where possible. The WiMAX antennas are used for connecting hospitals where the optic fiber has not reached yet and 802.11 hotspots are used for wireless devices (PDAs, notebook PCs etc.)

Due to the sufficient bandwidth of WiMAX, it is used to cover most of the needs of our telemedicine system. WiMAX is a telecommunication technology aimed at providing broadband wireless data connectivity over long distances. It is based on the IEEE 802.16 standard. The high bandwidth and increased reach of WiMAX make it suitable for providing a wireless alternative to cable and DSL for last mile broadband access. We tested the performance of both fixed outdoor and fixed indoor WiMAX antennas and the results are very promising, since both provided robust connections. Latest systems built using 802.16e-2005 and the OFDMA PHY™ as the air interface technology are called "Mobile WiMAX" and are expected to provide broadband connections while the client is moving.

Within the city limits of the capital Skopje there is a functional fiber optic Metro Ethernet network. The fiber optical connection enables fast and robust connectivity for provision of advanced telemedicine services like high quality video streaming of surgical procedures, medical visualization etc. Even when the fiber optical lines are used for communication, the WiMAX wireless lines could be used for backup in case of disrupted cable communication. While cables

can be physically cut, the WiMAX connections are stable even in severe weather conditions.

A wireless backbone network is established throughout the country, and hospitals in different cities are (or will be) connected to the network. Antennas are placed on hills overseeing cities, and coverage with the radio signal is good and robust. The backbone network is depicted in *Figure 2*, while one antenna in Skopje.

Implemented Services and Functionalities

In the initial stages we included two hospitals in the pilot project: The Institute for respiratory diseases in children-Kozle and the University clinical center in Skopje. Due to the lack of a modern Medical Information Systems (MIS) in the hospitals, we developed a prototype of a modular MIS that can later be distributed to all the hospitals. The main database is centralized, since the data for approximately 2.000.000 inhabitants in the Republic of Macedonia can easily be handled by the contemporary database

Figure 2. Optical network in Macedonia

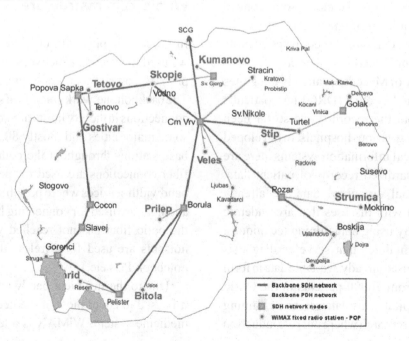

engines. Because of the idea for centralization of the database and since some hospitals cannot afford to maintain an IT department, the MIS is hosted on the Internet Service Provider's (ISP) servers. Knowing that connectivity speeds are high enough when using WiMAX, there is no need to host the MIS locally at the hospital. The MIS is developed as a web application that can be accessed by a common Internet browser. Querying data in the web based MIS is possible using multiple criteria. Data can be searched from other patients with similar symptoms in order to learn from other previous experiences. Entire patient history is accessible online, with strong regard to privacy issues. While patient identity details are available to the physician in charge of the particular case, for other medical personnel with lower access privileges, only medical information is available, without disclosing the identity of the particular patient.

The developed system includes software components specialized for use by PDA devices. Both patients and staff can wirelessly access different software modules. Physicians can access patient's data, results from laboratory analyses, forums and chats, web sites with medical scientific papers. Patients can access their results from different analyses, make appointments, and check the availability of certain physicians. We paid great attention to the usability of the user interface in the PDA applications. Due to the resolution and dimension limitations, significant effort was made to maximize the utilization of the given space on the small screens and to enable easy navigation through the user interface. We adopted a policy of gradual increase of details presented on demand, since scrolling and navigating large texts is unpleasant on a PDA device.

The system includes a Short Message Service (SMS) gateway that is used for SMS notifications for both physicians and patients. Current functionalities include confirmation of appointments for patients, notification for completed laboratory analyses, SMS emergency calls for physicians

on stand-by etc. The system can even notify the patient for the upcoming time for therapy or treatments. WiMAX is also used for Voice over IP (VoIP) services. PSTN telephone bills are drastically reduced as a result of the use of VoIP for communication among hospitals.

A vital part of a telemedicine system is the sharing of knowledge, experience and expertise. The implemented MIS includes a forum and a virtual chat room where physicians can consult each other. The forum enables posting various laboratory results and even video and audio sequences from various diagnostic procedures for the consultations to be supported by appropriate information. Since the system is centralized, consultations are possible among physicians from all hospitals included in the system. Posted materials in the virtual chat room cannot be connected to the patient identity.

Our system incorporates modules that enable laboratory results and other analyses to be submitted for review to the specialists. Physicians working in smaller towns can access the system using their accounts and can submit questions along with supporting materials electronically. Special web application software modules are developed for submitting images (MRI, X-Ray, CAT scan) from remote hospitals in the country to the specialist working in the capital. Also results from blood analysis are filled in online forms. Specialists review the results and can post their reply to the sender. This system enables reduction of transport costs, response times are drastically smaller and patients do not have to suffer through long trips to the specialist. We introduced a system of grading each submitted material giving it different priority according to the contents and level of urgency demanded by the sender. Extremely urgent submissions can even cause the SMS gateway to notify the specialist for the incoming request. We tested streaming video through the WiMAX connections and we set up a system where experts from one hospital can oversee complex surgical operations performed by the surgeons elsewhere.

Also, students at the University hospital in Skopje will be able to learn from the live feed from surgeries performed elsewhere.

We performed several video streaming experiments from a paramedic's vehicle to the hospital. In the first experiment we used a vehicle equipped with a WiMAX antenna and an MPEG coding device. A continual video stream was established, and used for transmitting live feed from the patient in the ambulance to the hospitals. The video link enables specialists to give advice to first aid workers on the scene of an accident, based on real time video feed from the patient's condition. Paramedics could be supervised by experienced medical personnel while performing necessary life support interventions. In the second experiment we used a 3G mobile telephony device for the same use, but the bandwidth was insufficient for a higher quality video. Due to current limitations of WiMAX, the ambulance must not move while being connected online. However new equipment based on Mobile WiMAX (802.16e-2005) is expected to overcome this issue. The equipment used in the experiment was SCOM® MPEG-2 Digital Video Encoder/Decoder. The used WiMAX antennas support 2-10 Mbit/s. The particular experiment used 2 Mbit/s, but an acceptable video quality is achieved even with a 512 Kbit/s connection. A third experiment was conducted using a personal computer instead of a specialized MPEG coding device; however a noticeable delay was evident in the video stream. The later architecture is applicable for a smaller spectrum of services.

The small indoor antennas were also used for video telephony experiment. We tested a scenario where an older woman suffering from strong pain in the back and almost immobilized, had to communicate with her doctor for consultation. Since transportation of the patient was difficult and painful, we brought the WiMAX antennas and IP video phones at both locations (the patient's and doctor's) and established a video link that they used for consultation. We also used the video phones for establishing sign language communication for

patients with impaired hearing. We used Leadtek® IP broadband videophones (BVP8882). They use H.323 protocol for high performance and good quality video communication. The quality of the video stream using only 256 Kbit/s was sufficient for the common sign language to be used and understandable by the communicating parties.

The video signal that we used in most of the testing originated from a digital video camera. Another even more import feature is streaming of digitalized video signals received from analogous endoscopy equipment. We worked on digitalization of an analogous signal from a fluoroscopic camera using a Plextor® MPEG encoder. The digital output from the encoder was easily streamed. The received live video could be used to consult subspecialists not present at the location where the exam is performed. Using VoIP and chat on PDA devices, the specialist could provide feedback and guidance to the person performing the exam in the field or in the remote hospital.

The implementation of the system consists of three main parts: the database, the online web and PDA applications and a standalone application that performs batch data processing and performs scheduled jobs and maintenance functionalities. Most of the applications are developed in Microsoft® .NET technology, using SQL Server 2005® as a database engine, and some are coded in PHP and hosted on Apache servers using MySQL databases.

OUR MEDICAL EXPERT SYSTEM

A crucial module in the integrated system was a decision support subsystem that would provide useful advice to users based on information gathered from the medical information system in use. For that purpose we developed several expert subsystems, the main of which is a diagnostic module.

The goal of the web medical expert subsystem presented here is to serve as a consultant to physicians when setting a diagnosis. The physician logs in the system and chooses the appropriate input form that suite the test data that he/she is going to enter. We have previously collected training data from various patient histories from hospitals and training datasets from the UCI machine learning repository™ (http://archive.ics.uci.edu/ml/data-sets.html). By using the training data we trained classifiers using the SA Tabu Miner algorithm. After the doctor inputs the patient's data and submits the form, the classifier assigns a class (disease) to the patient. The classifier also presents the percent of its predictive certainty, hence the certainty of its diagnosis.

The data entered by the physician is stored. Later, when the diagnosis is confirmed and the entered data is rechecked, the confirmed records are added to the training data for a new training cycle of the classifiers, each time with more data. The training cycle is repeated in different intervals for different classifiers, since not all diagnostic forms are used with the same frequency. The tendency is to run the training when new training cases exceed 5% of the previous number of training records.

The training process is based on a well-known 10-fold cross-validation procedure (Weiss & Kulikowski, 1991). Each data set is divided into 10 mutually exclusive and exhaustive partitions and the algorithm is run once for each partition. Each time a different partition is used as the test set and the other 9 partitions are grouped together and used as the training set. The predictive accuracies (on the test set) of the 10 runs are then averaged. Eventually the training is performed with the entire dataset so that the generated rules are based on the entire knowledge available. These final rules have significantly more impact in the deciding process when the system is in use. The rules generated in each iteration are stored. When deciding, the different groups of rules vote for the final classification of the new case with different impact, dependant on the predictive accuracy. The system adopts the weighted majority vote ap-

proach to combine the decision of the rule groups. The average predictive accuracy is necessary to estimate the reliability of the system when used as a diagnosis consultant.

Extracting Knowledge in Expert Systems, Rule Induction

Some efforts were made to implement an expert system entirely using the ID3 algorithm (Mingers 1986, Quinlan 1986), while other expert systems use combination of data mining and human knowledge verification (Holmes & Cunningham, 1993).

Empirically derived knowledge is commonly represented by classification rules, gained using specific algorithms. A number of induction methods were devised for extracting knowledge from the data, and most common known are decision trees (Breiman et al., 1984), rough set theory (Tsumoto et al., 1995), artificial neural networks, etc.

This text describes an algorithm for rule induction called SA Tabu Miner (Simulated Annealing and Tabu Search based Data Miner). The goal of this rule induction algorithm is a type of data mining that aims to extract knowledge in form of classification rules from data. Simulated Annealing (SA) (Kirkpatrick et al., 1982) and Short-term Tabu Search (TS) algorithm (Zhang & Sun, 2002; Sait & Youssef, 1999; Glover, 1989) are used to develop the algorithm since the rule discovery problem is NP-hard. To the best of our knowledge, the use of SA and TS algorithms for discovering classification rules in data mining is still unexplored research area.

Despite the accuracy of the discovered knowledge, it is equally important for the derived rules to be comprehensible for the user (Fayyad et al., 1996; Freitas & Lavington, 1998). Comprehensibility is very important especially when the discovered knowledge will be used for supporting a decision made by a human user. Comprehensible knowledge can be interpreted and validated by a human. Validated knowledge will be trusted and actively used for decision making. When deriving rules for classification, comprehensibility is achieved with discovering rules that contain less terms in the "if" part. Also, fewer rules are easier to comprehend.

An Overview of Rule Induction Algorithms

Several methods have been proposed for the rule induction process such as ID3 (Quinlan, 1986), C4.5 (Quinlan, 1993), CN2 (Clark & Boswell, 1991), CART (Breiman et al., 1984), AQ15 (Holland, 1986) and Ant Miner (Parepinelli et al., 2002). All mentioned algorithms can be grouped into two broad categories: sequential covering algorithms and simultaneous covering algorithms. Simultaneous covering algorithms like ID3 and C4.5 generate the entire rule set at once, while the sequential covering algorithms like AQ15 and CN2 learn the rule set in an incremental fashion.

The algorithm ID3 (Iterative Dichotomiser 3) is used to generate a decision tree. The ID3 algorithm takes all unused attributes and evaluates their entropy. It chooses the attribute for which the entropy is minimal and makes a node containing that attribute. Always using the attribute with minimal entropy rule can lead to trapping in local optima.

C4.5 is an extended version of ID3. It implements a "divide-and-conquer" strategy to create a decision tree through recursive partitioning of a training dataset. The final tree is transformed into an equivalent set of rules, one rule for each path from the root to a leaf of the tree. Creating decision trees means using quite a lot of memory which grows exponentially when the number of attributes and classes increases.

CN2 works by finding the most influential rule that accounts for part of the training data, adding the rule to the induced rule set, removing the data it covers, and then iterating this process until no training instance remains. The most in-

fluential rule is discovered by a beam search, a search algorithm that uses a heuristic function to evaluate the promise of each node it examines. Always using the most influential rule can also lead to trapping in local optima.

Heuristic Search Algorithms in Data Mining and Rule Induction

Ant Colony Optimization (ACO) has recently been successfully used for rule induction by Parepinelli et al. (2002). He developed an ACO based algorithm that managed to derive classification rules with higher predictive accuracy than CN2. Also, the ACO derived rules were quite simpler and more comprehensible for humans.

Some general use of Simulated Annealing and Tabu Search in data mining applications can be found in literature. Zhang has used TS with short-term memory to solve the optimal feature selection problem (Zhang et al. 2002). Tahir et al. (2005) also propose a feature selection technique using Tabu Search with an intermediate-term memory. TS is used (Bai, 2005) for developing a Tabu Search enhanced Markov Blanket (TS/MB) procedure to learn a graphical Markov Blanket classifier from data sets with many discrete variables and relatively few cases that often arise in health care. Johnson and Liu (2006) have used the traveling salesman approach for predicting protein functions.

Unlike SA and TS, Genetic algorithms (GA) can be found related to classification more often. Bojarczuk et al. (2000) use genetic programming for knowledge discovery in chest pain diagnosis. Weise et al. (2007) developed a GA based classification system to participate in the 2007 Data-Mining-Cup Contest, proving that combinatorial optimization heuristic algorithms are emerging as an important tool in data mining. Other cases of algorithms for deriving classification rules using Genetic Algorithms are referenced in Gopalan et al., (2006); Otero et al., (2003); Yang et al., (2008); Podgorelec (2005).

SA Tabu Miner - Algorithm for Rule Induction

The SA Tabu Miner algorithm incrementally constructs and modifies a solution - a classification rule of the form:

```
IF < term1 AND term2 AND ...> THEN
<class>
```

Each term is a triple <attribute, operator =, value>. Since the operator element in the triple is always "=", continuous (real-valued) attributes are discretized in a preprocessing step using the C4.5 algorithm (Quinlan, 1993).

A high level description of the SA Tabu Miner algorithm is shown in Algorithm 1. The algorithm creates rules incrementally, performing a sequential process to discover a list of classification rules covering as many as possible training cases with as big quality as possible.

Algorithm 1: SA Tabu Miner, the rule induction algorithm.

```
TrainingSet = {all training cases};
DiscoveredRuleList = [ ]; /*initialized
with an empty list*/
While (TrainingSet > Max_uncovered_cases)
Calculate entropy and hence probability
Start with an initial feasible solution S
∈ Ω.
Initialize temperature
While (temperature > MinTemp)
    Generate neighborhood solutions V* ∈
N(S).
    Update tabu timeouts of recently
used terms
    Sort by (quality/tabu order) desc
sol-s S* ∈ V*
    S* = the first solution ∈ V*
    While(move is not accepted or V* is
exhausted)
        If metrop(Quality(S) - Quality(S*))
then
            Accept move and update best solu-
tion.
            Update tabu timeout of the used
term
            break while
        End if
        S* = next solution ∈ V*
    End while
    Decrease temperature
End While
Prune rule S
Add discovered rule S in DiscoveredRuleList
TrainingSet = TrainingSet - {cases cov-
ered by S};
End while
```

where

- Ω is the set of feasible solutions,
- S is the current solution,
- S* is the best admissible solution,
- Quality(S) is the objective function,
- N(S) is the neighborhood of solution S,
- V* is the sample of neighborhood solutions.

At the beginning, the list of discovered rules is empty and the training set consists of all the training cases. Each iteration of the outer WHILE loop of SA Tabu Miner, corresponding to a number of executions of the inner WHILE loop, discovers one classification rule. After the rule is completed, it is pruned from the excessive terms, to exclude terms that were wrongfully added in the construction process. The created rule is added to the list of discovered rules, and the training cases covered by this rule are removed from the training set. This process is iteratively performed while the number of uncovered training cases is greater than a user-specified number called Max_uncovered_cases, usually 5% of all cases.

The selection of the term to be added to the current partial rule depends on both a problem-dependent heuristic function (entropy based probability), a tabu timeout for the recently used attribute values and the metropolitan probability function based on the Boltzman distribution of probability. The algorithm keeps adding one term at a time to its partial rule until one of the following two stopping criteria is met:

- Any term to be added to the rule would make the rule cover a number of cases smaller than a user-specified threshold, called Min_cases_per_rule.
- The control parameter "temperature" has reached its lowest value.

Every time an attribute value is used in a term added to the rule, its tabu timeout is reset to the number of values of the particular attribute. In the same time, all other tabu timeouts of the other values for the particular attribute are decreased. This is done to enforce the use of various values rather than the most probable one, since often the difference in probability between the most probable one and the others is insignificant. Therefore the final solution might not include the most probable values in the rule terms, but a combination of less probable ones.

The entropy based probability guides and intensifies the search into promising areas (attribute values that have more significance in the classification), therefore intensifying the search. The tabu timeouts that recently used attribute values are given, discourage their repeated use, therefore diversifying the search. The metropolitan probability function controls the search, allowing greater diversification and broader search at the beginning, while the control parameter temperature is big, and later in the process, when the control parameter temperature is low, it intensifies the search only in promising regions.

An important step in the rule construction process is the neighborhood function that generates the set V* of neighborhood solutions of the current rule S. The neighborhood contains as many rule proposals as there are values of attributes in the dataset. Let $term_{ij}$ be a rule condition of the form $A_i = V_{ij}$, where A_i is the i-th attribute and V_{ij} is the j-th value of the domain of A_i. The selection of the attribute value placed in the term is dependent on the probability given as follows:

$$P_{ij} = \frac{\phi_{ij}}{\lambda \times TabuTimeout_{ij}} \quad (1)$$

where

$$\phi_{ij} = \frac{\log_2 k - H_{ij}}{\sum_{j=1}^{b_i}(\log_2 k - H_{ij})} \quad (2)$$

where:

- b_i is the number of values for the attribute i.
- k is the number of classes.
- H_{ij} is the entropy $H(W|A_i=V_{ij})$.
- $TabuTimeout_{ij}$ is a parameter for the attribute value V_{ij}, reset to the number of values b_i of the attribute A_i, when V_{ij} is used in a term.
- λ is a multiplier of the tabu timeout used to increase/decrease the influence of the tabu timeout to the probability of using the particular attribute value.

For each $term_{ij}$ that can be "added" to the current rule, SA Tabu Miner computes the value H_{ij} of a heuristic function that is an estimate of the term quality, with respect to its ability to improve the predictive accuracy of the rule. This heuristic function is based on the Information Theory (Cover & Thomas, 1991). More precisely, the value of H_{ij} for $term_{ij}$ involves a measure of the entropy (or amount of information) associated with that term. The entropy of each term$_{ij}$ (of the form A$_i$=V$_{ij}$,) is given in the formula:

$$H_{ij} \equiv H(W | A_i = V_{ij}) = -\sum_{w=1}^{k} (P(w | A_i = V_{ij}) \cdot \log_2 P(w | A_i = V_{ij}))$$

(3)

where:

- W is the class attribute (i.e., the attribute whose domain consists of the classes to be predicted).
- P(w|A$_i$=V$_{ij}$) is the empirical probability of observing class w conditional on having observed A$_i$=V$_{ij}$.

The higher the value of the entropy H(W|A$_i$=V$_{ij}$), the classes are more uniformly distributed and so, the smaller the probability that term$_{ij}$ would be part of the new solution. If the entropy and the tabu timeout are smaller, the more likely the attribute's value is going to be used. H(W|A$_i$=V$_{ij}$) of term$_{ij}$ is always the same, for a constant dataset. Therefore, to save computational time, the H(W|A$_i$=V$_{ij}$) of all term$_{ij}$ is computed as a preprocessing step to every while loop.

If the value V$_{ij}$ of attribute A$_i$ does not occur in the training set, then H(W|A$_i$=V$_{ij}$) is set to its maximum value of log$_2$k. This corresponds to assigning the lowest possible predictive power to term$_{ij}$. Second, if all cases belong to the same class then H(W|A$_i$=V$_{ij}$) is set to 0. This corresponds to assigning the highest possible predictive power to term$_{ij}$. This heuristic function used by SA Tabu Miner, the entropy measure, is the same kind of heuristic function used by decision-tree algorithms such as C4.5 (Quinlan, 1993). The main difference between decision trees and SA Tabu Miner, with respect to the heuristic function, is that in decision trees the entropy is computed for an attribute as a whole, since an entire attribute is chosen to expand the tree, whereas in SA Tabu Miner the entropy is computed for an attribute-value pair only, since an

attribute-value pair is chosen to expand the rule. The tabu timeout given to recently used attribute values servers as diversifier of the search, forcing the use of unused attribute values.

Each time an attribute value V$_{ij}$ is used, its tabu timeout TabuTimeout$_{ij}$ is reset to the number of values b$_i$ of the attribute A$_i$. In the same time, the tabu timeouts of all remaining values of the attribute A$_i$ are decreased by 1. The parameter λ serves to increase or decrease the influence of the tabu timeouts to the probability of using the particular attribute value. The usual value of λ is one, but in certain datasets, its value may vary to achieve better results.

Once a solution proposal is constructed, it is evaluated using the quality measure of the rule. The quality of a rule, denoted by Q, is computed by the formula: Q = sensitivity • specificity (Lopes et al., 1998), defined by:

$$Q = \frac{TP}{TP + FN} \cdot \frac{TN}{FP + TN}$$

(4)

where:

TP - true positives, FP - false positives, FN - false negatives, TN - true negatives.

Q's value is within the range 0 < Q < 1 and, the larger the value of Q, the higher the quality of the rule.

The quality of the rule is the "energy" parameter of the SA metropolitan function that decides if the new solution proposal will be accepted as the next solution. As soon as our algorithm completes the construction of a rule, the rule pruning procedure is invoked. The term whose removal most improves the quality of the rule is effectively removed from it, completing each iteration. This process is repeated until there is no term whose removal will improve the quality of the rule.

The most outer while loop of the algorithm will execute r times, r being the number of discovered rules. This number is highly variable depending on the particular dataset. Before a new rule is constructed, the algorithm calculates the probability of using each attribute value as a preprocessing step. This step has the complexity of $O(n \times a)$, where n is the number of instances in the training dataset, and a is the number of attributes. The inner while loop will execute t times, where t is the number of temperature decrements. Its contents have the complexity of: choosing a probable attribute value of each attribute - $O(a \times v^2)$ and calculating the coverage and quality of each solution proposal - $O(a \times n \times a)$, bubble sorting the solution proposals and choosing the most probable - $O(a^2)$.

The rule pruning initially consists of evaluating k new candidate rules, derived by removing each one of the k terms from the rule. The next pruning iteration will evaluate k-1 new candidates etc., until pruning makes no improvement. k^2 is the worst case scenario. Every evaluation has the

complexity of $O(n \times k)$, hence the pruning process has the complexity of $O(n \times k^3)$.

Therefore the entire algorithm complexity is $O(r(n \times a + t \times a \times v2 + t \times n \times a^2 + t \times a^2 + n \times k^3))$. Since the average number of values per attribute v is insignificant compared to n, it can be excluded. Some of the other components can collapse, so the final complexity is $O(r \times n \times [t \times a^2 + k^3])$.

Experimental Results and Discussion

We compared the performance and results of our SA Tabu miner with the results derived by CN2, C4.5 and Ant Miner (Parepinelli et al., 2002). We used the CN2 version integrated in the WEKA™ package (http://www.cs.waikato. ac.nz/ml/weka), and for the Ant Miner we de-

Table 1. The predictive accuracy of the SA Tabu Miner algorithm compared with the predictive accuracy of CN2 and Ant miner.

Data Sets	Predictive accuracies (%)			
	SA Tabu Miner	CN2	Ant Miner	C45
Ljubljana breast cancer	65,1	67,69	75,28	73,22
Wisconsin breast cancer	90,3	94,88	96,04	93,28
tic-tac-toe	84,7	97,38	73,04	61,81
Dermatology	91,3	90,38	94,29	91,43
Hepatitis	89,2	90,00	90,00	83,33
AllBP	96,91	97,2	94,99	97,33
ANN	92,71	92,07	92,72	93,64
BUPA	63,70	58,53	57,23	59,12
New Tyroid	92,44	93,79	87,96	91,43
Echocardiogram	54,40	53,33	54,36	53,00
Haberman	74,86	66,33	73,32	72
Mamography	79,4	80,84	83,23	81,58
Transfusion	75,56	77,3	74,33	74,87
Nursery	43,7	74,08	86,38	82,72
Pima	68,4	67,5	67,96	66,58
PostOp	68,9	73,75	58,89	73,61
Heart disease	52,55	53	56,26	57,24
Parkinson	88,65	88	80,08	90

veloped our source code based on the description in the published materials. We coded versions in C#.NET and in Pyton. The performances were evaluated using public-domain datasets from the UCI (University of California at Irvine) machine learning repository™ (http://archive.ics.uci.edu/ml/datasets.html).

The comparison was performed across two criteria, the predictive accuracy of the discovered rule lists and their simplicity (hence comprehensibility). Predictive accuracy was measured by a well-known ten-fold cross-validation procedure (Weiss & Kulikowski, 1991).

The comparison of predictive accuracies after the 10-fold cross-validation procedure is given in Table 1.

Figure 3. Graphical representation of the predictive accuracy of SA Tabu Miner algorithm compared with the CN2, Ant miner and C4.5

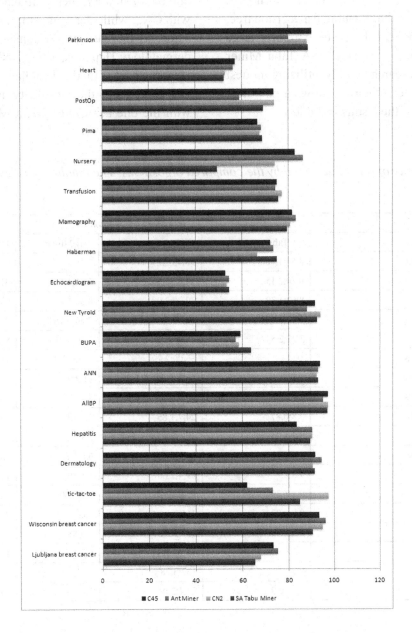

As shown in the Table 1, SA Tabu Miner achieved better predictive accuracy than CN2 in the Dermatology dataset, ANN, BUPA, Echocardiogram, Haberman and better accuracy than Ant Miner in tic-tac-toe, AllBP, BUPA New Tyroid, Echocardiogram and Haberman sets. In the other cases, the predictive accuracy is almost equal or slightly smaller than the other two. Despite the insignificantly smaller accuracy on some of the datasets, the advantage of SA Tabu Miner is in the robustness of the search, and its independence from the dataset size and number of attributes. While other algorithms that build a decision tree, might need exponential time or extremely large portions of memory to work, SA Tabu Miner can perform its search quickly, utilizing modest memory resources. Figure 3 shows a graphical representation of the results in Table 1.

An important feature of classification algorithm is the simplicity of the discovered rule list, measured by the number of discovered rules and the average number of terms (conditions) per rule. Simplicity is very important for any use of the rules by humans, for easier verification and implementation in praxis. The results comparing the simplicity of the rule lists discovered by SA Tabu-Miner, CN2 and Ant Miner are reported in Table 2.

SA Tabu Miner achieved significantly smaller number of simpler rules in all datasets compared with CN2, while deriving simpler rules than Ant Miner in the case of Wisconsin breast cancer, dermatology, Hepatitis, AllBP, ANN, New Tyroid, Haberman etc. In the Ljubljana breast cancer and tic-tac-toe, the simplicity is very similar with the one achieved by Ant Miner. Figure 4

Table 2. Simplicity of rules discovered by the compared algorithms. The number of rules and terms per rule

Data Set	# of Rules; Conditions per Rule			
	SA Tabu miner	CN2	Ant Miner	C45
Ljubljana breast cancer	8,55;1,70	55,40;2,21	7,10;1,28	9,7;2,56
Wisconsin breast cancer	6,10;2,15	34,67;1,94	12,6;1,07	37,9;1,85
tic-tac-toe	8,62;1,30	39,70;2,90	8,50;1,18	95;5,76
Dermatology	6,92;4,08	18,50;2,47	7,30;3,16	31;5,1
Hepatitis	3,21;2,54	7,20; 1,58	3,40;2,41	8;1,88
AllBP Thyroid disease	1:1	66,00;2,29	12,00;2,9	13;1,92
ANN Thyroid disease	1;1	86;3,45	11;2,99	27;3,19
BUPA liver disorders	9,9;0,95	98;3,03	8,2;0,98	24,4;2,91
New Tyroid gland data	5,8;0,87	24,7;1,85	7,2;1,07	13,5;1,40
Echocardiogram	8,3;1,25	40,7;2,33	6;1,55	11;1,91
Haberman's survival	6,4;0,85	76,7;2,40	6,6;0,85	3,8;1,37
PostOp	7;1,23	29,4;2,68	5;1,80	19,89;0,35
Nursery	9,2;1,39	298,5;5,09	5,4;1,00	328;7,43
Pima	9,8;0,90	166,2;2,94	8,6;2,76	47,4;2,91
Mamography	8,5;0,89	117,3;2,87	9;0,88	17,9;1,86
Transfusion	8,8;0,90	43,2;2,43	6,3;1,21	12,9;1,79
Heart disease	8,3;1,06	132;3,28	11,1;1,84	94,20;4,11
Parkinson	7,80;0,9	23,1;2,05	5,9;1,14	33,8;3,92

shows a graphical representation of the results in Table 2.

The parameters of the meta-heuristic algorithms used (SA, TS) have significant impact on the result quality. The given results are achieved by using a SA starting temperature of n×a/4, n being the number of training samples and a being the number of attributes. The temperature decrement and the final temperature were set to 1. The dependency of the SA parameters from the dataset size in not linear and aside from some nonlinear functions that we derived, different values can be derived empirically for each dataset.

Figure 4.Graphical representation of the rule simplicity of SA Tabu Miner algorithm compared with CN2 and Ant miner

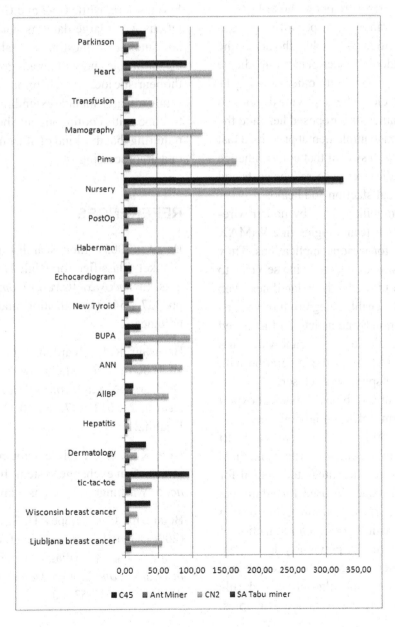

CONCLUSION

This chapter describes the basic framework of an integrated system for e-medicine. The prototype of the system is described along with its most essential modules. Using the contemporary communication and software technologies we tried to define ways to significantly improve medicine and health care. Most of the essential modules were developed, implemented and practically tested. Also, the performances of the used telecommunication technologies were put to the test.

The proposed framework especially applies to a growing information society like the one in the Republic of Macedonia. In such places, e-medicine should follow step along with other growing IT areas in order to close the gap with developed countries. The framework proposed here and the steps already taken to implement it promise a fast trip toward a modern system that could enhance the quality of medical services, reduce costs and increase patients satisfaction and health.

The quality of mobility offered by modern wireless communication technologies like WiMAX enforce their use for various applications. They enable the provision of telemedicine services to places previously unreachable by landlines. Web services and XML enable integration of various Medical Information Systems into an Integrated System for E-Medicine. High bandwidth and reliability of WiMAX helps the integration with bringing remote hospitals ever closer.

We also present a web based medical expert system that performs self training using a heuristic rule induction algorithm. The system has a self training component since data inserted by medical personnel while using the integrated system for e-medicine is subsequently used for additional learning. For the purpose of training, the system uses a hybrid heuristic algorithm for induction of classification rules that we previously developed. The SA Tabu Miner is inspired by both research on heuristic optimization algorithms and rule induction data mining concepts and principles.

We have compared the performance of SA Tabu Miner with CN2, C45 and Ant miner algorithms, on public domain data sets. The results showed that, concerning predictive accuracy, SA Tabu Miner obtained similar and often better results than the other approaches.

Since comprehensibility is important whenever discovered knowledge will be used for supporting a decision made by a human user, SA Tabu Miner often discovered simpler rule lists. Therefore, SA Tabu Miner seems particularly advantageous. Furthermore, while CN2 and C4.5 have its limitations when large datasets with big number of attributes are in question, SA Tabu Miner can still be applicable and will obtain good results due to the heuristic local search. Important directions for future research include extending SA Tabu-Miner to cope with continuous attributes, rather than requiring that this kind of attribute be discretized in a preprocessing step.

REFERENCES

Bai, X. (2005). Tabu Search Enhanced Markov Blanket Classifier for High Dimensional Data Sets. In *The Next Wave in Computing* (*Vol. 29*, pp. 337–354). Optimization, and Decision Technologies.

Bashshur, R. L., Reardon, T. G., & Shannon, G. W. (2000). Telemedicine: A New Health Care Delivery System. *Annual Review of Public Health, 21*, 613–637. doi:10.1146/annurev.publhealth.21.1.613

Bird, K. T. (1971). Telemedicine; a new health information exchange system. In *Annual Report no. 5*. Washingon: Veterans administration.

Bojarczuk, C. C., Lopes, H. S., & Freitas, A. A. (2000). Genetic programming for knowledge discovery in chest pain diagnosis. *IEEE Engineering in Medicine and Biology Magazine, 19*(4), 38–44. doi:10.1109/51.853480

Breiman, L., Friedman, J. H., Olshen, R. A., & Stone, C. J. (1984). *Classification and Regression Trees*. Belmont, CA: Wadsworth.

Brewlow, L. A., & Aha, D. W. (1997). Simplifying decision trees: a survey. *The Knowledge Engineering Review, 12*(1), 1–40. doi:10.1017/S0269888997000015

Chorbev, I., Mihajlov, D., & Jolevski, I. (2009). Web Based Medical Expert System with a Self Training Heuristic Rule Induction Algorithm. In *DBKDA 2009, The First International Conference on Advances in Databases, Knowledge, and Data Applications*, Cancun, Mexico: IEEE

Chorbev, I., & Mihajlov, M. (2008). Wireless Telemedicine Services as part of an Integrated System for E-Medicine. In *MELECON08, The 14th IEEE Mediterranean Electrotechnical Conference* (pp. 264-269), Ajaccio, France: IEEE

Clark, P., & Boswell, R. (1991). Rule Induction with CN2: Some Recent Improvements. In Y. Kodratoff (Ed.), *Fifth European Conference on Machine Learning* (pp. 151-163). Berlin, Springer-Verlag.

Fayyad, U. M., Piatetsky-Shapiro, G., & Smyth, P. (1996). From data mining to knowledge discovery: an overview. In Fayyad, U. M., Piatetsky-Shapiro, G., Smyth, P., & Uthurusamy, R. (Eds.), *Advances in Knowledge Discovery & Data Mining* (pp. 1–34). Menlo Park, CA, US: American Association for Artificial Intelligence.

Fontelo, P., DiNino, E., Johansen, K., Khan, A., & Ackerman, M. (2005). Virtual Microscopy: Potential Applications in Medical Education and Telemedicine in Countries with Developing Economies. *38th Hawaii International Conference on System Sciences*.

Freitas, A. A., & Lavington, S. H. (1998). *Mining Very Large Databases with Parallel Processing*. London, UK: Kluwer.

Glover, F. (1989). Tabu search - Part I. *ORSA Journal on Computing, 1*(3), 190-206.

Gopalan, J., Alhajj, R., & Barker, K. (2006). Discovering Accurate and Interesting Classification Rules Using Genetic Algorithm. In *International Conference on Data Mining, DMIN 2006* (pp. 389-395). Las Vegas, Nevada: CSREA Press

Holland, J. H. (1986). Escaping brittleness: the possibilities of general purpose algorithms applied to parallel rule-based systems. In Michalski, R. S., Carbonell, J. G., & Mitchell, T. M. (Eds.), *Machine Learning, an AI Approach* (*Vol. 2*, pp. 593–623). San Mateo, California: Morgan Kaufmann.

Holmes, G., & Cunningham, S. J. (1993). Using data mining to support the construction and maintenance of expert systems. In *Artificial Neural Networks and Expert Systems*. (pp. 156-159). First New Zealand International Two-Stream Conference.

Johnson, O., & Liu, J. (2006). A traveling salesman approach for predicting protein functions. *Source Code for Biology and Medicine, 1*(3), 1–7.

Kirkpatrick, S., Gelatt, C. D. Jr, & Vecchi, M. P. (1983). Optimization by Simulated Annealing. *Science, 220*(4598), 671–680. doi:10.1126/science.220.4598.671

Lopes, H. S., Coutinho, M. S., & Lima, W. C. (1998). An evolutionary approach to simulate cognitive feedback learning in medical domain. In Sanchez, E., Shibata, T., & Zadeh, L. A. (Eds.), *Genetic Algorithms and Fuzzy Logic Systems: Soft Computing Perspectives* (pp. 193–207). Singapore: World Scientific.

Maheu, M. M., Whitten, P., & Allen, A. (2001). *E-Health, Telehealth, and Telemedicine*. John Wiley and Sons.

Mingers, J. (1986). Expert Systems-Experiments with Rule Induction. *The Journal of the Operational Research Society, 37*(11), 1031–1037.

Olariu, S., Maly, K., Foudriat, E. C., & Yamany, S. M. (2004). Wireless support for telemedicine in disaster management. *Tenth International Conference on Parallel and Distributed Systems* (pp. 649-656).

Otero, F. E. B., Silva, M. M. S., Freitas, A. A., & Nievola, J. C. (2003). Genetic Programming for Attribute Construction in Data Mining. In *Genetic Programming* (pp. 384–393). Berlin, Heidelberg: Springer. doi:10.1007/3-540-36599-0_36

Parepinelli, R. S., Lopes, H. S., & Freitas, A. (2002). An Ant Colony Algorithm for Classification Rule Discovery. In Abbass, H. A., Sarker, R. A., & Newton, C. S. (Eds.), *Data Mining: Heuristic Approach* (pp. 191–208). Hershey, PA: Idea Group Publishing.

Podgorelec, V., Kokol, P., Molan Stiglic, M., Heričko, M., & Rozman, I. (2005). Knowledge Discovery with Classification Rules in a Cardiovascular Database. *Computer Methods and Programs in Biomedicine, 80,* S39–S49. doi:10.1016/S0169-2607(05)80005-7

Quinlan, J. R. (1986). Induction of deciscion trees. *Machine Learning, 1*(1), 81–106. doi:10.1007/BF00116251

Quinlan, J. R. (1987). Generating production rules from decision trees. In *International Joint Conference on Artificial Intelligence: Vol. 1. Knowledge Representation* (pp. 304-307). San Francisco: CA: Morgan Kaufmann.

Quinlan, J. R. (1993). *C4.5: Programs for Machine Learning.* San Francisco, CA: Morgan Kaufmann.

Sait. S. M., & Youssef, H. (1999). *General Iterative Algorithms for Combinatorial Optimization.* Los Alamitos, California, USA: IEEE Computer Society.

Shortliffe, E. H., & Cimino, J. J. (Eds.). (2006). *Biomedical Informatics: Computer Applications in Health Care and Biomedicine (Health Informatics).* Springer.

Tahir, M. A., Bouridane, A., Kurugollu, F., & Amira, A. (2005). A Novel Prostate Cancer Classification Technique Using Intermediate Memory Tabu Search. *EURASIP Journal on Applied Signal Processing,* (14): 2241–2249. doi:10.1155/ASP.2005.2241

Tulu, B., & Chatterjee, S. (2005). A Taxonomy of Telemedicine Efforts with respect to Applications, Infrastructure, Delivery Tools, Type of Setting and Purpose. *38th Hawaii International Conference on System Sciences* (pp. 147.2).

Vogel, L. H., & Perreault, L. E. (2006). Management of Information in Healthcare Organizations. In Edward, H., & Cimino, J. J. (Eds.), *Biomedical Informatics; Computer Applications in Health Care and Biomedicine* (pp. 476–510). Berlin, Heidelberg: Springer.

Weise, T., Achler, S., Göb, M., Voigtmann, C., & Zapf, M. (2007). Evolving Classifiers – Evolutionary Algorithms in Data Mining. [KIS]. *Kasseler Informatikschriften, 2007,* 1–20.

Weiss, S. M., & Kulikowski, C. A. (1991). *Computer Systems that Learn.* San Francisco, CA: Morgan Kaufmann.

Yang, Y. F., Lohmann, P., & Heipke, C. (2008). Genetic algorithms for multi-spectral image classification. In Schiewe, J., & Michel, U. (Eds.), *Geoinformatics paves the Highway to Digital Earth: Festschrift zum 60* (pp. 153–161). Geburtstag von Prof. M. Ehlers.

Zhang, H., & Sun, G. (2002). Feature selection using tabu search method. *Pattern Recognition, 35*(3), 701–711. doi:10.1016/S0031-3203(01)00046-2

Zielinski, K., Duplaga, M., & Ingram, D. (2006). *Information Technology Solutions for Health Care, Health Informatics Series.* Berlin: Springer-Verlag.

ADDITIONAL READING

Chorbev, I., & Mihajlov, D. (2007). Integrated system for eMedicine in a developing information society. In International Multiconference. Ljubljana, Slovenija: Information Society

Cooke, C. D., Santana, C. A., Morris, T. I., DeBraal, L., Ordonez, C., & Omiecinski, E. (2000). Validating expert system rule confidences using data mining ofmyocardial perfusion SPECT databases. [Cambridge, MA, USA]. *Computers in Cardiology, 2000,* 785–788.

Cover, T. M., & Thomas, J. A. (1991). *Elements of Information Theory.* New York: John Wiley & Sons. doi:10.1002/0471200611

Dhillon, H., & Forducey, P. G. (2006). Implementation and Evaluation of Information Technology in Telemedicine. *39th Hawaii International Conference on System Sciences.*

Holopainen, A., Galbiati, F., & Voutilainen, K. (2007). Use of smart phone technologies to offer easy-to-use and cost-effective telemedicine services. *First International Conference on the Digital Society* (p. 4).

Hu, P. J. (2003). Evaluating Telemedicine Systems Success: A Revised Model. *36th Hawaii International Conference on System Sciences*

Kohavi, R., & Sahami, M. (1996). Error-based and entropy-based discretization of continuous features. In *2nd International Conference Knowledge Discovery and Data Mining* (pp. 114-119). Menlo Park, CA: AAAI Press.

Lach, J. M., & Vázquez, R. M. (2004). Simulation Model Of The Telemedicine Program, *Winter Simulation Conference* (Vol. 2, pp. 2012-2017).

LeRouge, C., & Hevner, A. R. (2005). It's More than Just Use: An Investigation of Telemedicine Use Quality. *38th Hawaii International Conference on System Sciences* (pp. 150b - 150b).

Maia, R. S., von Wangenheim, A., & vNobre, L. F. (2006). A Statewide Telemedicine Network for Public Health in Brazil. *19th IEEE Symposium on Computer-Based Medical Systems* (pp. 495-500).

Okuyama, F., Hirano, T., Nakabayasi, Y., Minoura, H., Tsuruoka, S., & Okayama, Y. (2006). Telemedicine Imaging Collaboration System with Virtual Common Information Space. *Sixth IEEE International Conference on Computer and Information Technology*

Olariu, S., Maly, K., Foudriat, E. C., & Yamany, S. M. (2004). Wireless support for telemedicine in disaster management. *Tenth International Conference on Parallel and Distributed Systems* (pp. 649- 656)

Paul, D. L. (2005). Collaborative Activities in Virtual Settings: Case Studies of Telemedicine. *38th Hawaii International Conference on System Sciences.*

Sadat, A., Sorwar, G., & Chowdhury, M. U. (2006). Session Initiation Protocol (SIP) based Event Notification System Architecture for Telemedicine Applications. *5th IEEE/ACIS International Conference on Computer and Information Science and 1st IEEE/ACIS International Workshop on Component-Based Software Engineering, Software Architecture and Reuse (ICIS-COMSAR '06)* (pp. 214-218).

Yamauchi, K., Chen, W., & Wei, D. (2004). 3G Mobile Phone Applications in Telemedicine - A Survey. *The Fifth International Conference on Computer and Information Technology (CIT'05).* J. Mauricio Lach, Ricardo M. Vázquez. Simulation Model Of The Telemedicine Program, *2004* Winter Simulation Conference (pp. 956-960).

Zielinski, K., Duplaga, M., & Ingram, D. (2006). *Information Technology Solutions for Health Care. Health Informatics Series.* Berlin: Springer-Verlag.

Chapter 7
Web 2.0 Approaches for Active, Collaborative Learning in Medicine and Health

Eleni Kaldoudi
Democritus University of Thrace, Greece

Stathis Konstantinidis
Aristotle University of Thessaloniki, Greece

Panagiotis D. Bamidis
Aristotle University of Thessaloniki, Greece

ABSTRACT

In recent years, advances in information and communication technology and especially the Internet have acted as catalysts for significant developments in the sector of health care, having a strong impact in supporting medical diagnosis, enabling efficient and effective patient and healthcare management and reforming medical education. There is currently an international trend to involve computers and the Internet heavily in medical curricula, in continuing life-long medical learning, as well as in general health education of the public. However, effective technology-supported interventions are usually created when there is a successful alignment of the specific requirements with the potential end use of technology. And it is just such a juncture we are currently facing with the emergent paradigm of Web 2.0. This chapter elaborates on the potential of Web 2.0 for active and, potentially, effective learning in medicine and in health and reviews current practices and trends in the field. The discussion focuses on research directions and emerging applications that fully exploit the potential of Web 2.0 for advancing medical education. Finally, the envisaged merit of merging with Web 3.0 technologies is also discussed.

INTRODUCTION

Current innovations in information systems and communication services mark the switch from an "information society", characterized by mass information seeking and based on the distribution of pre-defined and standardized data, to a "knowledge society", that is, a society based on knowledge as a value. This emphasizes the cognitive advancement

DOI: 10.4018/978-1-61520-777-0.ch007

Copyright © 2010, IGI Global. Copying or distributing in print or electronic forms without written permission of IGI Global is prohibited.

and involvement of each individual. The growing use of Internet not only modifies quickly and habitually the way people work but it also leads the race in this educational revolution.

The penetration of technology and the Internet in medical education, and in education in general, created a new situation where the teacher as mediator to knowledge can often be bypassed while the individual strives for knowledge based on their own efforts and aided by the vast amount of information and educational activities presented in the Web. When new technologies where first introduced in education about two decades ago (although experimental attempts date back to 1970s), there was a considerable hype about the emerging electronic teacher, which fortunately soon enough subsided to reveal serious limitations of the computer-to-student education model (Dertouzos, 1997). The emerging Web 2.0 paradigm however is promising to bring about yet another new situation, where the conventional human mediator as well as the electronic mediator in the form of the Internet and the Web is replaced by virtual dynamic communities of peers that learn and advance together.

This chapter will elaborate on the potential of Web 2.0 for active and, potentially, effective learning in medicine and health and review current practices and emerging advances in the field, providing an indicative overview of various projects were Web 2.0 is used to support health and medical education. The chapter will also present some example emerging application areas where Web 2.0 is expected to find its full implementation by enabling new online educational experiences not previously possible to achieve, including full support of active learning, new ways of assessment and evaluation, content sharing educational communities and content repurposing in medical education.

BACKGROUND

Education in Medicine and Health

Medical education is drawing much attention, due to its special characteristics. Firstly, it is a field that encompasses not only the fundamental issue of education, but also the sensitive issue of health and health care services. Furthermore, education in medicine is multidisciplinary and rather long, involving a good number of academic years and extending to life-long continuing updating and learning. Additionally, medical education is traditionally based on a two-fold model: theoretical instruction based on textbooks and clinical practice with one-to-one interaction. Finally, one should stress the current enormous expansion in medical and biomedical knowledge, which constitutes a fundamental challenge in medical education (Papaioakeim et al, 2006). As a result, two main issues arise in medical education: (a) the necessity for overspecialized learning material and educators; and (b) the trend towards a disease-based approach, rather than the more intuitive patient centered view.

In order to address these problems, medical education is embracing tools and approaches from two different fields. On one hand, alternative educational approaches have long been introduced in medicine. These include integrative curricula delivered via active, self-directed, student-centered, experiential learning. One the other hand, information technologies are also being employed to harness information explosion and support teaching in various ways. Ultimately, these two different fields could combine their contributions, with information technology effectively supporting active learning in medicine.

Traditionally, medical education requires students to sit through hours of lectures on basic sciences, while discussion takes place in large groups, sometimes with the whole class present. Advances in our understanding of learning processes now suggest that such techniques may be suboptimal, and that learning should evolve from learning by acquisition to learning by participation. Thus, new educational approaches build on concepts of adult education. They rely on situational learning and are active, self-directed, student-centered, and experiential (National Research Council, 1999). Learning is perceived as a qualitative change of one's conception of phenomena and ideas (Marton et al, 1977) and, consequently, knowledge must be actively processed by the student. A fundamental idea is that learning is organized in small student groups, i.e. tutorial groups, and not around lecture meetings. In the tutorial group students actively work with reality-based situations to formulate problems and learning needs that will guide their further studies. The teacher's role is that of facilitating learning rather than transferring knowledge. In the tutorial group, the students discuss and defend their choices and standpoints. Using library resources, text books, databases, laboratory work, field studies, lectures and other forms of faculty resources, they are urged to find answers to and perspectives on their problems and learning needs. The aim is also to develop problem-processing skills, self-directed learning skills and group competence (Ehlers, 2007; Fyrenious, 2005). In response, professional organizations worldwide have called for increased emphasis on training in life-long, self-directed learning. The emerging view is of learning as an active, constructive, social, and self-reflective process (Berliner & Calfee, 1996). These basic research findings on learning suggest the need for educational environments that are learner-centered and knowledge-rich, guided by assessment, and situated in a community of learners (Schuable & Glaser, 1996). In higher medical education, educational programs increasingly include case-based or problem-based learning and other small group instructional models, collaborative organizations to support student-faculty interactions, and technology-enhanced educational tools (Jones et al, 2001).

Here, we should also stress tacit or personal knowledge, as articulated by Polanyi (1958, 1998). Tacit knowing refers to the taken-for-granted knowledge at the periphery of attention that allows people to understand the world and discern meaning in it. In this respect, knowing and doing involve practical knowledge that depends on humans' ability to learn from experience. Medical knowledge is simultaneously explicit and implicit with certain aspects already well known and easily transferable, and others that are not yet fully known and must still be learned (Sturmberg & Martin, 2008). Thus, current academics prompt for attention not to exclude tacit knowledge and the means for its attainment (e.g. observation of task performance, and recursive practice) from medical education (Henry et al, 2007; Heiberg Engel, 2008).

Information & Communication Technologies in Health and Medical Education

Like many other cognitive domains, medical education can be considered in terms of a number of levels of increasing complexity and importance (Davenport & Prusak, 2000): information (i.e. processed facts), knowledge (i.e. information with a purpose), and understanding (i.e. conscious knowledge, achievement of explanation and grasp of reasonableness). This refers and includes both explicit knowledge (those aspects of mental activities that are verbal and conscious), as well as tacit knowledge (a prerequisite to discern meaning of a situation).

Technology has been employed in diverse ways to support different levels of the educational process. Supporting the dissemination of information is the easiest and most straightforward achievement of information and communication technologies. They have extensively and successfully been used to give quick, easy and cheap access to information sources, such as books, textbooks, atlases, medical and biological databases, research journals, etc. Structuring and organizing information with a particular educational purpose refers to knowledge. On the other hand, understanding implies experience as well as inquiring (Williamson et al, 2002). Managing and supporting these levels of the educational process is a rather complex issue. Technology can certainly help by providing digital teaching files for the medical student to practice, together with tools that support continuous self-evaluation and mediate teacher-learner exchange. Of major importance is the potential of hypertext technology to provide interconnected pieces of information, and link questions with explanations within the wider scope of a particular medical task.

However, in order to promote knowledge and understanding in medical education, information technology, and especially the Internet and the Web, should embrace and support active learning approaches. It has been argued that computer mediated communication can be used to enhance collaboration and interaction within learner's groups. Especially, asynchronous discussion boards give the opportunity to analyze interaction and learning, measuring participation levels and interaction patterns. A comprehensive review of general research and practices in the area is presented by Finegold and Cooke (2006).

In retrospect, it is possible to identify three generations of information technology supported learning, which usually come under the collective term of "e-learning". The first generation is based on multimedia technology support, such as videos, CD-ROMs or other stand-alone educational software. The second generation employs telematic technologies and it is basically set up as teaching via the Web, where conventional educational material, and entire educational courses, is delivered via the network to remote students. The last, emerging generation, is about web based learning, where the Internet is used as a means to create active, context based, personalized learning experiences. This last generation of e-learning shifts the emphasis from 'teaching' to 'learning' and from the notion of technology as a didactic mediator to the notion of a sociable, peer-supported, involved learner.

Web and Web 2.0

The Internet and the Web were initially a static structure with passive viewers. Moreover, they were mainly targeted to human users, with the central role of information distribution – programs had little to do in this environment. Currently the Web is changing towards a second generation of dynamic services and communication tools that emphasize on peer-to-peer collaboration, contributing and sharing, both among humans as well as programs. This revolution is usually known under the collective term Web 2.0. In Web 2.0 the user is seen as a contributor, rather than a recipient. Content is created by participation and collaboration as an emergent product of human interactions. In the core of Web 2.0 lies an ensemble of standards, protocols, technologies and software development architectures and approaches that enable the seamless communication of third party programs thus creating the communities and networks of services that bring people together. One can argue that a major characteristic of Web 2.0 is the fact that it continually improves and grows in size, function, complexity and approach, thus making the term even more uncertain and difficult to define. An incomplete attempt to summarize what Web 2.0 refers to is given in

Initially, the term Web 2.0 was coined by O'Reilly (2005) as an attempt to emphasize the fact that promising new features such as 'social software technologies' were emerging. Web 2.0 is not a program or an upgrade or a single concrete piece of technology, it is rather a more fully implemented Web. It is based on the same infrastructure and standard protocols, and on well-proven technologies and tools of the Internet and the Web. However, the term Web 2.0 encompasses a whole new meaning and a collective emergent behavior of the use of these technologies, tools

Figure 1. A pictorial summary of what Web 2.0 refers to

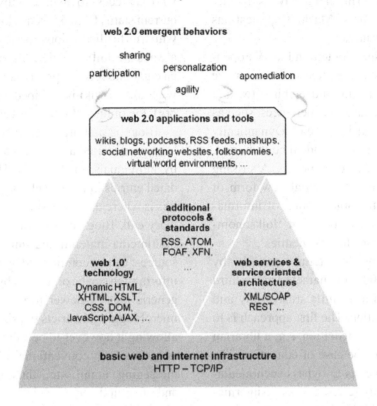

and applications that create networks and communities of users (both humans and programs) that enhance and promote:

- **Collaboration and Sharing**: Together with collaboration comes sharing of information and personal attitudes. For example social bookmarking, where not only links and services are shared, but their collaborative tagging and rating gives a new dimension to information organization.
- **Participation**: People of any background, culture, age etc. can participate without the need to understand the underlying technologies. Participation is perceived equally as accepting and as providing information (including adding new information items, as well as commenting and feedback on existing information). Core examples include wikis, blogs and personal profiles.

- **Reuse**: Content and information is discovered, used and re-used via notions such as content syndication and supporting technologies that allow programs and humans to build their own content aggregates and distribute them.
- **Openness**: Information is freely shared among humans and programs, thus promoting the notion that knowledge cannot be owned. Intellectual property rights do carry over from conventional publishing to online information sharing as supported conventionally on the Web. However, the participative character of Web 2.0, with emphasis on user generated content and on content sharing among peers, is currently leading to a paradigm shift.
- **Agility**: Function and content from many sources (personal and third party alike) are combined to create new added value

for individuals. This can always be readily shared with others. Mashup applications are a major example.

- **Personalization**: Content and service openness and reuse make it easier to customize information, function and their intertwining to create personalized experiences, such as personalized curricula, etc. Dynamically interlacing all this individual contribution, a 'wisdom of crowds' emerges. A striking example is the controversial new form of metadata for the organization of information, coming under the term 'folksonommies', as opposed to 'taxonomies'.

- **Apomediation**: A term coined by Eysenbach (2007) to characterize the third way for users to identify trustworthy and useful information. The first approach is to use some sort of mediation, e.g. a librarian or a teacher, in the case of education. The second approach is to bypass such mediation (commonly referred to as disintermediation), and this has been the basic role of conventional Web, with students seeking additional information on a variety of web-based information sources. In this third approach, enhanced and realized by Web 2.0, the user seeks information with peer guidance, as a result of networked collaborative filtering processes.

All this emergent behaviour that characterizes Web 2.0 is enabled one way or the other by a variety of applications and tools that form the core of Web 2.0 and in their turn are empowered by an ensemble of technology, embracing both familiar technologies from the early days of the Web as well as innovations. Among common Web 2.0 tools that are being explored for their possible use in education are wikis, blogs, podcasts, social networking tools and virtual worlds (Alexander, 2006).

Wikis are dynamic, group-developed websites that can be edited, updated or changed by anyone who has access to them (usually any visitor). The current status for wiki technology includes pages with fruitful discussions on each entry and there is always the ability to view the evolving history of an entry and recover previous versions. The most well-known wiki is Wikipedia (www.wikipedia. org), the online editable encyclopaedia.

Blogs is a short form of the term Weblogs, because it started as online diaries (logs) written by individuals on the Web. They are basically dated entries in reverse chronological order, and this is where the similarities with a conventional diary end. Blog entries can contain a variety of multimedia material and links to other web resources; can be commented by other users, while information can be organized by user defined and generic tags. A newer form of blog, known as microblogging, restricts the size of each posting, allowing it however to be submitted by a variety of means, e.g. conventional blog entry, instant messaging, email, etc., thus allowing for easy and often updates.

Mashups are web applications that merge data from one or more sources and present it in new ways. In many cases this is made possible by data providers that develop application programming interfaces (APIs) for their data. These APIs follow standard web service protocols and/or generic internet formats to represent data (such as RSS) and can easily be implemented in different programming languages. At the same direction notification services offer continuous updates of web sites in a standardized way for use in mashups and in a variety of other applications. Usually under the term "RSS feed" borrowed from the commonly used data representation standard RSS (meaning Really Simple Syndication or, as renamed, Rich Site Summary), they include summarized text and respective metadata and they can be read either by standalone special purpose software or by software embedded in commonly used internet tools (e.g. web browsers, mail clients, etc). RSS feeds and similar syndication technology is also used to distribute streams of audio and video data files to personal computers and portable media players – what is known under the term podcasting.

Social networking websites focus on creating online communities of individuals who publish their content and activities while exploring others content and activities. Such sites cover a variety of topics and provide most of web 2.0 tools and technologies for users to interact. Therefore an astonishing number of simple or more sophisticated social networking sites are currently emerging ranging from mere casual social networking to collaborative web bookmarking and searching, school teacher rating, collaborative document and spreadsheet editing, etc.

Virtual worlds are simulated environments were individual users participate via fictional avatars. Their implementation on the Internet provides a unique way to realize fictional communities for individuals to freely meet others, communicate, participate in a variety of activities and eventually learn.

Most often web 2.0 sites combine more than one of the above applications, and have in common a variety of tools and features that enhance participation and collaboration such as search engines, links to other resources, ability for the user to add content and/or comments, tools for organizing content (e.g. tags, extensions by similarity, rating, etc), and signals for updates (McAfee, 2006). Web 2.0 tools and applications make use of a range of technologies, mainly based on common internet and web technologies, that is the HTTP protocol and the suite of web development technologies, such as all variations of HTML and XHTML and CSS, XML and XSLT, Javascript, etc. Currently, the core of this basic suite of technologies comes under the collective term AJAX (Asynchronous Java Script and XML), an interrelated group of web technologies used to develop interactive web pages that process user requests immediately.

However, it can be argued that the real predecessor of web 2.0 notions and technology is the programming paradigm of web services and service oriented architectures. Web services are

a middleware technology for developing service-oriented architectures (SOAs). A SOA refers to a collection of interconnected software entities (services) that provide some capability through exchange of messages, and can be described, discovered and invoked over a network. Web services are loosely defined as self-contained, self-describing, modular applications that can be located and invoked over the Internet. Web services are based on open internet standards: built on the HyperText Transfer Protocol (HTTP), they use XML for data presentation while messaging is described in an XML-based messaging protocol, SOAP (Simple Object Access Protocol). Web services describe themselves through a standardized Web Service Description Language (WSDL) document, and can be published to one or more Intranet or Internet repositories for potential users to locate through a standard Universal Description, Discovery and Integration (UDDI) registry. A whole suite of additional standards have been developed to formally address issues such as security, reliability, transactions, etc. REST is a technologically simpler approach to web services that bypasses the SOAP communication protocol and concentrates on getting information content of a web page from its published XML file that contains desired information via the HTTP protocol. This core technology that supports Web 2.0 is continuously evolving and growing, as new specialized formats, standards, and protocols emerge. Examples include the RSS data/metadata XML format, the FOAF (Friend of a Friend) and XFN (XHTML Friends Network) protocols involved in social networking applications.

As a final remark, it should be noted that quality control takes up a new meaning in Web 2.0, and can mainly be ensured and applied via a model pretty much different from that in Web 1.0 and other conventional information sharing channels. As already stated, the major characteristic of Web 2.0 is open participation of everybody. Thus, here the role of the conventional moderator is usually taken up by the collective group of participants, rather than a single authority. The collective body of participants is responsible as a whole to reject or amend, alter, etc. content and behaviour that is not proper and of good quality. In the case of employing Web 2.0 in the educational setting, the group is usually limited to the identifiable participants of the specific educational experience/activity, and thus their contribution is not anonymous and certainly has the corresponding repercussions to their educational evaluation and overall outcome. However, in general such a structure of the collective, participative nature of Web 2.0 can indeed be problematic in terms of information quality. Thus, one should be aware of this and limit the use of such technology and the corresponding paradigm to certain situations where it is really suited. As with any technological breakthrough, Web 2.0 is not a panacea, and should not (and will not) replace everything else. It is merely a different form of technology and approach, which should (and hopefully will) find its proper use and place in medical education, and in general.

WEB 2.0 IN MEDICAL EDUCATION

Initial involvement of the Web to support education was based on the metaphor of a virtual classroom, where by the web application follows the model of a real classroom conducting a conventional lecture, discussion, workshop and other educational activities (Cronje, 2006). In 2001, after a systematic and critical meta-analysis of more than 330 studies comparing technology enhanced versus conventional education, Russell concluded that there is no significant difference between various learning/teaching methods (Russell, 2001). Nowadays, it is widely accepted that this is an inappropriate comparison, as the use of technology not only changes the way education is deployed, but has a profound effect in the pedagogy itself. Therefore, it turns out that the discussion is about how technology and the Web

in particular, can stimulate a new learning culture and find novel, alternative ways to advance learning (Ehlers, 2007). Thus, one should concentrate and highlight whatever unique characteristics a new technology exhibits and strive to exploit in full such characteristics, changing the conceptual paradigm along with the technological one.

As presented in the previous section, web 2.0 salient characteristics include, among others:

- effortless communication and collaboration among peers,
- ample access to alternative sources of information, usually customarily combined at a meta-level,
- reporting and rating of information within open communities of peers,
- potential for different representations of the same content (for people with special needs, with different cultural backgrounds, different ages, different background), and
- context based organization of resources and activities.

However, despite all the above unique and exciting characteristics, in its early days Web 2.0 is still used in the majority of cases to hold and provide content (albeit created dynamically and via peer participation and collaboration) and then systematically deliver it to students. The following paragraphs give an indicative overview of such projects where Web 2.0 is used to support health and medical education, while the next section presents some example cases where this evolving web paradigm is or can be exploited for completely novel educational experiences.

Current Web 2.0 Applications in Medical Education

Nowadays, blogs are used in various educational settings and in many different ways, but mainly as a replacement of other forms of asynchronous computer mediated communication, merely because of their additional functionality such as updates via feeds, notion of ownership, decentralization, tagging, archiving and the reverse chronological order organization of content (Kim, 2008). In educational settings, usually blogs are limited to a particular audience, e.g. participants of a course. Thus, blogs in education are mainly used to publish articles and other educational material, as well as to keep track of class activities, often spanning across semesters and years of studies. Various medical schools worldwide have incorporated blogs in their web-based learning management systems, for instructors to post their comments and get students to submit their questions and suggestions, and in general to serve as reflective diaries for various educational experiences (McGee & Begg, 2008). They have even been used to post personal assignments (e.g. Cobus, 2009). Medical blogs may also include discussions about clinical cases, images and special clinical interest topics, thus supporting continuous education amongst medical experts; such an example involves using blogs for an online version of the conventional medical journal club (Genes & Parekh, 2009). Current literature includes a number of projects where blogs have been used to recreate almost any kind of conventional educational activity, ranging from personal educational experience recording, to posting of assignments and exams, to communication amongst peers and between instructors and students, to collaboration within learners groups. It is evident that the ease, with which one can publish content on a blog, makes blogs good candidates for any kind of educational use. However, it is also evident that most of the time the only good reason for using a blog in all those cases is this very ease to publish, despite the fact that a blog may not always be the best suited technology for the particular task. Indeed, blogs are yet to find their most pertinent application in medical education.

Wikis are increasingly used in medical education, as an ideal tool for collaborative work done by both students and teachers. At first, educational wiki implementations involved the mere development of material in the form of an online encyclopaedia with free contribution from anyone. This created a number of medical Wikipedia like (www.wikipedia.org) websites, which at some point were put under scrutiny for their lack of contributors' authentication and the quality of the content while addressing the sensitive area of health and medical education (Pender et al, 2008); although there have been proposals to overcome such shortcomings, e.g. by developing technological solutions that enable authorship tracking of each bit of information (Hoffmann, 2008). Additionally, such wiki applications do not fully exploit the web 2.0 paradigm for peer collaboration, engagement and participation when the educational process is considered. Currently new applications are emerging where wikis are used as a classroom metaphor for students collaborating on a group report, compiling data or sharing the results of their research, while faculty might use the wiki to collaboratively develop the curriculum of a course. Tonkin (2005) argues that different educational uses of wikis can include single-user wiki, used more like a blog without the date format, to hold and edit over time personal thoughts and output of the educational endeavour. Collaborative wikis can also be used along the metaphor of a lab book, collaborative writing assignment, or with the aim to produce a knowledge base, and a comprehensive review of published work supporting this is given by Parker & Chao (2007). Yet, wikis can find their place in medical education when used not as a substitute for the handing in of paper reports or the in-class conventional collaboration, but rather when their potential for distributed peer educational engagement is fully exploited. An interesting example involves use wikis for initial ice-breaking collaboration among students during the initialization phase of a course (Augar et al, 2004). More fully implemented applications employ wikis to support collaborative learning, for example in the case of the social learning within communities of practice (Wenger, 2000), that is, networks of individuals and institutions that share common practices, goals and problems about a certain topic. In this case, wikis can act as an evolving knowledge platform where members can share pieces of information, discuss and collaborate (Schaffert et al, 2006). Some more examples are presented in the next chapter.

Podcasting can be used for archiving and distributing lectures in video or audio format. It can especially enhance the learning experience in demanding hands-on educational environments such as in medicine (Boulos et al, 2006). Although such podcasting uses are closer to traditional passive learning and web paradigms, they can free class time to be used for problem-solving, project sessions and other active learning activities (Kurtz et al, 2007). An example of using podcasting to support collaborative and active learning can be found in the initiative of the Duke University, where podcasts are created both by teachers and students, covering not only formal educational material, but discussions as well as feedback comments on assignments etc. (Belanger, 2005). A number of medical professional associations and other related bodies are increasingly distributing educational podcasts, while many scientific medical journals are now offering content in the form of podcasts (Agrawal, 2007; Wilson et al, 2009).

Teachers and learners are also turning to video-sharing sites (such as www.teachertube.com) to share educational videos. Social networking sites are also used in various educational settings. Collaborative writing is supported by a number of respective websites that offer tools for collaborative text editing (such as www.thinkfree.com and docs.google.com). A striking example that fully realizes the web 2.0 paradigm is del.icio.us (http://delicious.com/), a collaborative bookmarking web site, that allow users to share their bookmarks, creating their own tags and organizing dynamically bookmarks (on any possible topic and within any context, including educational subjects and contexts), thus creating a vibrant bookmark folksonomy that evolves over time.

Finally, virtual worlds on the web are increasingly used to create fluid learning communities which can be engaged in real world didactic situations, collaborate to approach solutions to problems, seek knowledge, and communicate and interact with peers – a comprehensive review is given by De Lucia et al (2009). Although there is a large number of virtual worlds dedicated to learning, when generic virtual world web environments are used, such as Second Life (http://secondlife.com/) and There (http://www.there.com/) there is the additional advantage of the vast size of the community that participates and can potentially engage in learning activities (Kelton, 2008). A review of such applications in medical education is given by Boulos et al (2007).

Nowadays most of the above applications and tools are combined and intertwined within the same web site or service to give hybrid added value applications, enhancing the web 2.0 paradigm and the corresponding emergent behaviors mentioned above. A representative example is presented by the NHS Scotland e-Library (http://www.elib.scot.nhs.uk/) where various web and web 2.0 tools and techniques are employed and combined to create managed knowledge networks (Caldwell et al, 2008). In this case, web technology is used to link resources, services and people in a multitude of ways with the aim to provide a structure that supports the complete information cycle from recognizing the need for information, locating information, and then sharing knowledge to the benefit of the wider community using technology, which ensures seamless access to explicit and tacit knowledge at point of need.

As a final comment, it should be stressed that recent research shows an impressive web 2.0 awareness and penetration amongst medical students and qualified medical practitioners when casual personal use is considered (Sandars et al, 2008). What remains to be seen in the near future is the most appropriate application of web 2.0

technologies and their true penetration in medical and health education.

Challenges and Emerging Applications

Web 2.0 tools have crossed Moore's chasm, easily reached early maturity and are currently under rapid development and evolution (Ebner et al, 2007). However, the idea of social learning software itself, especially in educational scenarios, is not as far developed as one might expect, since too few innovators and early adopters are actually using Web 2.0 to enhance existing curricula designs and learning behaviours. What is also true is that web 2.0 technologies have led to a flood of new healthcare applications and services, with the potential to revolutionise the entire spectrum of health and medicine. With areas such as consumer-led preventive medicine, public health, home care, telemedicine, clinical care and biomedical research strongly affected and enriched by the use of Web 2.0, it is mandatory that health and medical education should also follow and exploit this media, content and collaboration rich revolution.

The introduction of Web 2.0 affects all levels of medical education, namely: undergraduate, postgraduate and continuing medical education (or profession development), as well public education and awareness. In all these levels the tools to be used may be similar, but the way of using them is usually different, so as to conform to the diverse skills and learning outcomes envisaged and mandated by the particular curricula or portfolio designs. For example, in undergraduate medical learning emphasis might be placed upon the skill of recognizing information taught in a traditional classroom and attempting its sideways expansion so as to ease comprehension and knowledge acquisition. For postgraduate learners the focus is shifted more towards skills related to analyzing and/or synthesizing different facets of information from contexts of existing formal and/or tacit knowledge. In continuing lifelong learning

or professional development, the need is shifted towards familiarization with new technology and/or new (evidence based) knowledge in a specified area as well as the exchange of peer experiences, activity or practice based training, and point of care or pervasive learning. In public education (or else communicating science and medicine to the public) challenges are associated with the wide diversity of the public scientific background and their differences in pursuing knowledge and health welfare.

As presented in the previous section, the majority of current exploitations of web 2.0 notions and technologies in medical education involve using this new medium to deliver education in the conventional way. However, there definitely exist those niches in the medical education era where Web 2.0 is expected to make a difference, by enabling new online educational experiences not previously possible to achieve. The following paragraphs present the authors' views about some indicative examples of such application areas.

Supporting Problem-Based Learning

In medical education, educational programs increasingly include case-based or problem-based learning and other small group instructional models, collaborative organizations to support student-faculty interactions, and technology-enhanced educational tools. The origins of active learning and problem-based learning (PBL) date way back in the 1940s (Lam, 2005), when the idea that students may learn better by doing and by thinking through problems was first introduced (Dewey, 1944). After its introduction in medicine at the McMaster University, Faculty of Health Sciences, in 1969 (Spaulding, 1969), PBL and active learning in general has been applied in numerous curricula in health sciences, and has been the centre of debate and comparative studies. Recent evidence from various disciplines suggests that active learning may work better than more passive approaches in health science education, e.g. (Michael, 2006; Schmidt et al, 2006). In a recent study, Kaldoudi et al (2008) proposed the combined use of various web 2.0 technologies, namely wikis, blogs and forums to support deployment of PBL sessions solely on the Web. In these PBL sessions, instruction is performed by an interdisciplinary team of experts from remote institutions, while the group of learners can be students from the same or different institutions. Instructors collaboratively develop a problem in a wiki. Discussion is initiated via a problem's blog or forum, where students and instructors collaborate to analyse the problem, identify conquered knowledge and plan actions for problem solving. Then students search (via the Web and not only there) for required information and collaborate to solve the case via the wiki. Student activities, progress and more importantly gained experience and competences are recorded, shared and commended on via their personal blogs. The entire learning episode and all its steps (with the final problem/answer deployment) are recorded, commended on and monitored via the wiki (final

and intermediate versions) and the participants' blogs.

Figure 2 shows typical screens from such an example PBL session, which in this case is presented as an individual course in a generic open source learning management system (Moodle, http://www.moodle.org). The didactic problem in this case is a multi-stage PBL session on "DICOM basics" offered to students in an MSc in Medical Informatics (http://iris.med.duth.gr/elearning/). Once the session is initialized, the students are encouraged to spend some time to get accustomed with the environment and the procedure. This familiarization phase always spawns interesting side discussions on technical issues around web 2.0 technologies as well as on educational notions and approaches, which are conducted via a second forum devoted to technical and procedural issues. Then, the first step of the problem is deployed and initial discussion is conducted via the forum. The students are encouraged to list unknown words and notions in the wiki (under a "Problem Deployment" area) and perform personal or collaborative

Figure 2. The front page of the PBL course in DICOM basics, a wiki page stating the first step of the didactic problem and the initial wiki page of the answer deployment

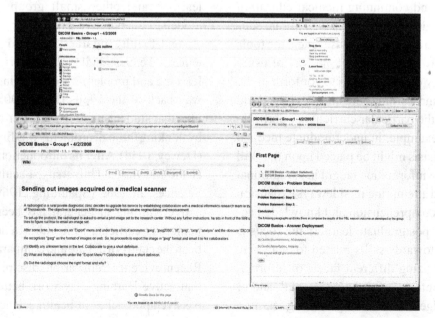

inquiries in order to resolve them. Final conclusion for each wiki entry is reached via a discussion for the specific wiki entry. Instructors participate in all discussions with comments and cues.

An important feature of this approach is that it enables various expert instructors (remotely located) to comment on and participate in the discussions providing highly specialized knowledge and experience in their individual field of expertise. Another interesting issue is that tacit knowledge can be recorded, archived and mined, via the blog entries of the participants. Using the provided blog, instructors can record interesting and important steps in addressing questions, thus implicitly recording their expertise in scientific problem solving. On the other hand, students can record their own process of tackling the problem, searching literature, resolving ambiguities etc. These blog entries can then be viewed collectively as PBL session entries to reveal the progression of problem solving procedure or as individual participant blog entries that may help evaluate personal progress and especially reveal skills mastered by each participant. This use of Web 2.0 has been deployed to support undergraduate and graduate medical education (Bamidis et al, 2008), as well as for dissemination of science to the public (Antoniou et al, 2008).

New Possibilities for Assessment and Evaluation

All this collaborative and participative emergent behaviour in Web 2.0 brings about and enables a novel approach to assessment and evaluation. Peer participation is enhanced and the conventional hierarchical relationship between teacher and student gives way for peer networks, with the individual on the spotlight. It logically follows that conventional student assessment mainly by comparing the individual with their peers on any given educational assignment, should be amended by other more appropriate approaches.

Luckily, web 2.0 technology can fully support this turn. For example, wikis and other social software are increasingly used for development of collaborative projects. Thus, individual wiki activities and appropriate clustering of wiki pages can be analysed in order to evaluate individual contribution to group projects (Trentin, 2009). A step beyond producing descriptive statistics, such as the number of postings per learner, number of replies, etc., one should turn towards analyzing interaction patterns in wiki discussions, in forums, and in blogs (and their comments) and see how this progresses over time, and from task to task, or from one educational goal (or problem stage) to the next, while using semantics to distinguish the purpose and outcome of interaction.

Probably, the most important advancement would come by using web 2.0 technology to help the individual analyze their own achievements both in knowledge and in competencies, either medicine specific or generic. In this case, appropriately tagged personal blogs that follow the educational progression of the individual over time, can highlight and reveal progress, strengths and weaknesses, and can be used to transfer the process of attaining the skills to achieve knowledge (rather than the achievement of knowledge itself). Thus putting focus to individual assessment as opposed to one's own history of achievement, rather than as opposed to peers' achievements. Via personal blog entries tacit knowledge can be recorded, archived and mined. Thus, experts and instructors can record interesting and important steps in exploring and appraising information, acquiring knowledge and addressing educational problems, and implicitly recording their expertise in scientific problem solving. On the other hand, learners can record their own process of tackling information, searching literature, resolving ambiguities, etc. These personal or group entries may help evaluate personal progress and especially reveal skills mastered.

Content Sharing in Medical Education

Continuous advances in medicine and biological sciences lead to an ever expanding core knowledge relevant to the medical practice (Papaioakeim et al, 2006). Thus, medical academic institutions are increasingly required to invest in order to enrich their curricula by developing overspecialized courses and corresponding educational content. It is evident that such an overspecialized expertise cannot be readily available in any medical academic institution, thus external experts have to be involved. Moreover, it cannot be easily available for professional medical doctors in their life-long continuous education. Although there is an abundance of up-to-date overspecialized medical educational content available in individual academic institutions, such content cannot at the moment be easily discovered, retrieved, re-used and thus shared across institutions and among medical teachers and students.

In order to support the emerging integrative curricula structures and exploit the over-specialized knowledge available by different experts, Web 2.0 technologies can be employed to develop virtual communities of educators and learners that share their pools of autonomous specialized educational modules and provide the mechanisms for searching, retrieving, evaluating and rating, adapting and revising educational content in medicine and life sciences (Kaldoudi et al, 2008b & 2009). Such educational content sharing communities may enhance the conceptual background and support the realization of the '5th freedom', that of free movement of knowledge (added to the four original principles of free movement of persons, capital, services and goods in the European Union) newly introduced by the heads of EU states and governments on March 14, 2008 in a statement following their traditional spring summit (European Council, 2008).

USA government and academia with the "Advanced Distributed Learning Initiative", a non-profit "Corporation for National Research Initiatives – CNRI", "Learning Systems Architecture Lab – LSAL" developed an open, standards-based model for designing and implementing software systems for the purposes of discovery, sharing and reuse of learning content through the establishment of interoperable federations of learning content repositories, the so called Content Object Repository Discovery Registration/Resolution Architecture (CORDRA) (Rehank et al, 2005). Although supported by prestigious international bodies, it seems that CORDRA architecture has not yet been widely adopted. Effective technology-supported interventions are usually created when there is a successful alignment of the specific requirements with the potential and the use of technology. Therefore, requirements for flexible, adaptive and ubiquitous online content sharing should evoke notions, practices and technologies from respective state-of-the-art evolutions in the Web.

Alternative content sharing solutions can be developed based on web 2.0 technologies (Kaldoudi et al, 2009). One such approach can be based on traditional isolated learning content management systems (LCMS), loosely associated via commonplace web 2.0 technologies. Each academic institution participating in such a virtual educational community publishes their content in their own LCMS. Notification and updates of newly published content in other affiliated LCMSs are performed by RSS feed mechanisms. Subscription to the RSS feeds can be open to institutions, educators and students alike. Independent mashup platform/repositories can store educational content, both as assets and as aggregation objects. All community participants can upload and download educational content to use on their isolated LCMS. Another alternative approach draws from the semantic web paradigm and is based on a federated architecture of LCMSs which is founded on a reference semantic web services architecture for search, interchange and delivery of learning objects.

Content Repurposing via Collaborative, Social Networks

Considering the state-of-the-art nature of medical educational content, it is imperative that such content can be repurposed, enriched, and embedded effectively into respective medical and other related scientific curricula, clinical practice and continuing education, as well as public dissemination and awareness.

Although many higher medical education institutions often use educational resources written in non-native languages (mainly English), the rule is that higher education is and should be delivered mostly in the native language. This is especially a mandate in healthcare, as acquired knowledge should be finally communicated to the patient. Additionally, common experience shows that there is also a demand for content localization. In the case of medical, and scientific content in general, this mainly refers to different legislation and local medical regulations, different lab tests norms, reference values and units as well as different medical requirements of various ethnic groups. Moreover, we should also consider the cultural differences among different user groups within the same national healthcare system. Healthcare education addresses a multitude of professions, ranging from medical doctors to nurses and lab technicians, to basic life scientists and even healthcare administrators. Thus, the same educational content often needs to be adapted in order to be delivered to an audience of a different background. Finally, we should also note the different pedagogical cultures present in healthcare education, which range from the conventional lecturing to clinical practice and a variety of active learning methodologies. All of these educational approaches would require the same content to be presented in a different way, e.g. a lecture presentation and notes for the conventional teaching approach should be restructured to be presented as, for example, a list of questions and answers or as a series of real world problems,

or a collection of interactive teaching files in the case of a more active learning episode.

Therefore, when medical educational content sharing is considered, the notion of re-purposing becomes a central requirement. The term re-purposing is used here to collectively refer to all instances that require any change and re-making of a particular educational content item to account for reasons such as those discussed in the previous paragraph. Content enrichment should also be considered as a requirement to all kinds of repurposing and involves adding new content and media in the form of other learning objects in order to add educational value. Standards based metadata is customarily used to describe learning objectives, learning outcomes, delivery methods, etc. Re-purposing of educational content can thus be described using such metadata which can be edited collaboratively in a social network, either by the instructor, or the student or even software itself.

The structure of an educational object that is repurposed may not necessarily change, but the key differences should be emphasized, described and organized in terms of a variety of tags, including time evolution, and other attributes. This brings in web 2.0 technologies. For example, consider a wiki used to create and hold the metadata that describes the repurposing history of a learning object and the various versions of the repurposed object itself (Figure 3) as they evolve through different uses within a community of medical educational content sharing.

FUTURE RESEARCH DIRECTIONS

Effective online learning experiences require a successful alignment of the learning approach with the technology used. Such an inherent alignment exists between the notion of active, collaborative learning and the paradigm of Web 2.0, as they both rely on and emphasize social skills (such as

Figure 3. Using wikis for metadata creation simultaneous with educational content repurposing

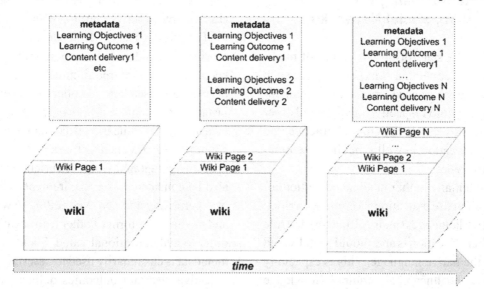

collaboration, interaction and peer activity) as opposed to mere content. Within this framework, it is expected that future work will put emphasis to individual's competences for knowledge management, rather than knowledge itself. Work in progress elaborates on mechanisms to process and analyze the learning process as recorded in personal blogs, wikis and social networks so as to extract meaningful information about capturing expert's practical skills competences and share this with the novice (Kaldoudi et al, 2008).

Additionally, the current enormous expansion in knowledge (including expert competences and tacit knowledge as well) constitutes a fundamental educational challenge. Higher academic institutions are increasingly required to invest in order to enrich their curricula with courses given by external experts, while experts working within an academic institution often restrict their state-of-the-art knowledge to a very limited audience (Papaioakeim et al, 2006). In order to support the emerging integrative curricula structures and accommodate the over-specialized knowledge available by different experts, web 2.0 applications can be employed to develop virtual distributed pools of autonomous specialized educational

modules and provide the mechanisms for searching, retrieving, evaluating and rating, adapting and revising educational content in medicine and life sciences (Kaldoudi et al, 2009). This is the scope of the European mEducator Best Practice Network (http://www.meducator.net/, grant no. ECP-2008-EDU-418006, funded under the eContent*plus* EU programme), which aims to enable seamless content sharing in medical formal education. Specifically, mEducator addresses a comprehensive collection of different types of health educational material. These include conventional educational content types also used in other areas (e.g. lecture notes, books, exam questions, practicals, graphs, images/videos, algorithms and simulators, etc), educational content types unique in medical education (e.g. teaching files, virtual patients, evidence based medicine forms, clinical guidelines, anatomical atlases, etc,) and alternative educational content types, either reflecting active learning techniques (extensively used in health education) and/or stemming from newly introduced web 2.0 technologies (e.g. problem/case based learning sessions, serious games, web traces, wikis, blogs/discussion forums, etc). Additionally, mEducator focuses on implementing and comparing two alternative solutions for educational content discovery and retrieval on the web. The first solution is based on traditional isolated learning content management systems (LCMS), loosely associated via commonplace web 2.0 technologies, using RSS feeds for notification and updates of newly published content. The second solution is based on a federated architecture which is founded on a reference Semantic Web Service (SWS) architecture for search, interchange and delivery of learning objects.

Such current research focusing on data semantics, ultimately leads to a further interesting advancement that is currently emerging and shows potential to grow into a next generation of Web, what is commonly referred to as Web 3.0. The notion and the prediction of this evolution are attributed to the founders of Web, Berners-Lee and colleagues (2001), almost a decade ago. However, the explosion of Web 2.0 has really prepared both technology and users for the semantic networking of information and services, thus the Web 3.0 is currently arising with a promising potential for educational applications (Bratsas et al, 2008).

While Web 2.0 is seen as the evolution of the web of information dissemination towards the web of human participation and information sharing, Web 3.0 emphasizes on machine-facilitated understanding of information so as to provide a context based, intuitive user experience. Although commonly referred to as a third generation of web technology (thus the 'version' number 3.0) we would argue that it should be more appropriate to use the descriptive term "semantic Web", to address the enabling of contextual and semantic information (mainly based on appropriate metadata) to both conventional web and web 2.0 applications. Moreover, the semantic web should not be seen as opposed to Web 2.0 nor as its mere evolution, but as complimentary. A fuller implemented Web is expected to arise by the appropriate merging of notions, technologies and approaches in all 'versions' of the Web. Recently Precia & Motta (2007) showed an interesting approach of

merging notions of web 2.0 collective behavior with semantics. In their work, they use collaboratively created tags used in social networking sites to automatically create groups of concepts and partial ontologies, thus merging folksonomies with the semantic Web.

In 2008 the World Wide Web Consortium (W3C) (http://www.w3.org/) has established the Semantic Web for Health Care and Life Sciences Interest Group (HCLS IG) (http://www.w3.org/2001/sw/hcls/) to develop and support the use of semantic web technologies to improve collaboration, research and development, innovation, and adoption in the domains of Health Care and Life Sciences. During the last five years, there is a considerable increase of adoption of semantic web technologies in health sciences, especially for discovering and managing the vast amount of scientific information available on the Web, e.g. (Vandervalk et al, 2009; Dumontier& Villanueva-Rosales, 2009; Manning et al, 2009). A foreseen application and impact in the case of education is to enable more efficient information search and retrieval using conventional web content, as well as the ability to construct personalized information searches tailored to a specific educational objective; further administration and semantic linking of educational content amongst institutions and degrees is also to be expected (Ohler, 2008).

Among other things, the semantic Web is about making information and services more meaningful to individuals as well as programs. Such an environment is expected to shift focus from 'finding information' to constructing 'meaningful and relevant information maps', leading to personal learning agents that will eventually support individuals in maintaining and administering their personal education and personal learning network. Thus, collaborative, participative learning within Web 2.0 will be transformed to a context based personalized learning shared within a network society. Web 2.0 applications such as wikis, blogs, mashups and RSS feeds will contain context related 'intelligence' and the problem will not be to find relevant information, but to identify information of quality and to learn how to use it best. Last but not least, for the aforementioned developments to be well accommodated within educational systems and curricula, the pivoting importance of standardising content sharing should be understood and exploited. In other words, much work will need to be carried along the paths of describing in standard ways the content to be shared and the various learning attributes associated with it (i.e. the context).

CONCLUSION

The last few years showed an increasing adoption of Web 2.0 for active and, potentially, effective learning in medicine. As with any new technology and technology paradigm shift, initial applications of Web 2.0 were mostly mere use of new technology in its most profound manner to support conventional practices, i.e. the metaphor of a virtual classroom, mainly supporting information dissemination. However, most interesting is to see how Web 2.0 can stimulate a new learning culture and find novel, alternative ways to advance medical education, by highlighting whatever unique characteristics this new technology exhibits and striving to exploit in full such characteristics, changing the conceptual paradigm along with the technological one. The real value of Web 2.0 in medical education will be revealed by those emerging application areas that enable new online educational experiences not previously possible to achieve, including full support of active learning, new ways of assessment and evaluation, content sharing educational communities and content repurposing in medical education. If it is to play a key role in education, emphasis with Web 2.0 should be geared along collaboration and participation and not the mere provision of content. The slow but sure emergence of semantic Web in combination with Web 2.0 creates even greater hopes and anticipations.

REFERENCES

Alexander, B. (2006). Web 2.0. A new wave of innovation for teaching and learning? *EDUCAUSE Review, 41*(2), 32–44.

Antoniou, P., Delidou, E., Aggeioplasti, K., & Kaldoudi, E. (2008) Astronomy Education for the Public via Web 2.0 technologies. In *Proceeding of ICERI2008 – International Conference of Education, Research and Innovation*, Madrid, Spain.

Argawal, V. (2007). Podcasts for psychiatrists: a new way of learning. *Psychiatric Bulletin*, col 31, 270-271.

Augar, N., Raitman, R., & Zhou, W. (2004). Teaching and learning online with wikis. In R. Atkinson, C. McBeath, D. Jonas-Dwyer & R. Phillips (Eds.), *Beyond the comfort zone: Proceedings of the 21st ASCILITE Conference* (pp. 95-104). Perth.

Bamidis, P. D., Constantinidis, S., Kaldoudi, E., Maglaveras, N., & Pappas, C. (2008). The use of Web 2.0 in teaching Medical Informatics to postgraduate medical students: first experiences. Published as Multimedia Appendix in G. Eysenbach (Ed.). Medicine 2.0: Social Networking, Collaboration, Participation, Apomediation, and Openness. *Journal of Medical Internet Research, 10*(3), e22. Retrieved from http://www.jmir.org/2008/3/e22/ doi:10.2196/jmir.1022-23

Belanger, Y. (2005). *Duke University iPod first year experience final evaluation report*. Durham, NC: Duke University. Retrieved November 14, 2008, from http://www.duke.edu/ddi/ipodfye.html

Berliner, D., & Calfee, R. (Eds.). (1996). *Handbook of educational psychology*. New York: Macmillan.

Berners-Lee, T., Hendler, J., & Lassila, O. (2001). The semantic web. *Scientific American, 184*(5), 34–43. doi:10.1038/scientificamerican0501-34

Boulos, M., Maramba, I., & Wheeler, S. (2006). Wikis, blogs and podcasts: A new generation of web-based tools for virtual collaborative clinical practice and education. *BMC Medical Education, 6*, 41. doi:10.1186/1472-6920-6-41

Boulos, M. N. K., Hetherington, L., & Wheeler, S. (2007). Second Life: and overview of the potential of 3-D virtual worlds in medical and health education. *Health Information and Libraries Journal, 24*(4), 233–245. doi:10.1111/j.1471-1842.2007.00733.x

Bratsas, C., Bamidis, P. D., Kaimakamis, E., & Maglaveras, N. (2008). Usage of Semantic Web Technologies (Web-3.0) Aiming to Facilitate the Utilisation of Computerized Algorithmic Medicine in Clinical Practice. Published as Multimedia Appendix in G. Eysenbach (Ed.), Medicine 2.0: Social Networking, Collaboration, Participation, Apomediation, and Openness. *J Med Internet Res, 10*(3), e22. Retrieved from http://www.jmir.org/2008/3/e22/ doi:10.2196/jmir.pp1038-39

Caldwell, L., Davies, S., Stewart, F., Thain, A., & Wales, A. (2008). Scottish toolkit for knowledge management. *Health Information and Libraries Journal, 25*(2), 125–134. doi:10.1111/j.1471-1842.2007.00747.x

Cobus, L. (2009). Using blogs and wikis in a graduate public health course. *Medical Reference Services Quarterly, 28*(1), 22–32. doi:10.1080/02763860802615922

Cronje, J. C. (2001). Metaphors and models in internet-based learning. *Computers & Education, 37*(3-4), 241–256. doi:10.1016/S0360-1315(01)00049-5

Davenport, T. H., & Prusak, L. (2000). *Working Knowledge: How Organizations Manage What They Know*. Boston, MA: Harvard Business School Press.

De Lucia, A., Francese, R., Passero, I., & Tortora, G. (2009). Development and evaluation of a virtual campus on Second Life: The case of Second-DMI. *Computers & Education, 52*(1), 220–233. doi:10.1016/j.compedu.2008.08.001

Dertouzos, M. (1997). *What will be* (pp. 175–189). London, UK: Judy Piatkus Ltd.

Dewey, J. (1944). *Democracy and Education*. New York: Free Press.

Dumontier, M., & Villanueva-Rosales, N. (2009). Towards pharmacogenomics knowledge discovery with the semantic web. *Briefings in Bioinformatics, 10*(2), 153–163. doi:10.1093/bib/bbn056

Ebner, M., Holzinger, A., & Maurer, H. (2007). Web 2.0 Technology: Future Interfaces for Technology Enhanced Learning. In C. Stephanidis (Ed.), Universal Access in HCI, Part III, HCII 2007 (LNCS 4556, pp. 559-568). Berlin, Germany: Springer-Verlag.

Ehlers, U. (2007). The new pathway for e-learning: From distribution to collaboration and competence in e-learning. *Association for the Advancement of Computing in Education Journal, 16*(2), 187–20.

European Council. (2008). Presidency Conclusions of the Brussels European Council, 13/14 March 2008. Retrieved January 28, 2009, from http://www.consilium.europa.eu/ueDocs/cms_Data/docs/pressData/en/ec/99410.pdf

Eysenbach, G. (2007). From intermediation to disintermediation and apomediation: new models for consumers to access and assess the credibility of health information in the age of Web2.0. *Studies in Health Technology and Informatics, 129*(Pt 1), 162–166.

Finegold, A. R. D., & Cooke, L. (2006). Exploring the Attitudes, Experiences and Dynamics of Interaction in Online Groups. *The Internet and Higher Education*, *9*, 201–215. doi:10.1016/j.iheduc.2006.06.003

Fyrenious, A. (2005). Lectures in problem-based learning—Why, when and how? An example of interactive lecturing that stimulates meaningful learning. *Medical Teacher*, *27*(1), 61–65. doi:10.1080/01421590400016365

Genes, N., & Parekh, S. (2009). Bringing journal club to the bedside in the form of a critical appraisal blog. [article in press, epub ahead of print]. *The Journal of Emergency Medicine*, (Jan): 24.

Heiberg Engel, P. J. (2008). Tacit knowledge and visual expertise in medical diagnostic reasoning: implications for medical education. *Medical Teacher*, *30*(7), e184–e188. doi:10.1080/01421590802144260

Henry, S. G., Zaner, R. M., & Dittus, R. S. (2007). Viewpoint: Moving beyond evidence-based medicine. *Academic Medicine*, *82*(3), 292–297. doi:10.1097/ACM.0b013e3180307f6d

Hoffmann, R. (2008). A wiki for the life sciences where authorship matters. *Nature Genetics*, *40*(9), 1047–1051. doi:10.1038/ng.f.217

Jones, R., Higgs, R., de Angelis, C., & Prideaux, D. (2001). Changing face of medical curricula. *Lancet*, *357*(9257), 699–703. doi:10.1016/S0140-6736(00)04134-9

Kaldoudi, E., Bamidis, P. D., Papaioakeim, M., & Vargemezis, V. (2008). Problem-based learning via Web 2.0 technologies. In *Proceedings of CBMS2008: The 21th IEEE International Symposium on Computer-Based Medical Systems, Special Track: Technology Enhanced Learning in Medical Education*. (pp. 391-396). Jyväskylä, Finland: IEEE Computer Society.

Kaldoudi, E., Bamidis, P. M., & Pattichis, C. (2009). Multi-type content repurposing and sharing in medical education. In *Proceedings of INTED2009: International Technology, Education and Development Conference*, Valencia, Spain: International Association of Technology, Education and Development.

Kaldoudi, E., Papaioakeim, M., Bamidis, P. M., & Vargemezis, V. (2008b). Towards expert content sharing in medical education. In *Proceedings of INTED2008: International Technology, Education and Development Conference*, Valencia, Spain: International Association of Technology, Education and Development.

Kelton, A. J. (2008). Virtual worlds. Outlook good. *EDUCAUSE Review*, *43*(5), 5–22.

Kim, H. N. (2008). The phenomenon of blogs and theoretical model of blog use in educational contexts. *Computers & Education*, *51*(3), 1342–1352. doi:10.1016/j.compedu.2007.12.005

Kurtz, B., Fenwick, J., & Ellsworth, C. (2007). Using podcasts and tablet PCs in computer science. In *Proceedings of 45th ACM South East Conference* (pp. 484-489). Winston Salem, NC: ACM.

Lam, T. P. (2005). *The origin of problem based learning. Medical Teacher, 27(5), 473.* Letter to the Editor.

Manning, M., Aggarwal, A., Gao, K., & Tucker-Kellogg, G. (2009). Scaling the walls of discovery: using semantic metadata for integrative problem solving. *Briefings in Bioinformatics*, *10*(2), 164–176. doi:10.1093/bib/bbp007

Marton, F., Dahlgren, L.-O., Svensson, L., & Saljo, R. (1977). Inlarning och omvarldsuppfattning. Stockholm, Sweden: Almqvist och Wiksell forlag AB.

McAfee, A. (2006). Enterprise 2.0: The dawn of emergent collaboration. *MIT Sloan Management Review*, *47*(3), 21–28.

McGeee, J. B., & Begg, M. (2008). What medical educators need to know about "Web 2.0". *Medical Teacher*, *30*(2), 164–169. doi:10.1080/01421590701881673

Michael, J. (2006). Where's the evidence that active learning works? *Advances in Physiology Education*, *30*(4), 159–167. doi:10.1152/advan.00053.2006

National Research Council. (1999). *How people learn*. Washington, DC: National Academy Press.

O'Reilly, T. (2005). *What is Web 2.0: Design patterns and business models for the next generation of software*. Retrieved February 1, 2008, from http://www.oreillynet.com/pub/a/oreilly/tim/news/2005/09/30/what-is-web-20.html

Ohler, J. (2008). The semantic web in education. *EDUCAUSE Quarterly*, *31*(4), 7–9.

Papaioakeim, M., Kaldoudi, E., Vargemezis, V., & Simopoulos, K. (2006). Confronting the problem of ever expanding core knowledge and the necessity of handling overspecialized disciplines in medical education. In *Proceedings of ITAB 2006: IEEE International Special Topic Conference on Information Technology in Biomedicine*. Ioannina, Greece: IEEE.

Parker, K. R., & Chao, J. T. (2007). Wiki as a teaching tool. *Interdisciplinary Journal of Knowledge and Learning Objects*, *3*, 57–72.

Pender, M. P., Lasserre, K., Kruesi, L., Del Mar, C., & Anuradha, S. (2008). Putting Wikipedia to the test: a case study. In *Proceedings of the Special Libraries Association Annual Conference*. Seattle, Washington.

Percia, L., & Motta, E. (2007). Integrating folksonomies with the Semantic Web. In Lecture Notes in Computer Science, vol. 4519, The Semantic Web: Research and Applications (pp. 624-639). Berlin/Heidelberg: Springer.

Polanyi, M. (1958, 1998). Personal knowledge. Towards a post critical philosophy. London: Routledge.

Rehank, D. R., Dodds, P., & Lannom, L. (2005). A model and infrastructure for federated learning content repositories. In *Proceedings of the 14th International World Wide Web Conference, Chiba, Japan: W3C et al.*

Russell, T. L. (2001). *The no significant difference phenomenon*. Montgomery, USA: IDECC.

Sandars, J., Homer, M., Pell, G., & Croker, T. (2008). Web 2.0 and social software: the medical student way of e-learning. *Medical Teacher*, *83*(986), 759–762.

Schaffert, S., Bischof, D., Buerger, T., Gruber, A., Hilzensauer, W., & Schaffert, S. (2006). Learning with semantic wikis. In *Proceedings of the First Workshop on Semantic Wikis – From Wiki To Semantics (SemWiki2006)* (pp.109-123). Budva, Montenegro.

Schmidt, H. G., Vermeulen, L., & van der Molen, H. T. (2006). Longterm effects of problem-based learning: a comparison of competencies acquired by graduates of a problem-based and a conventional medical school. *Medical Education*, *40*(6), 562–567. doi:10.1111/j.1365-2929.2006.02483.x

Schuable, L., & Glaser, R. (Eds.). (1996). Innovations in learning. New Jersey: Mahwah.

Spaulding, W. B. (1969). The undergraduate medical curriculum (1969 model): McMaster University. *Canadian Medical Association Journal*, *100*(14), 659–664.

Sturmberg, J. P., & Martin, C. M. (2008). Knowing-in medicine. *Journal of Evaluation in Clinical Practice*, *14*(5), 767–770.

Tonkin, E. (2005). Making the case for a wiki. *Ariadne*, 42. Retrieved November 14, 2008, from http://www.ariadne.ac.uk/issue42/tonkin/

Trentin, G. (2009). Using a wiki to evaluate individual contribution to a collaborative learning project. *Journal of Computer Assisted Learning, 25*(1), 43–55. doi:10.1111/j.1365-2729.2008.00276.x

Vandervalk, B. P., McCarthy, E. L., & Wilkinson, M. D. (2009). Moby and Moby 2: Creatures of the Deep (Web). *Briefings in Bioinformatics, 10*(2), 114–128. doi:10.1093/bib/bbn051

Wenger, E. (2000). Communities of practice and social learning systems. *Organization, 7*(2), 225–246. doi:10.1177/135050840072002

Williamson, K. B., Kang, Y. P., Steele, J. L., & Gunderman, R. B. (2002). The Art of Asking: Teaching Through Questioning. *Academic Radiology, 9*(12), 1419–1422. doi:10.1016/S1076-6332(03)80669-4

Wilson, P., Petticrew, M., & Booth, A. (2009). After the gold rush? A systematic and critical review of general medical podcasts. *Journal of the Royal Society of Medicine, 102*(2), 69–74. doi:10.1258/jrsm.2008.080245

ADDITIONAL READING

Adams, S.A. (2009). Blog-based applications and health information: Two case studies that illustrate important questions for Consumer Health Informatics (CHI) research. *International Journal of Medical Informatics.*

Armstrong, K., & Retterer, O. (2008). Blogging as L2 writing: A case study. *Association for the Advancement of Computing in Education Journal, 16*(3), 233–251.

Bond, S. T., Ingram, C., & Ryan, S. (2008). Reuse, repurposing and learning design – Lessons from the DART project. *Computers & Education, 50*(2), 601–612. doi:10.1016/j.compedu.2007.09.019

Booth, A. (2007). Using evidence in practice, Blogs, wikis and podcasts: the 'evaluation bypass' in action? *Health Information and Libraries Journal, 24*(4), 298–302.

Burns, T. M. (2007). The forecast for podcasts: Sunny skies but not necessarily with clear visibility. *Neurology, 68*(15), E19–E20. doi:10.1212/01.wnl.0000259068.95721.dc

Chen, H., Ding, L., Wu, Z., Yu, T., Dhanapalan, L., & Chen, J. Y. (2009). Semantic web for integrated network analysis in biomedicine. *Briefings in Bioinformatics, 10*(2), 177–192. doi:10.1093/bib/bbp002

Cheung, K.-H., Prud'hommeaux, E., Wang, Y., & Stephens, S. (2009). Semantic web for health care and life sciences: a review of the state of the art. *Briefings in Bioinformatics, 10*(2), 111–113. doi:10.1093/bib/bbp015

Cheung, K.-H., Yip, K. Y., Townsend, J. P., & Scotch, M. (2008). HCLS 2.0/3.0: Health care and life sciences data mashup using Web 2.0/3.0. *Journal of Biomedical Informatics, 41*(5), 694–705. doi:10.1016/j.jbi.2008.04.001

Cobus, L. (2009). Using Blogs and Wikis in a Graduate Public Health Course. *Medical Reference Services Quarterly, 28*(1), 22–32. doi:10.1080/02763860802615922

Devedzic, V. (2004). Education and the Semantic Web. *International Journal of Artificial Intelligence in Education, 14*, 39–65.

Duffy, P., & Bruns, A. (2006). The Use of Blogs, Wikis and RSS in Education: A Conversation of Possibilities. In *Proceedings Online Learning and Teaching Conference 2006* (pp. 31-38), Brisbane.

Eaton, K. A., Reynolds, P. A., Grayden, S. K., & Wilson, N. H. F. (2008). A vision of dental education in the third millennium. *British Dental Journal, 205*(5), 261–271. doi:10.1038/sj.bdj.2008.736

Ellaway, R., & Martin, R. D. (2008). What's mine is yours-open source as a new paradigm for sustainable healthcare education. *Medical Teacher, 30*(2), 175–179. doi:10.1080/01421590701874058

Evans, C. (2008). The effectiveness of m-learning in the form of podcast revision lectures in higher education. *Computers & Education, 50*(2), 491–498. doi:10.1016/j.compedu.2007.09.016

Falkman, G., Gustafsson, M., Jontell, M., & Torgersson, O. (2008). SOMWeb: A Semantic Web-Based System for Supporting Collaboration of Distributed Medical Communities of Practice. *Journal of Medical Internet Research, 10*(3), e25. doi:10.2196/jmir.1059

Friedman, L. H., & Bernell, S. L. (2006). The importance of team level tacit knowledge and related characteristics of high-performing health care teams. *Health Care Management Review, 31*(3), 223–230.

Greenhalgh, J., Flynn, R., Long, A. F., & Tyson, S. (2008). Tacit and encoded knowledge in the use of standardised outcome measures in multidisciplinary team decision making: A case study of in-patient neurorehabilitation. *Social Science & Medicine, 67*(1), 183–194. doi:10.1016/j.socscimed.2008.03.006

Hall, W., De Roure, D., & Shadbolt, N. (2009). The evolution of the Web and implications for eResearch. *Philosophical Transactions of the Royal Society A, 367*(1890), 991-1001.

Hammond, M. (2006). Blogging within formal and informal learning contexts: Where are the opportunities and constraints? In *Proceedings of the International Research Conference on Networked Learning 2006*, Lancaster, UK.

Henry, S. G. (2006). Recognizing tacit knowledge in medical epistemology. *Theoretical Medicine and Bioethics, 27*(3), 187–213. doi:10.1007/s11017-006-9005-x

Insch, G. S., McIntyre, N., & Dawley, D. (2008). Tacit knowledge: a refinement and empirical test of the academic tacit knowledge scale. *The Journal of Psychology, 142*(6), 561–579. doi:10.3200/JRLP.142.6.561-580

Mazzolini, M., & Maddison, S. (2007). When to jump in: The role of the instructor in online discussion forums. *Computers & Education, 49*(2), 193–213. doi:10.1016/j.compedu.2005.06.011

Philip, C. T., Unruh, K. P., Lachman, N., & Pawlina, W. (2008). An explorative learning approach to teaching clinical anatomy using student generated content. *Anatomical Sciences Education, 1*(3), 106–110. doi:10.1002/ase.26

Sandars, J., & Morrison, C. (2007). What is the Net Generation? The challenge for future medical education. *Medical Teacher, 29*(2), 85–88. doi:10.1080/01421590601176380

van der Pol, J., van den Berg, B. A. M., Admiraal, W. F., & Simons, P. R. J. (2008). The nature, reception, and use of online peer feedback in higher education. *Computers & Education, 51*(4), 1804–1817. doi:10.1016/j.compedu.2008.06.001

Wang, K. T., Huang, Y.-M., Jeng, Y.-L., & Wang, T.-I. (2008). A blog-based dynamic learning map. *Computers & Education, 51*(1), 262–278. doi:10.1016/j.compedu.2007.06.005

Whitehead, D. E. J., Bray, D., & Harries, M. (2007). Not just music but medicine. Podcasting surgical procedures in otolaryngology. *Clinical Otolaryngology, 32*(2), 3–6. doi:10.1111/j.1365-2273.2007.01351.x

Wilson, P., Petticrew, M., & Booth, A. (2009). After the gold rush? A systematic and critical review of general medical podcasts. *Journal of the Royal Society of Medicine, 102*(2), 69–74. doi:10.1258/jrsm.2008.080245

Chapter 8
Integrating Medicinal Learning Objects with Daily Duties

Juha Puustjärvi
Helsinki University of Technology, Finland

Leena Puustjärvi
The Pharmacy of Kaivopuisto, Finland

ABSTRACT

Lifelong learning is a term that is widely used in a variety of context. The term recognizes that learning is not confined to the classroom, but takes place throughout life and in a range of situations. The authors of this chapter have analyzed lifelong learning in healthcare sector, where the fast development of drug treatment requires special knowledge that needs to be renewed frequently. This chapter analyzes various ways of ensuring that the employers of medicinal organizations are aware of the relevant medicinal instructions such as medicinal learning objects and guides. In particular, the authors consider three complementary ways for the dissemination of medicinal instructions: (i) by providing keyword-based searching, (ii) by providing ontology-based searching, and (iii) by automatic integration of medicinal instructions to employers' day-to-day work tasks. The integration can be based either on the similarity of the metadata descriptions of the tasks and learning objects, or on the ontology which specifies the relationships of the tasks and instructions. The authors' argument is that integration is most preferable as medicinal instructions are provided just-in-time and tailored to their specific needs. In addition, a notable gain of ontology based integration is that employees will be aware of the existence of the all relevant instructions.

INTRODUCTION

The role of continued education and lifelong learning is becoming still more important as the fast development of technologies requires specialized skills that

DOI: 10.4018/978-1-61520-777-0.ch008

need to be renewed frequently. E-learning adopts well for continued education as it can be done in parallel to other work. However, e-learning sets new requirements for organizations: they have to build global learning infrastructures, learning material has to be in digital form, and learning material has to be distributed. In addition, organizations need

Copyright © 2010, IGI Global. Copying or distributing in print or electronic forms without written permission of IGI Global is prohibited.

learning processes that are just-in-time, tailored to their specific needs, and ideally integrated into day-to-day work patterns.

Healthcare is a field where the fast development of drug treatment and the introduction of new drugs require specialized skills and knowledge that need to be renewed frequently (Puustjärvi & Puustjärvi, 2006). As each drug has its unique indications, cross-reactivity, complications and costs also the prescribing medication as well as the distribution of medicinal products becomes still more complex (Jung, 2009). As a result, also the amount of new instructions concerning new medication increases rapidly. An interesting question arising from this reality is how medicinal instructions should be organized and retrieved in order to ensure that the employees are aware of the relevant medicinal instructions.

Ideally, the (medicinal) information retrieval system should be able to retrieve all the medicinal instructions, which are relevant while retrieving as few non-relevant instructions as possible. This kind of quality of information retrieval system is usually measured by two fractions, called recall and precision (Baeza-Yates & Ribeiro-Neto, 1999). *Recall* is the fraction of the relevant documents (e.g., medicinal instructions), which has been retrieved. *Precision* is the fraction of the retrieved documents, which is relevant. The values of these fractions are highly dependent on the way the query and the content of medicinal documents are presented.

Though the high quality in retrieving medicinal instruction is of high importance, our ultimate goal has been the integration of learning processes and daily duties in a way that searching educational material does not require extra efforts. That is, with respect to the dissemination of instructions, we have adopted the push technology instead of the pull technology, which is generally used with e-learning systems. In general, *push technology* describes a style of communication where the request for a given document originates with the publisher. It is contrasted with pull technology,

where the request for the transmission of documents originates with the receiver.

A notable gain of integration is that by integrating learning objects as well as all other relevant information (or their links) with daily task is that we can ensure that employees will be aware of the existence of all the relevant material. This has turned out to be crucial as the volume of information coming in from a variety of information sources such as pharmaceutical companies, medicinal wholesalers, social insurance institutions and other authorities is increasing all the time.

In the following sections, we restrict ourselves on this topic. In particular, we consider three complementary ways for the dissemination of medicinal information: (i) by providing keyword-based searching, (ii) by providing ontology-based searching, and (iii) by integrating the medical learning objects to employers´ daily duties. Our argument is that integration is most preferable as medical learning objects are provided just-in-time, tailored to their specific needs, and integrated into daily duties. However, as we will show, automating the integration of learning objects to daily work patterns is not an easy task as it requires the management of medicinal ontologies and the deployment of business processes.

LEARNING OBJECTS AND METADATA BASED SEARCHING

Learning Objects

During the past few years the term learning object (LOM, 2004) is widely used in the discussion concerning educational information systems. Generally the term is understood to be a digital entity deliverable over Internet such that any number of learners can use them simultaneously. For example, a study course, a course book and a lecture are typical learning objects. By the term *medicinal learning objects* we refer to learning objects that deal medicinal information.

There are four commonly accepted functional requirements set on learning objects.

- First, learning objects should be usable in different instructional contexts, i.e., learning objects should be reusable.
- Second, learning objects should be independent of the delivery media and learning management system, i.e., learning objects should enable the interoperability of learning management systems.
- Third, learning object should be designed in the way which allows the combination of learning objects.
- Fourth, learning objects should provide appropriate metadata (annotation) in order to allow easy searching facilities.

Our research is focused on the fourth requirement. Particularly we restrict on learning objects metadata and on the ontologies that give the semantics for the metadata items.

In general, annotations are comments, notes, explanations, or other types of external remarks that can be attached to a learning object or to a selected part of it. As they are external, it is possible to annotate any learning object independently, without needing to edit the document itself. From a technical point of view, annotations are usually seen as metadata, as they give additional information about an existing piece of data.

One interesting question is who should annotate the learning object or documents? Our approach is based on the assumption that the sources of the information entities are responsible for the annotation, i.e., the communicating parties are committed to use the same taxonomies and ontologies. As the sources of information entities are medicinal authors, medicinal wholesalers and pharmaceutical companies, we assume that the documents they deliver are annotated in an appropriate way.

The representation and organization of documents (e.g., learning objects) should provide an easy access to the documents. Ideally the system should be able to retrieve all the documents, which are relevant while retrieving as few non-relevant documents as possible (Figure 1).

This kind of quality of information retrieval system is usually measured by the following fractions (Baeza-Yates, 1999):

- *Recall:* the fraction of the relevant documents, which has been retrieved.
- *Precision*: the fraction of the retrieved documents, which is relevant.

The values of these fractions are highly dependent on the way the query and the content of document are presented. As we will show, by ontology based integration of learning objects and daily duties we can achieve the ideal case where

Figure 1. Relevant learning objects and retrieved learning objects

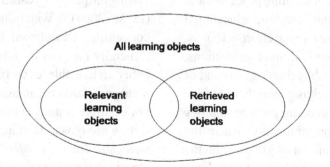

the sets of retrieved learning objects and relevant learning objects are equal.

Learning Objects and Metadata

The notion of metadata (Najjar et al., 2003) has variable interpretations depending upon the circumstances in which it is used. Fundamentally, *metadata* is data about data. It describes certain important characteristics of its target. Equally metadata can be described by meta-metadata, which is descriptive information of the metadata itself. The typical types of metadata that can be attached to documents include document's author, publisher, publication date, language and keywords.

Educational metadata describes any features of a learning object. Such descriptions facilitate educational institutions to provide suitable information about their course supply and facilitate learners in retrieving learning objects (Lamminaho, 2000). Educational metadata can be classified into syntactical metadata and semantic metadata. *Syntactical metadata* describes the structural characteristics of learning object, such as the format, language, technical requirements, target group, and the author of the learning object. Further, *learning object content models* extend

syntactical metadata by identifying different kind of learning objects and their components. So, learning object content models are taxonomies of learning objects' structure. They provide precise ways to specify the internal structure of learning object. Their main goal is to encourage learning object reusability. For example, Duval and Hoddings (Duval & Hodgins, 2009) have developed a taxonomy, which is comprised of the following levels: Raw media elements, Information objects, Learning objects and Aggregate assemblies.

Raw data media elements include smallest units such as sentences, paragraphs illustration and animation. Further, *Information objects* are set of raw media elements. These two levels are application domain independent meaning that they can also be deployed for example in the field of technical documentation. A collection of information objects comprises a learning object. Hence, here learning object appears in a more restrictive sense than in the LOM standard. *Aggregate assemblies* (e.g., lessons or chapters) are collections learning objects. Further, these can be assembled into a large *collection* like courses and curricula.

However, neither content models nor syntactical metadata address the issue of learning object's content (Puustjärvi, 2004). Instead *semantic*

Figure 2. A learning object content model

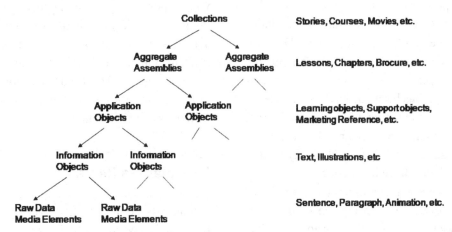

metadata describes the semantic content of the learning object (Puustjärvi & Pöyry, 2003). For example, the keywords attached to learning objects represent semantic metadata. Further, in order to standardize semantic metadata certain domain specific taxonomies and ontologies are introduced. They give the semantics for the semantic metadata, and so they provide a shared and common understanding of the metadata items.

Metadata Standards

The idea behind standardization is to achieve interoperability between systems from different origins. An important point in standardization is that it does not impose a particular implementation but rather a common specification which establishes an opportunity for collaboration by diverse groups.

There are many organizations which standardize metadata. Next we will consider two well known standards namely Dublin Core and LOM.

Dublin Core (Dublin Core, 2009) is a widely known metadata standard that has been developed since 1995. The metadata elements of the Dublin Core represent syntactical metadata, i.e., they do not describe the content of the target. Originally, they are intended to facilitate the discovery of electronic resources from the Web. It includes 15 metadata elements that describe the content, the intellectual property rights and the instantiation of the object. For example, the standard includes the following elements: Creator, Date, Description, Subject, and Language. Even though, the Dublin Core does not include educational metadata elements, it has been used as basis for many educational metadata projects. On the other hand, proposals to extend the standard by educational elements (e.g., Audience, Interactivity type, and Interactivity level) have been done.

Dublin Core also includes metadata attributes that can be used in specifying the relationship between resources. Thorough these attributes it is possible to define for example that a lecture is a part of a course (IsPartOf), a course is a version of another course ((IsVersionOf), a laboratory work requires certain software (IsRequiredBy), and a course is based on another course (IsBasedOn).

LOM (Learning object metadata standard) (LOM, 2004) defines the structure of a meta-data instance for a learning object. A learning object is regarded as any entity, digital or non-digital, that may be used for learning. In addition, the standard facilitates the sharing and exchange of learning objects by enabling the development of catalogues and inventories while taking into account the diversity of cultural contexts in which the learning object will be exploited. The goals of the LOM are to enable the learners to search and use learning objects and enable computer agents to automatically compose learning objects to individual learners.

Using the LOM it is possible to specify for example the teaching or interaction style of a course, the grade level of a course, the difficulty of a course, typical learning time of a course, the prerequisites of a course and the relationships of learning objects.

In LOM the metadata elements describing a learning object are grouped into different categories. The categories that relates to metadata are the General category and the Classification category: The *General category* groups the general information that describes the learning object as whole. For example the metadata elements title, language and keywords belong to this category. The *Classification category* describes the learning object in relation to a particular classification system, e.g., to ACM-classification. To define multiple classifications, there may be multiple instances of this category.

Annotating Documents by Metadata Items

Documents content is traditionally represented through keywords, which are extracted from the document. It is also possible to represent the document by first automatically eliminating its articles, connectives, adjectives, adverbs and verbs and then extracting its all remaining words to keywords. In this approach we say that the content of a document is represented by full text indexing.

Assume now that full text indexing is applied to learning objects descriptions. Hence, the description of each learning object is a set of keywords. Now, if a learner is interested in learning objects focusing on WWW, he or she enters the keyword "WWW". Then the search engine returns all the learning objects were the keyword "WWW" is stated.

Probably the quality of this retrieval is not very good. For example, the document having statement "World Wide Web" will not be returned. It is obvious that there are a lot of documents discussing World Wide Web but without explicitly stating that term. So the probability of missing many relevant documents is rather high.

Within full text indexing a reason for missing many relevant documents is that the keywords used with queries and documents descriptions are not standardized. In order to standardize semantic metadata specific taxonomies, which describe certain topics, are introduced in many disciplines. We next illustrate the use of medicinal taxonomies in searching medicinal information.

TAXONOMY- AND THESAURUS - BASED SEARCHING OF MEDICINAL LEARNING OBJECTS

Taxonomy

Taxonomy is a way to classify or categorize a set of things into a hierarchy. It is a tree like structure consisting of a root and branches where each branching point (i.e., a node) is a node is an information entity. In the context of information technology taxonomy is generally understood as the classification of information entities in the form of a hierarchy, according to the presumed relationship of real-world entities that they represent (Daconta et al., 2003).

The logic behind taxonomy is that when one goes up the taxonomy toward the root, the information entities become more general, and respectively when one goes down towards the leaves the information entities become more specialized. We can also state this in a more formal way: depending on the direction of the link each link between a parent and a child node represents a subclassification relation or superclassification relation. For example, *oral pain drug* is a subclassification of a *pain drug*, and *drug* is a superclassification of a *pain drug*. Similarly, *taxonomy* is a subclassification of *ontology* and *ontology* is a superclassification of *taxonomy*.

A simple drug taxonomy is presented in Figure 3. The idea behind this classification is that the medicinal instructions can be annotated by the metadata items (the branching points and the leaves) represented in the tree. A user can then query medicinal instructions by Boolean expressions (Baeza-Yates & Ribeiro-Neto, 1999) comprising of operands and operations. The operands are the used keywords (which are taken from the taxonomy) and the operands are typically "and", "or", and "not". For example, by using the taxonomy of Figure 1 the keywords attached to the medicinal instruction "New warnings of using pain drugs in topical use with children" could be "Pain drugs for topical use" and "Prescription based pain drug".

Now assume that a pharmacist has to check the instructions concerning pain drugs, and so she enters the Boolean expression: *Prescription based pain drug* and *Pain drug for topical use*. Now assume that the result includes at least the instruction "New warnings of using pain drugs in topical use with children". After reading the instruction the pharmacist is interested to read the previous medicinal instruction of the same topic. The pharmacist may also be interested to know the medicinal products that are under this new warning. Unfortunately by using keyword based searching (i.e., Boolean expressions) the pharmacist has no hope for finding the answers for such queries.

Thesaurus

A thesaurus differs from a taxonomy in that the relationships between terms are clearly displayed and identified by standardized relationship indicators. The relationships are equivalence, homographic, hierarchical and associative.

The primary purpose of equivalence and homograph in the context of e-learning systems is to manage semantic heterogeneity, i.e., the cases where different terms are used in the same meaning and vice versa. For example, it may be necessary to state that "Tablet" is equivalent with "Pill" (equivalence) or that the guide "Psychiatric treatment" within the material of physicians and within the material of patients is not the same guide (homographs).

Hierarchical relationships can be used to specify the relationships between a parent and its children (hierarchic parent of), or between a children and its parent (hierarchic child of). For example, we can specify that the term "Medical treatment" is broader than "Medicinal treatment", or that "Medicinal treatment" is narrower than "Medical treatment". Associative relationship between two terms means that there are some unspecified relationships between the two terms. For example, a drug may be associated with prescription.

The motivation for developing thesaurus is based on the idea of using controlled vocabulary for the indexing and searching. A controlled vocabulary gives many advantages such as normalization of indexing terms and retrieval based on concepts rather than words. These advantages are particularly important in specific domain such as in medicine as there is already a large amount of knowledge compiled.

There are different tools, e.g., MetaMap (MetaMap, 2009), and ways available for automatic or semiautomatic creating of thesauri, e.g., different kinds of statistical co-occurrence analyses, the concept space approach, and by representing the terms as Bayesian networks. Constructing a thesaurus is however, outside the scope of this article, and thus we have not analyzed which way of creating thesaurus would be most appropriate in the domain of medicinal learning objects.

In the next section we will consider an ontology-based (Gruber, 1993; Antoniou & Harmelen, 2004) searching. The advantage of ontologies is that they have stronger expression power than taxonomies or thesaurus has, and so they can be used among other things for modeling taxonomies and thesaurus.

ONTOLOGY–BASED SEARCHING

A Medicinal Ontology

The term ontology originates from philosophy where it is used as the name of the study of the nature of existence. In the context of computer science, the commonly used definition is "An ontology is an explicit and formal specification of a conceptualization" (Gruber, 1993). So it is a general vocabulary of a certain domain. Essentially the used ontology must be shared and consensual terminology as it is used for information sharing and exchange. On the other hand, ontology tries to capture the meaning of a particular subject domain that corresponds to what a human being knows about that domain. It also tries to characterize that meaning in terms of concepts and their relationships.

In order that the information retrieval system could answer for the queries presented in previous section we have to extend the search functionalities by querying features. This requires the deployment of an ontology.

Each ontology describes a domain of discourse. It consists of a finite set of concepts and the re-

Figure 3. Medicinal product categories in taxonomy

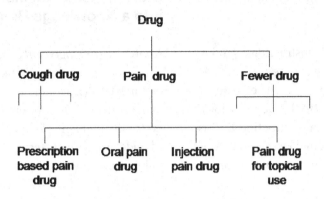

lationship between the concepts. Our developed medicinal ontology models the medicinal instructions as well as their relationships to other relevant medicinal concepts such as patient, physician, patient record, drug, and e-prescriptions. In addition the ontology models the associations of medicinal instructions to the tasks of the day-to-day work tasks. Part of this ontology is graphically presented in Figure 4.

In the figure ellipses represent classes and boxes represent properties. The ontology includes for example the following information:

- Medicinal product category is a class and each instance of the category may have a parent, which is also an instance of medicinal product category, i.e., among other things, the ontology models the taxonomy presented in Figure 1.

- Each medicinal instruction relates to zero or more medicinal products (e.g., Aspirin), and each medicinal product includes one or more drugs and has one or more substitutable medicinal products.

- Each medicinal instruction is associated to zero or more tasks which are parts of a workflow. That is, each medicinal instruction is associated to a task and a workflow which represents functionalities in a day-to-day work patterns.

Figure 4. A medicinal ontology

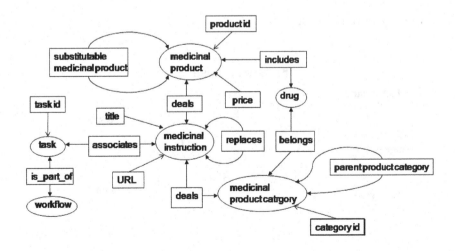

The medicinal ontology allows making queries such as:

- Give me medicinal instructions having keywords *Prescription based pain drug* and *Pain drug for topical use* (i.e., a query that corresponds to a Boolean expression).
- Give me the medicinal instruction that is replaced by the medicinal instruction *"New warnings of using pain drugs in topical use with children"*.
- Give me the names of the medicinal products that relate *to the medicinal instruction "New* warnings of using pain drugs in topical use with children".
- Assuming that the result includes the medicinal products *A* and *B*, then it allows querying (browsing by clicking the edges) the substitutable medicinal products and prices for *A* and *B*, as well as the drugs that are included to these medicinal products.

In the next section, we illustrate how our used ontology can be stored in a knowledge base and can be specified by an ontology specification language.

Storing Medicinal Instructions into a Knowledge Base

Knowledge management concerns with acquiring, accessing and maintaining knowledge within an organization (Daconta et al., 2003). Knowledge management system refers to a computer based system for managing knowledge in organizations. The idea of such system is to enable employees to have ready access to the organization's documented base of facts, sources of information, and solutions. Hence, knowledge management systems also provide a natural framework for storing medicinal instructions.

A gain of knowledge management system is that it provides unified means for data management for various kinds of applications such as CRM (Customer Relationship Management) system, SCM (Supply Chain Management) system, Content management system and Learning content management systems. Conceptually a knowledge base is a single data store which includes all the relevant information that is stored and accessed in the organization.

In our case, the workflow engine which integrates the instructions with daily tasks accesses the medicinal ontology through the knowledge base. The idea of a knowledge base and a shared ontology is illustrated in Figure 5.

Figure 5. The users of knowledge base

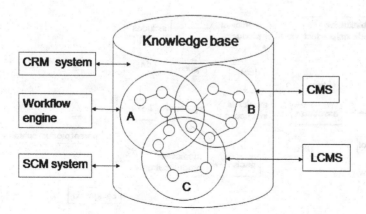

The information entities (small circles) inside circle *A* are accessed by the Workflow engine, the information entities inside circle *B* are managed by the CMS, and the information entities inside circle *C* are managed by the LCMS, i.e., circle *C* represents the learning object ontology. The edges between the information entities represent the associations between them. Such associations are illustrated in the *Information entity* ontology the part of which is presented in Figure 6.

The ontology includes for example the following information: *Regulation* is a subclass of the class *information entity*, each instance of the subclass regulation has property *validity*, and it may replace some other regulation. Further, each regulation is published by a *medicinal author*.

Further, the class *Information entity* has four subclasses, which are *regulation*, *announcement*, *recommendation* and *learning object*. Each subclass represents information that is used in specific tasks. The relationship of the tasks and information entities is presented by the property *relatesTo*. When the workflow engine coordinates the execution of a task it uses the Information entity ontology in querying the information entities that are associated (relatesTo) to that task.

For example, in coordinating the task "Check the dose" the workflow engine submits a query "Give the URLs of the information entities that are associated to the task Check the dose", and then after the query is processed, the links of the related instructions are provided for the user. Then the user may open the entities by clicking the provided URLs. The location of an information entity may be in any organization. Further, the entity may be in a human readable form such as in HTML (Daconta et al., 2003), or in machine readable form such as in XML (Daconta et al., 2003).

Using OWL for Presenting Ontologies

The OWL Web Ontology Language OWL (OWL, 2003) is intended to be used when the information contained in documents needs to be processed by applications, as opposed to situations where the content only needs to be presented to humans. OWL can be used to explicitly represent the meaning of terms in vocabularies and the relationships between those terms. This representation of terms and their interrelationships is called an ontology.

Figure 6. Information entity ontology

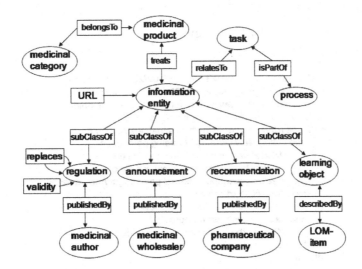

OWL has more facilities for expressing meaning and semantics than XML, RDF and RDF Schema (RDFS, 2000), and thus OWL goes beyond these languages in its ability to represent machine interpretable content of the ontology (Mattocks, 2009). In particular, it adds more semantics for describing properties and classes, for example relations between classes, cardinality of relationships, and equality of classes and instances.

The instances in OWL-ontologies are presented by RDF-descriptions, and thus we can query them by query languages developed for RDF, e.g., by SPARQL (SPARQL, 2008), which is standardized by the RDF Data Access Working Group (DAWG) of the World Wide Web Consortium, and is considered a component of the semantic web. On January 2008, SPARQL became an official W3C Recommendation.

There are various ways in capturing knowledge with RDF, e.g., as natural language sentence, in a simple triple notation called N3, in RDF/XML serialization format, and by as a graph of the triples (Davies et al., 2002). For example, the statement

"New warnings of using pain drugs in topical use with children deals the medicinal products Pain drugs for topical use."

is a natural language sentence that can be presented by RDF/XML serialization format (Figure 7) by using the vocabulary (ontology) presented in Figure 4. This description also states that the new instruction identified by *Instruction123* replaces the instruction identified by *Instruction122*. In addition, the description associates *Instruction123* to task named "Check the dose". How this association is presented in our used business process specification language is the topic of Section 5.

Storing Ontologies in Relational Database Systems

In a relational database, all data is stored and accessed via relations. A relation is defined as a set of tuples that have the same attributes. A tuple usually represents an object and information about that object. A relational database management system is a database management system that is based on the relational model.

We use relational database management system (Oracle) for storing our used ontologies, i.e., implementing the knowledge base. In principle, we represent each RDF-description element by a tuple of a relation. However, as we will see, in many cases due to the normalization requirements of the relations, we have to split each RDF-description into more than one relation.

Figure 7. An RDF-statement in a medicinal ontology

```
<rdf:RDF
      xmlns : rdf="http://www.w3.org/1999/02/22-rdf-syntax-ns#"
      xmlns : xsd="http://www.w3.org/2001/XMLSchema#"
      xmlns : mo="http://www.lut.fi/ontologies/medicinal_ontology#">
      <rdf:Description rdf:about=" # Instruction123">
      <rdf:type rdf:resource="&mo;medicinal_instruction"/>
         <mo : title> New warnings of using pain drugs
            in topical use with children </mo : title>
         <mo : deals>Pain drugs for topical use</mo : deals>
         <mo : deals> Prescription based pain drugs</mo : deals>
         <mo : replaces> rdf: resource
               Instruction122</mo : replaces>
         <mo : associates> rdf: resource
               Check_the_dose</mo : associates>
      </rdf : Description>
</rdf:RDF
```

First we have to transform the OWL ontology into a relational schema, which specifies the logical structure of the database. The schema specifies the names of the relations, their attributes, key constraints and constraints in general.

We follow the following rules in transforming the ontologies into relational schemas:

1. The name of the class is the name of the relation.
2. Each property of the class is an attribute of the relation.
3. The key of the relation is comprised of the identification of the class and of the identification of those classes that are in a multivalued relationship to the class.

In order to illustrate this consider the Information entity ontology presented in Figure 4. Information entity is a class in the ontology, and so the relation InformationEntity is created. According to the above rules its schema is the following: InformationEntity (URL, title, replaces, productId, categoryId, taskId)

The underlined attributes constitute the key of the relation. For example, product_id is underlined as the information entity may deal many medicinal products, i.e., it represents a multivalued relationship. In principle, we could insert the RDF_description of Figure 7 in this relation, but it would include redundant data as it is not in BCNF (Boice-Codd Normal Form) (Ullman & Widom, 1998). Therefore we have to normalize the relation before we can store the RDF-description. As a result of the normalization the original relation schema is partitioned into following four schemas, which are in BCNF.

InformationEntityA (URL, title, replaces,)
InformationEntityB (URL, productId,)
InformationEntityC (URL, categoryId)
InformationEntityD (URL, taskId)

Note that no relation schema itself does contain any semantics about the relationships of its attributes. To find such relationships one has to go to look the conceptual schema (ontology) from which the schema was derived. For example, the schema InformationEntityD contains attributes URL, and taskeId, but it indicates nothing about their relationships. However, from the ontology (Figure 4) we can see that the task which is stored at a given URL is associated to the given tasks.

ATTACHING LEARNING ONJECTS TO DAILY DUTIES

Using BPMN in Specifying Medical Processes

Though the original goal of using Business Process Modeling Notation (BPMN) (White, 2006; BPMN, 2009) is the automation of the coordination of business processes, we use it to model medicinal processes as well as their tasks associations to medicinal instructions.

The BPMN defines a Business Process Diagram (BPD), which is based on a flowcharting technique tailored for creating graphical models of business process operations. These elements enable the easy development of simple diagrams that will look familiar to most analysts. In addition BPMN allows an easy way to connect documents (e.g., medicinal instructions) and other artifacts to flow objects, and so narrows the gap between process models and conceptual models. Also, a notable gain of BPMN specification is that it can be used for generating executable BPEL (Business Process Execution Language) (BPEL, 2007) code.

We now give an overview of the BPMN. We first shortly describe the types of graphical objects that comprise the notation, and then we show how they work together as part of a BPD (White, 2006). After it, we give a simplified pharmaceutical process description using BPD.

In BPD there are tree Flow Objects: Event, Activity and Gateway:

- An Event is represented by a circle and it represents something that happens during the business process, and usually has a cause or impact.
- An Activity is represented by a rounded corner rectangle and it is a generic term for a task that is performed in companies. The types of tasks are Task and Sub-Process. So, activities can be presented as hierarchical structures.
- A Gateway is represented by a diamond shape, and it is used for controlling the divergence and convergence of sequence flow.

In BPD there are also three kind of connecting objects: Sequence Flow, Message Flow and Association.

- A Sequence Flow is represented by a solid line with a solid arrowhead.
- A Message Flow is represented by a dashed line with an open arrowhead and it is used to show the flow of messages between two separate process participants.
- An Association is represented by a dotted line with a line arrowhead, and it used to associate data and text with flow objects.

Attaching Learning Objects into Tasks

We have analyzed the automatic integration of medicinal instructions to business processes in two ways:

(i) by using medicinal ontologies that specify the associations of the instructions and the tasks, and

(ii) by analyzing the similarity of the instructions and tasks' metadata descriptions.

In order to illustrate the former approach, we first illustrate (Figure 8) how the process of producing electronic prescription can be represented by a

BPD, and how we use BPD's Association object to attach instructions to Activities and Gateways. For example, *Instruction A* is associated to activity "Produce prescription", and *Instruction B* is associated to gateway "Check negative effects".

The integration of instructions in this BPD is based on the medicinal ontology presented in Figure 4, where the associations of instructions and tasks are specified.

We can also use a more expressive ontology than then medicinal ontology presented in Figure 4. Its Information entity has subclasses Regulation, Announcement, Recommendation and Learning object. Therefore, if we use that ontology, then we do not attach just Instructions to tasks but rather information entities that are regulations, announcements, recommendations or learning objects. Such a case is illustrated in Figure 9.

The associations between information enti-

Figure 8. Attaching medicinal instructions to a BPD

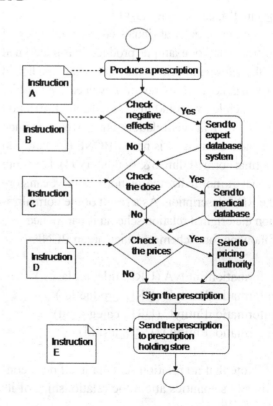

ties and tasks in a BPD are not determined by the business process designer but the workflow engine, which coordinates the execution of the process. In attaching instructions the workflow engine makes a query to the Knowledge base and requests the information entities that are attached to the task, and then based on the response the attaching (i.e., presenting the links of the actual entities for user) is done. From user point of view the association embodies in the links provided for the user. The user can then open the instruction(s) by just clicking the link(s).

If we do not have an ontology that specifies the associations of tasks and medicinal instructions then the integration of tasks and instructions can be made by comparing the similarities of the metadata descriptions of the instructions and the tasks. This requires that the metadata items of the workflow tasks are picked up from the same taxonomy that is used for annotating medicinal instructions. Hence we can conclude that an instruction is relevant for

Figure 9. Attaching information entities to a medicinal process

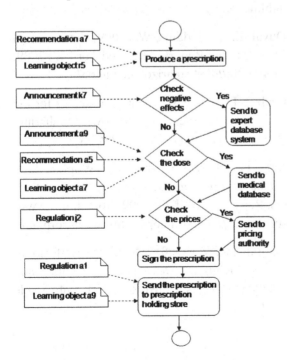

the task, if they have similar metadata description. That is, it is appropriate to integrate *Instruction I* to *Task T*, if they have somehow similar keywords. To illustrate this, assume that *Instruction I* has m keywords and *Task T* has m keywords, then they have at most min$\{m,n\}$ common keywords. So we can assume that the higher the number of the common keywords is, the better the *Instruction I* match for the *Task T*. Hence, we order the instructions of the *Task T* according to the number of their common keywords.

CONCLUSION

Healthcare is a field where the fast development of drug treatment and technologies requires specialized skills and knowledge. Also medical knowledge as well as the amount of new instructions concerning new medication is expanding all the time. As a result neither the physicians nor other workers in the health care sector can keep up without the help of modern information and communication technology. How to ensure that healthcare staff is aware of the new instructions is not an easy task. However, applying computing technology for retrieving and disseminating medicinal information this complexity can be alleviated in many ways.

We have investigated various ways to acquire the information that is required in daily work patterns. We first considered taxonomy-based and ontology-based retrieving of medicinal instructions. It is turned out that by deploying ontology-based retrieving method the expression power of searching expressions can be increased. Further the quality of information retrieval can be improved by ontology-based retrieval. On the other hand, the drawback of ontology-based searching is that the ontology must be updated whenever a new medicinal instruction is published. However, such an update can be done by medicinal authorities, and thus it does not burden the medicinal organizations that use the ontology.

We have also investigated how the dissemination of medicinal instructions can be carried out by integrating the learning objects and other relevant information entities with daily tasks. The gain of this approach is that dissemination processes are integrated in a natural way into day-to-day work patterns, and thereby minimize the extra time required for retrieving the instructions. In particular we consider keyword-based integration and ontology-based integration. Which of these methods is appropriate depends on whether there is an ontology that specifies the associations between tasks and information entities. It is obvious that by using ontology-based integration the quality of integration is much better, i.e., less non relevant entities are associated and less relevant entities are omitted to integrate.

An important requirement of ontology based solutions is that the used ontology must be shared and consensual terminology as it is used for information sharing and exchange. In our analyzed case it means that the communicating parties such as pharmacies, medicinal authors, medicinal wholesalers and pharmaceutical companies have to commit to the same ontology. It, however, does not require, the introduction of a universal ontology for the healthcare sector. This situation is analogous with natural languages: a pharmacy, or any medicinal organization, may communicate in Finnish with medicinal authorities and in English with pharmaceutical companies. Just as there is no universal natural language, so there is no universal ontology.

The introduction of a new technology in retrieving and disseminating medicinal instructions is also an investment. The investment on new ICT-technology includes a variety of costs including software, hardware and training costs. Introducing and training the staff on new technology is a notable investment, and hence many organizations like to cut on this cost as much as possible. However, the incorrect usage and implementation of a new technology, due to lack of proper training, might turn out to be more expensive in the long run.

REFERENCES

Antoniou, G., & Harmelen, F. (2004). *A semantic web primer*. The MIT Press.

Baeza-Yates, R., & Ribeiro-Neto, B. (1999). *Modern Information Retrieval*. New York: Addison Wesley.

BPEL. (2007). *Business Process Execution Language for Web Services*. Retrieved April 22, 2009, from, http://www.ibm.com/developerworks/library/specification/ws-bpel/

BPMN. (2009). *Business Process Modeling Notation (BPMN)*. Retrieved April 22, 2009, from http://www.bpmn.org/

Daconta, M., Obrst, L., & Smith, K. (2003). *The semantic web*. Indianapolis: John Wiley & Sons.

Davies, J., Fensel, D., & Harmelen, F. (2002). *Towards the semantic web: ontology driven knowledge management*. John Wiley & Sons.

Dublin Core. (2009). The Dublin Core Metadata Initiative. Retrieved April 22, 2009, from, http://dublincore.org/

Duval, E., & Hodgins, W. (2009). International LOM Survey: Report. Retrieved April 22, 2009, from, http://dlist.sir.arizona.edu/403/

Gruber, T. R. (1993). Toward principles for the design of ontologies used for knowledge sharing. *Padua workshop on Formal Ontology*.

Jung, F. (2009). XML-based prescription drug database helps pharmacists advise their customers. Retrieved April 22, 2009, from, http://www.softwareag.com/xml/applications/sanacorp.htm

Lamminaho, V. (2000). Metadata specification: Forms, Menus for Description of Courses and All Other Objects. CUBER project: Deliverable D3.1

LOM. (2004). *Learning Object Metadata*. Retrieved April 22, 2009, from, http://ltsc.ieee.org/wg12/

Mattocks, E. (2009) Managing Medical Ontologies using OWL and an e-business Registry / Repository. Retrieved April 22, 2009, from, http://www.gca.org/xmlusa/2004/slides/mattocks&dogac/Mattocks%20-%20Managing%20Medical%20Ontologies%20using%20OWL%20and%20an%20e-business%20Registry%20%20Repository.ppt

MetaMap. (2009). *Meta Map Portal*. Retrieved April 22, 2009, from http://metamap.nlm.nih.gov/

Najjar, J., Ternier, S., & Duval, E. (2003). The Actual Use of Metadata in ARIADNE: an Empirical Analysis. *3rd Annual Ariadne Conference*, K.U.Leuven, Leuven, Belgium.

OWL. (2003). *WEB Ontology Language*. Retrieved April 22, 2009, from http://www.w3.org/TR/owl-ref/

Puustjärvi, J. (2004). Integrating e-Learning Systems. *Proc. of the International Conference on Web-Based Education* (pp. 417-421).

Puustjärvi, J., & Pöyry, P. (2003). Searching learning objects from virtual universities. In *Proc. of the International Workshop on Multimedia Technologies in e-Learning and Collaboration (WOMTEC)*.

Puustjärvi, J., & Puustjärvi, L. (2006). The challenges of electronic prescription systems based on semantic web technologies. In *Proc. of the 1st European Conference on eHealth* (pp. 251-261).

RDFS. (2000). *Resource Description Framework (RDF) Schema Specification 1.0*. Retrieved April 22, 2009, from http://www.w3.org/TR/2000/CR-rdf-schema-20000327/

SPARQL. (2008). *SPARQL Query Language for RDF*. Retrieved April 22, 2009, from http://www.w3.org/TR/rdf-sparql-query/

Ullman, J., & Widom, J. (1998). *Principles of Database Systems*. Prentice Hall.

White, A. (2006). *Introduction to BPMN*, Retrieved April 22, 2009, from http://www.bpmn.org/Documents/Introduction%20to%20BPMN.pdf

Chapter 9
Personal Health Information in the Age of Ubiquitous Health

David Wiljer
University Health Network, Canada

Sara Urowitz
University Health Network, Canada

Erin Jones
University Health Network, Canada

ABSTRACT

We have long passed through the information age into an information perfusion in health care, and new strategies for managing it are emerging. The ubiquity of health information has transformed the clinician, the public, and the patient, forever changing the landscape of health care in the shift toward consumerism and the notion of the empowered patient. This chapter explores essential issues of ubiquitous health information (UHI), beginning with its origins in the explosion of health information and the advent of new technologies. Challenges of UHI include privacy issues, change management, and the lack of basic infrastructure. However, benefits for patients include improvements in access to information, communication with providers, prescription renewals, medication tracking, and the ability to self-manage their conditions. Benefits at the organizational level include increased patient satisfaction, continuity of care, changes in costing models and improved standardization of care as organizations streamline processes to address this change in clinical practice.

INTRODUCTION

In health care the "information age" has long passed and we have entered into the era of information perfusion. The ubiquity of health information has transformed the clinician, the public, and the patient. As technology progresses and we see exciting and innovative strategies for managing it emerge, ubiquitous health information (UHI) has brought on a tectonic shift that will forever change the landscape of health care.

This chapter explores the essential issues of UHI: the debates and controversies, the risks and benefits, and efforts that must be made to manage them. To begin, we trace the origins of UHI – the rise and explosion of several genres of health information in

DOI: 10.4018/978-1-61520-777-0.ch009

Copyright © 2010, IGI Global. Copying or distributing in print or electronic forms without written permission of IGI Global is prohibited.

conjunction with the evolution of new technologies. We look at the definition and components of UHI, the types of health information that are available, and the methods for their exchange. We also explore the rise of consumerism and the notion of empowered patients within the context of ubiquitous health information.

The chapter also examines the role of UHI in the changing landscape of health care. We investigate the growing number of social, economic, cultural, ethical and legal issues, as technologies allow for the dissemination and exchange of personal health information. The impact of the perfusion of information on the public and patient is explored, as well as its impact on health professionals and the type of care delivered, and the new and alternative environments in which it is carried out. The benefits and the risks of UHI are discussed, including the educational, clinical and research opportunities. And finally, we offer a consideration of future research directions, and potential frameworks for the evaluation and assessment of UHI.

BACKGROUND

Ubiquitous Heath Information Today: Towards a Definition

The perfusion of health information today can be overwhelming. Health information is now everywhere, all the time. We see messages about our health from television, radio, newspapers, the Internet, billboards and advertising. Health services and health products are an enormous industry, and controlling the messages is an ongoing battle between multiple interest groups that is being waged at the expense of those individuals who need it most – the public and the patients. Media and web sites are becoming battlegrounds over major health issues of the twenty-first century, ranging from circumcision and vaccinations to novel and alternative treatments. The social and financial stakes are high, and information flows at a rate that is almost incomprehensible.

As new strategies for navigating this sea of information develop, so our ability to generate more information increases, contributing to this state of UHI. The emergence of new technologies, and the changing expectations of health care consumers have each influenced the explosion of UHI, both in their own right, and through an intricate relationship to each other.

It is evident that healthcare has experienced a shift toward consumerism and the notion of the empowered patient. Patients and the public are no longer satisfied with the status quo and a growing wave of public and patient expectation is mounting (Ball, Costin, & Lehmann, 2008; Hassol et al., 2004; Leonard, Casselman, & Wiljer, 2008; Leonard & Wiljer, 2007; Pyper, Amery, Watson, & Crook, 2004; Wiljer et al., 2006). The traditional health care system that was characterized by the physician driven model, an insular system of practice that neither had the means nor the inclination to share expert knowledge, is now a thing of the past. Today, patients are acknowledged as expert consumers. Health care providers work in partnership with their patients to make shared decisions, and there is the growing global trend of adopting legislation to ensure that patients are able to access, review, and amend their medical record (Beardwood & Kerr, 2005; Blechner & Butera, 2002; Chasteen, Murphy, Forrey, & Heid, 2003; Dietzel, 2002; France & Gaunt, 1994; Harman, 2005; Ishikawa et al., 2004; Jones, 2003; Kluge, 1993; Mathews, 1998; Mitchell, 1998; Pyper, Amery, Watson, Crook, & Thomas, 2002). As a result, the information asymmetry that once existed between health care professionals and the health care consumer is now significantly diminished and UHI is pervasive.

At the same time, technology is advancing. The role of information and communications technologies (ICTs) in health care is growing, and evidence of this trend is all around us. Research has shown that the number of MEDLINE citations for "Web-based therapies" showed a 12-fold increase between 1996 and 2003 (Wyatt & Sullivan, 2005). There are virtual health networks and electronic health records (EHRs) being used to coordinate the delivery of services, and knowledge management ICTs used to establish care protocols, scheduling, and information directories. ICTs are also increasingly seen as a key element of consumer-based health education, and the delivery of evidence-based clinical protocols (Branko, Lovell, & Basilakis, 2003). Health care teams are finding increases in efficiency and efficacy when new technologies help to manage patient data and provide a method of coordinating team members' interactions (Wiecha & Pollard, 2004).

There are many potential benefits to be realized by effective use of UHI. Patient benefits include better access to health information, increased ability to self-manage chronic health conditions, increased medication tracking, safer prescription renewals, and improved connections for patients and providers (Ball, Smith, & Bakalar, 2007; Tang, Ash, Bates, Overhage, & Sands, 2006). Potential benefits at the professional level include increased patient satisfaction, continuity of care, changes in costing models and improved standardization of care as organizations streamline processes and information to address this change in clinical practice (Ball et al., 2007; Tang et al., 2006). There are still a number of barriers to overcome, including privacy and security issues, change management issues, and the lack of basic infrastructure such as EHRs (Tang et al., 2006).

UHI has transformed the entire concept of health, and we are seeing rapid changes in the health delivery system. One prominent idea is the prospect of chronic disease management and self-managed care, facilitated through UHI. This ambition has inspired a growing interest in harnessing the power of EHRs beyond the point of care delivery. Health care organizations are also realizing the potential benefits of patient accessible health records (PAEHRs), including improving

the patient experience, supporting patients with chronic conditions, improving transparency, increasing referral rates, and ensuring the continuity of care beyond the hospital walls.

THE HISTORY OF UHI: HOW DID WE GET HERE?

Health Care Consumerism

The role of the patient has been impacted by societal influences, starting with the Civil Rights movement and continuing through the 1980's and beyond. Expectations are changing, and patients are no longer seen to be passive recipients of health care information, but rather are considered to be health care consumers who actively seek out, and more recently, create knowledge (Cresci, Morrell, & Echt, 2004; Urowitz & Deber, 2008).

Shared Decision Making

As consumers of health care, people are more invested in actively participating in their care and making informed health care choices. This is commonly referred to as shared decision making (Charles, Gafni, & Whelan, 1997; Deber, Kraetschmer, Urowitz & Sharpe, 2005; Deber, Kraetschmer, Urowitz & Sharpe 2007).

Effective shared decision-making requires that people are able to access and understand large amounts of complex medical and health related information. Once, this would have been a daunting task for most individuals. It would require trips to specialized libraries, an understanding of professional textbooks, and synthesizing large amounts of information from both traditional and non-traditional sources. Now, the pervasiveness of technology-supported health information has simplified shared decision-making. Video, CD-ROMs and the Internet have brought health information more into the public domain, making expert information available to the masses.

Decision aids are one possibility for supporting health care consumers through this process. Decision aids provide health information to help people understand their options, and to consider the personal importance of possible benefits and harms (O'Connor et al., 2002). Like in prostate cancer, they are most helpful when there is more than one medically reasonable option. Information in decision aids was traditionally delivered through pamphlets and more recently through videos, CDs and Internet based programs. For instance, the Ottawa Health Research institute offers a decision aids page (http://decisionaid.ohri.ca) that allows the public to search their inventory of decision aids, or download a generic decision strategy sheet, which can be applied to the process of making any health decision.

Shared decision making has been greatly facilitated by the introduction of the Internet, which has enabled health care consumers to independently seek out information that ranges from the layperson's to the expert's level. The National Library of Medicine in the United States has a section of their web page (www.nlm.nih.gov) designated "especially for the public" where users can find current and accurate health information for patients, families and friends.

The Chronic Care Model and Chronic Disease Management

The welcoming of patients' participation in their own care, combined with the abundance of health related information available through the Internet, is continuing to drive a shift in the delivery of health care and increasing the demand for accessible, timely and relevant health information. We are moving away from the clinician driven model of care toward a patient centred model, in which empowered patients are encouraged to play an active role, not only in the decision making process, but in their own care management. This model is particularly relevant to the growing segment of the population living with long-term chronic illnesses that require ongoing monitoring and treatment. The aging population and advances in modern medicine have resulted in larger numbers of people living longer and experiencing more chronic illnesses, many dealing with multiple conditions at the same time (Orchard, Green, Sullivan, Greenberg, & Mai, 2008; Ralston et al., 2007). Whereas a disease such as cancer once had a high probability of mortality, people are now living longer, disease-free lives, even after a diagnosis of this once fatal condition (Hewitt & Ganz, 2006). The Chronic Care Model (CCM) and the paradigm of chronic disease management (CDM) are responses to the changing health care needs of the population.

The Chronic Care Model suggests that optimal functional and clinical outcomes can be achieved in a system that supports productive interactions between informed clients, which includes patients, their families, and knowledgeable providers, who are working as part of a team with a client-centered focus (Wagner, 1998). CDM espouses the importance of people who are living with chronic illness taking responsibility for effectively managing their illness. People need to see themselves as active partners in their care with a keen understanding of what is best for them and their bodies, who can make behaviour changes through goal setting, but also know when to ask for help. Adopting this approach to disease management can result in overall improvements in long-term health (Lorig, Sobel, Ritter, Laurent, & Hobbs, 2001).

There are 5 steps to effective CDM 1) Identification of a problem 2) Goal setting 3) Planning ahead and considering obstacles to achieving goals 4) Determining confidence level for achieving the goal, and 5) Following up and staying connected with the health care team. Applying these 5 steps is an effective approach to changing behaviours. Since behaviour changes can be difficult to effect, access to UHI can facilitate knowledge sharing, education, and an understanding of the condition which are all factors in ensuring success (Wyatt & Sullivan, 2005).

CDM is most effective when coupled with personal empowerment interventions. These interventions might consist of education in improving individual decision-making, disease complication management, efficient use of health services, improved health behaviors, or life coping skills (Paterson, 2001; Wallerstein, 2006). Empowerment interventions aim to increase the capacity of individuals to make choices and transform those choices into desired actions and outcomes (Wallerstein, 2006). The empowerment facets of CDM include the promotion of new knowledge and skills, within a system that reinforces active participation (Lorig et al., 2001; Wallerstein, 2006), resulting in better health outcomes and improvements in quality of life for the chronically ill (Wallerstein, 2006).

UHI and the Management of Chronic Illness

The growth of technology and the appearance of UHI have had an impact on the rise of CDM, especially in terms of the increasing capacity to share information. Often, patients with chronic illnesses are seeing many physicians and specialists, who will all need access to their information. For example, a diabetes patient may be seeing his or her family doctor along with any number of specialists, including nephrologists, podiatrists, and ophthalmologists. All of these specialists may be prescribing various medications, ordering tests or making additional referrals to still other health care providers. Timely transmission of this information becomes key to maintaining good continuity of care, and now UHI is enabling the provision of this sort of care in a less fragmented manner (Anderson & Knickman, 2001).

In fact, the emerging goal for information technologies managing UHI is to be unobtrusive, seamlessly working in the background to provide users with value-added services (Pallapa & Das, 2007). As we approach this goal, technology is being more and more commonly applied to the home monitoring of vital signs for patients with chronic disease, and telemedicine is beginning to replace some home nursing visits (Branko et al., 2003). For example, remote patient monitoring for home haemodialysis utilized a system that that acquired, transmitted, stored and processed patient vital signs that were monitored according to algorithms that triggered alarms if intervention was required. In addition, the system included an IP-based pan-tilt-zoom video camera for clinical staff to observe remotely if the patient desired (Cafazzo, K.J, Easty, Rossos, & Chan, 2008). The hope is that UHI, coupled with the right technology, will be responsive to patient demand; ensuring that information can be personalized for the individual seeking it, and that services can be delivered at the time and the place they are needed (Wyatt & Sullivan, 2005).

Exchanging Health Information

The notion of technology assisted exchange of health information is not a new idea. It has been over four decades since physicians first started using interactive video as a way of providing and supporting health care when distances separated participants. This was one of the earliest forms of telemedicine, or the use of electronic information and communication technologies for the provision of health care. Most commonly telemedicine was restricted to the sub-specialities (Field & Grigsby, 2002), but as Internet technology progresses, and the growth of health consumerism increases, our expectations and information practices in health care are changing. Innovative means of communication that were once limited to sub-speciality health care providers are becoming more common place. Traditional ways of providing information are still in use in many health care institutions, but health care is slowly beginning to harness the power of the Internet to store, manage, exchange, and share information. More recently, the collaborative properties of Web 2.0 applications are making information sharing possible for a wide range of participants, including patients, providers, caregivers and researchers through the use of collaborative, adaptive, and interactive technologies (CAIT) that (1) facilitate collaboration among users in traditional or novel ways, (2) support adaptation of form, function, and content according to user needs or preferences, and (3) enable users to interact with the technology via mechanisms of explicit interaction (O'Grady et al., 2009).

Currently, there are already some guidelines in place for providing patients with information. Many jurisdictions have sophisticated legal requirements that protect not only the privacy of patients, but also their right to access this information in a timely and accessible manner (*Wiljer & Carter, In Press*). There are several obstacles to meeting these requirements using the traditional methods of delivering patient information; that is, locating a patient's file – either paper or electronic – and producing a hard copy of the information. There are often limited resources to dedicate to providing this information. Nurses and administrative staff already face a time crunch in dealing with the volume of their work. In addition, certain jurisdictions suggest that an explanation of medical terms be given along with the information (*Wiljer & Carter, In Press*). This is often not feasible for the same reasons: time constraints on overloaded staff, and a lack of infrastructure for providing the information. In some cases there may be pre-existing pamphlets or glossaries available; however, these resources contain very generic content which may or may not address the specific information the patient is looking for. The traditional methods of delivering information have always faced these barriers, but as information continues to proliferate, new strategies and, correspondingly, new challenges are coming to the fore.

Electronic Health Records (EHRs)

The pervasiveness of the Internet supports new methods for accessing patient information. Electronic Health Records (EHRs) are now increasingly being used to record and manage patient data. An EHR can be defined in its simplest form as a computerized version of a traditional health record. Detailed definitions can be more complex, however, as an EHR may contain patient's full medical record, or may be used only for recording certain aspects of care, such as lab results (Urowitz et al., 2008; Tang et al., 2006). EHRs can facilitate the sharing of information between health care providers and with in a health care system. This sharing of information is dependent upon the existence of interoperable systems. One promising approach is through the use of health level 7 (HL7), a message-based communication system implemented by an asynchronous common communication infrastructure between facilities with different EHRs (Berler, Pavlopoulos, & Koutsouris, 2004). HL7 is now commonly used as the standard interface for the exchange of health information.

The benefits of an EHR include that it can be made widely accessible, and that it can facilitate the integration of care by allowing all members of a particular patient's care team to access his or her information at need (Urowitz et al., 2008; Tang et al., 2006). However, the use of EHRs is still in its early stages in many health systems. A Canadian study in 2008 determined that over half of the nation's hospitals (54.2%) had some sort of EHR, but that only a very few had records that were predominantly electronic (Urowitz et al., 2008). In Japan, a similar study determined that most hospitals (92%) used computerized administrative systems, but few (21%) used electronic "official documents". Barriers to adoption became evident when professionals participating in the study reported that they expected efficiency and quality improvements from their EHR, but worried that the proposed system might be too complicated, threatening to slow down workflow or compromise patient privacy (Ishikawa et al., 2007). These types of barriers are of great interest, since having data in an electronic format is key to facilitating access to information.

Personal Health Records (PHRs)

The development of storing data in electronic formats opens up further opportunities to integrate information. As a compliment to EHRs, which increase accessibility for professionals, there are many proponents for the implementation of Personal Health Records (PHRs). Markle Foundation's Connecting For Health group, a public-private collaborative for interoperable health information structures, defined PHR as "An electronic application through which individuals can access, manage and share their health information, and that of others for whom they are authorized, in a private, secure and confidential environment" (Markle, 2003).

There is a broad spectrum of approaches to implementing a PHR. At its simplest, a PHR may allow a patient to enter, store, and access his or her own information in a stand-alone application. In a more integrated model, the PHR could allow patients to access the information stored in their provider's EHR, or even request appointments, renew prescriptions or communicate with their doctors online (Tang et al., 2006). PHRs can also provide a platform for communication between patients and health care providers. For example, Partners Group in Massachusetts supports the Patient Gateway. Patient Gateway allows patients to access an extract of their medical record and facilitates online communication through secure messaging with medical practices (Kittler et al., 2004).

The actual benefits of PHRs are being researched and documented. In a study by Wuerdeman et al (2005) it was found that medical records are often incomplete, missing data from certain test results, for example. Patient-reported data became

very useful in these situations, as practitioners who need comprehensive information must often ask the patient if they have had a certain test, or what the results were. While patients' ability to report specific numeric test results did prove less accurate than information found in the medical record, patients were more reliable in reporting the absence or presence of a test and whether or not it fell in the normal range. In addition, patients were able to report problems that may not have appeared in the symptom list of the official record, such as depression (Wuerdeman et al., 2005).

Sharing Personal Information and Web 2.0

Patients uploading their own information would not only enable the sharing of information with their doctors, but also with one another. Traditionally, patients who wished to share information about their illness joined support groups or found other ways of meeting face-to-face. This is changing with the spread of Web 2.0 culture. Web 2.0 is a somewhat nebulous concept that is coming to be defined as a general spirit of open sharing and collaboration (Giustini, 2006). Generally, the idea is that the web can act as more than a unidirectional method of publishing information. Information can travel back and forth, and users are able to both access what they need as well as contribute what they have to share. Wikipedia, an information resource that functions as an encyclopaedia that anyone can contribute to, is a well-known example of the Web 2.0 philosophy. The proliferation of these Web 2.0 technologies is adding a new exponential dimension to UHI.

We are seeing the use of Web 2.0 technologies in health care, especially wikis and blogs (a contraction of web logs). A wiki is a website that allows multiple users to enter information, acting as a repository of information from different resources, as well as a mode of discussion about the information added. For example, Healthocrates. com is a health care wiki that offers free membership and encourages anyone and everyone to join and become a collaborator. Healthocrates claims to be home to over 8,500 articles, adding 500 to 1,000 new items each month. "Articles" include all types of media, from video and images, to discussion forums and case reports.

A blog is another type of website, containing regular entries, much like an online diary. Blogs allow their authors to write articles, or even post personal videos, as well as have discussions with readers in the form of posted comments in a miniature forum, which generally appears below the day's entry. Patients and clinicians alike have been known to blog. One well known example is Ves Dimov's *Clinical Cases and Images*, which offers a reliable "one stop shopping" location for health news and research findings taken from the web daily (Giustini, 2006). Specialized and reliable sources like these can be helpful in reducing the time patients and professionals spend wading through ubiquitous health information on the web. The introduction of UHI, and collaborative technologies such as blogs and wikis is contributing to a new phenomenon of the democratization of health information. Information that was once firmly in the strong hold of the hierarchical health system is much more freely exchanged.

Types of Health Information

Even as our abilities to store, exchange, and seek out information change, the information itself is changing. As technology increases, our ability to manage large amounts of information, and as the value of different kinds of information is becoming recognized, we are seeing information that is increasingly specific and personalized joining stores of information that were once predominantly generic. Leonard et al. have argued that there is an identifiable information paradigm for patients who are actively managing their health, especially those patients managing chronic conditions (Leonard, Wiljer, & Urowitz, 2008). The paradigm encompasses several distinct informa-

tion types, including general health information, and personal health information and experiential health information.

General Health Information

General health information is very pervasive. A visit to a family physician can result in large amounts of information about a wide variety of health issues, from screening programs for a wide array of diseases to lifestyle choices and concerns. General health information covers a wide spectrum, and is usually basic information about a health issue (i.e. obesity), a condition, (i.e. diabetes), or medications, (i.e. diuretics or beta blockers). This information is intended to provide a starting point to give a layperson a basic understanding of a particular aspect of health. The literature shows that many patients are still most likely to seek information directly from physicians (Rutten, Arorab, Bakosc, Azizb, & Rowland, 2005). However, information is not always clear during a clinical encounter, which is often short and overwhelming, with large quantities of information being exchanged.

Traditionally, patients left their physician's office with the essential health information that they have heard from the physician or nurse reinforced by a pamphlet or a brochure. However, new technologies now provide important alternative sources of information. The Internet has changed the dynamic of general health information. The notion of searching for information, or turning to "Dr. Google", has been commonplace for many individuals. The pervasiveness of general health information is astounding; for example, type "diabetes" into Google and in a tenth of a second, 96,800,000 hits are returned, "asthma" 30,900,000, "cancer" 232,000,000. At that rate, if you looked at each page for a second, it would take 7 years to view all of the information on cancer. The amount of health information on the Internet alone is beyond ubiquitous and will only continue to grow at an astounding rate.

Figure 1. Caring to the end of life

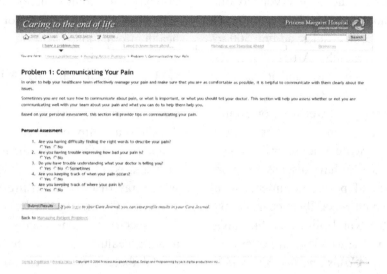

There are, of course, many different types of general information available on the Internet, and they vary greatly in quality and reliability. Many sites offer static content that is updated at regular or irregular intervals. Other sites have been developed to be more dynamic, offering tools and resources to help patients find information much more specific to their particular circumstances. For example, a palliative care site, www.CaringtotheEnd.ca, allows patients and family members to complete questionnaires based on a series of questions and then provides specific information to meet the needs of the user (Figure 1).

Several technologies have also been developed to enhance the exchange of general health information between patients and clinicians. For example, a patient education prescription system, known as PEPTalk, (Figure 2, 3) has been developed, that allows physicians to prescribe general health information to their patients (Atack, Luke, & Chien, 2008).

Personal Health Information

It is evident that general health information has become ubiquitous, and certainly the advent of new technologies has improved access to it. None-theless, this of type information is of a general nature and does not provide patients with access to the information that is directly relevant to their particular situation. One of the promises of new technologies is to provide people with access to their own information. As an example, this type of access has clearly revolutionized the banking industry with the advent of online banking. Yet the health care industry, overall, has been much more reluctant to embrace these types of technologies.

Over the last decade, however, there has been a growing interest in utilizing new technologies

Figure 2. PEPTalk - clinician view

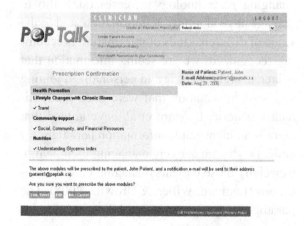

Figure 3. PEPTalk – patient view

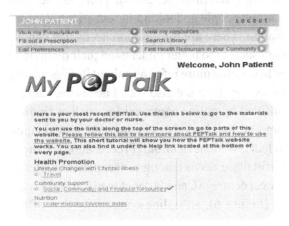

to improve access to personal health information. This type of information generally includes an individual's physical or mental health and family history, documentation of provided care, a care or service plan as well as administrative data (Cavoukian, 2004). For the moment, personal health information has the potential to be accessible anywhere the user is, but the promise has not yet been fully realized.

In 2005, a collaboration began in Canada between Shared Information Management System (SIMS) Partnership and the Weekend to End Breast Cancer (WEBC) Survivorship Program began. The project was a an online portal called

InfoWell, designed specifically to empower cancer patients to be active partners in their care, to participate in self-management activities and to find the support and resources they need in dealing with long-term consequences of their illness and treatment. Built using a commercially available patient portal as a foundation and customized by SIMS system engineers, InfoWell provides general health information as well as personal health information, which encompasses patient-generated information including a patient profile, medication lists, and treatment history (Figure 4). InfoWell also allows patients to view elements of their own EHR (Figure 5) (Leonard, Wiljer, & Urowitz, 2008).

Experiential Health Information

From an early age, many of us glean valuable health information from our parents, siblings, teachers, and physicians. We learn important life lessons about things like diet, nutrition, exercise, and personal hygiene. Some of this "experiential" information is based on scientific evidence, and some of it based on family folklore, but it will all have a large impact on our lifestyle choices. It is amazing how a story or experience that a family member has when we are young can influence the

Figure 4. InfoWell – patient-generated PHR

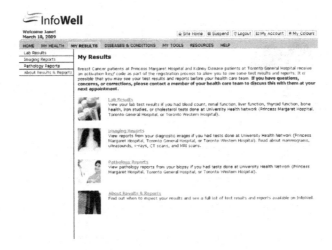

day-to-day decisions that we make. The ubiquity of health experience and health information informs the very essence of who we are, whether we are always conscious of it or not.

There is a specific type of experiential information that is of particular interest to most patients: the experiences and feelings of others with the same or similar conditions. Online communities are on the rise as a new way of finding and sharing this kind of information; 84% of Internet users participate in online groups, and 30% of these participants are members of medical or health related groups

(Johnson & Ambrose, 2006). There are several reasons people go looking for experiential information. There are information needs that can be met, such as to better understand their diagnosis, or to become more informed about its treatments. However, there are also social needs that can be fulfilled by online communities, such as finding support, helping others in the same situation, or to feel less alone or afraid (Preece, 2000). To help fulfill these needs among cancer patients, a large cancer centre in Canada developed CaringVoices. ca (Figure 6), an online community that offers

Figure 5. InfoWell, my health – access to EHR

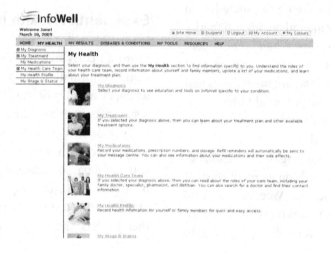

Figure 6. Caring voices

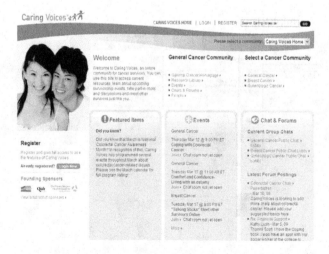

support for people living with cancer and their caregivers. CaringVoices.ca provides access to current educational resources, peer support, and advice and education from health care and community experts. There is also a people-matching function that allows members of the community to connect and share experiential information. A real-time chat function enables social networking between patients, as well as discussions hosted by health care professionals, volunteer cancer survivors, and staff from community cancer agencies.

There are several benefits to patients' participation in online communities. A major cause of non-compliance with a care plan is a lack of understanding of the treatment. Online communities offer patients a place to share information and foster a greater understanding of the process; they also offer a chance to connect for patients who are separated by distance or time. This is especially helpful to those who live in rural areas or may be homebound due to illness. The holistic approach to most online communities might also help to ease the burden on the health care system of patients who might otherwise over utilize the health care system. There are potential research benefits, as well. Observing interactions between large groups of patients provides an unobtrusive method of gathering information. Patterns in discussions may emerge, producing useful information about topics like adverse drug reactions, or clustering of disease types within age groups or geographical locations (Johnson & Ambrose, 2006).

The use of online communities can also have drawbacks. Especially viewed from a standpoint of ubiquitous health information, there is concern that patients may be unable to find reliable resources, and may even be mislead by inaccurate information. As a response to this, there are many communities that now offer question-and-answer periods with a real physician. However, it has been argued that these too are insufficient, as the doctors leading these sessions do not treat the patient, and have no information as to their

particular medical background (Preece, 2000). As such, it is important that patients have reliable means of way-finding through such vast expanses of ubiquitous information.

BENEFITS AND RISKS: WHERE ARE WE NOW?

We have traced the history of UHI and gained some insight into the different circumstance and events that have led to the vast amounts of information that surround us today. In our exploration, we have touched on the idea that one of the major benefits of growth in both technology and levels of information, is the potential to personalize. With the management of large amounts of personal information, however, also comes risk. It is important to critically examine both the risks and benefits that face us today in order to ensure that in the future we can properly take advantage of the opportunities as well as manage our risks.

Benefits of Personal Health Information

Once personal information has been captured, the benefits that can be realized from utilizing it correctly are substantial. Personal information is more and more commonly found in electronic format. This development opens up possibilities for technologies that can improve access and transportability of information, and in turn, help patients to engage as members of their own care team.

Access to Information

As the role of the modern patient continues to shift toward the idea of the empowered consumer, there is an increasing demand for access to, and control over, personal information. Leonard, Wiljer and Urowitz (Leonard, Wiljer, & Urowitz, 2008), estimate that 40- 45% of the population in the

United States and Canada are chronic illness patients with a strong desire for information on their condition. Members of this demographic group are knowledgeable about the health care system and eager to bypass the painstaking traditional methods of getting access to information. Wagner estimated that 40% of the population accounts for 70-80% of health care spending globally (Wagner, 1998). These numbers suggest that there are huge potential financial savings to be made by helping patients to manage their own health (Leonard et al., 2008).

It has been shown, however, that improving access to information can introduce benefits beyond cost reduction. In 2003 an award-winning project entitled *Getting Results* focused on the potential benefits of providing electronic access to laboratory results for haematology patients who spend long periods of time waiting in the hospital for these results. Patients and professionals alike saw benefits from the approach. Staff identified potential benefits such as improved workflow, decreased workload and a lower occurrence of unnecessary hospital visits (Wiljer et al., 2006).

Transportability

Another benefit of the electronic management of personal health information is that it becomes *transportable*. Information that is more easily transported, is also more easily shared. Some independent or "untethered" ways of storing data are quite physically transportable: smart card technology, USB drives, or CDs, for example (Tang et al., 2006).

Information that is "tethered" to a network, or stored online, can also be easy to share (Tang et al., 2006). The communication benefits of this can be seen in all types health care relationships; patient to provider, provider to provider, and patient to patient. Information that can be passed freely between patient and care provider changes care from episodic visits to a continuous process, and could dramatically reduce the

time taken to address medical problems (Tang et al., 2006). In the relationship between separate providers, interoperable systems could virtually eliminate the need for paper and make important patient records instantly available in any facility involved in treatment, resulting in efficiencies and quality improvements in care (Gloth, Coleman, Philips, & Zorowitz, 2005). Additional benefits are seen when information can be passed easily from patient to patient. With the advent of Web 2.0 technology, large numbers of people can now unite and collaborate (Deshpande & Jadad, 2006). Patients are able to find one another and create communities that allow them to feel less alone or anxious, offer each other support, and increase their understanding of the information they collect at a physician visit.

Self-Managed Care

Once information is personal (that is, specific to a given individual), and can be easily accessed by that individual as well as shared with care providers that need it, another avenue of patient empowerment opens up, through the possibility of self-managed care. Self-managed care involves the patient or non-professional caregiver (usually a close friend or family member) taking an active role in the patient's care. The degree to which a patient is involved can vary substantially from patient to patient: one patient may feel very comfortable in taking an active role, navigating the system and ensuring that they receive the care that is right for them. Another patient may want to participate in their care, but have much more involvement from their health care team.

The management of more clinical aspects of care, or self-care requires patients to have very specific knowledge and some training around a medical task. The type of self-care is, of course, often very specific to the type of disease that is being managed: for diabetes, it may be monitoring blood levels and taking insulin as required; for heart disease, it may be monitoring daily weight and controlling diet and intake of sodium; for breast cancer, it may monitoring activities to avoid infections and performing self-massage to control lymphedema. Advents in technology such as wearable monitoring technologies have made these tasks easier for people. As early as 1999, one set of researches have reported on a subminiature implantable device to provide remote monitoring of glucose levels and the ability to transmit the glucose concentration data to a corresponding receiver and computer (Beach, Kuster, & Moussy, 1999). Now monitoring devices connected to specialized computer modems are used to reliably measure and transmit physiological parameters including blood pressure, heart rate, blood glucose level, and pulse oximetry data (Field & Grigsby, 2002). Technologies such as portable monitoring devices, wearable sensors and even smart shirts can all be used for electronically support self-care (Tan, 2005).

RISKS OF UBIQUITOUS HEALTH INFORMATION

We have largely focused on the benefits and potential of UHI, but there are also risks to ubiquitous health information that can threaten an individual or their family, an organization or a community. UHI has the potential to lead to the loss of privacy for individuals, to security threats to organizations, and to the loss of social justice for communities and society. All of these risks have real implications and the use of electronic media pose risks at a much larger magnitude than paper. There have occasionally been errors in the safe disposal of paper records that lead to sensitive data appearing in inappropriate places, or the risk of losing a medical file, but the potential for wide scale breaches is much larger when dealing with electronic data. It is important therefore, to understand the risks and implications of the directions UHI is taking, in order to create protocols,

policies and procedures that will ensure that as the amount of health information grows, the risks are mitigated as much as possible.

In discussing the protection of information, it is useful to distinguish between the terms security, privacy, and confidentiality. Security, in all its contexts, refers to the notion of protection. In the case of sensitive information, it is the information itself that must be protected, by extension protecting the owner of that information. Security then, refers to the systems or means we use to ensure that access to protected information is appropriate. Privacy, in turn, deals with denying access that would not be appropriate, and determining policies for what information should be protected, and who should have access. Lastly, confidentiality refers to defining those situations where some access to personal data is appropriate (*Wiljer & Cater, In press*). Any person who is accessing data that they do not own is being held in confidence, and it is understood that they will use their access only in the manner and purpose that is intended (Schoenburg, 2005).

Risks to the Individual: Privacy

The greatest potential risks to the individual are around privacy issues. Awareness of these risks is increasing, and Internet users are beginning to protect their anonymity online. Members of the online community at PatientsLikeMe.com, who visit with the express purpose of sharing their information still tend to choose user names and avatars that represent them while keeping their identities anonymous. This may be especially desirable for patients living with illnesses such as HIV or mood disorders.

With respect to receiving care, the notion of privacy relates to the fiduciary relationship between the patient and individual members of their health care team. The majority of privacy issues relate to data in health records such as family history, diagnostic tests, treatment and medication records and clinical notes. In most circumstances the patient and provider relationship is a private one, nonetheless, there are complex ethical issues that, at times, can impact on an individual's right to privacy. Most jurisdictions have legislation that protect the rights of patients to privacy in general or specifically with respect to information pertaining to their health information. In the United States for example, the Health Insurance Portability and Accountability Act (HIPAA) protects personal health data.

Risks to Organizations: Security

UHI also has the potential to cause security risks for organizations. The potential for wide scale breaches is much larger when dealing with electronic data, than the risks involved with paper files; errors in the safe disposal of files or the risk of losing a medical record. It is because of this that is it so important to create protocols, policies and procedures that mitigate this risk as much as possible.

Data must be protected in three major domains: the server side, where information is stored; the network, through which it travels; and the client side, the place where the information is received and used (Schoenburg, 2005). Each of these domains will require different actions to protect the data. It is important to allot equal attention to creation of protocols for each domain, since a vulnerability at any point could be the area where a potential breach would occur. Yet it is also important to find a balance between security and the need to construct usable systems. Applications that are not easily understood and used, or that are not effective in the delivery of care invite "workaround" solutions from frustrated staff who have found more efficient ways to operate. Oftentimes, workaround solutions are indeed more efficient, but they may circumvent the security protocols that are in place, creating new vulnerabilities for information to leak through.

Risks to the Community: Social Justice and Equity

In addition to the issues affecting every day operations in health care, UHI has social implications on quite a broad scale. A survey in the United States (Brodie et al., 2000) shows that the Internet provides health information to large numbers of lower income, less-educated, and minority citizens. Nearly one-third of adults under age sixty are seeking such information online. And yet, there is still progress to be made. A digital divide still exists in terms of computer ownership. Lower income African Americans in the United States are far less likely than lower income whites to own a computer at home (Brodie et al., 2000) Once this barrier has been overcome, however, this study suggests that use of the internet to find health care information among computer-owners is similar across income, education, race, and age.

It is clear that online health information is key to closing these gaps and improving equity in access to information. When it comes to personal health information, however, there is a delicate balance between the desire for accessibility and the need for security. Breaches in security could result in the loss of social justice for entire communities. Delicate information that is not well protected can lead to financial threats, misinformation, fraudulent information, and even identify theft (Setness, 2003).

OPPORTUNITIES

The ubiquity of information is coming to be synonymous with increased accessibility, transportability, and capacity for detail. All of these important elements of information translate to health care opportunities on several levels. In education, personal data is enabling information to be tailored to the individual who needs it, making it more meaningful, and thereby improving learning. On the clinical level, personalized health and wellness programs are on the rise, offering the public the chance to engage as managers of their own health matters. And finally, in research, the opportunities for data mining the wealth of surrounding information are beginning to be realized, not only by health care professionals, but by patients who are eager for in-depth learning about their condition.

Opportunities in Education: Tailored Education

Health information is everywhere, but it can be delivered in a number of different ways, depending on who the target audience is and what the goals are for disseminating the information. The same basic kernel of information can evolve into several different key messages, when we are informed about who will be receiving it. For example, "don't smoke because it is harmful to your health" is a very generic piece of information. It applies to you whether you are male or female, 6 or 60, African American or Caucasian. One could argue it should be sufficient to influence behaviours. Yet, the United Nations predicts over 7.1 million tonnes of tobacco will be consumed in 2010 ("FAO Newsroom," 2004). Even with 6.7 billion people around the globe ("World Factbook," 2009), the number is staggering. So, the question arises whether or not a simple generic piece of information is sufficient to influence the behaviour of individuals.

Opportunities for the Clinic: Personal Health Programs

As developments like EHRs and Web 2.0 technologies allow us to make information more transportable, shareable, and specific to a particular individual, health care can become more and more personalized. Personal information gathered from health care professionals, and from patients themselves, can be combined with standard care

plans, transforming them into personal health programs.

An example of this type of synergistic effort can be found in employee wellness programs in the United States, where a partnership between CapMed and Staywell Health Management offers opportunities for managing personal health. CapMed offers PHR solutions that allow patients to monitor and manage their health information, while Staywell is a health assessment and disease management organization, creating wellness programs for employers. By adding the power of the personal information PHRs can capture, wellness programs can become personalized to a particular individual. Members will be able to access individually relevant patient education resources and set up health alerts and reminders. Additional health management tools are also available, including a drug interaction checker, data importer to collect information from remote health care systems, and authorizations that allow family members and caregivers to view all or part of the data a patient is storing ("CapMed and Staywell Health Managment Offer PHR/Wellness Program Presentations at AHIP 2008," 2008).

Opportunities in Research: Data Mining

It is difficult to consider the concept of ubiquitous health information in depth, without touching on the prospect of public health and surveillance. Public health is an issue that is currently booming, due to the events of the past decade. The anthrax threats that occurred after September 11th, and natural disasters such as hurricane Katrina and the Asian tsunami have raised awareness of the need for strengthened public health infrastructures (Kukafka, 2007). Spending has been increased for public health informatics in the United States, and research is showing that syndromes surveillance systems, which operate by collecting existing information by mining ubiquitous data are now capable of detecting some types of disease outbreaks quite rapidly. This trend of public health being increasingly tied to developments in informatics and the proliferation of health information and geographical information systems (GIS) (Tan, 2005) appears to be continuing as we move forward into the future. Prior to September 11th, 2001 a PubMed search for articles on "public health informatics" yielded only six results. In 2007, this same search resulted in over 600 articles (Kukafka, 2007).

The public health benefits of data mining go beyond prevention. There is also the potential for identifying areas for improvement in quality of care. As an example, a New York state initiative in 1979 began collecting data on all hospitalized patients (Setness, 2003). Ten years later, a report card was published giving comparisons of cardiac bypass surgery deaths, by hospital and surgeon. The statistics were a shock for staff at hospitals that did not score well in the report. This discovery led to the revamping of several cardiac surgery programs throughout the state.

Improvements to the system are not the only type of public health benefit; there are benefits to be seen on the level of the individual as well. Patients being treated for a wide spectrum of conditions are finding benefits from this capacity for data mining UHI. PatientsLikeMe.com, is a website open to the public, that offers patients being treated for a variety of illnesses the chance to form communities. The home page offers the visitor three options that sum up the motivations for seeking health information online: Share your experiences, find patients like you, and learn from others. The site also hosts message boards with postings on information on treatments and symptoms, although it is not clearly documented where the information originates from.

When they join, patients create their own PHR, by filling in information fields and posting their own data about their symptoms, treatments and outcomes. Of particular interest is the Research section of the site. The research team at

PatientsLikeMe have harnessed the self-reported information from the PHR aspects of the site. The data in these personal profiles is compiled and displayed graphically to the community in the form of symptom and treatment reports. Members can view these reports to gain a broader understanding of what an entire population of patients like themselves are experiencing. The site allows members to discuss these issues in forums, contact each other through private messaging, and post comments on each other's personal profiles (Frost, 2008).

Having such robust information has proved very valuable to patients. Being able to locate others with very specific experiences allows members to target information searching and sharing. Users could find the right person to ask a specific question to, and know who was likely to benefit most from hearing their own experiences. It became easier for patients to form relationships that were stronger and more edifying; when they were communicating with people they had much in common with (Frost, 2008).

FUTURE RESEARCH DIRECTIONS

The field of UHI is burgeoning. It is difficult to know which areas will really blossom as integral parts of the health care system. Certainly, the domain of EHRs and PHRs seems to be firmly taking root with the emergence of industry giants such as Google and Microsoft staking a claim to this virtual space. In other areas of social networking and information exchange, organizations such as *PatientsLikeMe* are transforming the paradigm for health information sharing in ways that are still not evident. What is clear is that there are many new and intriguing opportunities in this area. There are opportunities to implement solutions and services that will contribute to the empowerment of patients and their families and provide them with new opportunities to be active participants in control of their health care. Leadership in the health system is required to affect the required changes. Finally, research is essential to produce new evidence and new knowledge so that effective change can be made. Research is required into many, aspects of ubiquitous health information and this research needs to build on the growing literature in health informatics and information and communication technologies.

Benefits Evaluation and Research on UHI

Ubiquitous Heath Information poses several challenges to current models of the evaluation of health information. Many evaluation and research approaches of online resources and tools assume a relatively static, homogenous model. From this model, there are a series of assumptions made about the reliability and quality of the online resource. The very notion of ubiquitous information, however, suggests that this type of information is not only everywhere, but it is, at the same time, highly dynamic in nature. The current evaluation techniques, for the most part, depend on measuring a constant or static condition and, therefore, in the realm of ubiquitous health information, many of the current evaluation endpoints for online information must themselves be challenged and examined.

Evaluation and research models for online health information are based on the assumption that there is a "single" content provider. This may be one author, a group of authors, or an organization that can be identified as the source of content. Based on this assumption, a user of the information can employ a series of endpoints or parameters to assess the nature of the site. For example, the reliability of the site may be assessed based on the credibility of the source of the content. One may look at the credentials of the source, any conflicts of interest, publication record, and so on. However, if there are multiple authors who have no other association than being contributors to a collaborative site, such as a wiki

or community of practice, it is much more difficult to assess the "global" reliability of the content on a site. Each "fragment" of authored content must be assessed individually. Making matters somewhat more complex, it is not always easy to immediately identify the "voice" of an individual. For example, wiki technologies are designed to integrate the work of many authors into a single message within a set framework. Although many wiki sites track individual contributions, these unique contributions or content fragments are not always readily apparent to the reader. In the case of a wiki, assessing the reliability of the information may be more about assessing the ability of a wiki community to self-correct and self-monitor the quality of the information on its site than assessing the credentials or credibility of individuals generating the content.

Difficulties also arise when applying current assessment tools to the quality of an online resource. In assessing the usability of the site, there are often several distinct technologies stitched together in what are often referred to as "mashups". In assessing the usability of the platform or information communication technology, a new dimension of the evaluation may be required to assess not only the ease of use of the technology, but also the "integration" of information being aggregated from a number of sources. New models of evaluation are required that consider the exchange and flow of information.

These new models need to expand the parameters for evaluation and assessment. For example, the strength of an online community can be assessed by looking at the number of users, frequency of posting and quantity of collaboration. A shift in focus is also required to investigate health systems improvements that are linked to UHI. These improvements may include continuity of care, the quality of information provided, fewer duplicated tests and better surveillance. In addition, psychosocial outcomes need to be included, such as reductions in distress, anxiety and depression. Levels of patient empowerment, activation and participation also must be considered to incorporate adherence to guidelines and care plans, as well as improved self-efficacy and self-management.

CONCLUSION

Starting with general health information and the advent of the Internet, advances in technology and changes in the expectations of health care consumers have brought on a massive shift in the treatment of information in health care. We have moved from a focus on protecting and securing data to understanding how to provide equitable access to information in a safe and useful format. Health information is truly all around us, in many forms. The Age of the Internet has brought us dynamic social networking technologies and the spread of experiential health information, from video stories to the real-time exchange of health experiences.

Slowly, health care is beginning to enjoy the benefits of UHI, especially the potential to personalize care. Patients are seeing improvements in access to health information and communication with their providers, and beginning to take an active role in their care through easier prescription renewals, medication tracking, and the power of Internet technologies to empower those with chronic illness to self-manage their conditions. At the organizational level, we are starting to see increased patient satisfaction, better continuity of care, reductions in cost and improved standardization of care.

However, it is also important to properly manage the risks and opportunities that come with ubiquitous health information. We must remember the challenges, so that we may create policies that effectively manage the risks of privacy and security issues, and strive to overcome the barriers of change management and the lack of basic infrastructure in many areas. If we are to take full advantage of our opportunities and make sense of the "everywhere, all the time" presence of health information, researchers must create a roadmap for utilizing emerging technologies. This new map must plot a pathway that will ensure that these new, disruptive and transformative technologies will result in more effective and efficient health systems, in which patient outcomes and quality of life are dramatically improved.

REFERENCES

Anderson, G., & Knickman, J. (2001). Changing the chronic care system to meet people's needs. *Health Affairs*, *20*(6), 146–160. doi:10.1377/hlthaff.20.6.146

Atack, L., Luke, R., & Chien, E. (2008). Evaluation of Patient Satisfaction With Tailored Online Patient Education Information. *Computers, Informatics, Nursing*, *26*(5), 258–264. doi:10.1097/01.NCN.0000304838.52207.90

Bader, J., & Strickman-Stein, N. (2003). Evaluation of new multimedia formats for cancer communications. *Journal of Medical Internet Research*, *5*(5).

Ball, M. J., Costin, M. Y., & Lehmann, C. (2008). The personal health record: consumers banking on their health. *Studies in Health Technology and Informatics*, *134*, 35–46.

Ball, M. J., Smith, C., & Bakalar, R. S. (2007). Personal health records: empowering consumers. *Journal of Healthcare Information Management*, *21*(1), 76–86.

Beach, R. D., Kuster, F. V., & Moussy, F. (1999). Subminiature implantable potentiostat and modified commercial telemetry device for remote glucose monitoring. *Instrumentation and measurement. IEEE Transactions on*, *48*(6), 1239–1245.

Beardwood, J. P., & Kerr, J. A. (2005). Coming soon to a health sector near you: an advance look at the new Ontario Personal Health Information Protection Act (PHIPA): part II. *Healthcare Quarterly (Toronto, Ont.), 8*(1), 76–83.

Berler, A., Pavlopoulos, S., & Koutsouris, D. (2004). Design of an interoperability framework in a regional healthcare system. *Conference Proceedings. Annual International Conference of the IEEE Engineering in Medicine and Biology Society. IEEE Engineering in Medicine and Biology Society. Conference, 4*, 3093–3096.

Blechner, B., & Butera, A. (2002). Health Insurance Portability and Accountability Act of 1996 (HIPAA): a provider's overview of new privacy regulations. *Connecticut Medicine, 66*(2), 91–95.

Branko, C., Lovell, N., & Basilakis, J. (2003). Using information technology to improve the management of chronic disease. *The Medical Journal of Australia, 179*(5), 242–246.

Brodie, M., Flournoy, R., Altman, D., Blendon, R., Benson, J., & Rosenbaum, M. (2000). Health information, the Internet, and the digital divide. *Health Affairs, 19*(6), 255–265. doi:10.1377/hlthaff.19.6.255

Cafazzo, J. A. K.J, L., Easty, A., Rossos, P. G., & Chan, C. T. (2008). *Bridging the Self-Care Deficit Gap: Remote Patient Monitoring and the Hospital-at-Home.* Paper presented at the eHealth 2008.

CapMed and Staywell Health Managment Offer PHR/Wellness Program Presentations at AHIP 2008. (2008). Retrieved March 10, 2009, from http://www.bioimaging.com/assets/pdf/press_release/2008/2008-CapMed-Staywell-Collaborate.pdf

Cavoukian, A. (2004). *A Guide to the Personal Health Information Act.*

Charles, C., Gafni, A., & Whelan, T. (1997). Shared decision-making in the medical encounter: what does it mean? (or it takes at least two to tango). *Social Science & Medicine, 44*(5), 681–692. doi:10.1016/S0277-9536(96)00221-3

Chasteen, J. E., Murphy, G., Forrey, A., & Heid, D. (2003). The Health Insurance Portability and Accountability Act: practice of dentistry in the United States: privacy and confidentiality. [Electronic Resource]. *The Journal of Contemporary Dental Practice, 4*(1), 59–70.

Cresci, M., Morrell, R., & Echt, K. (2004). The Convergence of Health Promotion and the Internet. In Nelson, R., & Ball, M. (Eds.), *Consumer Informatics: Applications and Strategies in Cyber Health Care.* New York: Springer.

Deber, R. B., Kraetschmer, N., Urowitz, S., & Sharpe, N. (2005). Patient, consumer, client, or customer: what do people want to be called? *Health Expectations, 8*(4), 345–351. doi:10.1111/j.1369-7625.2005.00352.x

Deber, R. B., Kraetschmer, N., Urowitz, S., & Sharpe, N. (2007). Do people want to be autonomous patients? Preferred roles in treatment decision-making in several patient populations. *Health Expectations, 10*(3), 248–258. doi:10.1111/j.1369-7625.2007.00441.x

Deshpande, A., & Jadad, A. (2006). Web 2.0: Could it help move the health system into the 21st century? *Journal of Men's Health & Gender, 3*(4), 332–336. doi:10.1016/j.jmhg.2006.09.004

Dietzel, G. T. (2002). Challenges of telematics and telemedicine for health care: from e-Europe 2002 to the electronic health passport. *International Journal of Computerized Dentistry, 5*(2-3), 107–114.

Eysenbach, G. (2008). Medicine 2.0: Social Networking, Collaboration, Participation, Apomediation, and Openness. *Journal of Medical Internet Research, 10*(3). doi:10.2196/jmir.1030

Field, M. J., & Grigsby, J. (2002). Telemedicine and remote patient monitoring. *Journal of the American Medical Association, 288*(4), 423–425. doi:10.1001/jama.288.4.423

France, F. H., & Gaunt, P. N. (1994). The need for security--a clinical view. *International Journal of Bio-Medical Computing, 35*, 189–194.

Frost, J., & Massagli, M. P. (2008). Social uses of personal health information within Patients-LikeMe, an online patient community: what can happen when patients have access to one another's data. *Journal of Medical Internet Research, 10*(2), e15. doi:10.2196/jmir.1053

Giustini, D. (2006). Scrooge and intellectual property rights. *British Medical Journal, 333*, 179–1284.

Gloth, M., Coleman, E., Philips, S., & Zorowitz, R. (2005). Using Electronic Health Records to Improved Care: Will "Hight Tech" Allow a Return to "High Touch" Medicine? *Journal of the American Medical Directors Association*, 270–275. doi:10.1016/j.jamda.2005.05.003

Harman, L. B. (2005). HIPAA: a few years later. *Online Journal of Issues in Nursing, 10*(2), 31.

Hassol, A., Walker, J. M., Kidder, D., Rokita, K., Young, D., & Pierdon, S. (2004). Patient experiences and attitudes about access to a patient electronic health care record and linked web messaging. *Journal of the American Medical Informatics Association, 11*(6), 505–513. doi:10.1197/jamia.M1593

Hewitt, M., & Ganz, P. (Eds.). (2006). *From Cancer Patient to Cancer Survivor: Lost in Transition*. Washington, DC: The National Academies Press.

Ishikawa, K., Konishi, N., Tsukuma, H., Tsuru, S., Kawamura, A., & Iwata, N. (2004). A clinical management system for patient participatory health care support. Assuring the patients' rights and confirming operation of clinical treatment and hospital administration. *International Journal of Medical Informatics, 73*(3), 243–249. doi:10.1016/j.ijmedinf.2003.11.021

Ishikawa, K., Ohmichi, H., Umeatso, Y., Terasaki, H., Tsukuma, H., & Iwata, N. (2007). The guideline of the personal haelth data structure to secure safety healthcare: The balance between use and protection to satisfy the patients' needs. *International Journal of Medical Informatics, 76*, 412–418. doi:10.1016/j.ijmedinf.2006.09.005

Johnson, G., & Ambrose, G. (2006). Neo-Tribes: The Power and Potential of Online Communities in Health Care. *Communications of the ACM, 49*(1), 107–113. doi:10.1145/1107458.1107463

Jones, T. M. (2003). Patient participation in EHR benefits. *Health Management Technology, 24*(10).

Kittler, A. F., Carlson, G. L., Harris, C., Lippincott, M., Pizziferri, L., & Volk, L. A. (2004). Primary care physician attitudes towards using a secure web-based portal designed to facilitate electronic communication with patients. *Informatics in Primary Care, 12*(3), 129–138.

Kluge, E. H. (1993). Advanced patient records: some ethical and legal considerations touching medical information space [see comment]. *Methods of Information in Medicine, 32*(2), 95–103.

Kukafka, R. (2007). Guest Editorial: Public Health Informatics. *Journal of Biomedical Informatics, 40*, 365–369. doi:10.1016/j.jbi.2007.07.005

Leonard, K., Wiljer, D., & Urowitz, S. (2008). Yes Virginia, There Are System Benefits to be Gained from Providing Patients Access to Their Own Health Information. *Healthcare Quarterly (Toronto, Ont.), 11*(4), 66–70.

Leonard, K., Wiljer, D., & Urowitz, S. (2008). Yes, Virginia, There are System Benefits to Be Gained From Providing Patients Access to Their Own Health Information. *Healthcare Quarterly (Toronto, Ont.), 11*(4), 66–77.

Leonard, K. J. W., D., & Casselman, M. (2008a). An Innovative Information Paradigm for Consumers with Chronic Conditions: The value proposition. *The Journal on Information Technology in Healthcare.*

Leonard, K. J., Casselman, M., & Wiljer, D. (2008). Who will demand access to their personal health record? A focus on the users of health services and what they want. *Healthcare Quarterly (Toronto, Ont.), 11*(1), 92–96.

Leonard, K. J., & Wiljer, D. (2007). Patients Are Destined to Manage Their Care. *Healthcare Quarterly (Toronto, Ont.), 10*(3), 76–78.

Lorig, K. R., Sobel, D. S., Ritter, P. L., Laurent, D., & Hobbs, M. (2001). Effect of a self-management program on patients with chronic disease. *Effective Clinical Practice, 4*(6), 256–262.

Markle. (2003). Connecting for Health: A Public-Private Collaborative. http://www.connecting-forhealth.org/resources/final_phwg_report1.pdf. Accessed: 2008-09-22. (Archived by WebCite® at http://www.webcitation.org/5b24kHscL).

Mathews, S. (1998). Protection of personal data--the European view. *Journal of American Health Information Management Association, 69*(3), 42–44.

Mitchell, P. (1998). France gets smart with health a la carte. *Lancet, 351*(9104), 7. doi:10.1016/S0140-6736(05)78518-4

Newsroom, F. A. O. (2004). Retrieved March 10, 2009, from http://www.fao.org/english/news-room/news/2003/26919-en.html

O'Connor, A., Stacey, D., Entwistle, V., Llewellyn-Thomas, H., Rovner, D., Holmes-Rovner, M., et al. (2002). Decision aids for people facing health treatment or screening decisions. (Publication no. 10.1002/14651858.CD001431).

O'Grady, L., Witteman, H., Bender, J. L., Urowitz, S., Wiljer, D., & Jadad, A. R. (2009). Measuring the Impact of a Moving Target: Towards a Dynamic Framework for Evaluating Collaborative Adaptive Interactive Technologies. *Journal of Medical Internet Research, 11*(2), e20. doi:10.2196/jmir.1058

Orchard, M., Green, E., Sullivan, T., Greenberg, A., & Mai, V. (2008). Chronic disease prevention and management: implications for health human resources in 2020. *Healthcare Quarterly (Toronto, Ont.), 11*(1), 38–43.

Pallapa, G., & Das, S. (2007). *Resource Discovery in Ubiquitous Health Care.* Paper presented at the Advanced Information Networking and Applications Workshops

Paterson, B. L. (2001). The shifting perspectives model of chronic illness. *Journal of Nursing Scholarship, 33*(1), 21–26. doi:10.1111/j.1547-5069.2001.00021.x

Preece, J. (2000). *Online Communities: Designing Usability, Supporting Sociability.* Chichester, England: Wiley & Sons Ltd.

Pyper, C., Amery, J., Watson, M., & Crook, C. (2004). Patients' experiences when accessing their on-line electronic patient records in primary care. *The British Journal of General Practice, 54*(498), 38–43.

Pyper, C., Amery, J., Watson, M., Crook, C., & Thomas, B. (2002). Patients' access to their online electronic health records. *Journal of Telemedicine and Telecare, 2*, 103–105. doi:10.1258/135763302320302244

Ralston, J. D., Carrell, D., Reid, R., Anderson, M., Moran, M., & Hereford, J. (2007). Patient Web Services Integrated with a Shared Medical Record: Patient Use and Satisfaction. *Journal of the American Medical Informatics Association, 14*(6), 798–806. doi:10.1197/jamia.M2302

Rutten, L., Arorab, N., Bakosc, A., Azizb, N., & Rowland, J. (2005). Information needs and sources of information among cancer patients: a systematic review of research (1980-2003). *Patient Education and Counseling, 57*(3), 250–261. doi:10.1016/j.pec.2004.06.006

Schoenburg, R. (2005). Security of Healthcare Information Systems. In D. Lewis, G. Eysenbach, R. Kukafka, P. Z. Stavri & H. Jimison (Eds.), Consumer Health Informatics. New York: Springer Science+Business Media Inc.

Setness, P. (2003). When privacy and the public good collide. Does the collection of health data for research harm individual patients? *Postgraduate Medicine, 113*(5), 15. doi:10.3810/pgm.2003.05.1418

Tan, J. (2005). *The Next Health Care Frontier*. San Francisco: Jossey-Bass.

Tang, P. C., Ash, J. S., Bates, D. W., Overhage, J. M., & Sands, D. Z. (2006). Personal health records: definitions, benefits, and strategies for overcoming barriers to adoption. *Journal of the American Medical Informatics Association, 13*(2), 121–126. doi:10.1197/jamia.M2025

Urowitz, S., & Deber, D. (2008). How Consumerist Do People Want to Be? Preferred Role in Decision-Making of Individuals with HIV/AIDS. *Health Policy (Amsterdam), 3*(3).

Urowitz, S., Wiljer, D., Apatu, E., Eysenbach, G., DeLenardo, C., Harth, T., et al. (2008). Is Canada ready for patient accessible electronic health records? A national scan. *Journal, 8.* Retrieved from http://www.pubmedcentral.nih.gov/articlerender.fcgi?tool=pubmed&pubmedid=18652695

Wallerstein, N. (2006). *What is the evidence on effectiveness of empowerment to improve health?* Albuquerque: Europe's Health Evidence Network.

Wiecha, J., & Pollard, T. (2004). The Interdisciplinary eHealth Team: Chronic Care for the Future. *Journal of Medical Internet Research, 6*(3). doi:10.2196/jmir.6.3.e22

Wiljer, D., Bogomilsky, S., Catton, P., Murray, C., Stewart, J., & Minden, M. (2006). Getting results for hematology patients through access to the electronic health record. *Canadian Oncology Nursing Journal, 16*(3), 154–164.

World Factbook. (2009, March 5, 2009). Retrieved March 10, 2009, from https://www.cia.gov/library/publications/the-world-factbook/print/xx.html

Wuerdeman, L., Volk, L., Pizziferri, L., Ruslana, T., Harris, C., Feygin, R., et al. (2005). *How Accurate is Information that Patients Contribute to their Electronic Health Record?* Paper presented at the AMIA 2005.

Wyatt, J., & Sullivan, F. (2005). eHealth and the future: promise or peril? *Journal.* Retrieved from http://www.bmj.com/cgi/content/full/331/7529/1391

ADDITIONAL READING

Andersen, J., & Aydin, C. (Eds.). (2005). Evaluating the Organizational Impact of Healthcare Information Systems. New York: Springer Science+Business Media Inc.

Brender, J. (2006). *Evaluation Methods for Health Informatics*. San Diego: Elsevier.

Bruslilovsky, P., Kobsa, A., & Nejdl, W. (Eds.). (2007). *The Adaptive Web: Methods and Strategies of Web Personalization*. Pittsburgh: Springer.

Committee on Quality of Health Care in America. (2001). *Crossing the Quality Chasm: A New Health System for the 21ˢᵗ Century*. Washington, DC: National Academy Press.

Europe, W. H. O. (2006). *What is the evidence on effectiveness of empowerment to improve health?* Retreived March 13, 2009 from http://www.euro.who.int/Document/E88086.pdf

Gerteis, M., Edgman-Levitan, S., & Daley, J. Delblanco, T. (Eds.) (1993). Through the Patient's Eyes. San Francisco: Jossey-Bass.

Johnston Roberts, K. (2001). Patient empowerment in the United States: a critical commentary. *Health Expectations, 2*(2), 82–92. doi:10.1046/j.1369-6513.1999.00048.x

Kemper, D., & Mettler, M. (2002). *Information Therapy: Prescribed Information as a Reimbursable Medical Service*. Boise, ID: Healthwise.

Kreuter, M., Farrell, D., Olevitch, L., & Brennan, L. (Eds.). (2000). *Tailoring Health Messages: Customizing Communication with Computer Technology*. New Jersey: Lawrence Earlbaum Associates Inc.

Leonard, K. J., Wiljer, D., & Casselman, M. (2008). *An Innovative Information Paradigm for Consumers with Chronic Conditions: The value proposition*. The Journal on Information Technology in Healthcare.

Lewis, D., Eysenbach, G., Kukafka, R., Stavri, P. Z., & Jimison, H. (Eds.). (2005). Consumer Health Informatics. New York: Springer Science+Business Media Inc.

Picker, N. C. R. Eight Dimensions of Patient-Centred Care. Retrieved March 13, 2009 from http://www.nrcpicker.com/Measurement/Understanding%20PCC/Pages/DimensionsofPatient-CenteredCare.aspx

Preece, J. (2000). *Online Communities: Designing Usability, Supporting Sociability*. Chichester, England: Wiley & Sons Ltd.

Sands, D. Z. (2008). Failed Connections: Why Connecting Humans Is as Important as Connecting Computers. *Medscape Journal of Medicine, 10*(11), 262.

Sands, D. Z. (2008). ePatients: Engaging Patients in Their Own Care. *Medscape Journal of Medicine, 10*(1), 19.

Tan, J. (2005). *E-Health Care Information Systems: An Introduction for Students and Professionals*. San Francisco: Jossey-Bass.

Wagner, E. H. (1998). Chronic disease management: What will it take to improve care for chronic illness? *Effective Clinical Practice, 1*, 2–4.

Chapter 10
Healthcare Collaborative Framework Based on Web 2.0, Grid Computing and SOA

Wail M. Omar
Sohar University, Sultanate of Oman

ABSTRACT

Web 2.0 has been adopted by many as the best way for forming a collaborative framework e.g., sharing resources, experiences, information, knowledge and feedback. A collaborative framework for application to e-health is necessary to provide patients with the awareness that assists in improving their health. Moreover, collaborative framework can be used by physician to exchange experiences and discuss challenge cases. However, the use of Web 2.0 with healthcare applications is not simple as the use of Web 2.0 with other enterprise applications according to the privacy of healthcare applications, which requires high quality and security of data, availability of resources, maintainability of services, system security, and Quality of Services (QoS). To offer the required requirements, grid computing is proposed here. Grid computing supporting enterprise applications through offering massive resources through resources collaborative framework that is offering power computing, storage devices, and services. The use of grid computing by Web 2.0 requires robust model that is able to deploy, discover, invoke, and integrate resources in open standard format. Therefore, Service Oriented Architecture (SOA) is adopted as a model for managing the mixing between Web 2.0 and grid computing technologies. SOA for Web 2.0 and Grid Computing (SOAW2G) are used throughout this work to offer a fabric for e-health applications.

INTRODUCTION

Collaborative framework leverages the share of information, experiences, knowledge, resources and feedback among people in the field of interest. Like collaborative framework for distributed computing system, maintenance engineering, networking troubleshooting, entertainment, patients, physicians, and others. The collaborative framework is useful in decision making process, which is vital for many users like managers, physician, engineers and others. Healthcare collaborative framework is one of the

DOI: 10.4018/978-1-61520-777-0.ch010

Copyright © 2010, IGI Global. Copying or distributing in print or electronic forms without written permission of IGI Global is prohibited.

frameworks, that requires high level of cooperation. The healthcare collaborative framework is important in improving the patients' awareness and responsibilities towards their health, like what type of food and exercise is useful for diabetes patients, what type of tests are required for pregnant women in different trimester. Moreover, the healthcare collaborative framework facilitates the share of experience and knowledge between physician through exchanging medical experience, discussing challenges cases, sharing clinical insights, and trying new medicine. Healthcare management users also get benefit from the collaborative framework through getting the required information and experience from other management team for better decision making.

Online healthcare collaborative framework is not something new, and many are aiming to develop such framework science the mid of 90's, when the Internet be available in reasonable price and many places around the world. Advanced Research TEstbed for Medical InformaticS (ARTEMIS) is one of these environments that is aiming to build collaborative framework between the patients and physician (R Reddy, 1993; V Jagannathan, 1995). ARTEMIS aims to provide healthcare services to patients in large community. ARTEMIS is consisting of number of subsystems that are intended to overcome the barriers that inhibit the collaborative process. The subsystems include MONET (Meeting On the Net)--to provide consultation over a computer network, ISS (Information Sharing Server)--to provide access to multi-media information, and PCB (Project Coordination Board)--to better coordinate focused activities. For such system to be viable, it needs update information and resources to be feed to the system, which was difficult in the med of 90's with absence of the digital awareness and lake of the open standard format. However, with Web 2.0 technology the proposed system can be applied.

On the other hand, healthcare collaborative framework assists in overcoming the shortage of specialists, the high patient load on hospitals, the cost of health services, and the difficulty in getting treatment in rural and remote places. Most of the countries around the world are suffering from these problems. The healthcare collaborative framework can be considered as advisory system that is offering advices to patients as well as physician. The advices are feed to the system through physician or patients who have same disease.

However, this dream of having healthcare collaborative framework requires a massive resources (Vincent Breton, 2005) and control according to the privacy of the framework, which deals with human live. The resources like supercomputing, storage system, backup system, communication, and health services such as remote monitoring and video conferencing. The control and management system is required to ensure the quality of deployed information, availability of the system, quality of health services, and security of information. In addition, the collaborative framework is deployed over heterogeneous system, which requires the adoption of open standard format in exchanging medical information.

The healthcare collaborative framework would follow new concepts of enterprise applications, which are based on having the system as a number of services (Software as Services (SaS)). SaS requires model for managing the integration of services. Therefore, this chapter would discuss the development of model that is supporting the integration of services for forming health care collaborative framework and use massive resources from grid computing.

The chapter covers current attempt of using Web 2.0 in forming healthcare collaborative framework, the need for grid computing and SOA, SOAW2G model, scenario for using SOAW2G, case study for remote health monitoring system, conclusion and future works.

BACKGROUND

Web 2.0 for Healthcare Framework

Web 2.0 is the next generation of the Internet applications that depend on getting interaction with users. On other word, Web 2.0 is aiming to build collaborative framework that is considering users as active entity through participating in the framework by experience, knowledge, information and feedback. The framework will be improved with more users participating in the activities of the framework; like youtube (http://www.youtube.com), facebook (http://www.facebook.com), myspace (http://www.myspace.com), blogs and others.

Currently, Web 2.0 framework is available in different formats, such as blogs, wiki, podcasting, tags, and social networking. These formats are merged with different enterprise applications, like e-healthcare, e-business, e-science, e-government and others to offer a base for user collaboration framework. Such applications are reviewed by Hogg *et al.* (C. Schoth, 2007; R. Hogg, 2006). They conducted an in-depth investigation of 40 successful Web 2.0 applications. They summarized the range of characteristics to describe the phenomenon of Web 2.0 communities and to provide a systematic overview of current and emerging business models. Healthcare is one of the environments, that highly requires an establishing of collaborative framework. The following sections will describe the use of different Web 2.0 format in healthcare applications.

Healthcare Blogs

Blogs acronym is coming from Web Log. Blogs are digital content that are published through the Web by different types of person(s). Blogs are usually (but not always) written by one person and are updated regularly. The other persons can add comments, which encourage the participation in collaborative framework. Blogs are often (but not always) written on a particular topic – like blogs on business, education, health, and others. Blogs are consists of text, images, and multimedia files. The blogs are effective way for transferring the knowledge from person(s) to others. This includes the knowledge in healthcare. Therefore different blogs have been appeared in the area of healthcare. The blogs vary from patients to physician, like the blog that is discussing Swine flu and the latest news of it (http://well.blogs.nytimes.com/2009/04/28/the-symptoms-of-swine-flu/), and The Healthcare Blog (http://www.thehealthcareblog.com/) that is discussing the latest technology in IT for health sector.

Healthcare Wikis

Wiki is a web page that is allowing the users to freely create and edit Web page content using any Web browser. Wiki supports hyperlinks and has simple text syntax for creating new pages and crosslink between internal pages on the fly like the famous Wikipedia site (http://www.wikipedia.org/). Wikis have been employed in the healthcare environment to generate another mean for interaction with users. The physician as well as patients can use wiki for exchanging information. Examples of using wikis in healthcare are: flu wiki (http://www.fluwikie.com/) which provides a wealth of information about H5N1 and pandemic flu, and Ask Dr. Wiki (http://askdrwiki.com/) which allows doctors for publishing their review articles, clinical notes, pearls, and medical images on the site.

Healthcare Social Networking

Social networking is online community that is connecting people of sharing interests in one network. This assists users to communicate with others and get/pass knowledge to others. Like facebook (http://www.facebook.com) which is for general interests, and Café mom (http://www.cafemom.com) which provides advice, experience and information to mom and new mom. Social networking is also used in healthcare exchange of information, like Patientslikeme (http://www. Patientslikeme.com) and mycancerplace (http://www.mycancerplace.com/), which share information, give and receive support, and learn from the experiences of other patients. Patientslikeme and mycancerplace is more for patient social networking who are requiring support and advice. Sermo (http://sermo.com/) is social networking for physician. It provides collaborative framework for discussing challenging cases, sharing clinical insights, and improve patient care.

Healthcare Podcasting

Podcasting is to share multimedia files (audio and video) over the Internet. Podcasting is like radio and TV on-demand. The listener can select the time, place and content to listen to the program. Podcasting has been merged with healthcare applications to offer another way of creating multimedia collaboration framework among the users of the framework. Like continuing Medical Education (CME) Podcasting (http://www.cmepodcasting. com/list.asp), which is giving medical education courses, and Johns Hopkins medicine Podcasting (http://www.hopkinsmedicine.org/mediaii/ podcasts.html), which is a weekly podcast looking at the top medical stories of the week for people who want to become informed participants in their own health care.

Healthcare Web 2.0: What is Next?

There is no doubt about the important and benefit of using Web 2.0 framework with healthcare applications in order to create a collaborative framework specialist in healthcare services. Such healthcare collaborative framework improves the way of exchanging information, experience and knowledge between the users. This will take the healthcare applications to another generation through having knowledge flow up to the system by the users on-

fly. However, healthcare applications have privacy according to the sensitivity, security, scalability, and accuracy of the published information according to the fact that such information deals with human life. In addition, to get the full benefit of the published information, the information needs to be organized and managed based on number of characteristics, like the relativity, source, quality, and ranking of the published information.

Web 2.0 depends on the different activities and information that are supplied by the users. The published information will be improved with the increase of participants in Web 2.0 framework. Increasing users of framework causes the need for massive resources to keep the maintainability, Quality of Services (QoS), availability, and high performance of the framework. Therefore, we discuss the use of grid computing to offer the resources for web 2.0 healthcare applications in this chapter. Next section would discuss the grid computing and how it can be merged with Web 2.0 to support collaborative framework.

All these activities of Web 2.0 framework and the merging of grid computing with Web 2.0 require robustness model for managing the interaction between the Web 2.0 framework and resources. Furthermore, the suggested model would offer the fabric for providing all the required tools and facilities for improving the Web 2.0 framework. The model should be able to offer and guide the way of integrating different type of services that can form healthcare applications. Therefore, Service Oriented Architecture model is proposed here to facilitate the merging of Web 2.0 and grid computing as well as the integration of services and managing, controlling and monitoring the flow of information.

Web 2.0 and Grid Computing

Over the coming years, many are anticipating that grid computing infrastructures, utilities and services to become an integral part of future socio-economical fabric. The realisation of such a vision will be very much affected by many factors including; cost of access, reliability, dependability and security of grid computing services. Hoschek [29] defined grid computing as;

"... collaborative distributed Internet systems characterized by large scale, heterogeneity, lack of central control, multiple autonomous administrative domains, unreliable components and frequent dynamic change ... ".

Whereas, Berman *et al.* [3] defined grid computing as;

"...The Grid is the computing and data management infrastructure that will provide the electronic underpinning for a global society in business, government, research, science and entertainment..."

From the above definitions, the benefits of grid computing to support enterprise business application are accrued through collaborative distributed resources and information sharing including; software (services), hardware and associated content, to build one large system serving all subsystems and consumers.

As we can see from the concepts of the grid computing, it provides resources that assist in building enterprise applications. The resources are the collection of services and hardware. The services like monitoring systems, dictionaries, predication services, financial services, currency converter, weather broadcasting, load balance, autonomic computing and others services. The hardware consists of data storage, backup system, supercomputing and communication system.

Therefore, the merging of Web 2.0 and grid computing will draw the future vision of how to support the next generation of enterprise applications. Grid computing is proposed to be an attractive solution for offering different types of resources, that ensuring the availability of resources for operational framework.

Thus, this work is trying to focus on bringing the two technologies together in a way whereby each one boosts the other. Little work has been conducted to date regarding the linkage between grid computing and Web 2.0, but there have been some efforts to imitate Web 2.0 concepts and to try to adapt them into grid technology. S*emantic grid group (SematicGrid)* is one of the groups that works in this area. The main notion in Web 2.0 that can be extended is the *semantic web*, and hence their vision about the grid is called the semantic grid. It relies on concentrating the resources to a process able to deal with common knowledge that can be understood and dealt with by all parties taking part to create a specific grid, which will result in a drastic improvement in the dynamics of grid technology.

Conversely, grid computing has been applied for different types of enterprise applications including healthcare applications. For instant, Breton *et al.* (Vincent Breton, 2005) present a review of health grid technologies, by describing the current status of grid and E-Health systems, as well as analyzing mid-term developments including innovations and business opportunities. This review concluded with a listing of technical challenges in E-Health, namely: standardization of data, federation of databases, content-based knowledge extraction, and management of personal data. For community and public health, grid technology offers the opportunity to create a common working backbone for all stakeholders and dutyholders, to improve inter-operation and collaboration (Paindaveine, 2002). There are many other implementations for grid computing in healthcare applications, like Cancer Biomedical Informatics Grid-caBIG (caBIG), which is an information network enabling the cancer community – researchers, physicians and patients – to share data and knowledge, and Biomedical Informatics Research Network-BIRN (BIRN) is a geographically distributed virtual community aiming to advance the diagnosis and treatment of human disease.

Service Oriented Architecture (SOA)

After discussing the advantages of using Web 2.0 and grid computing in healthcare enterprise applications and collaborative framework, a model for managing the application framework operation is required. The model would facilitate the deployment, requesting, discovery, integration and invocation of resources, as well as the interaction with the users of the framework. SOA has been proposed through this work to be used for merging Web 2.0 and grid computing. SOA proves its efficiency in managing different large scale enterprise applications (Marks, 2006).

SOA is the model that is depending on the concept of Software as Services (SaS). Where, SOA is adopted to bring the Object Oriented (OO) mentality to the distributed large scale enterprise applications, where the new distributed applications are proposed to be structured from numbers of small object models (B. Borges, 2004), such objects can be web services. This is fitting with the concepts of the grid computing of offering resources as services. Web services are considered the basic operational units (resources) that offer services within the framework. SOA model is managing the integration of the web services to form large scale enterprise applications. This takes the enterprise applications to new generation of applications that is collecting services on-fly and on-demands. Simple Access Object Protocols (SOAP) (Thomas et al., 2001) and Hyper Text Transfer Protocol (HTTP) are the main protocols that are used for generating the request and response messages between the services and consumers within SOA model.

As has been described, SOA will serve the applications that are distributed in heterogeneous platform. Therefore, interoperability and the use of the open standard format are required to exchange messages between the components of the system. SOA would leverage the use of open standard format for developing services. Therefore, SOA adopts variety of standards to facilitate the inte-

gration and deployment of the applications, like Web Services Description Language (WSDL), SOAP, Universal Description Discovery and Integration (UDDI), HTTP, and eXtensible Markup Language (XML).

Consequently, SOA is anticipated to offer a generic model for implementing large scale enterprise applications (B. Borges, 2004; M. Endrei, 2004), such as e-health, e-commerce, e-science and e-government. SOA is a model for hiding the complexity of the usability of distributed services from the consumer in one hand, and provide a framework for services provider in the second hand (B. Borges, 2004; Fellenstein, 2005). Hence, SOA applications start to see the light in different fields including e-health. Chien *et al.* (Chien-Ming Tu, 2007) use SOA for a Newborn Screening Information System using the HL7 standard and state-of-the-art XML Web service. This is proposed to integrate the newborn screening procedures between phlebotomy clinics, referral hospitals, and the screening center. In addition to reducing the burden of manual operation, it speeds up the whole procedure and improves the accuracy of work, by ensuring quality control of the newborn screening. However, this initiative is still missing the interaction with physician to re-configure the system and to manage the resources.

The SOA model needs to be modified in order to occupy the demands of interacting with users at the top and use the grid computing resources at the button. The following section describes the merging of the two technologies (Web 2.0 and grid computing) in one model based on SOA, which is called Services Oriented Architecture for Web 2.0 and Grid (SOAW2G).

SOAW2G

SOAW2G is the model that is developed for facilitating the merge of the Web 2.0 and grid computing technologies in one framework, as previously described. The framework will be utilized for carrying out collaborative framework. To assist in developing the components of the system, the model is structured into a number of layers for smoothing the progress of the control and management of the functions and features of the system. The layers are categorized with the Customer Layer as the top layer, while the Resources Layer as the bottom layer, as shown in Figure 1. The rest of layers are between the two main layers, arranged in the following order: User Interface Layer, Support Function Layer, Control System, and Resources Management Layer. Furthermore, the research proposes an additional three layers for monitoring and controlling the operations of the framework, and ensuring the integration between services in a way that improves the Quality of Services (QoS), availability, fidelity, maintainability and reliability. The main duties of the extra layers are to control and manage the security, to manage interaction between layers, and to offer knowledge (ontology) for the different components of the system. The following sections describe the layers in details.

Resources Layer

The **resources layer** in SOAW2G covers all the required resources to structure Enterprise applications such as healthcare applications. The resources layer includes three main categories, which are Services, Computational and Data Processes. These categories consist of a variety of components, such as services, infrastructure, communication systems, monitoring resources, storage system, and controlling facilities.

Services are considered the basic unit that is responsible for offering service or function to the operational system. The services resources consist of all types of application and management services. Such services are health services (W. Omar, B. Ahmad, A. Taleb-Bendiab, 2006), financial services (B. Ahmad, 2006), dictionary services, monitoring services, controlling services and others.

Moreover, the resources layer provides the computational resources that are required for processing tasks. The tasks are requested from the services and/or users. Data storage and data

Figure 1. SOAW2G model

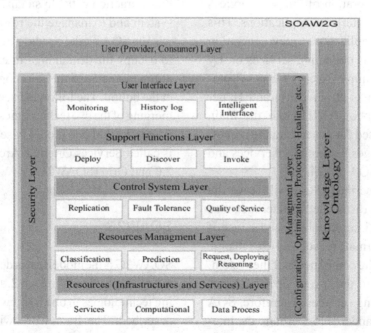

processing are also offered by this layer. Data mining, distributed data storage system, data grid (L. Ferreira, 2003), and others are examples of these resources.

As has been described previously, the new application is expected to follow the concept of integrating different services to form an application, like mashups (Jeffrey Wong, 2007; Rattapoom Tuchinda, 2008). Such services are expected to work as part of an interoperability system. Therefore, web services are proposed for establishing variety of services.

Resources Management Layer

This layer is responsible for classifying the resources that are deployed by the provider, according to the nature, functionality and behavior of resources. Such a classification process has been proposed to improve the functionality of the underneath layer, by enhancing the manageability and fidelity of selecting resources. Users' feedback is used to improve the classification processes. This layer consist of three main components (as shown in Figure 2) to accomplish the task of classifying resources. The three components are reasoning, prediction and classification. Reasoning receives the resources information from the resources providers as well as from the resources layer in

case there is an update for the existing resources. Moreover, reasoning will also use feedback from users to enhance the understanding of the features, behavior, and usage of resources. The reasoning provides the prediction component with the information that is used for predicting the type of the resources. The classification component uses the predicted type to classify the resources into one of the existing resources categories at the resources layer, or to generate a new resources category if the deployed resources are not matched to any one of the existing categories. This process categorizes the resources at the lower layer, which improves the manageability, efficiency and fidelity in discovering resources.

Control Layer

The control layer manages the operation of the resources at the resources layer in a way that offers high reliability, quality of services, availability, scalability and maintainability. To achieve these tasks, a number of tools and services are required to work together, such as replication, fault tolerance, load balancing, mirroring, monitoring system, and others. As shown from the type of services, this layer is concerning more regarding how to run services. For example, this layer is in charge of monitoring the load on the services

Figure 2. Resources management layer

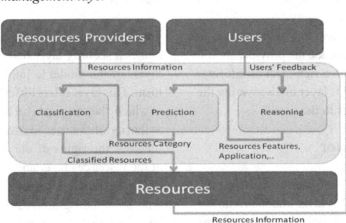

and detecting any overload on the services that can cause a reduction in the performance of the service and even failure in providing services. This layer then reacts accordingly, and finds the way for keeping the service alive and managing the load. This can be achieved through load balancing techniques, managing the access to service based on priority or first shortest job, and scheduling the service usage in advance, based on advanced and on-demand access (W. Omar, A. Taleb-Bendiab, Y. Karam, 2006).

Support Functions Layer

This layer is required for managing the processes of deploying, discovering and invoking resources based on requests from the upper layers. The deploy function coordinates the deployment of the resources from providers to resources container in the resources layer. The deployment service works with the resources management layer to ensure the manageability of the resources layer. The discovery function manages the process of discovering resources that are requested by the users. The discovery service depends on different parameters for discovering services, such as the application framework (e-health, e-government, etc.), services category, services load, Service Level of Agreement (SLA) for user and others. The invoke function controls and advises the method of accessing and utilizing resources in the lower layers. This also includes the required information for integrating services.

For this layer to offer high performance in achieving the required tasks, the provider should provide the system with a rich level of information in order to assist this layer in discovering the most suitable resources to the user.

User Interface Layer

This layer represents the gateway between the user and the system. This layer interacts with users through presenting the data in different forms

of Web 2.0 such as blogs, RSS, wikis, mashups and podcasting which show the interests of the users. In addition, this layer monitors the users' activities and records them in a user history log that can be used by the management layer for re-adjustment of the framework so that it is suited for the running application and for giving better services. This layer should be sufficiently flexible to include different rules and policies that describe the operations framework of the user, based on the nature of the applications (i.e. health, science, games and other frameworks). Moreover, the layer is in charge of monitoring collaborative framework and requests the required resources for ensuring the operation of the framework.

User Layer

The user layer represents the consumers as well as applications. The user in this framework is an active user and not a passive one. In another words, the user interacts with the system to improve the operation of the framework through providing the system with experiences, arguments (rules), policies, application specification and other information that assists in reconfiguring the framework to give better services. All the users' activities and behavior would be recorded by the lower layer. The user use variety formats of Web 2.0 in order to interact with the system.

Security Layer

To protect the system, the SOAW2G model includes a security layer that works with the other layers of the model to improve security mechanism. This layer offers different levels of security, in which, the security layer begins by checking the authority of the user to use the framework. This includes the rights of the user to use resources at the resources layer and/or add resources. The SLA is required to control and protect the users who have the right and privilege for deploying and using resources from those who do not have such access. A file system and user profile are proposed to be used in order to record the authority and SLAs for different users; and an encryption mechanism can be very useful to encrypt these files and protect them against sniffing and vandalizing activities.

The other level of the security is the admin level; the security at the control layer is used to manage the administrator access to control services. The security at this level will give more security management tools for the admin to control the security at the resources layer.

Finally, security at the resources layer is used to protect the layer from the different types of attacks including outside or inside attacks, which can be implemented in sourced or outsourced security systems (virus protection, worms' protection applications, etc.).

Management Layer

The management layer cooperates with all layers of the model for managing the Web2.0-grid computing framework. This layer consists of a number of capabilities, working together for managing the framework. Such capabilities are framework configuration, optimization, adaptation, healing, protection, organizing, and others which assist in improving the operational framework and moving it to on the demand framework (Fellenstein, 2005). All these capabilities should be selected, executed, blocked and destroyed in an automated way. Therefore, autonomic computing (IBM, 2003; Murch, 2004) can be attractive tools for this layer in order to have self-management system. Autonomic computing needs variety of services, like monitoring system, decision making system, prediction services, effectors, and other which are available at the resources container as shown in Figure 3.

Knowledge Layer

The knowledge layer in this model offers rich information to all layers of the system that would assist in efficient usage of the framework, as well

Figure 3. Functional details of the autonomic manager

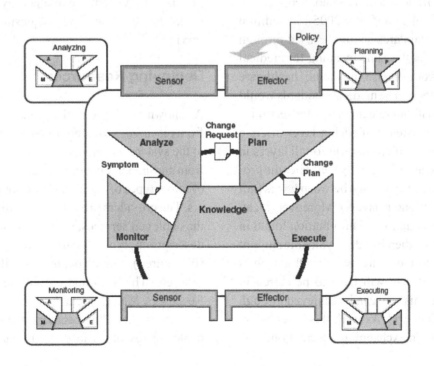

as facilitate interaction between the layers. This layer cooperates with all layers for gathering and providing information to each one of them. For example, it collects and provides information regarding the available control services to the control layer, the security policies and SLA to the security layer, user information and experiences to the user interface layer, classification and prediction service to the resources management layer, the available monitor resources (sensors, actuators, and loggers) to the monitoring system, gathering users' experiences and feedbacks from the user interface layer, providing and gathering medical information from physician and patients, and so on. Furthermore, this layer assists the user in selecting the services from the resources layer, based on the information provided by the resources management layer.

Because this layer is involved with all layers, it should use an open standard format that can be readable and understandable by all components. Therefore, different types of standards and description languages are used here to describe the processes, data and components of the system, such as Sensors and Actuators Description Language (SADL), and Monitor Session Description Language (MSDL) (W. Omar 2005). In addition open medical standards should be used through this layer to offer the same meaning for medical components from disease, medicine, healthcare services and others. The medical standards would be described with more details in later section.

Hence the existence of such a layer offers a storage and retrieval mechanism for all layers in the framework, and also greatly facilitates the process of information exchange between layers (not necessarily contiguous layers). Moreover, it can also act as a backup for the information found in each layer, which thereby adds a valuable amount of robustness to the entire system. Obviously a huge amount of data will have to be stored in some way, and this way can be achieved through utilizing the data grid. As well, this layer offers interoperability in exchanging information.

As described, the knowledge layer is considered as the heart of the model that provides every layer with the required information. Ontology is used to build the knowledge layer. Ontology offers the fabric for storing system information and its components in a semantic format, so as to offer a mechanism for the standard exchange of information between the layers of the system. As such, this increases the ability of the system to interact efficiently with the huge demands coming from the consumer, in intelligent and strategic ways. This work would provide a case study of how to use the ontology for describing medical resources at the resources layer.

SOAW2G IN ACTION

In this section, a vision of how the model will work to manage healthcare applications and collaborative framework is given. This vision includes deploying resources, managing resources, requesting and invoking resources, gaining knowledge from user experiences, managing interaction between layers of the system and other activities of the system. The vision is explained by providing a walkthrough scenario for requesting healthcare services.

Deploying Resources

As shown in Figure 4, the scenario commences from resources providers when provide resources to the system. Providers use the Deploy function from the Support Function Layer to upload services (or other types of resources) to resources containers. The providers provide information regarding the deployed services, such as the service name, description, type, location, input parameters (if required), output parameters (if any), SLA, cost, etc. This information will be used by the Resources Management Layer for understanding the functionality, behavior and nature of the deployed resources in order to categorize it to

Figure 4. SOAW2G in action

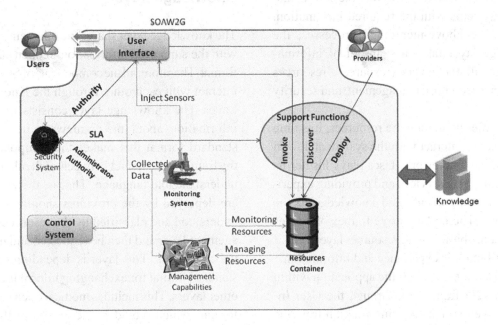

one of the sub-domains according to one of the three resource categories (services, computational and data processes). This process improves the functionality of the system towards the usability and manageability of the resources, which will be reflected in improving the reliability, performance, availability, maintainability and fidelity by selecting the most matched resources. For this layer to serve other layers in an efficient way, it provides the resources' information to other layers through the knowledge layer in open standard format.

Managing Resources

The resources layer needs a control system to manage its functionality and to ensure high availability, reliability and maintainability of the resources through managing the access to resources. This has done through the Resources Management Layer.

Therefore, a robust monitoring system is required to support the control system with data that is recording all activities of the resources container. According to the analysis of the monitored

data, the control layer manages the processes of replication, QoS, Fault Tolerance, load balancing and other control services.

Managing Security

The framework operation security is one of the important aspects that keep the framework running in a safe and protected mode. Therefore, the monitoring system provides the security system with security information regarding the security situation in the resources container. The security system specifies the security attributes and authorizations needed for the usability of resources in the resources layer as well as the administrator and user rights.

User Interaction and Collaborative Framework

To this end, we have resources deployed by the providers and categorized through the resources management layer inside the resources container. Such resources are monitored by the monitoring system, which in its turn provides the control and security systems with the required information. With all the above-mentioned processes, the knowledge layer takes a snapshot of information from all the layers (resources, resources management, control, management, and security layers).

Now, after deploying the resources, it is time for the user to interact with the system and form collaborative framework. User plays his/her/its role in requesting services and providing experiences, rules, arguments and knowledge to the framework. The collaborative framework saves the user contribution in the resources layer, even if the contribution is experience and information.

The user interacts with the application within the SOAW2G framework through the User Interface Layer, which takes information from the knowledge layer regarding the available resources, security levels, and other users' information. This information would be delivered to the users, so that the user would have a clear idea about the service and its functionality after sending a request and discovering the required resources before the invocation process. This assists in improving user time response, QoS and fidelity in selecting resources by requesting the most suitable and matched services to the user's needs, instead of invoking each resource and searching for the required one.

The user interface layer has another important job, which is recording the users' experiences, preferences, environment, characteristics, policies and applications features in order to adjust the framework to be more effective and useful for the user. This information is also used to manage and re-classify the underneath layer (resources layer) according to the user preference. After that, the user can call and use services from the resources container using the Invoke function from the Support Functions layer.

Knowledge Layer

The knowledge layer shares the other entire layer with the supported information in open standard format. Therefore, all the components of SOAW2G interact with each other through the Knowledge Layer. The knowledge layer consists of all the information about the framework in an open standard format that makes the components of the framework interact between each other in one understandable language. That is, the resources are deployed by the providers should be easily understood and classified by the resources management layer and then be requested and used by the consumers. This layer is depending on open standard format for exchanging information with other layers. This includes medical open standard format, which would be described in the next section.

MEDICAL OPEN STANDARD FORMAT

As has been mentioned in many places, this model will support the open standard format that facilitates the exchange of information between the components of the healthcare applications. This also applies for the medical standards that are using for exchanging medical data. Such standards are Systematized Nomenclature of Medicine--Clinical Terms (SNOMED CT), International Classification of Diseases (ICD-10), Health Level Seven (HL 7), MEDCIN (http://www.medicomp.com/), Clinical Data Interchange Standards Consortium (CDISC) (http://www.cdisc.org/) and Doctor Command Language (DOCLE) (http://www.docle.com.au/). The reason behind the use of these medical open standards is to unify the meaning of the clinical terms when clinicians and organizations use different terms. For example, the terms heart attack, myocardial infarction, and MI may mean the same thing to a cardiologist, but, to a computer, they are all different. Therefore, using unified medical terminology system is needed to interexchange medical data between different medical services and systems, which is required for the proposed model. Standardizing the meaning of the medical data is vital step towards semantic health services.

Two of these standards are described in brief here, which are SNOMED and ICD-10. SNOMED CT (IHTSDO; SNOMED-CT) is a comprehensive clinical terminology, originally created by the College of American Pathologists (CAP) and, as of April 2007, owned, maintained, and distributed by the International Health Terminology Standards Development Organization (IHTSDO). SNOMED CT is concept-oriented and has an advanced structure that meets most accepted criteria for a well-formed, machine-readable terminology, which make it a one of a good way for interoperability of medical information. SNOMED CT consists of collection of medical terminology covering most areas of clinical information such as diseases, findings, procedures, microorganisms, pharmaceuticals etc. It allows a consistent way to index, store, retrieve, and aggregate clinical data across specialties and sites of care. It also helps organizing the content of medical records, reducing the variability in the way data is captured, encoded and used for clinical care of patients and research.

ICD-10 was endorsed by the Forty-third World Health Assembly in May 1990 and came into use in World health Organization (WHO) Member States as from 1994 (ICD-10; Johann Eder, 2002; TriZetto). The ICD is the international standard diagnostic classification for general epidemiological, many health management purposes and clinical use. These include the analysis of the general health situation of population groups and monitoring of the incidence and prevalence of diseases and other health problems in relation to other variables such as the characteristics and circumstances of the individuals affected,

reimbursement, resource allocation, quality and guidelines (ICD-10)

The comparison between different medical standards is out of the scope of this chapter.

HEALTHCARE ONTOLOGY

The knowledge layer is considered as the heart of the model, which offers the guidelines for all the layers to work together and separately in an open standard framework. According to the importance of this layer, this chapter would try to give roadmap of how to implement this layer.

As has been described in many places through this chapter, the knowledge layer should provide meaning for the information that is delivered to layers. Therefore, Ontology is adopted throughout this work to build the knowledge of the model for healthcare applications, which can be extended to cover different types of other enterprise applications. The ontology for healthcare applications represents the knowledge base system that assists in the interaction between the system's components. The ontology will build the metadata that assists layers to query information regarding the resources functions, services, users' feedbacks and experiences. The ontology offers the data description and relationships. This is the base for semantic healthcare applications.

There are different methodologies for implementing the ontology; one of them is the Topic Maps. Topic Maps are used to design and implement the health ontology. The topic maps approach has been applied in a number of domains, including the definition of software application's ontology (Rath, 2003; S. Newcomb, August 2005), and the definition of the strategies for web site generation, management and navigation (NetworkedPlanet, 2005). For instance, topic maps are used to provide a site structural model, and the web content is generated through a combination of ontological models derived from the contents of the topic maps. For instance, Korthaus (A. Korthaus, 2003) present some basic considerations for the design and implementation of an open standards-based enterprise Knowledge Grid architecture using topic maps, the "Topic Maps Grid". In addition, Graauw (Graauw, 2002) has described the value of using Topic Maps to define the ontology in Business-To-Business applications. This article provides a comparison between topic maps and other methods for describing business ontology, as well as reasons as to why topic maps offer the best method for defining business concepts in a semantic format.

In this work, the Topic Maps technique describes and defines the healthcare ontology core components and their units in addition to the association between the players or components of the system. Ontopia software (Ontopia) has been used in this work for designing, developing and implementing Topic Maps for healthcare applications.

Healthcare Topic Maps is divided into numbers of categories for describing the components of E-health topic types, occurrence types, association types, role types, name types, and instances of the topic map. For further information regarding the concepts of the Topic Maps, the reader is referred to (Garshol, 2002; Graauw, 2002; Ontopia; Rath, 2003; TopicMaps.Org).

CASE STUDY: E-HEALTHCARE MONITORING SYSTEM (EHMS)

This case study discusses physician-patient collaborative framework through collecting readings from patient. Web 2.0 is used for getting physician's requests and sharing experience. Thus, EHMS is proposed as an example of the usability of the SOAW2G model with healthcare applications. EHMS represents the integration of services, infrastructure, monitoring system, knowledge system and others in one e-health enterprise application. EHMS is about collecting medical data from patients' side based on

physician demand. It is an implementation for on-deand and on-fly integration system. EHMS gathers users' (physician) experiences, feedback, rules and policies to re-configure the framework to be suited for the patient's monitored case. The system is also shared the experiences among the physicians as a way of collaborative framework. EHMS uses the knowledge layer (ontology) to provide information and guidance for other components of the system.

A remote EHMS monitors a patient's condition by, for example, taking a blood pressure, diabetes, cholesterol and other reading and relaying that information, as necessary, to hospitals or e-health applications. Such an approach would free hospital personnel from routine checks and visits, allowing them to concentrate scarce resources on more critical and difficult tasks. This would provide wider access to hospital and healthcare services, including rapid access to specialist care. In addition, EHMS increases the interaction with the user through offering 24/7 medical monitoring system, which has significant improvement on the quality of healthcare.

To best serve this scenario, we propose a grid computing overlay to support this EHMS. Merging a grid overlay with e-health services requires several components, as Figure 5 shows. The EHMS consists of several modules that represent the model's layers: knowledge layer, monitoring system, health monitoring system, autonomic computing, alert services, health consumers, and patients.

EHMS Scenario

A typical scenario for a remote e-healthcare monitoring system begins with a request from a hospital (physician), as Figure 5 shows. The hospital in this case represents the customer at the top layer. This request includes information regarding the required medical sensors, target (patient) information, and authorized agent (a digital signature, authorization number, or any secure identification

Figure 5. EHMS scenario

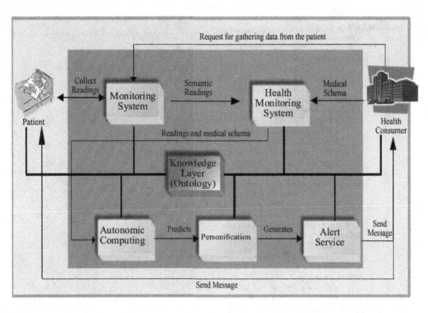

to indicate that the hospital has the right to make this particular request).This request should be in a standard format to be understood by the other parts of the system. One of the medical standards in addition to other open standards can be used here. Monitor Session Description Language (MSDL) (W. Omar 2005) is one such standards. MSDL is open format for requesting monitoring resources and dispatching requests from the hospital to the healthcare monitoring system. Figure 6 shows an example of MSDL for requesting services from EHMS. The details of the MSDL are beyond the scope of this paper and can be found in (W. Omar, 2005a, 2005b; W. Omar, A.Taleb-Bendiab, 2006; W. Omar 2005).

At the same time the health knowledge layer receives information from the health consumers such as the name of the consumer, SLA, address, and other information. The knowledge layer then provides the health consumer with the rich level of information that helps the physician and/or hospitals in selecting the health services, such as available services, health infrastructure, previous experiences, statistics, and so on.

The MSDL request goes to the monitoring system which analyzes the requirements in the

MSDL message. The monitoring system in cooperation with the knowledge layer starts the search for the available medical sensors that best match the consumers' requests in order to collect information from the patients. After that, the monitoring system injects the selected sensors into the target and starts the process of gathering information from the targets, taking into consideration the duration that the hospital has specified in the MSDL request message. The monitoring system stores these readings in the patient's log file inside the logger. The logger converts the formats of the readings into a semantic (open standard) format (an XML file). Subsequently, the monitoring system forwards the readings to the health monitoring system.

The health monitoring system receives messages from two sources. The first source is the monitoring system, as just described. The second source is the hospital, whose message includes the medical schema (ICD-10 or SNOMED CT) describing the medical concepts the system will use to interpret the collected readings. For example, the medical schema for patient X might include the thresholds for diabetes, blood pressure and cholesterol readings.

Figure 6. MSDL example

```
<MSDL>
    <MonitorSession Session_ID = "1">
    <Application>E-Health</Application>
    <Duration>
        <DurationStart>12/28/2004</DurationStart>
        <DurationEnd>21/1/2005</DurationEnd>
        <Interval>2</Interval>
    </Duration>
    <TargetInformation>
        <PatientID>33</PatientID>
        <HostName>SU_Wael</HostName>
        <WebAddress>192.168.1.248</WebAddress>
        <UserName>Wael</UserName>
        <Password>Aya</Password>
    </TargetInformation>
    <ContractInformation>
        <ContractID>33</ContractID>
        <ContractName>ww</ContractName>
        <LeaseTime>www</LeaseTime>
    </ContractInformation>
    <Sensors>
        <ID>2</ID>
        <Name>Hemoglobin</Name>
    </Sensors>
    <Sensors>
        <ID>4</ID>
        <Name>IRT</Name>
    </Sensors>
    </MonitorSession>
</MSDL>
```

The health monitoring system provides the autonomic computing (IBM, 2003; Partners, 2002; Wail M. Omar, 2006) with the required history data for finding the prediction model. Such history data and its concepts are provided through the medical schema. Autonomic computing, in its turn, uses this information for finding the model for each case according to the boundaries that are mentioned in the medical schema and then starts to predict the suggestion of diagnosis for the new case. The concept of autonomic computing is out of the scope of this chapter.

Ontology for HEMS

As shown in figure 8, healthcare Topic Maps consists of numbers of child Topic Maps; for example the supernode is the health consumer and the child topics are doctor or physician, hospital and medical center. Each child topic node inherits its specifications, parameters and characteristics from the supernode. Figure 8 shows most of the supernode and its subnodes for the components of an e-healthcare system.

Moreover, Figure 8 describes the types of associations between the topic types of the e-health and grid overlays, such as health consumer requests, health monitoring system, autonomic computing, tools comprising the monitoring system, and so on.

As a result of the above explanation, the healthcare Topic Maps offer rich information regarding the services, infrastructure, medical sensors, monitoring and controlling systems, in a metadata format that assists in integrating the different types of the components to form E-healthcare enterprise applications, according to SOA concepts. Moreover, healthcare Topic Maps describe the association between the different components of the system, as shown in figure 8. Such information is described in an open standard format based on the use of XML, and this description language is known as XML Topic Maps (XTM) (TopicMaps.Org). Figure 7

Figure 7. XTM example

```xml
<?xml version="1.0" encoding="utf-8"?>
<HRML>
  <Service ServiceID="12">
    <GeneralInformation>
      <ServiceName>CLARINASE REPETABS</ServiceName>
      <ServiceDescription>Provide information regarding CLARINASE REPETABS drug</ServiceDescription>
      <ServiceCategory>Drug Information</ServiceCategory>
      <Container>Schering-Plough Pty Ltd</Container>
      <Framework>Health</Framework>
      <Country>Oman</Country>
      <Price>$10</Price>
    </GeneralInformation>
    <UsedFor>
      <Treating>nasal and sinus congestion</Treating>
      <Treating>sneezing</Treating>
      <Treating>runny nose</Treating>
      <Treating>watery, itchy eyes</Treating>
    </UsedFor>
    <Ingredients>
      <Ingredient>loratadine</Ingredient>
      <Ingredient>pseudoephedrine</Ingredient>
    </Ingredients>
    <SideEffects>
      <Effect>trouble sleeping</Effect>
      <Effect>dry mouth</Effect>
      <Effect>headache</Effect>
      <Effect>sleepiness</Effect>
      <Effect>nervousness</Effect>
      <Effect>dizziness</Effect>
    </SideEffects>
    <SimilarDrugs>
      <Drug>Claritine</Drug>
      <Drug>Repetabs</Drug>
      <Drug>Claridine</Drug>
    </SimilarDrugs>
  </Service>
</HRML>
```

demonstrates part of the XTM for the E-Health Monitoring System (EHMS), which is explained in the next section.

More details regarding Topic Maps for HEMS, which represents the ontology that the system adopts for building the knowledge.

EHMS: Example

As an example of the developed ontology for EHMS, we applied the algorithm for the remote e-health monitoring system based on the use of grid overlay to monitor the status of pregnant women. The required tests for pregnant women are categorized into three major groups, according to pregnancy trimesters. Information about these tests comes from standard test specifications available at local hospitals; these specifications come from international test standards. The table in figure 8 lists the required tests.

The sensor container inside the monitoring resources consists of different types of medical sensors, which are provided by different providers. Such medical sensors can include blood sugar, blood pressure, hemoglobin sensors and others. The EHMS uses these deployed sensors to collect data from pregnant women. It is expected that smart home technology will be used in this case for installing the sensors in the patient's home.

Now, a simple example is demonstrated to show the usability of health ontology in finding the adequate monitoring resources (sensors) for collecting information from a pregnant woman. Topic map query language (TMQL) (Pepper, 2002; Rath, 2003) is used in this example for generating a query to the knowledge layer for providing the required information.

TMQL is a logic-based query language, which accesses the knowledge layer for obtaining information. Assertions in the knowledge layer consist

Figure 8. Table of health topic maps

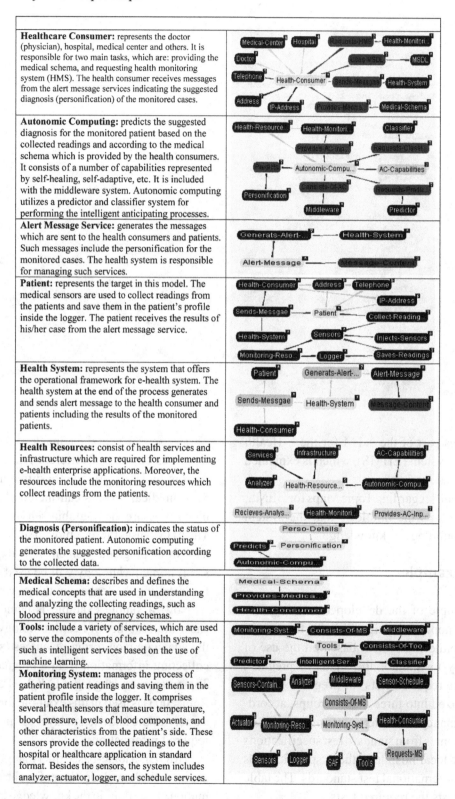

Healthcare Consumer: represents the doctor (physician), hospital, medical center and others. It is responsible for two main tasks, which are: providing the medical schema, and requesting health monitoring system (HMS). The health consumer receives messages from the alert message services indicating the suggested diagnosis (personification) of the monitored cases.	
Autonomic Computing: predicts the suggested diagnosis for the monitored patient based on the collected readings and according to the medical schema which is provided by the health consumers. It consists of a number of capabilities represented by self-healing, self-adaptive, etc. It is included with the middleware system. Autonomic computing utilizes a predictor and classifier system for performing the intelligent anticipating processes.	
Alert Message Service: generates the messages which are sent to the health consumers and patients. Such messages include the personification for the monitored cases. The health system is responsible for managing such services.	
Patient: represents the target in this model. The medical sensors are used to collect readings from the patients and save them in the patient's profile inside the logger. The patient receives the results of his/her case from the alert message service.	
Health System: represents the system that offers the operational framework for e-health system. The health system at the end of the process generates and sends alert message to the health consumer and patients including the results of the monitored patients.	
Health Resources: consist of health services and infrastructure which are required for implementing e-health enterprise applications. Moreover, the resources include the monitoring resources which collect readings from the patients.	
Diagnosis (Personification): indicates the status of the monitored patient. Autonomic computing generates the suggested personification according to the collected data.	
Medical Schema: describes and defines the medical concepts that are used in understanding and analyzing the collecting readings, such as blood pressure and pregnancy schemas.	
Tools: include a variety of services, which are used to serve the components of the e-health system, such as intelligent services based on the use of machine learning.	
Monitoring System: manages the process of gathering patient readings and saving them in the patient profile inside the logger. It comprises several health sensors that measure temperature, blood pressure, levels of blood components, and other characteristics from the patient's side. These sensors provide the collected readings to the hospital or healthcare application in standard format. Besides the sensors, the system includes analyzer, actuator, logger, and schedule services.	

Table 1.Required pregnancy test

Trimester	Test
First	Weight, hCG, Gonorrhea, Chlamydia, Syphilis, Urinalysis, UrineCulture, Rubella, IRT, StoolTrypsin, PapSmear, HIVAntibody, Hepatitis_B, Hemoglobin, SickleCell, CF_GeneMutation, SweatChloride
Second	Weight, Rubella, CVS, AFP_Maternal, hCG, nconjugatedEstriol, inhibin_A, Glucose, GTT, HIVAntibody, Urinalysis, Hemoglobin
Third	Weight, Rubella, Urinalysis, HIVAntibody, GroupB Streptococcus, Hemoglobin, PlateletCount, Gonorrhea, Chlamydia, Syphilis, fFN

of predicates, which are relationships between sets of values. A predicate can be thought of as a table of all the sets of values that make it true, and querying is done by matching the query against the table, and then returning all sets of values that match. This is shown in the simple example in Figure 9, which shows the query for requesting information regarding the required tests for the second trimester for the pregnancy case. The knowledge layer returns the predicates of all the resources required for accomplishing the task as shown in the figure. The predicate in this case represents the relation between the medical schema and the monitoring resources.

FUTURE WORK

The importance of collaborative framework for healthcare framework is clear, but it needs a lot of development and research. Till now there is no standard had been adopted in healthcare collaborative framework that is assisting in taking the collaborative framework to next level, which is semantic collaborative framework. The SOAW2G is first step towards the concept of semantic collaborative framework. SOAW2G provides model for controlling the collaborative framework and manage the use of resources in open standard format.

Figure 9. XTM example

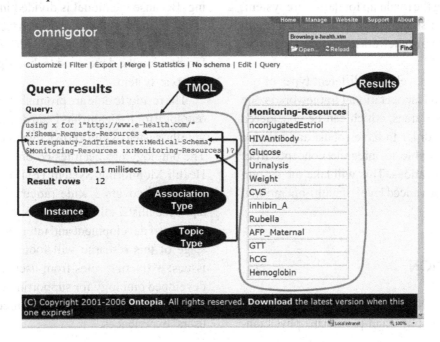

The SOAW2G model offers an operational framework for different types of enterprise applications. It is proposed initially for healthcare applications, but can be extended in the future to include a range of other applications. The specific type of application will assist in providing the framework with a roadmap on how to manage the resources layer, based on the priority of the framework. Additional cases studies and examples of developing healthcare applications using SOAW2G can be examined in the future, as can different smart classification methods, such as Self Organizing Maps, Neural Networks, Support Vector Machines, Multiple Regression Analysis, and others. All of the resources classification and management is established in the Resources Management Layer. Therefore, interaction between this layer and resource providers needs improvement, in order to have a common language between the system and providers, so as to facilitate the deployment and classification of resources on-fly.

System and data security is one of the major issues that need significant additional work in order to improve the level of security, e.g. through using a smart security system or a security agent that takes into consideration previous experience when drawing the roadmap for the secure system. Quality of published medical information through the collaborative framework needs to be monitored in the future.

Ultimately, developing different types of ontology based on an operational framework is one of the research areas, which can be considered the future, in order to have robust and reliable system that is able to integrate concepts from different applications. This will take the system to a new and advanced level of multi-operational framework.

CONCLUSION

This chapter discusses the healthcare collaborative framework for physician-physician, physician-

patient, and patient-patient interaction. The collaborative framework improves the responsibility of patients by providing patients with support, advice and services. Web 2.0 makes it possible to establish collaborative framework. However, such initiatives in early stage and needs a lot of support resources to run the enterprise applications.

Thus, the work in this chapter has presented a generic model for healthcare applications and collaborative framework, based on the integration of different technologies into one robust framework that uses SOA as a basis for managing the integration and interaction between components of the system. The developed model offers a resources manageable framework that is able to react to the changes in environmental behavior, in addition to applying users' experiences and knowledge for re-managing the operational framework to give better services and sharing framework. The SOAW2G model also offers a knowledgeable framework that assists the components of the system to obtain knowledge and information in an open standard format.

Different technologies are integrated through this model, including Web 2.0, Grid Computing, Ontology, Web Services, and autonomic computing. Because the model is divided into a number of layers, the development of each technology can be done separately. SOA provides the platform for merging the developed technologies together into one system.

The results to date are promising; in particular, ontology for E-Health has been developed to provide the system with a knowledgeable framework. The ontology has been tested on a prototype E-Health Monitoring System (EHMS). However, the model covers a wide range of applications and specialists, all of which needs a significant amount of development and integration. The next stage of this research will focus on two major issues: extracting rules from users based on the developed ontology for supporting collaborative framework; and managing resources based on users' experiences.

REFERENCES

Ahmad, B., Omar, W., & Taleb-Bendiab, A. (2006). *Intelligent Monitoring Model For Sensing Financial Application Behaviour Based On Grid Computing Overlay.* Paper presented at the Submitted to 2006 IEEE International Conference on Services Computing (SCC 2006), USA.

BIRN. (n.d.). http://www.nbirn.net/

Breton, V. (2005). *From Grid to Healthgrid: Prospects and Requirements.* Paper presented at the Healthgrid 2005. caBIG. (n.d.). https://cabig.nci.nih.gov/

Eder, J., & Koncilia, C. (2002). *Incorporating ICD-9 and ICD-10 Data in a Warehouse.* Paper presented at the 15th IEEE Symposium on Computer-Based Medical Systems (CBMS'02).

Fellenstein, G. (2005). *On Demand Computing: Technologies and Strategies.* IBM Press.

Ferreira, L., Berstis, V., Armstrong, J., Kendzierski, M., Neukoetter, A., & Takagi, M. (2003). *Introduction to Grid Computing with Globus.* IBM.

Garshol, L. (2002). *What Are Topic Maps?* Graauw, M. (2002). *Business Maps: Topic Maps Go B2B.*

Grid Services Provisioning. *Journal of Computer Sciences, 6*(2), 521-527.

IBM. (2003). Autonomic Computing. May 2004, from http://www.research.ibm.com/autonomic

ICD-10. (n.d.). http://www.who.int/classifications/icd/en/index.html.

IHTSDO. (n.d.). http://www.ihtsdo.org/.

Jagannathan, V., Reddy, Y. V., Srinivas, K., Karinthi, R., Shank, R., Reddy, S., et al. (1995). *An overview of the CERC ARTEMIS project.* Paper presented at the Symposium on Computer Applications in Medical Care.

Korthaus, A., & Hildenbrand, T. (2003). *Creating a Java- and CORBA-Based Enterprise Knowledge Grid Using Topic Maps.* Paper presented at the Workshop on Knowledge Grid and Grid Intelligence.

Marks, E. A. (2006). *Service-oriented architecture: a planning and implementation guide for business and technology / Eric A. Marks, Michael Bell.* Hoboken, NJ: Wiley.

Murch, R. (2004). *Autonomic Computing.* Prentice Hall.

NetworkedPlanet. (2005). Topic Maps in Web-site Architecture.

Newcomb, S., & Durusau, P. (August 2005). *Multiple Subject Map Patterns for Relationships and TMDM Information Items.* Paper presented at the Extreme Markup Languages 2005, Montréal, Canada.

Omar, W., Ahmad, B., & Karam, Y. (2006). Autonomic Middleware Services for Just-In-Time

Omar, W., Ahmad, B., & Taleb-Bendiab, A. (2006). *Grid Overlay for Remote E-Health Monitoring.* Paper presented at the The 4th ACS/IEEE International Conference on Computer Systems and Applications (AICCSA-06).

Omar, W., Ahmad, B., Taleb-Bendiab, A., & Karam, Y. (2005, 24-28, May). *A Software Framework for Open Standard Self-Managing Sensor Overlay For Web Services.* Paper presented at the 7th International Conference on Enterprise Information Systems (ICEIS2005), MIAMI BEACH- FLORIDA-USA.

Omar, W., & Taleb-Bendiab, A. (2006). E-Health Support Services Based On Service Oriented Architecture. *IEEE IT Professional, 8*(2), 35–41. doi:10.1109/MITP.2006.32

Omar, W., Taleb-Bendiab, A., & Karam, Y. (2005a, 27-28, June). *PlanetLab Overlay: Experimenting with Sensing and Actuation Support for Situated Autonomic Computing Services.* Paper presented at the 6th PG net2005 conference, Liverpool, UK.

Omar, W., Taleb-Bendiab, A., & Karam, Y. (2005b, 19-21,September). *PlanetLab Overlay: Experimenting With Sensing and Actuation Support For Situated Autonomic Computing Services For The Planetary- Scale System.* Paper presented at the iiWAS, Malaysia.

Omar, W., Taleb-Bendiab, A., & Karam, Y. (2006). Autonomic Middleware Services for Just-In-Time Grid Services Provisioning. *Journal of Computer Sciences, 6*(2), 521–527.

Ontopia. (n.d.). http://www.ontopia.net/.

Paindaveine, S. N. a. Y. (2002). *HealthGrid Terms of Reference.*

Partners, G. T. (2002). *The Autonomic Computing Report – Characteristics of Self Managing IT Systems.*

Pepper, S. (2002). The TAO of Topic Maps.

Rath, H. (2003). *The Topic Maps Handbook: empolis GmbH.* Germany: Gutersloh.

Reddy, R., Jagannathan, V., Srinivas, K., Karinthi, R., Reddy, S. M., Gollapudy, C., & Friedman, S. (1993). *ARTEMIS: a collaborative framework for health care.* Paper presented at the Annual Symposium on Computer Application [sic] in Medical Care.

SNOMED-CT. (n.d.). http://www.nlm.nih.gov/research/umls/Snomed/snomed_main.html.

TopicMaps.Org. (n.d.). XML Topic Maps (XTM) 1.0.

TriZetto. (n.d.). http://integratedhealth.trizetto.com/main/pages/TriZetto/IHMX/ShowCollateral.aspx?oid=26955&ssid=0&hid=0&sid=0&cp=1950.

Tuchinda, R., Szekely, P., & Knoblock, C. A. (2008). *Building Mashups by example.* Paper presented at the 13th international conference on Intelligent user interfaces, Gran Canaria, Spain.

Wong, J., & Hong, J. I. (2007). *Making mashups with marmite: towards end-user programming for the web.* Paper presented at the Human Factors in Computing Systems, San Jose, California, USA

Chapter 11
An Agent–Based Architecture to Ubiquitous Health

Daniel Ruiz Fernández
University of Alicante, Spain

ABSTRACT

Currently, evolution of health services is strongly influenced by the development of information and communication technologies. Distribution of health services brings new challenges to computer systems, with regard to processing capability as well as to communications, storage and security. The proposal explained in this chapter is an architecture design to be easily adapted to advances in healthcare decentralization. It is intended to provide the capability to implement a global distribution of healthcare, even reaching the patient's home, workplace or holiday hotel. This is a distributed architecture which is flexible to implement new functionalities and accessible from anywhere. The architecture is based on the paradigm of agents and defines the different types of agents that may form the system and their interactions.

INTRODUCTION

Information and communication technologies are essential pieces to the development of an enormous variety of knowledge areas such as those related to economics, engineering, advertising, education, etc. Furthermore, the fact that public organizations provide many services via the Internet has allowed computers to be increasingly present in homes.

Health is one of the areas with a high social impact to which computing can be applied. Despite the benefits that information technologies can bring to healthcare, the use of them is not direct and involves more difficulties than in other areas (Goldschmidt, 2005; Tan, 2005). First of all, it should be borne in mind that private information is being handled and must be protected to safeguard patients' privacy (Gritzalis, 2004). Along the lines of security, any transmission of personal health information must be protected to prevent accidental or deliberate interferences that may alter the data (Sulaiman, Sharma, Ma, & Tran, 2007). Moreover, a computer system to be used in healthcare environments should be flexible

DOI: 10.4018/978-1-61520-777-0.ch011

Copyright © 2010, IGI Global. Copying or distributing in print or electronic forms without written permission of IGI Global is prohibited.

enough to be adapted to new medical protocols or to any advance in the field of medicine.

In order to analyze to what extent information technologies can contribute directly to improve clinical activities, we need to understand the main objective of healthcare organizations. Thus, we are concentrating on their activity, which is aimed at maintaining population health. Health is defined in WHO Constitution as "a state of complete physical, mental and social well-being and not merely the absence of disease or infirmity" (WHO, 2006). Therefore, healthcare professionals' work extends beyond diagnosing and treating diseases. The computer systems to be used in healthcare must be tools that help professionals to ensure that patients reach a state of well-being as stated in the aforesaid WHO's definition.

According to the above definition and focusing on a health management system that is not interfered by economic or political factors, the activities of healthcare organizations can be divided into four main areas: prevention or health promotion, early detection and monitoring, treatment or cure, and maintenance. The improvement of healthcare and, therefore, the effectiveness in the performance of these activities, is limited by population growth, existing resources, both material and human, and scientific advances in medicine.

Population growth, due to both migration processes and increased birth rates and life expectancy, involves increasing healthcare needs. If these needs cannot be met, long-term care activities are usually sacrificed (e.g. prevention activities) in favor of a more direct care focused on diagnosis and treatment. In the same way, lack of material and human resources is tried to be solved: activities that maintain health status are restricted. For their part, advances in medicine are the most directly related to the improvements of healthcare that can affect citizens. Advances in medicine, especially in recent centuries, have greatly increased the body of knowledge, making the specialization of healthcare professionals necessary (Porter, 2006). This working sector does

not only include doctors and nurses but also those professionals who collaborate to reach the state of well-being defined by the WHO: psychologists, social workers, physiotherapists, etc.

Decentralization of health services is a strategy that can be followed in order to maximize existing health resources and to integrate the specialization arising from the increase of knowledge in health science into the health system. The most advanced health systems have gone from offering a variety of services in a hospital to distribute them amongst different entities and levels. Thus, there are *hospitals* that have professionals and the most advanced infrastructures to see the most complicated cases. In the next level, there are *specialty centers* that have specialized professionals who could see less serious cases using more limited resources. In the last level, there are *health centers* that are closer to patients and carry out healthcare with the aim of reaching the aforesaid state of well-being, more than treating serious health problems (which would be referred to specialty centers or hospitals) (Lisac, Blum, & Schlette, 2008).

However, it is still possible to define a lower level in health services that would bring healthcare to patients' home. Although there are already some activities that patients can carry out and, then, free health centers of these tasks (e.g. administration of insulin, blood pressure taking, etc.), these activities do not necessarily require professional supervision and are intended more for the patient's own control than for the monitoring of the doctor. The terms *home healthcare* and *hospital at home* refer to a wide range of services available thanks to the possibility of accessing the case history from home. This, for example, makes possible that the monitoring of blood pressure taken by a patient every day is recorded in his health record and reviewed by the doctor.

The decentralization of health services can even be adapted to diagnostic tasks so that a first remote diagnosis can be made through the advice via chat or by videoconference. This initial diagnosis may be useful to administer treatment more quickly or to establish a waiting list at the doctor's office depending on the seriousness of the situation (van Bemmel & Musen, 1997).

Other services that can be performed at home are related to dependence. The care of older people is not only restricted to prevent them from getting ill (and treat them when needed), but also to maintain good health status, i.e. to maintain a high degree of mental and social well-being. Therefore, any service with this objective can be included in the health information system. Among other services, the system could include rehabilitation applications that enable older people (who often have mobility problems) to do exercises at home. Information on the performance of the exercises would be instantly available to the doctor or physiotherapist who could monitor them (Martin Moreno, Ruiz Fernandez, Soriano Paya, & Berenguer Miralles, 2008).

One of the most important characteristics to be met by the systems that facilitate the decentralization of health services is flexibility. Excessive rigidity in the definition of the services or architectures would limit system expansion and implementation of new capabilities as advances in medicine and healthcare are made. Besides flexibility, availability of services and communication between the elements involved in the system are also aspects to take into account in the design. The decentralization of resources involves the need to transfer information; therefore, technology must be able to meet that need with high levels of reliability and security.

The paradigm of agents inherently meets the fundamental requirements of the architecture to be designed, such as the distribution of components and the needed flexibility. It also provides mechanisms for communication among the entities that will form the system. Another interesting feature of this paradigm is independence in the performance of the agents: each agent can have an independent functionality and, in certain circumstances, can cooperate with other agents to reach a common goal.

In this chapter it is explained, from a general a perspective, a distributed system based in the paradigm of agents oriented to satisfy the needs, in terms of ubiquity and decentralization, of health services. The purpose of the chapter is not to present concrete developments but to give a set of general needs and ideas which can be the base for further developments in the area of ubiquitous health or home health. The following sections present, firstly, an introduction to the paradigm of agents on which the designed architecture is based; next, we define a potential structure of a system with decentralized health services; after the structure, we put forward an application scenario and some ethical aspects related to the establishment of the system and, finally, conclusions on the subject are presented.

BACKGROUND

A review of literature on telemedicine provides an enormous variety of references from researches in pursuit of providing remote health services. Since communication technology was able to offer distance information transferring, researches have focused on harnessing these technologies for medicine (Wootton, Craig, & Patterson, 2006). The purpose of this chapter is not to be exhaustive in covering the history of telemedicine, nor to provide a detailed description of the developments and researches that are being undertaken nowadays. Instead, it is intended to provide a general overview of research on this area, in order to give the reader an idea of this issue and its different approaches.

Most investigations have been conducted focusing on specific problems or addressing just one specialty. In this respect, we find applications in all areas of medicine: neurology (Patterson, 2005), psychology (McGinty, Saeed, Simmons,

& Yildirim, 2006), cardiology (Nugent, Wang, Black, Finlay, & Owens, 2006), pneumology (Taylor, Eliasson, Andrada, Kristo, & Howard, 2006), pediatrics (Smith, 2007), etc.

One area in which a large number of research groups are working is medical image transfer. An example of these works is projects that try to integrate teleradiology into mobile systems (Georgiadis et al., 2007; Reponen et al., 2005). Other researches on teleradiology are focused on optimizing transfer and enhancing security (Alaoui et al., 2003; Puech, Chazard, Lemaitre, & Beuscart, 2007).

Besides, there have been developed projects related to medical diagnosis in which artificial intelligence techniques have been used to provide diagnosis-support systems (Greenes, 2007). Most of these systems also allow remote inquiries through the Internet. We can find clinical decision-support systems in many medical specialties such as cardiology (Yan, Jiang, Zheng, Peng, & Li, 2005), dermatology (Berenguer, Ruiz, & Soriano, 2008), oncology (Rossille, Laurentc, & Burguna, 2005), ophthalmology (Mitra, Lee, & Goldbaum, 2005), etc. There are some initiatives related to diagnosis support that use cooperative systems with several decision entities collaborating to provide a more accurate diagnosis (Ruiz, Soriano, Montejo, & Bueno, 2006).

We can also find projects related to medicine that tackle the development of knowledge networks. An example of this type of networks is OpenClinical project. OpenClinical is an international non-profit organization created and maintained as a public service with support from Cancer Research UK. One of the objectives of OpenClinical is to promote decision support and other knowledge management technologies in patient care and clinical research.

Other projects related to healthcare are those that try to bring sensor devices to homes (Leijdekkers, Gay, & Lawrence, 2007). These devices could be used to detect health problems or elderly people falling down and submit an alert message to a relative or to emergency services (Sixsmith & Johnson, 2004).

Finally, there are research projects in which agents are used to provide several health services, although, as mentioned before, they focus on solving specific problems. Intelligent agents are mainly used to implement diagnosis-support systems (Cervantes, Lee, Yang, Ko, & Lee, 2007; Moreno & Garbay, 2003).

AGENTS BASED ARCHITECTURE

The characteristics of the paradigm of agents make it an ideal base on which we can develop the distributed architecture, health-services-oriented, described on this chapter. An agent can be defined simply as an element that perceives the context and tries to modify it in a given direction, according to its objectives (Russell & Norvig, 2003; Wooldridge, 2000). Agents act with a certain degree of autonomy and independence in order to accomplish tasks without requiring the supervision of people or other agents. Besides the degree of autonomy, agents can also have different degrees of intelligence that determine their capabilities of decision and reaction to the environment (Tweedale et al., 2007). Depending on the degree of intelligence, the agents can be able to take initiatives or even to make inferences; therefore, symbolic rules can be defined (similarly to expert systems) or we can use heuristics based on artificial intelligence techniques like neural networks (Quteishat, Peng Lim, Tweedale, & Jain, 2009). An agent with a minimum degree of intelligence would agree with a reactive agent whose behavior is defined by perception-action rules.

Agents are able to work asynchronously and to modify their behavior according to the accumulated knowledge. This ability to learn provides agents with adaptability characteristics that have many applications in healthcare. For example, with regard to glycemic control in a person with diabetes, the agent responsible for this control

Table 1. Summary of the agent features in this architecture

Autonomy	It is not necessary a supervision of the activity to accomplish the objectives
Intelligence	To take initiatives and to make inferences.
Adaptability	Agents can adapt their behavior to a new environment
Veracity	Do not provide false information
Benevolence	They can help other agents
Rationality	To achieve the objectives in a rational way

should adapt the pattern of insulin administration according to patient's daily activity. In this case, agent's adaptation is essential, always within control ranks that ensure proper operation.

There are other characteristics that agents are held to present and that have a great importance in a medical environment (Cortés, Annicchiarico, & Urdiales, 2008; Moreno & Garbay, 2003; Moreno & Nealon, 2003). These characteristics are: veracity, which involves that an agent will not deliberately provide false information; benevolence, which means that an agent will help other agents provided that this will not come into conflict with its own objectives and goals, and rationality, which enables an agent to act in a rational fashion, trying to achieve its objectives, and prevents it from acting in a way contrary to them (according to its perceptions of the environment). Despite these features, and taking into account the area of application, we should asses the possible existence of malicious agents with objectives not in accord with those of the system. Table 1 shows a summary of the agent features of the architecture proposed in this chapter.

The union of several agents that interact to achieve an objective results in a multi-agent system (Tweedale et al., 2007; Weyns, Helleboogh, Holvoet, & Schumacher, 2009). In (Ferber, 1999), interaction is defined as a set of behaviors of a group of agents that collaborate to achieve an objective, focusing on their high or low resources availability and their individual profiles. This interaction will get more complex, as the problem-solving method will be more social and distribute

(Bai & Zhang, 2006; Shoham & Leyton-Brown, 2009). The form of interaction that best fits the operation we want in our system is cooperation in which each agent involved contributes in a different way, according its capabilities, to achieve a common objective (Ossowski, 2008; Zhang, Xi, & Yang, 2008). There are other forms of interaction between agents such as negotiation, but the clinical system presented does not include the aspects that require these other forms of interaction.

In order to unify communication between agents, Agent Communication Languages (ACLs) (Verdicchio & Colombetti, 2009) have been defined, which are standard formats to exchange messages between agents. One of the best known is KQML (Knowledge Query and Manipulation Language) (Finin & Labrou, 1997; Khazab, Tweedale, & Jain, 2009), based on the use of performatives (Abdalla, 2006). Also available is the standard defined by FIPA (Bagherzadeh & Arun-Kumar, 2006; FIPA, 2009), which includes features of KQML. In general, regardless the communication standard, it includes information on issuing and receiving agents, language used to transfer the body or content of the message, ontology on which communication will be based, and content. Those are the minimum necessary fields to make a controlled communication between agents. An example of a message using FIPA ACL can be:

```
(inform
  :sender (agent-identifier:idA12)
  :receiver (agent-identifier:idA23)
  :language XML
```

```
:ontology MED-DIABETES
:content (<measure>
  <value>105</value><date>20091230</
date><time>1235</time>
  </measure>))
```

The basic agent-based architecture that we use in this proposal is made up of a type of cognitive agents we named PCI (Perception-Cognition-Intention). These agents are based on BDI agents (Belief-Desire-Intention) (Novak & Dix, 2006; Padgham & Lambrix, 2005; Pokahr, Braubach, & Lamersdorf, 2005) but they overload the cognitive part. PCI agents are made up of a module called Perception (equivalent to Belief) that includes the set of functionalities that allow it to understand and classify significant states of the world, i.e. perceptions of the environment and beliefs arising from those perceptions. The cognitive module contains agent intelligence and represents the set of functionalities that makes task selection possible to achieve a particular objective. In this part of the agent, besides the desire to achieve a particular objective, we also include, for example, adaptability features and, therefore, the capability to modify agent's objectives. The knowledge and decision capabilities of the agent can be modeled using artificial intelligence methods as case-based reasoning, fuzzy logic or neural networks. Intention module is responsible for sending modification intentions to the environment, according to the decisions made. In addition, PCI also has the ability to memorize the states of the world and its own behavior, improving decision intelligence of the agent or allowing, for example, a continuous learning for cognitive functions based on artificial neural networks. Furthermore, a PCI agent can execute a sequence of actions in a previous established order known as a plan, in order to achieve an objective. The capacity to memorize internal and external states allows the agent to adapt its decision function and planning according to the results of previous intentions. In this way, if the agent faces a repeated situation can use the historical information stored to improve its decisions.

PCI agents are always in a cycle of perception, deliberation and execution of intentions. Figure 1 shows a diagram of the PCI agent.

Communication between PCI agents involves perceptions and intentions. Therefore, a perception may be a message coming from a system agent or from an external agent, or may be information from a sensor element that perceives a state of the environment (e.g. a device to measure vital signs like a tensiometer). Equally, intentions may be indications to devices (actuators) for the performance of particular actions (e.g. administration of an extra dose of insulin or call an emergency center). These messages may be sent to system agents or to external entities.

The architecture presented in this proposal is made up of several PCI agents that form a multi-agent system with the objective of providing the best health status of patients. As discussed above, when explaining communication, agents of a particular multi-agent system can also communicate with external agents, independent from their system. Hence, configuration of a multi-agent system is determined by the collection of agents that share the same objective or function and that work in a cooperative fashion. Several multi-agent systems can collaborate in certain situations, forming a super system.

Figure 1. Structure of a PCI agent

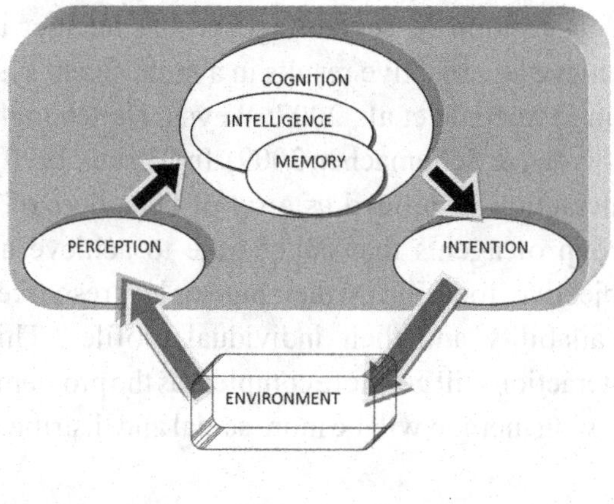

CLINICAL DISTRIBUTED SYSTEM

Once defined the basic architecture of our system, next we deal with a higher layer of abstraction to explain the functionalities of the different types of agents that form the system. To this end, we will explain first the performance of the global clinical distributed system.

Initial Considerations

The proposal outlined in this chapter aims to offer an architecture that can be used to provide ubiquitous health services and, thus, to meet technological requirements of healthcare decentralization as explained in the introduction. First of all, we classify the actors (human or artificial) that take part in healthcare:

- **Patients**: Direct targets of the system actions, oriented to improve health. It is important to highlight that, although the term "patient" is related to an ill person, this group includes ill users as well as healthy users that want to maintain or improve their health status.
- **Family**: This is a type of users that can provide useful information to the system and may be an essential part for the treatment needed to reach the best health status of a patient.
- **Healthcare staff**: This group involves all the people with health knowledge that work in any specialty with the objective of maintaining or improving the health status of patients. Users belonging to this group may also be present in other groups; then, their profile to access the system is modified according to the role they access with.
- **Administrative staff**: System users that accomplish tasks of system maintenance and administrative management. Among these tasks, we find the constant monitoring of the system to ensure proper operation.

- **Technical staff**: System users who are responsible for technically supervising the behavior of software agents and system devices.
- **Software agents**: Key elements of the system that form a health network which is able to provide several health services at anywhere and with the highest availability.
- **Devices**: Sensor and actuator elements required for software agents to obtain health information in order to make decisions and perform actions that are oriented to maintain or improve health.

All these groups of actors can be divided according to their participation in the system. This way, there are regular users that can be continually active in the system and casual users if they act in a sporadic or intermittent pattern. The same actor may be regular in some scenarios or for some patients and casual in other situations. For instance, a digestive specialist will be considered as a regular actor for a patient with a chronic digestive disease whereas, for a patient who gets indigestion, he will be a casual actor. The same will apply to software agents and devices. In figure 2 it is possible to observe a scheme of the system proposed.

After reviewing the types of system users, it is necessary to detail some system features, especially those that will determine in a way the system architecture and interaction of the components. These features are listed below:

- **Highest availability**: The system should provide the highest availability if it is possible. Some services may be available 24 hours a day, 7 days a week, while other services may have a lower availability due to either limited infrastructures in charge of the service (outside the system), or restricted schedules of staff seconded to the service. The first situation is the case of a dairy blood pressure taking when the sensor

Figure 2. Scheme of the actors in the system

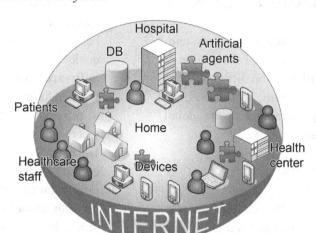

device breaks down. The second situation arises when telemedicine inquiries must stick to the doctor's schedule.

- **Autonomy**: Components providing different services must act with the highest possible autonomy by including self-correction routines (based on operating limits) in order to deal with situations of improper operation. Anyway, even though subsystems are interconnected, dependence relations must be minimized to prevent a problem in a particular service from causing a staircase effect. Addition of artificial intelligence techniques to agents will also increase their autonomy in terms of decision-making ability.

- **Accessibility**: Easy access to the system is another important feature. We should bear in mind that this is a complex system whose users have no technical knowledge. Moreover, the healthcare sector usually has well-defined protocols that determine its manner of working and, therefore, the system must be adapted to these protocols. Furthermore, we should consider that patients may be elderly people who are unfamiliar with information technology; indeed, we can find users who suffer from

any physical handicap such as vision or hearing problems. Taking into account this large diversity of users, usability and accessibility must be maximized.

- **Learning**: The system must be able to learn behaviors and situations, so that a highest degree of autonomy is reached. Such learning depends directly on the degree of intelligence given to the agents and may be a key in the improvement of the patients' quality of life. Providing health services which are able to learn patient's behaviors or emergency procedures is the ultimate expression of patient-oriented health care: an individualized healthcare for each patient.

- **Flexibility**: The system should allow relatively easy addition of new services along with maintenance and updating of existing services. Healthcare is continuously evolving, discovering new therapies or correcting existing therapies (due to advances or problem solving in terms of their application). All these changes should be quickly included in the services provided by the system.

Agents and Their Interaction

First of all, we would like to state that the types of agents presented here form a basic architecture, which must be adapted to every scenario, situation and service. Specific features for the agents are not described, but general behaviors that should be detailed in the specific implementations. Similarly, we explain general interactions among the different types of agents, without going into details.

We have chosen a functional classification of the types of agents, as we are going to stress this aspect. According to this classification, the system may have diagnostic agents, treatment agents, information agents, control agents and health agents. Figure 3 shows a diagram of these groups. Each group in turn will be divided into subgroups with more specific functionalities.

In the first place, diagnostic agents are those whose main function is to collaborate on diagnostic tasks. These tasks may refer to the whole diagnostic process or only a part. Depending on the activities they perform, there are agents responsible for retrieving useful information for the diagnostic

Figure 3. Types of agents

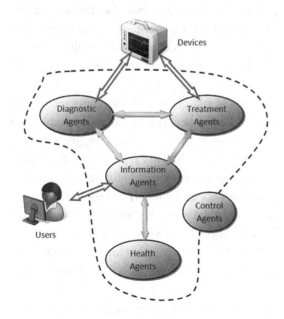

task and there are agents directly involved in the diagnostic decision-making process. In the first group, agents directly interact with medical sensor devices, such as an electrocardiograph or a pulsioximeter; besides, there are agents, belonging to this group, that control devices which are not considered medical devices, but they can certainly help in a diagnostic process, for example, a video camera to record the behavior of a person with Alzheimer's symptoms.

Agents involved in a diagnostic decision-making process may be agents that transmit a doctor's diagnosis as well as agents with a high degree of intelligence that include a clinical decision support system. Diagnostic agents have a minimum degree of intelligence and can be regarded as the interface of human specialists in relation to the system, as they give their expert opinions to the system with regard to a diagnosis. The degree of intelligence depends on the method used in the clinical decision support system implemented inside of the diagnostic agent (in the cognitive module). For example, it can be used an expert system based on rules or, if it is necessary more flexibility in the diagnosis task, a classification system based on neural networks can be implemented. Furthermore, measures from the decision support system as classification rate, specificity and sensibility can be used to set the reliability (in terms of diagnosis) for the diagnostic agent (Ruiz Fernandez & Soriano Paya, 2009). All these agents may act in isolation or collaborate in a cooperative diagnostic process consisting of a virtual meeting (as maybe they are not at the same place) of several entities (human and artificial) that issue possible diagnoses to achieve a single diagnosis agreed by consensus. In these cases, there is also a consensus agent (that belongs to the diagnostic agents group) responsible for handle negotiations in order to achieve the best possible diagnosis, according to previously established criteria (Ruiz et al., 2006). Moreover, these agents involved in diagnostic process will be able to send and receive inquiries to and from other diagnostic agents.

At this point, it is important to focus on the high degree of availability of the system in diagnostic processes, since, although when diagnosis is needed urgently and there are no doctors available for any reason, an artificial diagnostic entity will always be available for issuing a first urgent diagnosis. Ethical considerations that this action may involve will be discussed later.

In the second place, treatment agents are those intended for collaborating in administering or supervising treatment. Since the system aims to promote decentralization of health services and their extension to home care, the term treatment also refers to changes in behavior patterns the patient should make in is daily life. Therefore, there are treatment agents directly related to devices (such as an insulin pump), but there also are agents that are used for treatment validation or monitoring; although they are not directly related to treatment, they do contribute to asses development of a health problem. A simple example of this type of devices is a pedometer to record the number of steps in a patient with obesity problems who has been prescribed a two-hour daily walk.

We can consider that treatment agents that are monitoring a patient's activity are incurring violation of privacy rights of patients. In order to minimize this interference, monitoring results can be analyzed by an artificial diagnostic agent that, finally, will inform the doctor about the results of the treatment monitoring and not about specific data. In this way, all the data that can be considered "private" or "sensitive" is always inside the system and it is just possible to access to the medical results extracted from this information, not to the original data. If the original data are necessary, a patient can authorize a doctor to access. This will preserve patient's privacy rights to the maximum extent possible. For instance, in the case of monitoring a patient with cameras at home in order to determine whether a treatment for urinary incontinence is working or not, the treatment agent would inform an artificial agent (a decision-support system) about how many times

the patient goes to the bathroom and the diagnostic agent would determine whether the medicine is working or not, reporting the results to the doctor. Throughout this process, the doctor never would have access to recordings or to the number of times the patient goes to the bathroom (when needed, this information could be provided in ranges or specific information could be authorized by the patient). This mechanism to protect privacy is also used in collaboration when it is needed an interchange of information between agents (as well as the identification of the agents).

In the third place, information agents are those that provide users with any type of data, including health staff with medical information or patients with detailed information on a particular treatment. These agents collect and display information according to user access privileges and data protection levels. Furthermore, they provide other agents with the data necessary for them to undertake their functions. All this information can be gathered from system users (doctors and patients), other agents (e.g. agents connected to medical devices) or directly from electronic health records. Information agents are the only ones which have full access to patient's case history. Information agents are not only responsible for collecting information but also for storing new information of a patient in clinical databases: symptoms, diagnoses, treatment results, and so on. This type of agents is also the interface between users and the rest of agents.

In the fourth place, control agents accomplish tasks of system supervision. They are responsible for ensuring the whole system integrity and preventing intrusions. This type of agents includes security agents, responsible for intrusion prevention (unauthorized agents) and for validating the operation of the system agents. In order to perform this validation, there will be a database with information about the agents that form the system. This information on the agents will include an agent identifier, type of agent, access level, certification authority or authority responsible for the agent, status (indicating whether it is active or not) and a code for self-assessment. Periodically, security agents will ask the system agents to identify themselves as well as to perform self-assessment. Thus, a thorough control of agents and their operation is performed. Regardless of this control, critical agents can also include a self-assessment schedule every so often, so that the process does not require to be asked by a control agent.

Control agents will also be responsible for accepting or denying the new join of agents as well as for expelling or inhibiting agents with suspected malfunction. All these operations must be reported to technical and administrative staff in charge of the system. In fact, joins or inhibitions of agents considered to be critical must be granted by the system managers.

The last type of agents in the system is the group of health agents. These agents have no specific activity. Their objective is to discover undiagnosed health problems in patients. Therefore, these agents work with artificial intelligence techniques to analyze patient data, for instance, looking for potential risks situations that preventive treatment helps avoid. Health agents are also responsible for epidemiological studies and can use data mining techniques for that purpose.

Security

We must never forget that the proposed system is intended for healthcare environments in which information security is a crucial aspect (Xiao et al., 2008). Security can be addressed at two levels: a lower level, or structural, that must analyze security problems that may affect the architecture itself; and a higher level, or functional, directly related to the information that is transferred or displayed and its access restrictions.

At the functional level, security forces us to define a series of roles related to the types and subtypes of users with access to different information and system functionalities (for example, within the healthcare professional type, user "doctor"

and user "clinical assistant"). System access will require a valid user identification and password; in addition, we should consider, for some actions that involve a high degree of responsibility, the possibility of requiring an additional password, like the systems with dual password or signature used by some banks to operate through the Internet.

It is important to underline that, at no time we are distinguishing between human users and artificial entities (agents acting as system users). Therefore, those artificial entities trying to access the system as users will also have a role and authentication and user passwords will be required.

At the structural level of security, we should bear in mind that the architecture is based on agents that interact and that new agents may join the system or other agents may leave the system. In short, we are dealing with mobile agents that cause a security problem and pose a potential threat to the whole system. These security problems focus on two groups: information alteration and theft or unauthorized access to secured data. These problems are associated with significant risks like those described below:

- Confidential medical information on some patient could be maliciously published.
- User identifications and passwords could be published, completely threatening the information integrity.
- A modified agent could join the system with malicious objectives involving information destruction or unauthorized actions and, therefore, improper operation of the system.
- Control information or data that is being transferred could be obtained, modified and reintegrated into the system to cause unwanted situations or disinformation.

As we have seen, risks arising from security problems are very important and can affect the whole system integrity. Apart from controlling system access of agents acting as users (functional level), we should develop authentication policies for the agents (that guarantee the agent's identity) and access control system at the structural level.

One possible authentication policy is to apply encryption technologies based on public and private key algorithms (like RSA), so that the digital signature of the agent (encrypted text with the corresponding private key) includes a higher degree of security with regard to the information that it transfers (Rhee, 2003). Moreover, we can apply policies based on certificates, so that an agent joining the system should be certified by a higher control entity. This will minimize the risk that agents with malicious objectives will damage the system integrity by joining the system and performing unverified actions.

Certificates that show the validity of an agent can also include its degree of accessibility, i.e., depending on the certification authority of the agent and its level of reliability, the agent will have limitations on its ability to act and restricted functionalities. This may entail taking utility and operational ability from the agent, with the possibility of leaving it useless or unusable. Even though leaving an agent joining the system inoperative may seem a high risk of reducing global functionality, the system must be protected to the maximum extent from potential malicious agents. Regarding the type of information involved and the system functions, it is preferable to follow a conservative strategy in the admission of new agents to the system.

Furthermore, we should perform a continuous monitoring of operation of the agents forming the system in order to detect alterations in behavior and improper operations. These situations may be caused by the natural degradation of the agent functionality or by the alteration caused by an attack. Anyway, these situations must be detected and the malfunctioning agent must be immediately inhibited.

Another security aspect that arises is integrity and protection of private data, i.e. to prevent unauthorized staff from viewing private information or even modifying it and inputting false or wrong data into the system. This risk is mostly entailed by agent operations of data exchange and by information stored in databases. At this point, it is important to note that individual agent functionality must be considered as well as degree of achievement of objectives. Otherwise, an unexpected emergent behavior of several agents could alter achievement of goals. In this case, we should inhibit all the agents that work to achieve the objective and that are causing the wrong emergent behavior.

In order to prevent transfers between agents from being intercepted, apart from including both source and destination identifiers (fields that appear by default in ACLs), the information contained must be encrypted under an algorithm that not only encodes the message but that also detects any data integrity failure (e.g. algorithms like PGP). Moreover, all communications will be established through secure protocols like SSL and HTTPS.

With regard to databases, their content must also be encrypted and data must be dissociated as much as possible in relation to patients. This means that the data of patients should be related to them by random codes rather than using a name, a passport number or a health insurance number.

Database

Storing information in a system like this is an aspect of utmost importance. There are many database managers that can rigorously manage the storage of data which require high protection and integrity levels.

An alternative, used in the architecture implementation explained in the scenario, is to use XML databases (Powell, 2006). Such databases provide a total control over information and even allow agents to directly transfer parts of the database, without requiring processes for obtaining and transforming information. It is also possible to create distributed databases and easily generate small databases to work locally (e.g. a diagnostic agent monitoring a particular vital sign); later, this can be easily included in the global database.

Regarding the information stored in the system, in addition to the patients' health data that must be stored, user data should also be managed (including roles and access levels) as well as information on the agents forming the system. As an additional security measure and in order to make system audits easy, all actions involving any inquiry, information modification or deletion should be recorded.

Interfaces

The described architecture poses an access information system implemented on web technologies, where data are displayed using a structured graphic environment. This definition involves the use of the same interface to access the system from anywhere (ubiquity) and with a wide range of devices. The contents of the different pages displayed will be completed in a dynamic fashion, starting from the information provided by agents, which obtain the data from a database or directly from the devices.

Users may suffer from permanent or temporary disabilities that do not allow them to access the system in a normal way. For these users, it is possible to propose adapted environments that will enable them to enjoy the highest number of functionalities of the system. These environments can be based on visual and vocal recognition, so that the system can react to vocal or gesture commands and, in turn, can provide auditory information or light signal information.

Besides, we have mentioned the existence of elderly users or users with such a technological gap that they are not able to use a computer to access the Internet. For these users, we can think about implementing the interface in devices which may be closer to them like video game consoles (web browsers can be found in most of them) or DTT tuners (using MHP standard).

APPLICATION SCENARIO

This section presents a possible application scenario. We have implemented a particular agent-based architecture to accomplish an exhaustive monitoring of blood glucose levels and oxygen saturation (oximetry). Glycemic control is essential for diabetic patients, as the good control can reduce the number of problems associated with diabetes, especially among the elderly, like glaucoma or diabetic foot. Oximetry is a widely used assessment measure of the health status of patients in order to prevent oxygenation problems. Oxygenation monitoring is very important in patients with chronic lung diseases.

A system based on the said architecture is intended to be implemented so that it will improve quality of life of patients with diabetes and with lung diseases. In order to achieve this improvement, glycemic control and oximetry are to be performed without requiring the patient to come to the health center. In addition, we want to check that the patient does measure properly and with the frequency determined by the doctor.

The scenario is clearly shown in Figure 4. First, the sensors (a pulse oximeter and a glucometer in this case) capture patient information and transfer it to a PDA or a computer via Bluetooth. Second, the data are formatted into a SMS message, which is sent to the hospital via GSM band for mobile phones. The SMS, encrypted by the information agent, contains the type of measure, the responsible agent, the patient's code and the measure. Third, the text message is received at the hospital, thanks to a GSM modem and goes to the data processing center (hospital or health center server). Fourth, the received data are processed by a diagnostic agent in the data server, which analyzes informa-

Figure 4. Application scenario

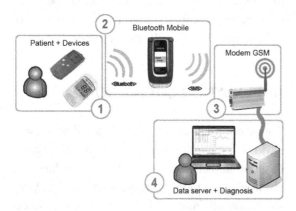

tion looking for anomalies (to alert the specialist assigned to the patient) and stores data.

There are two objectives in this development: first, to make life more bearable for patients and, second, to make doctors' task easier to the maximum extent possible, in order to improve the service provided to the former. In the development of the system software, we have implemented two information agents (one on the patient's side and another on the doctor's side), one control agent, one health agent (on the doctor's side) and three diagnostic agents. Out of the three diagnostic agents, two of them are responsible for data collecting in medical devices, on the patient's side, and the third one is located at the health center's server, analyzing the information. Next, it is explained with more detail the tasks of agents implemented.

On the patient's side we have defined a sensor network made up, initially, by a glucometer and a pulse oximeter connected to a laptop via Bluetooth interface. Diagnostic agents (one for each device) implemented on the laptop are responsible for collecting monitoring data. Diagnostic agents do not analyze this data; they just receive measure from the devices and send the data to the information agent implemented on the laptop. In this data, apart from the glycemic and oximetry values, it is also sent the identification of the patient and

of the diagnostic agent (for security reasons), the measure type (glycemic or oximetry), the date and the time. The information agent formats all this data into a SMS and submits it to the health center. For these transferences, GSM technology is applied, via mobile phone (connected to the laptop).

With regard to the health center, a more powerful infrastructure will be needed. A GSM modem will be provided and this will be managed by another information agent responsible for receiving data from different patients, processing this data and displaying it to healthcare staff in a clear and quick manner. This information agent is also the agent in charge of storing the data. To store data at the health center server, a XML database is used. Apart from receiving and storing data in the database, the information agent at the health center is also responsible for managing the interface with healthcare users.

We have implemented a diagnostic agent on the health center's server which analyzes the information received. Rule logic has been implemented in this diagnostic agent, equally to an expert system, in order to analyze blood glucose levels and oxygenation. If it detects values outside the range established for the patient (according to normality rules that depend on the treatment which is being administered), an alert is generated.

As an example, we have also implemented a health agent located at the health center's server which checks the database regularly, looking for any changes in the evolution of data that could represent an anomaly. In the case of finding any anomaly, an alert message is displayed, from which we can access the alert list, see the patient's medical history and contact him via SMS. The main difference between the diagnostic agent and the health agent located at the health center is that the former analyzes the data as receives them, only considering changes over the last 24 hours. However, the health agent analyzes all the data (not just the last 24 hours), looking for any abnormal pattern.

Control agent is responsible for validating other agents, according to the XML database implemented with information about the system agents. Although this scenario does not require these type of agents (as joining of new agents is not allowed and it is not an open network), they have been implemented too, in order to better adapt the scenario to the proposed architecture.

The interface for doctors' access (a patient access interface has not been designed this time) displays the information in two different ways (Figure 5). The first one allows us to check the patient's progress and consists of a list, similar to a medical history, as a data table, that shows: date and time of measures and the value obtained. The second one is a graph that only has the values (levels) obtained in the last controls of the patient. Thanks to this much more visual representation, patient's progress appears to be clearer.

With the designed architecture, once the infrastructure has been established, implementation of new clinical monitoring devices would be immediate, for example, pacemakers, blood pressure meters, scales, thermometers, and so on. This will broaden the range of patients that no longer would require coming to a health center for a routine check. Moreover, this infrastructure will allow emergencies to be directly reported to the emergency service, providing information on the alert and the patient's medical history in real time.

With the implementation of this scenario, we have tried to provide a small and concrete example for applying the architecture suggested in this chapter. The extension of this scenario with the recording of other medical measures or the addition of other specialties, doctors or even artificial diagnostic systems (clinical decision support systems) increases development complexity, especially with regard to interactions among all the elements that form the system.

ETHICAL ISSUES

The type of information handled by the system and the available functionalities force us to consider the related ethical issues. This section is not intended to provide ethical standards, but to raise questions and situations that may occur in the system operation and that require an ethical assessment. Nevertheless, many countries have already regulated by law some of the issues detailed below.

One of the problems that first arise is the access level to medical histories and their property. Medical histories contain information on patients so, a priori, it is logical to think that medical

Figure 5. Form containing medical data from a patient

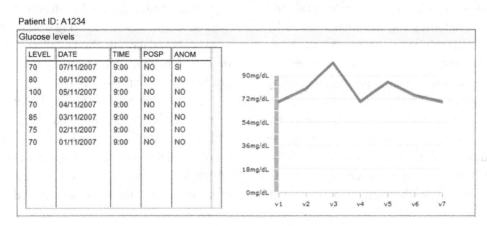

histories belong to patients and that they should have unlimited access to their data. However, the problem arises because healthcare staff is the one responsible for interpreting these data and, usually, the data are linked to that interpretation. Therefore, who is the owner of the data interpretation? Who is the owner of a diagnosis and its corresponding treatment?

In parallel with information property, there is the advisability that a patient should know or not know certain information about his health status. A situation may occur where a patient should not be fully aware of the extent of the disease, as the result would be a clinical depression that would increase the speed or severity of the disease development. In these situations, should we add system restrictions to limit the patients' access to their clinical history? Other cases may require the patient's relatives to care for him and they may need to know diagnosis data and treatment. Should the patient forbid his relatives to access his medical data when this is required for his care?

Another problem comes from the degree of automation in the system. If the issue of a medical diagnosis involves both human and artificial entities, how to decide which diagnosis prevails when they do not match? We face a decision problem in which the degree of certainty of each issued diagnosis is a variable, but how to assess diagnosis issued by a doctor? Furthermore, if there is an error in diagnosis, how to assess the part of responsibility that corresponds to the artificial entity? A possible solution is that a doctor should validate all diagnoses and treatments issued by the system. This solution solves the responsibility problem, but restricts the system functionalities (all diagnostic processes should be reassessed by a doctor) and increases the costs.

We must also consider responsibilities for problems related to data security. In a database with an administrator, it is easy to determine who is responsible for a security breach. However, in a system like this, in which information (which may sometimes be parts of a database) flows through communication networks, maybe with artificial agents acting as issuers and receivers, it is more difficult to determine who is responsible for the security problem.

Finally, we should bear in mind that an extensive system implementation can involve several regional governments and even countries, with different laws. Similarly to e-commerce systems in which seller and buyer may be in different countries and governed by different laws (which impose different obligations), a diagnosis issued by a doctor may have been requested by a patient in another country. Indeed, diagnosis may also be issued by an artificial agent developed in another country other than he is.

As noted above, ethical issues and arising problems are not unique to this proposal, but they are in line with those arising from similar proposals, such as e-commerce. With regard to the medical field, there are very strict laws in most countries, and it has a high social impact. These factors result in added difficulties when implementing such systems.

CONCLUSION

Throughout this chapter, we have described how an intelligent agent-based architecture may contribute to improve healthcare. The main contribution of this architecture is ubiquitous availability of medical services and, therefore, health decentralization. This decentralization can bring healthcare closer to patients and pay attention to other health questions which are difficult to study if healthcare is not brought to patients' homes.

Then, we have defined a set of users and system agents that can be involved in the system, as well as possible interactions between them. The typology of agents and users is a general proposal which must be adapted to each situation and detailed in specific implementations of the system.

In order to illustrate system operation, we have implemented a range of medical services that may be located at the patient's home.

Finally, design and development of the architecture described in this chapter involve a range of problems whose solution determines implementation. These problems include, therefore, technical questions as well as limitations by law and ethical issues.

REFERENCES

Abdalla, J. A. (2006). A communication model for structural design objects: Performatives and protocols. *Advances in Engineering Software, 37*(6), 393–405. doi:10.1016/j.advengsoft.2005.09.001

Alaoui, A., Collmann, J., Nguyen, D., Lindisch, D., Subbiah, R. T. N., Green, A., et al. (2003). *Implementing a secure Teleradiology system using the internet* Paper presented at the Computer Assisted Radiology and Surgery CARS 2003.

Bagherzadeh, J., & Arun-Kumar, S. (2006). Flexible Communication of Agents based on FIPA-ACL. *Electronic Notes in Theoretical Computer Science, 159*, 23–39. doi:10.1016/j.entcs.2005.12.060

Bai, Q., & Zhang, M. (2006). Coordinating Agent Interactions Under Open Environments. In Fulcher, J. (Ed.), *Advances in applied artificial intelligence*. IGI.

Berenguer, V. J., Ruiz, D., & Soriano, A. (2008). *Application of Hidden Markov Models to Melanoma Diagnosis*. Paper presented at the International Symposium on Distributed Computing and Artificial Intelligence (DCAI 2008).

Cervantes, L., Lee, Y.-S., Yang, H., Ko, S.-h., & Lee, J. (2007). Agent-Based Intelligent Decision Support for the Home Healthcare Environment (LNCS 4413, pp. 414-424).

Cortés, U., Annicchiarico, R., & Urdiales, C. (2008). Agents and Healthcare: Usability and Acceptance. In B. Basel (Ed.), Agent Technology and e-Health. Springer.

Ferber, J. (1999). *Multi-Agent Systems. An Introduction to Distributed Artificial Intelligence.* Addison-Wesley.

Finin, T., & Labrou, Y. (1997). KQML as an agent communication language. In Bradshaw, J. M. (Ed.), *Software Agents* (pp. 291–316). MIT Press.

FIPA. (2009). FIPA Agent Communication specifications. Retrieved May 5, 2009, from www.fipa.org

Georgiadis, P., Daskalakis, A., Nikiforidis, G., Cavouras, D., Sifaki, K., Malamas, M., et al. (2007). *PDA-based system with teleradiology and image analysis capabilities*. Paper presented at the Engineering in Medicine and Biology Society, 2007. EMBS 2007. 29th Annual International Conference of the IEEE.

Goldschmidt, P. G. (2005). HIT and MIS: Implications of Health Information Technology and Medical Information Systems. *Communications of the ACM, 48*(10), 69–74.

Greenes, R. A. (Ed.). (2007). *Clinical Decision Support. The Road Ahead.* Elsevier.

Gritzalis, S. (2004). Enhancing Privacy and Data Protection in Electronic Medical Environments. *Journal of Medical Systems, 28*(6). doi:10.1023/B:JOMS.0000044956.55209.75

Khazab, M., Tweedale, J., & Jain, L. C. (2009). Interoperable Intelligent Agents in a Dynamic Environment. In Nakamatsu, K., Phillips-Wren, G., & Jain, L. C. (Eds.), *New Advances in Intelligent Decision Technologies*. doi:10.1007/978-3-642-00909-9_18

Leijdekkers, P., Gay, V., & Lawrence, E. (2007). *Smart Homecare System for Health Tele-monitoring*. Paper presented at the Digital Society, 2007. ICDS '07. First International Conference on the.

Lisac, M., Blum, K., & Schlette, S. (2008). Health Systems and Health Reform in Europe. *Inter Economics*, *43*(4), 184–218. doi:10.1007/s10272-008-0253-z

Martin Moreno, J., Ruiz Fernandez, D., Soriano Paya, A., & Berenguer Miralles, V. J. (2008). *Monitoring 3D movements for the rehabilitation of joints in physiotherapy*. Paper presented at the 30th Annual International Conference of the IEEE Engineering in Medicine and Biology Society.

McGinty, K. L., Saeed, S. A., Simmons, S. C., & Yildirim, Y. (2006). Telepsychiatry and e-Mental Health Services: Potential for Improving Access to Mental Health Care. *The Psychiatric Quarterly*, *77*(4), 335–342. doi:10.1007/s11126-006-9019-6

Mitra, S. K., Lee, T.-W., & Goldbaum, M. (2005). A Bayesian network based sequential inference for diagnosis of diseases from retinal images. *Pattern Recognition Letters*, *26*(4), 459–470. doi:10.1016/j.patrec.2004.08.010

Moreno, A., & Garbay, C. (2003). Software agents in health care. *Artificial Intelligence in Medicine*, *27*(3), 229–232. doi:10.1016/S0933-3657(03)00004-6

Moreno, A., & Nealon, J. L. (Eds.). (2003). *Applications of Software Agent Technology in the Health Care Domain*. Springer.

Novak, P., & Dix, J. (2006). *Modular BDI architecture*. Paper presented at the 5th International Conference on Autonomous Agents.

Nugent, C. D., Wang, H., Black, N. D., Finlay, D. D., & Owens, F. J. (2006). ECG Telecare: Past, present and future. In Istepanian, R. S. H., Laxminarayan, S., & Pattichis, C. S. (Eds.), *M-Health. Emerging Mobile Health Systems* (pp. 375–388). Springer.

Ossowski, S. (2008). *Coordination and Agreement in Multi-Agent Systems*. Paper presented at the Cooperative Information Agents, 12th International Workshop.

Padgham, L., & Lambrix, P. (2005). Formalisations of Capabilities for BDI-Agents. *Autonomous Agetns and Multi-agent Systems*, *10*(3), 249–271. doi:10.1007/s10458-004-4345-2

Patterson, V. (2005). Teleneurology. *Journal of Telemedicine and Telecare*, *11*(2), 55–59. doi:10.1258/1357633053499840

Pokahr, A., Braubach, L., & Lamersdorf, W. (2005). *A BDI architecture for goal deliberation*. Paper presented at the 4th International Conference on Autonomous Agents.

Porter, R. (Ed.). (2006). *The Cambridge History of Medicine* (1st ed.). Cambridge University Press.

Powell, G. (2006). *Beginning XML Databases*. Wrox.

Puech, P., Chazard, E., Lemaitre, L., & Beuscart, R. (2007). *DicomWorks Teleradiology: Secure transmission of medical images over the Internet at low cost*. Paper presented at the Engineering in Medicine and Biology Society, 2007. EMBS 2007. 29th Annual International Conference of the IEEE.

Quteishat, A., Peng Lim, C., Tweedale, J., & Jain, L. C. (2009). A neural network-based multi-agent classifier system. *Neurocomputing*, *72*(7-9), 1639–1647. doi:10.1016/j.neucom.2008.08.012

Reponen, J., Niinimäki, J., Kumpulainen, T., Ilkko, E., Karttunen, A., & Jartti, P. (2005). *Mobile teleradiology with smartphone terminals as a part of a multimedia electronic patient record.* Paper presented at the CARS 2005: Computer Assisted Radiology and Surgery.

Rhee, M. Y. (2003). *Internet Security: Cryptographic Principles, Algorithms and Protocols.* Wiley.

Rossille, D., Laurentc, J.-F., & Burguna, A. (2005). Modelling a decision-support system for oncology using rule-based and case-based reasoning methodologies. *International Journal of Medical Informatics, 74*(2), 299–306. doi:10.1016/j.ijmedinf.2004.06.005

Ruiz, D., Soriano, A., Montejo, C. A., & Bueno, A. (2006). *Ubiquitous diagnosis: assurance through distribution and collaboration.* Paper presented at the Pervasive Health Conference 2006.

Ruiz Fernandez, D., & Soriano Paya, A. (2009). A Distributed Approach of a Clinical Decision Support System Based on Cooperation. In Olla, P., & Tan, J. (Eds.), *Mobile Health Solutions for Biomedical Applications* (pp. 92–110). Hershey, PA: IGI Global.

Russell, S. J., & Norvig, P. (2003). *Artificial Intelligence: A Modern Approach* (2nd ed.). Prentice Hall.

Shoham, Y., & Leyton-Brown, K. (2009). *Multiagent Systems. Algorithmic, Game-Theoretic, and Logical Foundations.* Cambridge University Press.

Sixsmith, A., & Johnson, N. (2004). A Smart Sensor to Detect the Falls of the Elderly. *IEEE Pervasive Computing / IEEE Computer Society [and] IEEE Communications Society, 3*(2), 42–47. doi:10.1109/MPRV.2004.1316817

Smith, A. (2007). Telepaediatrics. *Journal of Telemedicine and Telecare, 13*(4), 163–166. doi:10.1258/135763307780908021

Sulaiman, R., Sharma, D., Ma, W., & Tran, D. (2007). A Multi-agent Security Framwork for e-Health Services. In *Knowledge-Based Intelligent Information and Engineering Systems* (*Vol. 4693*). Springer. doi:10.1007/978-3-540-74827-4_69

Tan, J. (Ed.). (2005). *E-health care information systems: an introduction for students and professionals* (1st ed.). San Francisco, USA: Jossey-Bass.

Taylor, Y., Eliasson, A., Andrada, T., Kristo, D., & Howard, R. (2006). The role of telemedicine in CPAP compliance for patients with obstructive sleep apnea syndrome. *Sleep and Breathing, 10*(3), 132–138. doi:10.1007/s11325-006-0059-9

Tweedale, J., Ichalkaranje, N., Sioutis, C., Jarvis, B., Consoli, A., & Phillips-Wren, G. (2007). Innovations in multi-agent systems. *Journal of Network and Computer Applications, 30*(3), 1089–1115. doi:10.1016/j.jnca.2006.04.005

van Bemmel, J. H., & Musen, M. A. (Eds.). (1997). *Handbook of Medical Informatics* (1st ed.). Houten, the Netherlands: Springer-Verlag.

Verdicchio, M., & Colombetti, M. (2009). Communication languages for multiagent systems. *Computational Intelligence, 25*(2), 136–159. doi:10.1111/j.1467-8640.2009.00333.x

Weyns, D., Helleboogh, A., Holvoet, T., & Schumacher, M. (2009). The agent environment in multi-agent systems: A middleware perspective. *Multiagent and Grid Systems -. International Journal (Toronto, Ont.), 5*, 93–108.

WHO. (2006). Basic Documents. Constitution of the World Health Organization. 45. from http://www.who.int/governance/eb/who_constitution_en.pdf

Wooldridge, M. (2000). Intelligent Agents. In Weiss, G. (Ed.), *Multiagent Systems: A Modern Approach to Distributed Artificial Intelligence*. The MIT Press.

Wootton, R., Craig, J., & Patterson, V. (Eds.). (2006). *Introduction to Telemedicine* (2nd ed.). Rittenhouse Book Distributors.

Xiao, L., Vicente, J., Saez, C., Gibb, A., Lewis, P., Dasmahapatra, S., et al. (2008). *A Security Model and its Application to a Distributed Decision Support System for Healthcare*. Paper presented at the Third International Conference on Availability, Reliability and Security.

Yan, H., Jiang, Y., Zheng, J., Peng, C., & Li, Q. (2005). A multilayer perceptron-based medical decision support system for heart disease diagnosis. *Expert Systems with Applications*, *30*(2), 272–281. doi:10.1016/j.eswa.2005.07.022

Zhang, C., Xi, J., & Yang, X. (2008). *An architecture for intelligent collaborative systems based on multiagent*. Paper presented at the Computer Supported Cooperative Work in Design. CSCWD 2008.

Chapter 12
Semantic Web Architecture to Provide E-Health Content and Services

Mahmood Tara
Mashad University of Medical Sciences, Iran

ABSTRACT

This chapter is aimed at introducing the Semantic Web, the related common languages, and the Semantic Web Services Architecture as a hope for future information services architecture on the Web. In particular, the chapter will focus on the current and prospective (or practical and potential) contributions of the Semantic Web technologies in providing e-Health content and services to its potential users worldwide. To stay health-focused and to illustrate the potentials of the health related services, a real-life journey of a health consumer seeking health information services has been used as the context throughout this chapter. This consumer's journey will help the readers to comprehend the superior aspects of the Semantic Web technologies as an emerging upgrade to the current physical architecture.

INTRODUCTION

Steve is a 59-year-old carpenter working in the rural area of Victoria British Columbia, Canada. He lives with his wife, Sara, and his two daughters, Mary (16) and Kathy (14). Steve has a history of heart-related issues which first appeared as a heart attack ten years ago, when Steve was on a trip to Toronto. Steve was diagnosed with mild hypertension and a moderate blockage of two of his heart's vessels and, since that time, has been under the supervi-

sion of Dr. Roberts for the required treatments and follow-ups. Two months ago, after another episode of hypertension symptoms, Steve was advised by Dr. Roberts to take serious action to help lower his blood pressure. Mary, Steve's older daughter, suggested that Steve search the Internet. She encouraged her father to read online health guidelines to discover techniques to lower blood pressure. She also thought he might find stories about how others had been successful in lowering their high blood pressure. Following his daughter's advice, Steve entered "how to lower my blood pressure" in the Google search box. Approximately 48,000,000

DOI: 10.4018/978-1-61520-777-0.ch012

Copyright © 2010, IGI Global. Copying or distributing in print or electronic forms without written permission of IGI Global is prohibited.

information links were identified by Google as relevant material. Steve scanned the first few search results pages, checking several of the sites mentioned, but after about thirty minutes became quite frustrated. Steve wondered:

1. How to know if a Web site is a trusted one.
2. How to find stories regarding individuals' experiences of fighting hypertension.
3. How to locate the best and most practical advice among forty eight million Web pages.
4. If the Internet could help locate an online forum or club through which others discuss similar health issues.
5. If the Internet could help to find health-related resources such as health-related products or clinics, clubs, and health centers with services and facilities to help in individual cases.
6. ......

Very soon, Steve realized that he had overestimated the informational power of the current World Wide Web (WWW). He had entered into a facility which housed a billion (or more) books without an index, shelves, or indeed, book titles! Instead, the World Wide Web only offered an inadequate search machine that could only locate the books that had any mention of the keywords he entered. Therefore, locating 48 million related resources out of the existing billions was deemed a success!

The story above happens to perhaps millions of people who seek health-related content and services online every day. The state of information accessibility and availability on the World Wide Web is not what its founder, Tim Berners-Lee, originally planned (Berners-Lee, 1998). His original goal was to build a universal network of logically-related, meaningful content, called the Semantic Web (SW) in which the descriptions of online resources and their content could be understood by software agents processing users'

information requests such as those Steve made. However, contrary to this original goal, the first Web language introduced (Hypertext Markup Language (HTML)) —and the related protocol (Hypertext Transfer Protocol (HTTP)) allowed anyone, worldwide, to post almost any type of content, including health-related content, independent of its meaning and content structure. This simplicity in the health information domain very quickly resulted in a plethora of health and medical resources (documents, services, etc.) posted on the Web that were (and are) haphazardly interrelated through their physical machine address (i.e., IP address), making information retrieval inefficient and unsatisfactory.

To make the World Wide Web more efficiently usable, a global upgrade to the Semantic Web is inevitable. During such an upgrade, the physical Web currently functioning primarily as a global storage for health/medical-related resources should evolve into a universal provider of health information services, which will enable users worldwide to locate the information (and services) they need, to monitor their updates, and to compare and finally select the ones best match their preference. Such an improvement would make the current inaccessible *black box* of health information into a practical and handy Web of interrelated health resource and services within which discovering the quality and relevant resources regarding a health topic such as blood pressure would be a minor job.

The goal of this chapter is to review and discuss the various steps to be taken to make the Semantic Web happen. In this chapter, various aspects of the Semantic Web architecture (in its current vision) and the latest service models will be discussed using health resources and e-Health services as domains of context/example. Pursuing this goal, the chapter, after some introductory definitions, will begin with a discussion of the shortcomings of the current physical Web architecture in providing e-Health content and services and will continue with the description of the technologies (XML,

RDF, and OWL) required to enable the Semantic Web. All the explained technologies in this chapter and their potential contributions to the tomorrow's information world will be exemplified using the Steve's story.

FROM PHYSICAL WEB TO SEMANTIC WEB: A VITAL UPGRADE

The *Internet* is a network of hundreds of millions of *physically* interconnected computers scattered worldwide. Similar to the international telephone system, this web of interconnection has been made possible by assigning a unique machine address, called *IP* (*Internet Protocol*) *address*, to every connected computer worldwide. The Internet allows authorized users in any part of the network to connect to any other computer (inside the network) and browse (and perhaps further use) the contents made available by that computer. Until a couple of decades ago, such access to computers was a rather frustrating task, only done by computer/network professionals. If "Steve" had lived in those decades (with no Windows and no browsers) and was trying to locate "Your Guide to Lowering Blood Pressure" on an Internet-connected computer belonged to the National Institute of Health (NIH - US Department of Health and Human Services), he would have had to meet the following requirements:

1. Be a computer professional (which Steve was not)
2. Know if a computer on the Internet holding a guideline titled "Your Guide to Lowering Blood Pressure" existed. At that time, there was no public search engine to help Steve in this regard)
3. Know the IP address for that specific machine, (again, there was no directory or program providing IP addresses of organizations' computers, sorted by name)

4. Enter the National Health Institute's machine using a special network application
5. Discover the exact name of the guideline file (such as LowerBP.txt) and the exact directory in which it was located (hard to imagine how)
6. Transfer a copy of that file to a personal computer to open it and determine if it is helpful or not.
7. And if the guideline was not useful, repeat the entire process again and again until the right guideline shows up.

Well, luckily, the Internet access has changed dramatically. Among all changes, three have probably been the most significant: First, a new language (HTML) was created and accepted internationally to ease communication between computers. HTML is a simple presentation language that allows every computer to share text, images, audios, and other types of information in a format that is understandable/processable to/by most types of computers worldwide. HTML also introduced *Hypertext* technology. Hypertext enables the contents in HTML documents to be linked to other related HTML document/s worldwide, using HTTP protocol. This composite property of HTML, Hypertext, and HTTP enabled interconnection of all the Internet-available documents and resources, and made the *World Wide Web* of information happen. Second, user-friendly browser applications emerged to facilitate browsing and navigation through HTML files. Browsers allow users to jump from one page of information located, for example, in a *host computer* (an Internet-connected computer providing html documents and Web-based services) in Australia to another page (image, audio, or multimedia) residing in another host computer located in Canada. And third, DNS (Domain Naming Service) was created to allow each Web-available computer to be accessed through a user-friendly name and extension. For instance, instead of entering into the NIH Web site with a twelve-digit IP address, the Web site is now accessible to Steve by simply typing www.nih.gov into his browser's address bar. As result, finding information has definitely become easier for health information / service seekers worldwide, including Steve. The WWW, in its current state, allows each person with basic computer knowledge worldwide, an Internet-ready computer, and an Internet connection to browse the seemingly infinite world of information on the Web and to acquire helpful information regarding his or her health-related issues.

However, although finding information no longer seems difficult, finding the *right health information* (the health information which matches the particular and actual needs of a health information seeker) remains a challenge. Consider Steve's story of information research. As mentioned earlier, one out of the millions of host computers currently providing relevant information regarding blood pressure is the host computer for the NIH. The NIH computer holds a variety of guidelines on heart-related diseases and issues, including the one titled "Your Guide to Lowering Blood Pressure." For Steve to discover this particular guideline in the current state of WWW, he would have to pursue one of the following methods:

1. Know and type the exact physical Web address of the computer in which the guideline is located into a Web browser. For instance, Steve might have come across a poster titled "Lower Your Blood Pressure Today" on a bulletin board in a local clinic and copied the Web address provided.
2. Use a search engine that provides the links to such physical Web addresses using user-entered keywords. In this case, Steve would be lucky to come across the correct link among the (approximately/over) seven million listed!
3. Find a portal or gateway maintained by a group or organization that has already conducted research and has provided a list of manually searched-and-selected Web sites

identified as useful in relation to a specific topic such as hypertension.

Although, the above routes to access online health information may not seem to be efficient, with the current powerful search engines, it is now much easier for a patient like Steve to find a specific guideline with a clear topic. The challenge occurs as Steve becomes interested in finding more relevant information. For instance, while reading through the above mentioned guideline, Steve became eager to learn more about his own health status: what he should or should not do, what diets he could try, what medicinal supplements he could take, what aerobic/physical activities he could do, what helpful places could he visit, and what people could he to talk to. With the current volume of health information and resources on the Web, it is reasonable to think that such information is most likely available. However, three major shortcomings of the current Web architecture have made the broad access to quality health information, resources, and services a complicated task:

Lack of Universally-Uniformed Syntax for Data

Uniformed Data Syntax is also required to enable medical knowledge sharing. Data from basic medical research and clinical guidelines of best practices need to be shared across a country (or internationally) in order to improve local to global quality of care. Unlike the traditional medicine, the knowledge regarding the diagnosis, treatment, and prevention of disease is no longer considered as a personal matter of knowledge eventually evolved through individual attempts of try and errors on patients which used to be only transferred heart to heart from the ancestors of medical expertise to their limited circle of trusted successors. In other words, in (today's and) tomorrow's medicine,

"Curing and preventing disease requires a synthesis of understanding across disciplines." ((Ruttenberg, et al., 2007), p. 1). This synthesis is

also what the NIH RoadMap for medical research in the 21st century has emphasized under the notion of translational research according to which the *"discoveries from basic research"* should be eventually translated into *"application at the clinical level"* (Zerhouni, 2003). While the need for such a knowledge-translation environment is doubtless, the enablers are still lacking.

Lack of Metadata Descriptions for Online Health Resources

A main shortcoming of the World Wide Web is its lack of *metadata descriptions* for its contained *health resources* (health information, knowledge, and related services). Metadata (data about data or information about information (NISO, 2004)) is additional information about a resource, a piece of data or information, or about almost anything that helps the external viewers better understand the item. For instance, 150/90 is a piece of data that may not mean much to an external viewer. However, the dialog below reveals how this piece of seemingly meaningless data eventually becomes meaningful:

Speaker 1: 150/90

Speaker 2: What is this?

Speaker 1: **Blood pressure**

Speaker 2: Blood pressure of whom?

Speaker 1: of **Steve Jameson**

Speaker 2: When was it measured?

Speaker 1: on **08-04-99**

Speaker 2: What time?

Speaker 1: **4:50pm**

Speaker 2: Who took it?

Speaker 1: **Nurse Elena Colbert**

Speaker 2: Which unit it is based on?

Speaker 1: **mgh**

Speaker 2:.....

Every question regarding 150/90 is a request for an additional information *element* such as its measuring unit, which in return brings a piece of information *value* (highlighted in bold) which for instance here is mgh. This basically infinite list of additional element-value information regarding a piece of data or information is all metadata descriptions about that item or resource. Such descriptions could be provided for a health Web site, a clinic, or a new drug, for example.

No single person has ever read through or sorted and indexed all the health/medical resources available on the Web, if ever possible. It also is doubtful that any single individual could ever be aware of the plethora of online information and services that could potentially improve Steve's health status. Fortunately, search engines are designed to assist human search endeavours. Search engine systems have software components that could crawl all over the Web and take an electronic copy of all the Web pages posted and later index them for search enquires. However, due to the lack of uniform structure or machine-understandable descriptions for online health resources, search engines are not able to recognize whether a PDF document suggested to health consumers like Steve (in search results) is a scientific paper or a page of randomly ordered words. For the same reason, the search engines also are NOT able to provide Steve with the list of nearby cardiologists, clinics, rehab centers, and additional resources that might be extremely helpful to Steve. For example, when Steve entered a search phrase like how to empower your heart into the search box, the only thing the search engines might identify is the list of pages that contain one or more instances of such keywords. Therefore, Google provides Steve the pages that contains each or all of the words <u>how</u>, <u>to</u>, <u>empower</u>, <u>your</u>, <u>heart</u>, regardless of their degree of scientific quality, integrity, or relevance.

Lack of Universal Information Service Engines

Finding the "right" health information services on the Web is rather a cumbersome task. This is particularly true when a health consumer's needs require the services from several providers to be combined. A common example is trip planning. Suppose Steve needed to go on a three-day trip to Vancouver, to have some cardiac tests. Susan and Mary, his wife and daughter, would like to accompany him on this trip and spend some quality family time altogether. Steve needs to buy tickets for ferry, reserve the hotel room, inquire information on some of the entertaining places they can visit or the festivals they might participate in, check the bus and sky train routes

to their destination, and come back at the end of the third day. In the current Web state, Steve has to first find most of these services individually through a search engine (after trying tens of different links) and then proceed with the procedures required by each service provider. Although much easier than it used to be, the process still seems a bit frustrating.

The reason for the above complexity to plan such a simple and small trip is the current independent, non-standardized service provision by the related providers on the Web. At the moment, most of the online information services are performed by independent applications in server computers spread around the world. These machines provide services through a *Web interface*, a Web page containing user interface to the application. As shown in Figure 1, in order for Steve to get air tickets, to make a hotel reservation, and to check the city transit routes, he has to navigate the related Web interface of the desired service provider (after researching which provider will best meet his needs), to submit his request, to receive the appropriate response, and then, to move on to the

Figure 1. A common health information seeking process. the user has to evaluate all resources separately

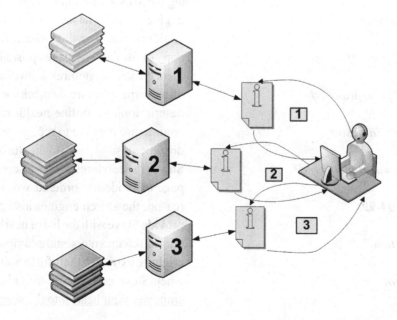

next provider, one after another (Illustrated in Figure 1 as Stages 1 to 3). After he has completed all three, Steve has to integrate the responses for all three service providers as one trip plan and to check that there are no conflicts of for example time, or location between the descriptions he was given. For instance, Steve would need to be sure whether or not the sky train schedule would match his plan to visit the Science Museum before his cardiac test.

The main reason for the above complex and time-consuming procedure is the lack of a standard for service descriptions and service procedures. If all of the three machines shown in Figure 1 shared the same service language, it would then be quite possible to design an application, *an information service engine*, to automatically mediate all the human-computer communications for Steve, in a faster, easier, and more accurate way. This is one of the features the Semantic Web is expected to accomplish.

VITAL TRIPLE UPGRADE TO HEALTH/MEDICAL SEMANTIC WEB ARCHITECTURE: IMPROVING ACCESSIBILITY OF HEALTH RESOURCES

To improve the accessibility/availability of health resources, a triple action is required. *First*, universal data syntax for health/medical data should be designed and adopted universally to enable interoperability across enterprises and information systems. This syntax should encompass all variants of medical data, including labs, imaging, patient, drugs, and virtually any type of data that are currently being used in health information systems worldwide. *Second*, a standard description language must be available to enable description of health resources (information, knowledge, and services) on the Web. This language would help the health resource providers worldwide to describe their posted resources in a universally-understand-

able description language. The language would also help the third-party bodies (e.g., communities, groups, societies, and libraries) to provide external descriptions to health-related resources such as accreditation information regarding a health Web site. *Third*, a standard information service language should be available worldwide in order to automatically process users' information/service requests worldwide. This language should be compatible with the resource description standard in order to find the best available health resource which matches a user's particular requests as well as with the standard data syntax to interpret the semantics of the data to efficiently process requests for data exchange.

In the next few sections, you will see how several worldwide initiatives, from more than a decade ago, have pursued the fulfillment of the above three prerequisites, with the hope of eventually upgrading the current physical Web architecture into *Semantic Web architecture*.

HTML TO XML: PROVIDING UNIVERSAL DATA SYNTAX

The origin of the Semantic Web likely dates back to the introduction of the first *content markup language*, XML (extensible markup language), in the mid-1990s. XML is perhaps one of the most outstanding technical upgrades of the original HTML-oriented Web architecture. XML is a *meta markup language*, a general purpose language to create special purpose markup languages. The unique property of XML is its universal under-standability. As result, a piece of medical data with standard XML-based data syntax could, potentially, be shared with almost every health information system, regardless of its platform, without the need of multiple conversions.

To understand the substantial contribution of XML to the world of data communication, including medical data, an example is given from Steve's medical history. Steve's cardiologist, Dr.

Roberts, needed Steve's past medical history in regard to his previous heart attack. At the time of his original heart attack, Steve was taken to Simon Rose Hospital, located in Toronto, Ontario, the city he used to live in. Dr. Roberts sent an official request to the hospital and requested a copy of Steve's medical record. Assuming that Simon Rose Hospital maintained electronic patient records, to send a copy of Steve's medical record to Dr. Roberts would require one of the following methods:

1. Print off Steve's medical record and send it to Dr. Roberts using mail or email. In this case, Dr. Roberts has to scan the paper record and attach it to Steve's electronic medical record. However, this piece of valuable information is not searchable (by subject or specific field) and also is not indexable (e.g., sorting all of the Steve's ECG result in one page).

2. Send the record using a database file, assuming that Dr. Roberts has exactly the same database application with which to open the record and use it (given the plethora of records keeping programs, this is an unlikely scenario).

3. Send the record using a standard HTML-based Web page. Figure 2a shows Steve's medical record (just the first page), and Figure 2b shows the html code behind it.

Although the above record may seem simple, clear and organized, is only usable by a human reader, supposing Dr. Roberts already knows what IBR, IHR, or IRR stands for and what their measuring units are (medical terminology/abbreviations and measurement units might vary from one region to another). This means that the above record looks only like a page of random text characters to a computer, thus reflecting the weakness of HTML.

In the above HTML code (Figure 2b), a combination of a header (with the page title) and a body, as represented by the <HEAD> and <BODY> *tags*, is all the *content structure* an HTML code can provide to every Web page. But these two tags plus their *subtags* such as <BR> for breaks, <P> for paragraphs, etc are *presentation structure* tags that are applied to almost every Web pages regardless of their actual content. That is why HTML is generally known as a presentation language. Therefore, for Dr. Roberts to discover the name of the cardiologist whom Steve had first visited, he has to scan through all the pages one after

Figure 2. (left) A view of steve's record in a standard browser, (right) the HTML code carrying steve's record

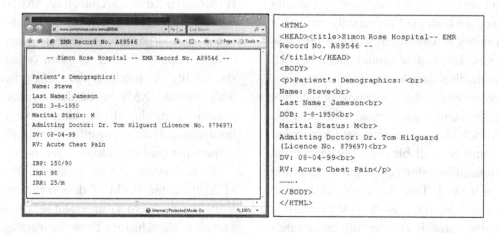

another. The only help his computer would offer is to search the pages for some keywords, supposing they are the right keywords. Furthermore, Dr. Roberts would not be able to easily add Steve's medical data to Steve's electronic medical record that he maintains in his clinic. For instance, the particular medicines Steve was treated with during his first heart attack are not extractable from the record to be appended to the list of all medicine Steve has received so far (for further follow-up) in Dr. Roberts office's record.

4.   Send the record using a standard XML format. Figure 3a shows the same medical data sent to Dr. Roberts in a standard XML-based code. The included *content tags* (or *elements*) such as <patientName>, <reasonofVisit>, <initialRespRate>, etc., tells an *XML parser* (an application that analyzes XML-based document to understand its structure) what the patient name is, or what the reason for Steve's visit was. Therefore, XML formatted data are meaningful to computers. For

instance, Dr. Roberts can easily query the received record for the name and license number of the admitting doctor (the licenseNo stands as *attribute* to the element <AdmittingDr>) or for the findings in the initial physical examination.

XML documents are independent of formatting and thus can be represented in a variety of presentation formats based on the users' preference. As shown in Figures 3b and 3c, the same XML-based data have been represented in two completely different formats. Figure 3b shows Steve's record organized in a standard screen format with information blocks, fields, and the actual data, and Figure 3c shows the record, this time in a story-like case report format generated by computer. For the latter, a report generator has used a report template built based on standard tags for medical data and has replaced the tags with their content extracted from Steve's record.

Who defines or enforces the set of XML elements to be used to describe for example a

Figure 3. (left) the XML code carrying steve's record (right-up) a view of steve's record in a standard application with XML viewer, (right-down) another view of steve's record written in natural language (produced by computer)

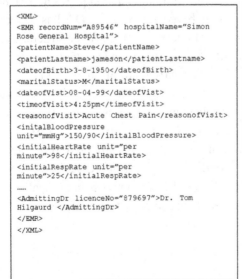
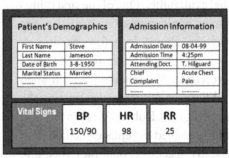

patient record? As emphasized earlier, XML has general specifications to generate standard markup languages suitable for every discipline or field of science/business. One of the initial steps in creating a particular XML-based language for a specific domain, such as a patient record, is to declare a set of standard elements and attributes plus its range of possible data using controller schemas such as DTDs (Document Type Definition) and XML schemas (http://www.w3.org/XML/Schema). These schemas help the XML-based systems to validate the element-attribute-value set and to ensure the integrity of document/data set produced.

How does the application know if the element <initialRespRate> equals RR (in Figure 3b) or Respiratory rate (in Figure 3c)? This assessment is done by anther property of XML called XML NameSpace or XMLns (http://www.w3.org/TR/REC-xml-names/). Using this feature, the people who design a particular XML-based language, should also develop a set of terms that are allowed in the produced documents. For instance, a standard committee would decide if they prefer <patName>, <givenName>, <name>, or <patient-Name> as the standard tag holding a patient's first name. The set of the standard tags finally selected by such committees are ultimately posted on the Web for global availability. One of the first things the XML parser applications (such as the one on Dr. Roberts' machine) do before parsing an XML document is to check the related namespace standard (a reference is contained within such documents). After recognizing and extracting the content for such tags, Dr. Roberts' system has also been particularly trained to replace such content name with locally accepted/common terms, e.g. Respiratory rate instead of initialRespRate. These are the magic features of XML: making computers understand the data semantics and speaking to them in local languages.

XML is now accepted by most data-related application designer vendors and companies as universal data standard. Even the word processor used to compose this chapter (Word 2007) has XML as one of its save options. XML has also been adopted as the selected data syntax in the field of medical information from the very first days of its emergence. Below, three examples of the XML-based standard for medical data syntax, HL7, MML, and DICOM-SR will be briefly explained.

HL7

HL7 (Health Level 7 – www.hl7.org) is one of the oldest and most universally-accepted standards for medical data communication worldwide. HL7 is a multi-facet data standard that encompasses the entire spectrum of the data cycle within the health information system, from concepts to documents. To construct standards for health/medical information system, various conceptual models of the real-life system have been developed under Reference Information Models (RIMs) (Smith & Ceusters, 2006). RIMs are then used as models to design the required data/presentation structures for clinical documents in XML. These predefined structures are called Clinical Document Architectures (CDA, formerly known as Patient Record Architecture (PRA))(Dolin, Alschuler, Boyer, & Beebe, 2000). CDA-based pages are standard electronic versions of actual pages in patient records built based on XML. CDA has several levels. Level one has a three-layer structure consisting of a *header*, *body*, and *content section*. The actual patient data (called data messages) is carried within the content section of the body. The syntax for medical messages has been defined in HL7 messaging standard (currently v.3). HL7 standards, if implemented globally, will bring semantic life to all existing health/medical data and will ease worldwide automated communications between healthcare information systems.

MML

MML (Medical Markup Language) is a standard medical data syntax designed and maintained by the Special Interest Group of the Japan Association for Medical Informatics the "Electronic Medical Record Research Group"(Guo, et al., 2004). MML was designed based on SGML (Standard Generalized Markup Language - the mother language of HTML and XML) in 1995, before XML was officially born. MML had first defined nine modules of medical documents such as patient information, basic medical information, surgery information, and then proposed a standard two-layer (header and body) structure for all the related documents (Araki, et al., 2000). MML also adopted XML from its inception, and the governing consortium chose the name MedXML. The newest version, MML v.3, has been enhanced in many ways to improve compatibility with HL& v. 3.

DICOM-SR

DICOM (Digital Imaging and Communication in Medicine – http://medical.nema.org) is the most common standard for electronic images and their communications developed and maintained by NEMA (National Electrical Manufacturers Association – www.nema.org). The DICOM standard consists of a standard file format and a communication protocol with which DICOM-based files should be exchanged. The contribution of XML to DICOM is to its new version called DICOM-SR (DICOM Structured Reporting). The SR classes allow DICOM images (or any part of them) to be annotated by free or structured text and therefore *"bridges the traditional gap between imaging systems and information systems"* ((Hussein, Engelmann, Schroeter, & Meinzer, 2004) p.1). As SR is a user-controlled addition to DICOM, many XML-based initiatives to govern the SR structure (particularly through HL7 standards) are underway.

RDF AND RDF SCHEMA TO DESCRIBE HEALTH RESOURCES

As emphasized earlier, a major shortcoming of the current Web architecture is the lack of machine-understandable descriptions for the resources posted on the Web. As result, users have to trust the power of search engines to identify the relevant resources on the basis of the keyword entered. However, this method could be inefficient for most information service requests. For instance, Steve is looking for *a consumer health guideline* on *how to lower the blood pressure* from *a trusted institute,* which is *written for the general public* (and not for a specific health or age group). These four conditions are general descriptions of the resource/s Steve is looking for. Now, if such description items (*type, subject, trust-level,* and *target- user*) were available for all the resources posted on the Web, and the search engines would be able to support description-based searches, Steve would have found the guideline of his preference in less than a second. This is what RDF is designed to do.

RDF (Resource Description Framework- http://www.w3.org/RDF/) provides a framework to *annotate* (or to *assert*) Web resources, including health-related resources, located at different URIs, worldwide. In general, Web-accessible or referable items are interchangeably called resources, documents, or objects (Berners-Lee, 1997). In the health domain, a health Web site, a consumer health or clinical practical guideline, or an application service listing nearby clinics and doctors are all examples of resources available on the Web. To uniquely describe online resources, a unique reference to each resource, called URI (Uniformed Resource Identifier - http://www. w3.org/Addressing/) is assigned. The common term URL (Uniform Resource Locator) is also a type of URI that locates a resource through its machine address using HTTP. Another common type of URI is URN (Uniformed Resource Name- http://www.w3.org/TR/uri-clarification/),

Table 1. Description of URI

Subject	Predicate	Object
The URI	is an instance of a	consumer health guideline
The URI	has title of	Your Guide to Lowering Blood Pressure
The URI	is created by	National Institute of Health
The URI	is written for	general public

which refers to the universal unique name of a resource, e.g., ISBN (International Standard Book Number).

To describe a resource, additional information (i.e., statements) is provided and associated with the resource. These descriptions are similar to the predicate statement used in knowledge-representation languages such as description logics (Horrocks, Patel-Schneider, & van Harmelen, 2003) consisting of a subject, predicate (property or element), and object (or value). For instance, one of the consumer health guidelines matching Steve's request is the one published by the National Institute of Health (US Department of Health and Human Services) and titled "Your Guide to Lowering Blood Pressure." This guideline is posted on the URI (a URL in this case) http://www.nhlbi.nih.gov/health/public/heart/hbp/hbp_low/hbp_low.pdf described below.

Each of the above statements about the resource being discussed could be shown in a Graph Data model using nodes (subjects and objects) and arcs (property), as below (Figure 4).

The above graph data model is called an *RDF triple*, referring to its three contained components: subject, predicate, and object. If all the RDF triples associated with a resource are merged, for

example for the above guideline, an *RDF network/ graph* such as the one illustrated in Figure 5 will be created.

To post RDF descriptions on the Web, *RDF language* is crucial. RDF language uses XML namespace syntax to represent the above graph in a markup language. Namespace (or *qualified name*) provides uniqueness to a property, class, or other names being used to describe a resource by associating them with a unique URI. For instance, to describe the above guideline in RDF markup language, use an assumptive four-element description vocabulary provided by Hinfomed Group (abbreviated as hm) as namespace. The resulting RDF code is presented below:

```
<rdf:RDF xmlns:rdf="http://www.
w3.org/1999/02/22-rdf-syntax-ns#"
xmlns:hm="http://www.hinfomed.com/vocab">
<rdf:Description rdf:about="http://www.
nhlbi.nih.gov/health/public/heart/hbp/
hbp_low/hbp_low.pdf ">
<hm:title> Your Guide to Lowering Blood
Pressure</hm:title>
<hm:instance_of>Consumer Health Guide-
line</hm:instance_of>
<hm:creator>National Institute of
Health</hm:creator>
<hm:written_for>general_public</
hm:written_for>
</rdf:Description>
```

Similar to object-oriented languages, the elements used to describe resources may consist of classes, subclasses, properties, and subproperties.

Figure 4. A graph data model with nodes

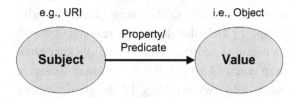

244

Figure 5. Network of four RDF triples associated with a particular URI (our example consumer health guideline)

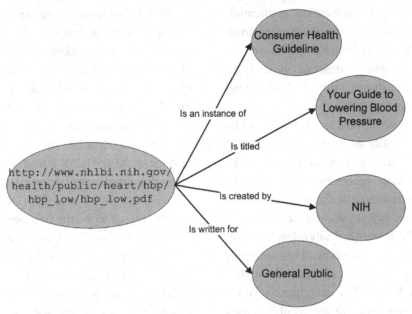

For instance, the above resource provides an example of class Consumer Health Guideline, which is in turn a subclass of health_guideline. In addition, properties' values can also be instances or subclasses of other classes. For instance, general_public can be a value for property written_for is a subclass of class consumer.

Compared to XML documents, in which the original data object or resource contains metadata information (i.e., internal metadata), RDF data are mostly maintained and handled independently (external metadata) from their associated resources. This capability allows *knowledge brokers* or *information mediators* (such as third party groups, associations, or organizations) that mediate the provision of information created by other parties) to provide potentially infinite set of descriptions for the same resource according to the particular information needs of the target users.

The emergence of RDF opened a broad area of software contributions boosting the eventual upgrade to Semantic Web. The RSS (Really Simple Syndication – formerly RDF Site Summary) is a minor but well-known example. RSS is piece

of software that provides its users an updated description of the latest articles/information entries to a subscribed Web site. For instance, for Steve to be kept posted regarding the latest news and articles on hypertension, he only needs to subscribe to a consumer health Web site providing such information through his Mozilla Firefox (assuming it already provides RSS service). RSS reader software (built into the browser software) communicates with Steve's favorite Web site every once in a while, (update intervals could be adjusted by Steve) and updates the list of feeds available to Steve. RSS is now a very common and practical tool to bring the latest health information news to health consumers worldwide. Now, Steve habitually checks out the heart-related news and articles every morning.

For RDF to describe all types of resources worldwide, two requirements should be fulfilled: a *unique set of names* that could be used as element names in descriptions and a *schema* that determines the set of elements and possible values, their classes and subclasses, and their order. The set of names for RDF elements, as described earlier, is defined according to XML Namespace. The uniqueness property of this naming technique prevents confusion of information application when comparing two descriptions coming from two different sources. In addition, it avoids conflict that might happen when a description aggregator agent tries to aggregate multiple descriptions regarding a specific resource.

The *RDF schema*, which seems like an addition to RDF, is actually an entirely new category of semantic Web languages. A main drawback to syntax as a knowledge-representation framework for real-world instances of description is its built-in tolerance to incompleteness and inconsistency (W3C, 2004). Therefore, it not only allows varying description sets for the same type of resource, but also tolerates missing values or blank nodes within the descriptions. Such ad hoc descriptions would confuse the automatic intelligent agent that tries to compare the descriptions of some resources against a user's description of her/his desired resource. To enforce consistency of meaning and also range of possible values in the classes and properties, the descriptions must be clearly declared in a schema (i.e., RDF schema) which will be elucidated in the next section.

RDF Schema

Similar to DTDs (Document Type Definition) and XML schemas—which declare and validate the components (element-attribute-value) and structure of an XML document—the validity of the RDF descriptions is controlled through RDF schema (RDFS) as a *description language*. RDF Schema (http://www.w3.org/TR/rdf-schema/) is a description language to define a hierarchy of possible classes and subclasses, properties, and the range of appropriate values (i.e., constraints) that must be shared between a series of similar resources (in a particular domain or across the Web). Such definitions ensure interoperability between applications exchanging machine-understandable descriptions about the resources on the Web. This

is a major building block toward establishing the Semantic Web.

RDF Schema allows the definition of description sets for any resource worldwide. In the health context, such descriptions are used for a wide variety of health-related entities, from health Web sites, guidelines, journals and books, to clinics, doctors, and drugs and to other health-related products. A very well-known example of such descriptions is Dublin Core Metadata Initiative (DCMI - http://dublincore.org). DCMI introduced a set of fifteen cross-domain standard elements, called the Dublin Core Metadata Element Set (DCMES), that are widely agreed to be the best general description of Web resources. These elements are: Title, Creator, Subject, Description, Publisher, Contributor, Date, Type, Format, Identifier, Source, Language, Relation, Coverage, and Rights. This standard has been approved by many professionals and organizations worldwide (Hillmann, 2005) and was accredited by the ISO (International Standard Organization) in 2003 as ISO standard 15836 (ISO, 2003). Although DCMES was developed prior to the introduction of the RDF Schema, it was based on the same concept and structure described later for RDFS. After RDFS was approved by the World Wide Web Consortium (W3C -www.w3c.org) as a standard description language for the Semantic Web, it was adopted by Dublin Core by defining their element set in RDFS (http://dublincore.org/schemas/rdfs/). Although, DCMES is not specific to health domain, it has been adopted by several health-related initiatives. An example of such an approach was HIDDEL. HIDDEL was developed through MedPICS, MedCERTAIN (Eysenbach, et al., 2001) and the MedCIRCLE project to allow self- and third-party labeling of health Web sites (Eysenbach, et al., 2001). The HIDDEL vocabulary was focused on attributes of quality in health resources and consisted of more than 300 elements in four levels (of classes and subclasses). The quality element set proposed by HIDDEL was later followed by the Quatro (Archer, 2005) and MedIEQ (Mayer, et al., 2006) projects, each which continued the work of the previous one to improve the usability and usefulness of the element set. MedIEQ, in its AQUA system, provides an RDF tool to describe the Health Web resources using controlled criteria (available in RDFS).

Another initiative in this category is CISMeF (Catalogue and Index of French-speaking Medical Sites) (Darmoni, et al., 2000; Thirion, Loosli, Douyere, & Darmoni, 2003), a project by Rouen University Hospital-France. CISMeF provides a health-resource catalogue that uses a combination of Dublin Core as its main vocabulary (and MeSH thesaurus as its terminology standard) and HIDDEL for additional elements to provide a ranking description of the health resources collected. HealthCyberMap (M. N. Boulos, Roudsari, & Carson, 2002; M. N. K. Boulos, 2004), another example, is an online portal maintained by the W3C Semantic Web group as a novel universal health-information registry using a visual metaphor as its interface. HealthCyberMap uses DC standard as its main vocabulary while adding several extra elements for resource quality and geographical provenance (and UMLS Knowledge Source Server as a source of concepts for the DC subject element). Another example, PrimeAnswers (Ketchell, St Anna, Kauff, Gaster, & Timberlake, 2005), an NLM-funded initiative by the University of Washington, is a primary-care reference portal (for health professionals) to evidence-based resources annotated and stored on a metadata registry. The PrimeAnswers' vocabulary consists of elements from Dublin Core in addition to extra, home-added elements for evidence ranking. Finally, "Virtual Staff" by is a cooperative diagnosis environment based on RDFS which allows the descriptions for medical cases (e.g., patients) to be aggregated and networked for later use in decision support (Dieng-Kuntz, et al., 2006).

To understand the contribution of RDFS, imagine all the health-related resources worldwide described with DCMES and a couple of elements borrowed from other element sets such as quality rating and target reader and their descriptions made globally available. If that were to happen, it would be easy for Steve's computer (the client software agent processing Steve's request) to query the description registry for the all the quality consumer health guidelines that have been published/revised in the last two years, with the subject of hypertension and ways of lowing blood pressure, targeted to general public, and written in English. Although the contribution of Semantic Web services is greater than what is predicted in this example, even this level of contribution, if developed, would be still outstanding.

WEB ONTOLOGY LANGUAGE (OWL) TO ENABLE SEMANTIC WEB SERVICES

"*Semantics is a prerequisite for reasoning support* ((Antoniou & Van Harmelen, 2004) p.2)," and enabling such reasoning in computers is what the Semantic Web hopes to enable. To achieve this advancement, the seamlessness of the semantic description tools must be primarily ensured. Unfortunately, the description powers of RDF and RDF Schema, although handy in many cases, are still very limited. RDF has no control. A resource such as a consumer health guideline can be described in RDF with almost any number or types of meaningful or meaningless properties and values. RDFS, which is supposed to control RDF's openness, has its own shortcomings. For instance, it cannot limit the number of values a property can be assigned (i.e., *cardinality*). Therefore, RDFS cannot enforce a clinic (as a resource being described) to have only one physical address or a consumer health guideline to have only one title. It also cannot define *disjointness* between properties. For instance, it is not semantically powerful enough to force the type of a particular guideline to be either professional OR consumer and NOT both. For such limitations and much more whose comprehension is out of the scope of this chapter, RDFS has been enhanced with a powerful language called OWL (Web Ontology Language).

OWL is the latest generation of logic description languages (Horrocks, et al., 2003). The goal of such languages, and particularly OWL, is to enable intelligent and automated processing of service requests and reasoning between multiple resources and services across the Web, which is the highest level of the Semantic Web envisioned by Tim Berneres Lee, its founder (Berners-Lee, 1998). The origin of such high level semantic activities goes back to AI (artificial language)-inspired content (knowledge representation) markup languages such as SHOE (Heflin, Hendler, & Luke, 1999) and OIL (ontology interface language) (Fensel, van Harmelen, Horrocks, McGuinness, & Patel-Schneider, 2001), which were continued by DAML (DARPA Markup language) and its successors, such as DAML+OIL (McGuinness, Fikes, Hendler, & Stein, 2002) and the most current OWL (http://www.w3.org/TR/owl-features/). The goal of all those languages, and again particularly OWL, has been to provide a complementary vocabulary description language to RDF schema through which to include an additional and detailed logical description about classes and properties and their relationships, such as cardinality constraints (i.e., the number of possible values), interclass or inter-property relations such as *equality* and *inequality*, and *symmetry*.

The main contribution of OWL is to enable *Semantic Web Services (SW Services)*. Once the Semantic Web is created (i.e., all the available resources are described), the associated Semantic Web services should be defined. SW Services are a set of service operations (and information) whose description and access information are Web-available through standardized XML messaging (Burstein, et al., 2005; Charif & Sabouret, 2006; McIlraith, Son, & Honglei, 2001). The Semantic Web Services use the same layers of metadata architecture described for the Semantic Web (XML/RDF, RDFS and OWL), utilizing an ontology characterized to fit the Web service concepts. In this ontology, the Web services offered are considered as main class, *Service*, and its instances of service is comprehensively described using OWL (called *OWL Services* or OWL-S). Service operations are processed during interactions between three major stakeholders of SW services: service requester, service provider, and service broker (Sollazzo, Handschuh, Staab, & Frank, 2002) (also called *Semantic Matchmaker* (Burstein, et al., 2005)).

OWL and OWL-S help service providers not only to describe *the resources* they have available, but also *the information services* they offer. Every instance of service is described by a *Service Profile* that contains *Provider* information (description, contact), *Function* information (preconditions, required input, available outputs, etc.), and *Feature* information (category, quality, and parameters)(Martin, et al., 2004). Service Profiles are made publically available to service requesters or service brokers, through a service registry or similar tool. As demonstrated in Figure 6, to invoke a service, the service profile of one or more providers is reviewed by the service requester (mostly a client agent) to discover the best matching service, and a service request, as an input query, is sent to the preferred provider/s. After negotiating the preconditions and other related tasks, service provision is granted (or refused) and service execution is monitored until successful (or unsuccessful) result/s are achieved (Burstein, et al., 2005). In a higher level, OWL and OWL-S also provide a foundation that allows service users to check the proof (digital signature) and trust (reliability of content) of the provided information and services (da Silva, McGuinness, & Fikes, 2006; Golbreich, Zhang, & Bodenreider, 2006; Lu, Dong, & Fotouhi, 2002).

To explain a stepwise view of Semantic Web service operations, an example is given from our health-related context. The steps below show the procedure through which Steve's request to find a nearby hypertension clinic is processed and replied to:

Figure 6. A brief view of semantic web services operation

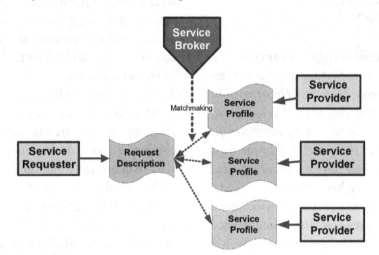

1. **Service Description Publishing (or advertisement):** The service provider/s (e.g., local health authorities, national medical societies) publish the description of their information services (service profiles) e.g., clinics information, doctors information, etc, including the type of information they offer regarding their contained resources. Such information might be available directly through the provider (e.g., a consumer-health Web site) or posted on a service registry provided by a service broker (e.g., health-information portal).

2. **Service Request:** The Web user (e.g., Steve: a health consumer) has various paths to use such services. In the first path, he might be already knowledgeable about the services provided by a particular service provider (although this level of knowledge would be somewhat unusual) and directly submit his request (using search query protocols). More often, he may submit his request to a service broker or matchmaker (e.g., a meta-search engine for clinics and doctors), which composes a well-defined request package according to the request received from the user.

3. **Service Discovery, Negotiation, and Agreement:** Whether the request is submitted directly by the user or through a client agent or matchmaker, the request is examined (negotiated) by the service provider against the service constraints and preconditions (e.g., such as service fees for the guideline subscription, eligibility, security, etc.). Negotiation may also happen in parallel. For instance, in cases in which a service broker or client agent submits the request to multiple providers, the broker or the agent exchange negotiation messages and compare the weight of available service offers to decide which one to commit to and which others to ignore (e.g., the agent automatically decides which clinic best matches the one Steve is looking for).

4. **Service Enactment and Management:** After agreement is achieved between requester and provider, the service is initiated, monitored, and terminated (e.g., Steve downloads the clinic information and is satisfied with the service).

COMPOSITE SERVICE (SERVICE FLOW)

Find me a nearby dietitian's office with experience with cardiac diets! Also, find some guidelines on DASH (Dietary Approaches to Stop Hypertension) diets with Canadian recipes in it! Don't forget to get the appointment, just check my calendar if I would be available at that time! And by the way, which stores around here have a low-cal section? Yes, this is Steve telling his computer his needs, only a few years from now! Processing the above service requests requires a handful of intelligence and automation power. The new Semantic Web is a thing of beauty compared to the current Web, particularly in its envisioned capability to handle composite service request along a workflow (i.e., *service flow*)A high level beauty of Semantic Web (Charif & Sabouret, 2006).

Unlike a single request, the handling of composite requests is mostly based on interactions between automated service-processing agents and appropriate service brokers and/or providers. During this process, *syntactic* and *semantic* knowl-edge between the available choices of service descriptions and the service-request description are matched, and a workflow called *service flow* is composed. Lee and Geller (2006), in a study and implementation of service flow composition cases, found need for an additional knowledge—referred to as *contextual* or *pragmatic*—that provides the rules and constraints related to the specific context or flavor of the requester. For instance, if more than one cardiac dietitian is available and each has a different set of appointment sessions available, the agent can refine the query so that the earliest session from the closest clinic that matches Steve's availability and his residence address appears. In addition, among the dietitians available, the agent may choose the one whose range of fees is affordable, according to Steve's determination of his economic status, or the one whose background and quality of service is worth a longer drive. Pragmatic knowledge is person-alized knowledge and thus should be seen as a dynamic knowledge. Therefore, a predefined set of generic contextual rules (such as a preference for closer, more affordable health services) may

Figure 7. A modern composite service operation process. An automated Web service engine splits the user's request into several requests and process each independently. At the end, it discovers and returns the most relevant resource/s

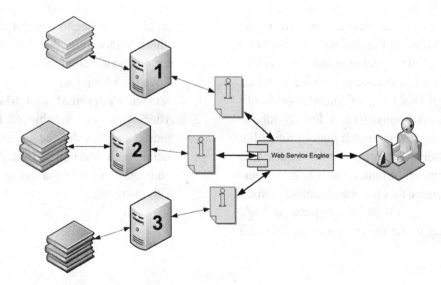

not apply to all varieties of consumers. Figure 7 depicts the above procedure.

SEMANTIC WEB (AND SERVICES) ARCHITECTURE

Semantic web architecture sits on top of the current Web architecture (rather than being a revision). According to this architecture, demonstrated in Figure 8, Web-available data objects (health-related resources or medical documents), in XML, XHTML and other formats, are described using the RDF data model controlled under RDF schema and stored in an RDF database. RDFS can further be enhanced by OWL to include a more detailed logics description. This allows RDF data to be used as pieces of Web-processable knowledge, making the Web an information/knowledge space (rather than the current data space). Finally, the holders or owners of an RDF database can provide varieties of information/knowledge services using OWL-S. Through this layer, service descriptions (profiles) are listed or made accessible through Web registries, allowing automated client agents to compare, negotiate, and engage selected services, while confirming their proof and level of trust. Overall, it is hoped that the Semantic Web will turn the Web space into an interactive knowledge

Figure 8. Five layers of semantic web (and services) architecture

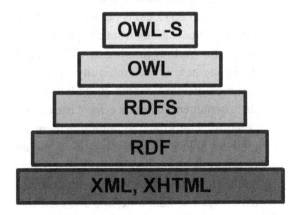

space whose every piece of content or services is transparently described and made machine processable.

MAJOR CHALLENGES AND FUTURE RESEARCH DIRECTIONS

It has been more than a decade from the inception of the Semantic Web notion, but due to several challenges, the pace of adoption, especially in the health domain, is still sluggish. Some of the major challenges are discussed below and the routes to the potential solutions will be pointed as the directions for future research.

1. **Requirement for high-level formalism**: One of the main challenges the Semantic Web is facing is the high reliance of the related technology on formal schemes of descriptions. As explained earlier in this chapter, RDFS and OWL were developed to profoundly formalize the resource descriptions. This level of formalization is required in order to make the computer agents to unmistakably understand the content and services without least confusion and conflicts. However, similar to the domain of AI (*Artificial Intelligence*) applications, the more formality the descriptions turn into, the farther they become from the continuous, fuzzy, and uncertain world of reality; and thus will be eventually destined to fail. Unfortunately, the Semantic Web and its main languages (especially OWL and OWL-S) are principally based on predicate logic formalism which requires a great deal of crisp agreement among the related developers and describers. Achieving this level of formalism is expensive, resource and time consuming and complicated. This complexity explains why the competing but mainly-informal initiatives such as the *Web 2.0* (a second generation of the Worldwide

Web based on collaboration and sharing) have spread much wider in a shorter period of time. The research studies have proposed a variety of potential solutions. Some of the research studies have been focused on ways to soften the Semantic Web formalism. These studies have suggested potential methods to support uncertainty and fuzziness in OWL and the other Semantic Web (ontology/taxonomy-based) languages (Chau, Smith-Miles, & Yeh, 2006; Chau & Yeh, 2005; Holi & Hyvonen, 2004; Lukasiewicz & Straccia, 2008). A recent track of research has also focused on mash-up solutions between Web 2.0 and Semantic Web architectures in order to complete each other's strength (Ankolekar, Krötzsch, Tran, & Vrandecic, 2008; Battle & Benson, 2008; Bojars, Breslin, Finn, & Decker, 2008; Greaves & Mika, 2008). These studies propose combinatory solutions to reuse the large volume of content shared and annotated everyday by the social networks' users using automatically-produced descriptions. A relevant example (in the health context) is the attempt by Cheung et al. (2008). In their study, Cheung et al. combined several Web 2.0 services (Yahoo! Pipes, Google Maps, and GeoCommons) and created a combinatory service that could integrate and visualize public health data based on their geographical information.

2. **Cumbersome description of the current informal and chaotic Web content**: A second challenge that impedes the implementation of the Semantic Web technologies is the lack of competent methods to address the current (huge and chaotic) mass of the Web content. As elucidated earlier (in this chapter), the first step to enable the Semantic Web is to describe all of the Web resources (such as health information and the related services) and to make such descriptions available to the Semantic Web automated agents. However, this ambition is quite unattainable for two

main reasons: First, it is far from reality to expect the provider of the Web resources to rebuild their resources according to a new set of standards (based on the Semantic Web); and second, it is more or less impossible to manually review and describe every single one of the available Web pages. Thus, the practicality of the Semantic Web concept as an upgrade solution to the current Web content is questionable. Various solutions have been proposed. A proposed solution is to describe and formalize only the resources that are better organized/structured. Several attempts of this type have been made in regard to the available medical resources. Two relevant examples are the approaches by Chang et al (2009) to formalize ICD (International Classification of Diseases) and by Frey (2009) to describe lab information. A second solution is to use the *Semantic Web mining* (Stumme, Hotho, & Berendt, 2006) techniques (such as *ontology learning* and *instance learning*) to analyze and extract both the content and structure of the Web resources. A key limitation of such approaches is their need to human engineering and supervision which makes them less practical. Future research is recommended to discover more practical solutions.

3. **The dynamic user-determined notion of "trust" and "quality" (for health resources):** Providing the health consumers with the quality and trusted health information (and services) is perhaps one of the primary expectations from the prospective Semantic Web technologies. The major challenge here is the ambiguity of the description elements which could best act as the consumers' hallmarks for "trust" and "quality." Unfortunately, although there is a plethora of articles on the matter of quality in online health information, few research studies have investigated the potential contribution of semantic description elements

in enhancing the health consumer's feel of quality in her searches for health information. Of eighteen health/medical search engines listed by a recent study very few provide users with the semantic description of the resources retrieved (as search result). In addition, search engines such as WRAPIN (the search engine by the Health on the Net Foundation), although they claim (Gaudinat, et al., 2006) to have quality elements as the basis of their indexing and retrieval methods, are disappointing in practice. In an actual retrieval, for instance, WRAPIN, it only shows the quality seals of the links listed. Even Healia, (Eng, 2006) as one of the latest and most sophisticated consumer health search engines, only uses metadata to filter the content based on target audience (age, gender, and race), reading level, and quality seals. However, the original index includes only the health Web sites that have been already approved according to some criteria. Few practical solutions are available across the published research. A recent study (Tara, 2007) propose a knowledge requirements engineering framework using which the information regarding the quality elements for a health Web site are aggregated from various sources, including literature, existing Web sites, and interviews with local health professionals and health consumers and weighted for final selection. The study showed that adding the information regarding only three pieces of metadata elements (from the discovered elements), in the search results, enabled the consumers to choose the Web sites they actually liked. A superior feature of this method is that it does not filter the online health resources and thus does not objectively exclude the health Web sites or pages with content possibly useful for consumers (but with low third party quality rating). Therefore, it actually empowers the health consumers by providing awareness and helping them make decisions (rather than making decisions for them). Further research in the area of quality is required to determine the likely area of global agreement on quality elements.

CONCLUSION

For a long time, the Semantic Web seemed to be an ambitious universal conjunction point between artificial intelligence, computer science, and information science. However, through hard work and compromise, seemingly unbeatable technical problems have largely been overcome, and services are emerging one after another. The Physical Web happened through a great deal of physical networking actions and a few primary standards. The establishment of the ultimate Semantic Web with full services would definitely be much more difficult. Semantic Web requires a global movement toward acceptance of standards for syntax, descriptions, and service exchange. Therefore, the Semantic Web has already started, but every single one of us determines the speed at which it evolves and rises.

REFERENCES

W3C (2004). Concepts and Abstract Syntax. *Resource Description Framework (RDF)*. Retrieved June 5, 2009, from http://www.w3.org/TR/rdf-concepts/

Ankolekar, A., Krötzsch, M., Tran, T., & Vrandecic, D. (2008). The two cultures: Mashing up Web 2.0 and the Semantic Web. *Web Semantics: Science. Services and Agents on the World Wide Web, 6*(1), 70–75.

Antoniou, G., & Van Harmelen, F. (2004). Web ontology language: Owl. *Handbook on ontologies, 2*, 45-60.

Araki, K., Ohashi, K., Yamazaki, S., Hirose, Y., Yamashita, Y., & Yamamoto, R. (2000). Medical markup language (MML) for XML-based hospital information interchange. *Journal of Medical Systems, 24*(3), 195–211. doi:10.1023/A:1005595727426

Archer, P. (2005). *Quatro – a metadata platform for trustmarks*. Paper presented at the International Conference on Dublin Core and Metadata Applications: Vocabularies in Practice, Madrid, Spain.

Battle, R., & Benson, E. (2008). Bridging the semantic Web and Web 2.0 with Representational State Transfer (REST). *Web Semantics: Science. Services and Agents on the World Wide Web, 6*(1), 61–69. doi:10.1016/j.websem.2007.11.002

Berners-Lee, T. (1997). *Axioms of Web Architecture: Metadata*. Retrieved June 5, 2009, from http://www.w3.org/DesignIssues/Metadata

Berners-Lee, T. (1998). *Semantic Web Road Map*. Retrieved June 5, 2009, from http://www.w3.org/DesignIssues/Semantic

Bojars, U., Breslin, J. G., Finn, A., & Decker, S. (2008). Using the Semantic Web for linking and reusing data across Web 2.0 communities. *Web Semantics: Science. Services and Agents on the World Wide Web, 6*(1), 21–28. doi:10.1016/j.websem.2007.11.010

Boulos, M. N., Roudsari, A. V., & Carson, E. R. (2002). Towards a semantic medical Web: Health-CyberMap's tool for building an RDF metadata base of health information resources based on the Qualified Dublin Core Metadata Set. *Medical Science Monitor, 8*(7), MT124–MT136.

Boulos, M. N. K. (2004). A first look at HealthCyberMap medical semantic subject search engine. *Technology and Health Care, 12*(1), 33.

Burstein, M., Bussler, C., Finin, T., Huhns, M. N., Paolucci, M., & Sheth, A. P. (2005). A semantic Web services architecture. *Internet Computing, IEEE, 9*(5), 72. doi:10.1109/MIC.2005.96

Charif, Y., & Sabouret, N. (2006). An Overview of Semantic Web Services Composition Approaches. *Electronic Notes in Theoretical Computer Science, 146*(1), 33. doi:10.1016/j.entcs.2005.11.005

Chau, R., Smith-Miles, K., & Yeh, C. (2006). *Ontology Learning from Text: A Soft Computing Paradigm (. LNCS, 4234, 295.*

Chau, R., & Yeh, C. H. (2005). *Enabling a Semantic Smart WWW: A Soft Computing Framework for Automatic Ontology Development.*

Cheung, K.-H., Yip, K. Y., Townsend, J. P., & Scotch, M. (2008). HCLS 2.0/3.0: Health care and life sciences data mashup using Web 2.0/3.0. *Journal of Biomedical Informatics, 41*(5), 694–705. doi:10.1016/j.jbi.2008.04.001

da Silva, P. P., McGuinness, D. L., & Fikes, R. (2006). A proof markup language for Semantic Web services. *Information Systems, 31*(4-5), 381. doi:10.1016/j.is.2005.02.003

Darmoni, S. J., Leroy, J. P., Baudic, F., Douyere, M., Piot, J., & Thirion, B. (2000). CISMeF: a structured health resource guide. *Methods of Information in Medicine, 39*(1), 30–35.

Dieng-Kuntz, R., Minier, D., Ruzicka, M., Corby, F., Corby, O., & Alamarguy, L. (2006). Building and using a medical ontology for knowledge management and cooperative work in a health care network. *Computers in Biology and Medicine, 36*(7-8), 871–892. doi:10.1016/j.compbiomed.2005.04.015

Dolin, R. H., Alschuler, L., Boyer, S., & Beebe, C. (2000). *An update on HL7's XML-based document representation standards*. Paper presented at the AMIA Symposium.

Eng, T. (2006). Healia, a search engine for finding high quality and personalized health information. *Journal of Men's Health & Gender, 3*(4), 418–419. doi:10.1016/j.jmhg.2006.09.005

Eysenbach, G., Kohler, C., Yihune, G., Lampe, K., Cross, P., & Brickley, D. (2001). A metadata vocabulary for self- and third-party labeling of health web-sites: Health Information Disclosure, Description and Evaluation Language (HIDDEL). In *Proc AMIA Symp* (pp. 169-173).

Fensel, D., van Harmelen, F., Horrocks, I., McGuinness, D. L., & Patel-Schneider, P. F. (2001). OIL: an ontology infrastructure for the Semantic Web. *Intelligent Systems, IEEE, 16*(2), 38. doi:10.1109/5254.920598

Frey, J. G. (2009). *The value of the Semantic Web in the laboratory.* Drug Discovery Today.

Gaudinat, A., Ruch, P., Joubert, M., Uziel, P., Strauss, A., & Thonnet, M. (2006). Health search engine with e-document analysis for reliable search results. *International Journal of Medical Informatics, 75*(1), 73–85. doi:10.1016/j.ijmedinf.2005.11.002

Golbreich, C., Zhang, S., & Bodenreider, O. (2006). The foundational model of anatomy in OWL: Experience and perspectives. *Web Semantics: Science. Services and Agents on the World Wide Web, 4*(3), 181–195. doi:10.1016/j.websem.2006.05.007

Greaves, M., & Mika, P. (2008). Semantic Web and Web 2.0. *Web Semantics: Science. Services and Agents on the World Wide Web, 6*(1), 1–3. doi:10.1016/j.websem.2007.12.002

Guo, J., Takada, A., Tanaka, K., Sato, J., Suzuki, M., & Suzuki, T. (2004). The development of MML (Medical Markup Language) version 3.0 as a medical document exchange format for HL7 messages. *Journal of Medical Systems, 28*(6), 523–533. doi:10.1023/B:JOMS.0000044955.51844.c3

Heflin, J., Hendler, J., & Luke, S. (1999). *SHOE: A Knowledge Representation Language for Internet Applications* (No. Technical Report CS-TR-4078): Department of Computer Science, University of Maryland.

Hillmann, D. (2005). Using Dublin Core Retrieved June 5, 2009, from http://dublincore.org/documents/usageguide/

Holi, M., & Hyvonen, E. (2004). *A method for modeling uncertainty in semantic web taxonomies.* Paper presented at the Proceedings of the 13th international World Wide Web conference on Alternate track papers & posters.

Horrocks, I., Patel-Schneider, P. F., & van Harmelen, F. (2003). From SHIQ and RDF to OWL: the making of a Web Ontology Language. *Web Semantics: Science. Services and Agents on the World Wide Web, 1*(1), 7. doi:10.1016/j.websem.2003.07.001

Hussein, R., Engelmann, U., Schroeter, A., & Meinzer, H. P. (2004). *DICOM Structured Reporting Part 1. Overview and Characteristics 1* (*Vol. 24,* pp. 891–896). RSNA.

ISO. (2003). The Dublin Core metadata element set *ISO 15836:2003.* Retrieved June 5, 2009, from http://www.iso.org/iso/en/CatalogueDetailPage.CatalogueDetail?CSNUMBER=37629&scopelist=PROGRAMME

Jiang, G., Pathak, J., & Chute, C. G. (2009). Formalizing ICD coding rules using Formal Concept Analysis. *Journal of Biomedical Informatics, 42*(3), 504–517. doi:10.1016/j.jbi.2009.02.005

Ketchell, D. S., St Anna, L., Kauff, D., Gaster, B., & Timberlake, D. (2005). PrimeAnswers: A practical interface for answering primary care questions. *Journal of the American Medical Informatics Association, 12*(5), 537–545. doi:10.1197/jamia.M1601

Lee, Y., & Geller, J. (2006). Semantic enrichment for medical ontologies. *Journal of Biomedical Informatics*, *39*(2), 209. doi:10.1016/j.jbi.2005.08.001

Lu, S., Dong, M., & Fotouhi, F. (2002). The Semantic Web: opportunities and challenges for next-generation Web applications. *Information Research*, *7*(4), 7–4.

Lukasiewicz, T., & Straccia, U. (2008). Managing uncertainty and vagueness in description logics for the Semantic Web. *Web Semantics: Science. Services and Agents on the World Wide Web*, *6*(4), 291–308. doi:10.1016/j.websem.2008.04.001

Martin, D., Burstein, M., Hobbs, J., Lassila, O., McDermott, D., McIlraith, S., et al. (2004). Semantic Markup for Web Services. *OWL-S*. Retrieved June 5, 2009, from http://www.w3.org/Submission/OWL-S/

Mayer, M. A., Karkaletsis, V., Stamatakis, K., Leis, A., Villarroel, D., & Thomeczek, C. (2006). MedIEQ–Quality Labelling of Medical Web Content Using Multilingual Information Extraction. *Press Medical and Care Compunetics*, *3*, 183–190.

McGuinness, D. L., Fikes, R., Hendler, J., & Stein, L. A. (2002). DAML+OIL: an ontology language for the Semantic Web. *Intelligent Systems, IEEE*, *17*(5), 72. doi:10.1109/MIS.2002.1039835

McIlraith, S. A., Son, T. C., & Honglei, Z. (2001). Semantic Web services. *Intelligent Systems, IEEE*, *16*(2), 46. doi:10.1109/5254.920599

NISO. (2004). Understanding Metadata Retrieved June 5, 2009, from http://www.niso.org/standards/resources/UnderstandingMetadata.pdf

Ruttenberg, A., Clark, T., Bug, W., Samwald, M., Bodenreider, O., & Chen, H. (2007). Advancing translational research with the Semantic Web. *BMC Bioinformatics*, *8*(Suppl 3), S2. doi:10.1186/1471-2105-8-S3-S2

Smith, B., & Ceusters, W. (2006). HL7 RIM: An incoherent standard. *Studies in Health Technology and Informatics*, *124*, 133.

Sollazzo, T., Handschuh, S., Staab, S., & Frank, M. (2002). *Semantic Web Service Architecture -- Evolving Web Service Standards toward the Semantic Web*. Paper presented at the the15th International FLAIRS Conference, Pensacola, Florida.

Stumme, G., Hotho, A., & Berendt, B. (2006). Semantic Web Mining: State of the art and future directions. *Web Semantics: Science. Services and Agents on the World Wide Web*, *4*(2), 124. doi:10.1016/j.websem.2006.02.001

Tara, M. (2007). Development and evaluation of a knowledge requirements engineering model to support design of a quality knowledge-intensive eHealth application. Canada, Victoria.

Thirion, B., Loosli, G., Douyere, M., & Darmoni, S. J. (2003). Metadata element set in a quality-controlled subject gateway: a step to a health semantic Web. *Studies in Health Technology and Informatics*, *95*, 707–712.

Zerhouni, E. (2003). The NIH roadmap. *Science*, *302*(5642), 63–72. doi:10.1126/science.1091867

Section 3
Management Issues

Chapter 13
Mobile Virtual Communities in Healthcare
The Chronic Disease Management Case

Christo El Morr
York University, Canada

ABSTRACT

The number of citizens with chronic diseases is increasing and is expected to grow more in the next few decades; consequently, the cost of healthcare delivery will increase, and it becomes vital for societies to investigate ways to decrease healthcare cost. On the other hand, mobile technologies are becoming widespread; besides, virtual communities (VCs) are evolving and are taking advantage of users' mobility. This chapter explores the ways in which mobility within virtual communities can play an important role in facing the current and future healthcare challenges, suggests that mobile VCs (MVCs) can help patients with chronic disease to self-manage their health, shows the many advantages of this approach, particularly in terms of enhanced healthcare delivery and reduced healthcare cost, and discusses the challenges that this approach faces.

INTRODUCTION

Chronic Diseases

Worldwide, chronic diseases (e.g. cardiovascular diseases, cancer, chronic respiratory diseases, diabetes) are on the rise. Global chronic disease related deaths were estimated to be 35 million out of 58 million annual deaths in 2005; besides, the number of people that die annually from cardiovascular diseases is almost twice the number of people who die from all infectious diseases combined (i.e. AIDS, tuberculosis, malaria) (World Health Organization, 2005). By 2015, and for the first time in its history, Canada will have more people having an age of 65 and above, than people having an age under 15 (Institute of Aging-University of British Columbia, 2007) which will eventually cause the number of patients with chronic diseases to rise. Nevertheless, chronic diseases are not the monopoly of elderly nor of developed countries; indeed, they strike a high percentage of adults, adolescents and children.

DOI: 10.4018/978-1-61520-777-0.ch013

Copyright © 2010, IGI Global. Copying or distributing in print or electronic forms without written permission of IGI Global is prohibited.

For example, 46 million U.S.A. adults (about 1 in 5) were reported with doctor-diagnosed arthritis, and 1 in 250 children has some form of arthritis or related condition (Marks, 2008); besides, diabetes and asthma are dominant chronic diseases; to be sure, 32.8% of males and 38.5% of females in U.S.A. born in 2000 will develop *diabetes* in their lifetime (Narayan, Boyle, Thompson, Sorensen, & Williamson, 2003); and the prevalence of *overweight* has increased from 15% in 1981 to 35.4% in 1996 among boys, and from 15% to 29.2% among girls; while the prevalence of obesity in children went from 5% to 16.6% for boys and from 5% to 14.6% for girls (Public Health Agency of Canada, 2002).. Furthermore, up to 17 percent of the population in the United States and Canada suffers from Asthma (International Study of Asthma and Allergies in Children (ISAAC) Steering Committee, 1998; Public Health Agency of Canada, 1999), the number of Asthma patients is approximately 5 million in the US alone (Mannino, et al., 2002). In Canada, about 20% of boys and 15% of girls aged 8 to 11 have been diagnosed with asthma (Secretariat of the Commission for Environmental Cooperation (CEC), 2006). Comparable data can be found in developing countries(Yach, Hawkes, Gould, & Hofman, 2004; Yusuf, Reddy, Ounpuu, & Anand, 2001), for instance the populations in developing countries suffer from chronic diseases (World Health Organization, 2003); in fact, the number of deaths from cardiovascular diseases (CVD) in developing countries is twice the same number in developed countries, and more than three-quarters of deaths related to diabetes occur in developing countries (World Health Organization, 2005). Similar observations can be found in Latin America regarding chronic obstructive pulmonary disease (Menezes, et al., 2005) and obesity (Uauy, Albala, & Kain, 2001). In India research findings point to the fact that chronic diseases, such as cardiovascular diseases, cancer, hypertension, contribute to an estimated 53% of deaths and 44% of disability-adjusted life-years(Reddy, Shah, Varghese, & Ramadoss, 2005).

Self Managed Care

In 2006, Canada spent $148 billion on health services, which is more than three times the expenditure on health services in 1975 after taking inflation into account (Canadian Institute for Health Information, 2007). Worldwide, the rising cost of healthcare is pushing governments to find more efficient and less costly ways to deliver care.

In this context, self-managed care appears to be one aspect of the solution. Self management of one's health condition, increases autonomy and improves care quality as part of a managed care policy(Meuser, Bean, Goldman, & Reeves, 2006). While homecare is an important part of healthcare strategies, millions of people in the developed countries will be sick while they are studying or working outside their homes; therefore, finding ways to help people manage their health while they are on the move and away from a point of care, becomes an important part of the solution.

Supplied by telemonitoring functionalities, self management of chronic disease permits patient autonomy and allows daily activities to continue with minimal intervention of healthcare professionals at a point of care (hospitalization, emergency department, nurse visits, etc.) allowing intervention to take place only when needed.

While telemedicine applications exit and are diverse in application (patient care and monitoring, tele-cardiology), few telemedicine applications are mobile and targeting chronic diseases (Xiao & Chen, 2008). From a telemedicine perspective self managed care through mobile technology constitute a kind of an extension of telemedicine services.

Nowadays, youth use the internet and mobile phone on a daily basis; besides, youth are the "social network" generation, a fact confirmed by the massive adoption of social networking services (e.g. Facebook®, MySpace®, etc.) and the different applications and research directions evolving in the social networking field (Brendel & Krawczyk,

2008). Capitalizing on the former two aspects, i.e. mobility and social networking, we suggest that mobile virtual communities (MVCs) can play an important role in self-managed healthcare policies. Mobile virtual communities are systems that allow people to gather as a community using mobile technologies, in order to achieve common aims and goals. The MVC concept is an extension to the VC concept that emerged at the beginning of the 1990's with the proliferation of the World Wide Web.

In the next paragraphs, we will explore virtual communities (VCs) as well as the MVCs; then we will outline how chronic disease management can profit from mobility in virtual communities, and discuss the advantages and challenges of such approach.

VIRTUAL COMMUNITIES AND MOBILITY

Virtual Communities

In the 1990's and due to the internet phenomena, a particular kind of communities was born: the Online Community, also known as VCs (VCs). VCs varied in the technologies they use and the wide domain of applications. In the 1990's mobility emerged in the telecommunication industry and had a remarkable impact of VC research; particularly on the design, the infrastructure to use, the services to offer, the usability of the interface, the security, and the users' privacy.

VCs advantages and challenges have been investigated in the health field in applications. Health Virtual Communities can be defined as a group of people using information and communication technologies to deliver health care services; they cover a wide range of clinical specialties, technologies and stakeholders (Demiris, 2005). Studies have showed that the information (symptoms and preferences) provided by patient to their doctors is effective in improving patient

care (Cornelia, Thomas, Marguerite, Gilbert, & Samir, 2003); thus, virtual communities have been developed in order for a virtual team to provide care for patients at home (Pitsillides, et al., 2004), to provide care for dying patients (Demiris, Parker Oliver, Porock, & Courtney, 2004), and to provide support for patients with cancer, HIV and coronary artery diseases (Gustafson, et al., 2001, 2002).

Mobility in VCs

Exploring mobility within virtual communities was a logical next step that has taken shape following the proliferation of mobile technology since the mid 1990's, which led the way to the concept of Mobile Virtual Communities (MVCs). Researchers in MVCs investigated different aspects of mobility and their implications in virtual communities in order to find solutions to the many challenges it faces; for instance to find appropriate *technologies that support un-interrupted services* (Wang, Green, & Malkawi, 2002), appropriate *user interface* that overcome the small screen limitations (Axup, Viller, & Bidwell, 2005; Glissmann, Smolnik, Schierholz, Kolbe, & Brenner, 2005). The MVCs *applications* ranged from leisure (Brown, Chalmers, Bell, Hall, & Rudman, 2005) to health and human rights (El Morr, Subercaze, Maret, & Rioux, 2008). Besides, challenges related to *security* (Halpert, 2005), *privacy* (Häkkilä & Chatfield, 2005) and *trust (Ali Shaikh & Omer, 2005)*, as well as to finding profitable business models were investigated (Schubert & Hampe, 2005). Finally, an effort has been made to classify MVCs based on the degree of *virtualization* they permit, the degree of *mobility* they empower and the degree of *cooperation* they allow (El Morr, 2007).

Health Virtual Communities

Health Virtual Communities can be defined as a group of people using information and communication technologies to deliver health care services;

they cover a wide range of clinical specialties, technologies and stakeholders(Demiris, 2005). The stakeholders and participants of Health VCs are health care providers, educators, patients, health professionals (e.g. nurses). Health VCs can be divided into three types depending on the objectives they aim to achieve; a VC can be (1) Patient Centered, (2) General Public Centered, or (3) Professional Centered.

Examples of *professional centered* VCs include knowledge exchange and research teams. Members in these communities are health professionals that interact and work in virtual teams in order to exchange knowledge and create new knowledge if possible (Davies, Duke, & Sure, 2003; Maret, Hammoud, & Calmet, 2004). Indeed, Medical tele-consultations among peers, medical personnel can significantly improve the quality of diagnosis and treatment. Professional centered VCs are made available for professionals in order to build a knowledge network (KN) (Clark, 1998; Willard, 2001). Members in KNs capture, access, use, create, and define knowledge (Merali & Davies, 2001). The use of professional centered VCs for knowledge networking has been a subject of research interest from different aspects (Davies, et al., 2003; Maret, et al., 2004). Health professional researchers use VCs in an effort to cooperate and collaborate, exchange knowledge and create it. Professional centered VCs aim to support researchers by providing them with tools that allow them to coordinate their work, to create and disseminate knowledge, as well as to educate the public and non-governmental organizations (El Morr, et al., 2008).

Patient centered VCs involve usually patients, their family members, and a health professional delivers health care services to community members. Patient centered VCs permit professional-to-patient and patient-to-patient communication. Indeed, health care professionals can form virtual teams to provide care and support in disease management; individuals diagnosed with the same chronic or life threatening disease, or undergoing

the same treatment, can exchange and share health information and personal stories. Thus, patient centered VC can support continuity of care through the exchange of messages and resources. The most known example in of this type of communities is the Comprehensive Health Enhancement Support System (CHESS) research project that addressed cancer and HIV patients (Gustafson, et al., 2001, 2002; Temesgen, Knappe-Langworthy, Marie, Smith, & Dierkhising, 2006). Other VCs addressed drinking problems (Cheng & Arthur, 2002). COSMOS is a VC dedicated for cancer patients (Arnold, Daum, & Krcmar, 2004; Arnold, Leimeister, & Krcmar, 2003).

General public centered VCs are open and include educational services, discussion forums, and access to health information, offering public health informational services; they are dedicated for a specific segment of the population, such as women (@neWorld, 2008; The Center for Health Enhancement Systems Studies, 2008; Women's Health Matters Network, 2008).

Opportunity

Information and Communication Technologies (ICT) provide the opportunity to implement mobile self managed care. Mobile phones and Internet, have a high penetration rate - this phenomenon is not limited to developed countries but extends to developing countries as well. Indeed, the penetration rate of both the Internet and mobile communication is higher in developing countries: the number of internet users in Africa increased by 66.6% between 2003-2004, the highest growth in the world (United Nations, 2005), similar phenomenon can be observed in the mobile phone field in all developing countries combined(United Nations, 2005). Therefore, the solutions provided for mobile self-managed care can tend themselves to patients in developing countries.

To implement self-managed care we can build on the knowledge and experiences in VCs, and particularly in MVCs, to suggest a solution for an efficient and less costly healthcare delivery, away from the point of care, relieving healthcare resources (hospitals, doctors, nurses) in order to take care of more urgent and more complex health situations. Research on telemonitoring has shown that care delivery is more efficient when nurses can serve remotely patients since home based telemonitoring reduces the number of days spent in hospital and lead to cost savings compared to nurse telephone support (John G.F. Cleland, 2006; John G. F. Cleland, Louis, Rigby, Janssens, & Balk, 2005). Comparable results could be expected by implementing a patient centered MVC for self-management of chronic diseases.

RESEARCH PERSPECTIVES IN CHRONIC DISEASE MANAGEMENT

The projects involving virtual communities' applications in healthcare covered a wide range of health cases and tackled a variety of aspects. Different virtual communities were developed to support practitioners (Luiz Olavo Bonino da Silva, Renata, & Marten van, 2005; Santos, Guizzardi, & Sinderen, 2005), or support cancer patients (Krcmar, Arnold, Daum, & Leimeister, 2002). Aspects like trust (Ebner, Leimeister, & Krcmar, 2004), sociability and usability (Becker, 2004; Maloney-Krichmar & Preece, 2005), roles and relationships inside a community (Maloney-Krichmar, 2002) were also studied. Besides, some researchers traced the development of internet based healthcare communication (Denis, 2002), as well as the virtual communities applications in healthcare (Demiris, 2005; Siau & Shen, 2006) and in chronic disease management in particular (Winkelman & Choo, 2003). Mobility also started to be undertaken quite recently for cancer patients' support (J.M. Leimeister, Daum, & Krcmar, 2002; J. M. Leimeister, Daum, & Krcmar, 2003; Moreno & Isern, 2002) and telemonitoring through mobile phones (Hubert, 2006).

Chronic disease management is two folds, **caregiver to patient** and **patient to patient**. The

caregiver to patient relationship can be supplemented by the communication through a virtual community, while patient to patient relationship can be created through a VC that enables peer support. A systematic review of peer to peer (patient to patient) interaction showed no evidence of virtual communities harming patients, though conditions under which mutual support can be more effective in a VC needs more investigation (Eysenbach, Powell, Englesakis, Rizo, & Stern, 2004). The patient-patient relationship involves the exchange of knowledge between patients based on their experience of their health conditions. Moreover, beside mutual moral support, the information and knowledge that patients generate represent a wealth of information that can be made available to researchers who can thus have insight into aspects of the patients' health that wouldn't be available otherwise, such as patient suffering, coping strategies, behaviour, etc. This knowledge can provide practitioners and researchers with precious information that could be used to enhance healthcare delivery protocols, and make longitudinal prospective or retrospective studies.

Building a MVC for self management of chronic diseases (1) needs a versatile design that can be used for a wide variety of diseases, and (2) should enable caregiver-patient as well as patient-patient relationships. In the following paragraph, we will present a model for a MVC for self management of chronic diseases and present the aforementioned two features, based on Kawash-El Morr-Itani Model (K.E.I.) model (El Morr, 2007; Kawash, El Morr, & Itani, 2007).

A Versatile MVC Model for Chronic Disease Management

In order to build a versatile MVC that allows self management of chronic diseases, we propose a model built around the service oriented architecture concept. The center of this model is a platform that offers several services that can be used by the community members. A member can discover the

Figure 1. The general architecture of a mobile virtual community platform for chronic disease management

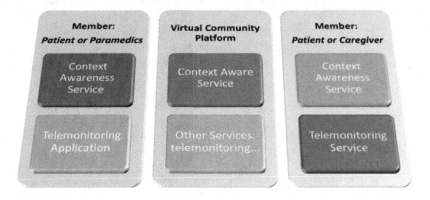

services available on the MVC and use them.. The central service being the Context Awareness Service; it provides the VC members with the ability to discover members' contextual information (e.g. location based services). The telemonitoring service is the second core service in the design; it provides disease-specific telemonitoring services. Figure 1 illustrates this model.

Mutual Support: Patient to Patient Communication

Kawash-El Morr-Itani (K.E.I) mobile virtual community model has already been proposed as a versatile model built around a producer and consumer roles; each member of the MVC can play both roles by producing information or consuming it. The MVC platform can track users and generate a snapshot of the community as presented in figure 2. The snapshot represents members as spot circles in a geographical area (e.g. location of a member in a city). The size of the member spot is defined by users and represents the user level of awareness; indeed, a member who needs a high level of awareness, i.e. to be aware of members (or actions happening) in a large geographical area, will assign a large radius to her/his circle.

Members can receive notifications of the presence of another member when their corresponding circles (representing their required awareness) overlap. In Figure 2, MVC members A and B are represented by 2 circles that are intersecting with D circle (representing member D). Therefore, members A and B will receive notification of the presence of D in their neighbourhood and D will receive notifications of the presence of A and B in her/his neighbourhood. The radii of A, B and D are different since each member defines a different awareness level; for instance, A was keen to meet members in a geographic area larger than B. The awareness level and other parameters can be defined by the each member using a platform's service.

The relationships between members' spots are calculated based on simple arithmetic. Two members can be in one of the following two major states:

- **Disjoint**: The members' spots are mutually exclusive; such is the case of A and C in figure 2
- **Intersect**: The members' spots have a common area; such is the case B and D as well as B and α in figure 2

Therefore, members can be aware of each other's presence in a simple and yet efficient way that does not require extensive computing power.

Figure 2. A mobile virtual community platform model. It shows a snapshot for the community showing four members A, B, C and α.

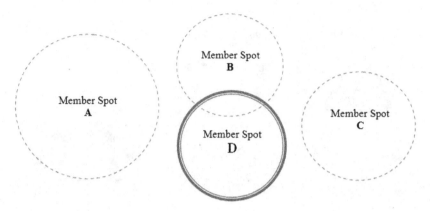

The platform can always map the members' positions and, using simple mathematics, compute the members' circles that intersect. Community members with intersecting spots will be notified of each other's presence. Obviously, each member can use an MVC membership management service to customize her/his member's parameters; for instance, a member can make her/his contextual information available to other members, or can hide this information. Besides, a member can choose to stop receiving alerts from the MVC, or decide on the time slots and the dates she/he wishes to receive these alerts. As previously mentioned, members can also use the mobile membership management service to tune the radius of their spots which represent the size of the geographic areas of interest to them, the center of which being their own position in the city at any time.

Using the MVC, members can be aware of each other's presence in the city, and consequently communicate and exchange information. Members with chronic diseases can therefore use the MVC to for mutual support by exchanging life experiences. Besides, each patient can communicate some information related to the chronic disease to other members of the community (e.g. a healthy recipe, a new scientific finding). The patients can also use the MVC to foster sociability in the com-

munity; thus, members can use a shared calendar service to set appointments with other members for a healthy dining, or a group jogging, or other kind of healthy activities.

Patient Monitoring: Patient to Caregiver Communication

The same MVC can be used to connect patients and caregivers. Once a patient situation needs attention (e.g. very high or very low glucose level in the blood, an elderly has fallen down), the device monitoring the patient's health, or the patient herself/himself, can generate an alert and propagate it to the nearest paramedic using the telemonitoring service on the VC platform. The MVC should have available a telemonitoring service that allows caregivers and patients to exchange securely health information and thus to monitor patients health. A context awareness service would be able to determine the position of the patient based on their GPS enabled mobile devices. Once an anomaly has been detected the telemonitoring service notifies the most available or nearest caregiver and/or the patient. The caregiver can take a corrective action: sending an ambulance, calling or notifying the nearest paramedic, calling the patient, etc. (see figure 3)

Figure 3. Communication between patient and health care professional using a dedicated chronic disease management MVC

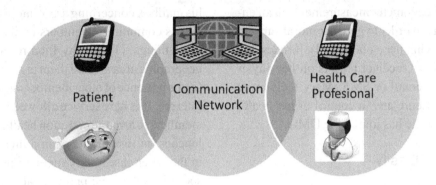

Mobile Chronic Disease Management Scenarios

We will illustrate in the next two scenarios how can Mobile VCs be of support for chronic disease management. The two scenarios are in relation with diabetes and obesity.

Scenario 1: Diabetes

Mary is a student at Knowledge University; she is diabetic. The accurate management of her health condition is centric to her well being and her daily life. She was very glad to participate in the new launch of the first Mobile VC for diabetes management at her university: The Diabetes Management Community or "DMC". She met a health professional in the on-campus clinic, discussed with her the practicality of her health situation and how she is managing her health daily; and then joined the DMC via a website that she could access in the clinic. Since then, Mary started receiving on her mobile/cell phone some daily health advice, as well as reminders to take her medications on time and to measure her blood glucose level; all these three services are of prime importance for to manage well her health. Furthermore, Mary could collect the measurement she takes using her blood sugar level measurement device, and send them through her Bluetooth enabled mobile phone to

the DMC; these measurements were received by one of the many health professionals moderating the DMC. In case of an anomaly, the DMC system generates an SMS notification/alarm that is sent to Mary as well as the healthcare professional who is managing her case; the latter will contact Mary by phone whenever she/he estimates necessary. In the case of an emergency, the healthcare professional can call an ambulance and send to it the exact location of Mary due to a location based service offered by the DMC. Mary is also given the choice to push a specific screen option, or a combination of buttons, that sends an SOS request with her location to the DMC system. The latter dispatches a message to the appropriate parties and sends the request to the ambulance nearest to Mary's location.

Besides, Mary has just joined a new service in the DMC that notifies her daily (though she could have chosen a different notification frequency) about healthy food recipes and moderate physical activities that suit her health situation. She could even download a video teaching her how to practice the physical activities. Lately, she bought a Bluetooth enabled pedometer that she is using during her daily jogging sessions to register the distance she traveled. When she ends her jogging session, she uses her Bluetooth enabled mobile phone to upload the pedometer data to a newly added DMC service that collects members' jogging related data (e.g. number of meters, date, time, etc.). The DMC healthcare professional reacts weekly to her pedometer measurements in an encouraging way in order to give her moral support (eventually giving her a phone call); besides, the system sends her succinct reports on her physical activity by email or SMS. Mary feels more comfortable, secure and in control of her health situation since she has joined the DMC.

Scenario 2: Obesity

Dico, a young computer professional is obese; he did try several times to stick to a one diet or the other without success. He tried formulae that were published in a local newspaper or that was televised in a show; but he could not always implement them either because they were not tailored to his needs or that he forgot few details; besides he really needed the moral support to continue a diet; and sometimes he felt he wanted to talk to people who are living the same experience. The issue that mostly frustrated him was finding each day a different recipe that is suitable for his diet!

Yesterday, Dico's family physician, discussed with him this new thing called "Diet Community" or DietC, established by a group of physicians and dieticians. He subscribed to DietC; he only needed to enter few parameters such as his mobile phone number, his name, his weight and height that allow the computation of his body mass index (BMI), and few other health indicators. His physician advised him with a specific diet that was also entered into his DietC profile. Since that moment Dico was receiving daily on his mobile 3 times a day 3 meal suggestions for breakfast, lunch and dinner that are tailored for his specific needs. Besides, each week, Dico is sending to the DietC his new weight measurement via SMS or mail or web. He had also the chance to go online to the DietC web based interface and display a chart showing how he is progressing, or search for new information or simply have a chat with some other fellows in DietC and discuss progress,

difficulties, and seek peer moral support. A year later, Dico was pleased to discover a message in his mailbox concerning a new mobile service that allows community members to discover, among other things: (1) healthy food restaurants in the geographic area around them at any moment, and (2) the presence of other members around an area of interest. This new service allowed Dico and other members to arrange common healthy dinners and lunches, in restaurants or in a member's house; in the latter case, every member used to bring a special food he/she prepared at home and share the meals. Dico found this feature particularly helpful and supportive. Besides, these common dinners and lunches helped strengthening his sense of belonging to a real community of people he now knows in person.

Finally, Dico's family physician could always go online to see how Dico is progressing and called him from time to time to give him advice and support him or propose an appointment for follow up; that particularly meant a lot for Dico since it added a personal touch to his relation with his family physician.

Dico and some other members even signed to participate in a study conducted by few psychologist who wanted to access DietC in order to understand the determinants of the members' behaviour and suggest improvements on DietC service.

DISCUSSION

Advantages

Mobility in the chronic disease management case would offer many advantages, the main ones being: improving patients' independence, enhancing patient productivity, providing continuity of care, decreasing healthcare cost, empowering patients, providing better health, increasing clinical knowledge, increasing information symmetry, and enhancing the quality of life.

Indeed, managing self health while in mobility increases patient independence, the patient is no longer bound to home or to a point of care, she/he can continue their activities while taking care of herself/himself. Since the loss of *independence* has a direct impact on the health related quality of life (HRQL) (Karin, et al., 2004) the increased independence would be expected to have a positive impact on the HRQL. Besides, with patient increased autonomy the patient *productivity* is improved, and his/her contribution in the society is increased as well, due to less absenteeism at work or college/school, and due to a better health that has a direct impact productivity (Tompa, 2002). On the other hand, mobility in chronic disease management will provide better *continuity of care* for patients since it allows healthcare professionals to reach out for patients when necessary and to advise them when needs be while these patients are distant, thus complementing the care given at a clinic or hospital. The overall approach would have a direct impact on the *cost* of healthcare; indeed, more autonomous and better supported patients will less likely visit emergency departments or hospitals, which would result in a decrease in the healthcare cost. Moreover, the whole framework *empowers patients*; indeed, patient members of such communities are supposed to take care of themselves and co-handle their health with a caregiver, it is known that patient empowerment has a *positive impact on health* (Angelmar, 2007). Furthermore, the direct implication of the patient in their care in a virtual community while they are continuing their daily activity, allows gathering a phenomenal amount of data related to their conditions and experiences, a situation that wouldn't have been possible without mobile VCs; therefore, clinical *knowledge* would grow as a result of analysis of the information gathered from the patients' experiences and behaviour. In addition, the patient is expected to have access to more information through her/his interactions with a health professional and access to information through knowledge dissemination mean in

the mobile VC; this would help to fill the gap of information between the patient and heath professional balancing to some extent the well known *information asymmetry* between both parties. Overall the patients are expected to experience a better *quality of life*.

Challenges and Limitation of Mobility

Nevertheless, this approach raises many challenges that should be overcome in order for it to be successful; the main challenges are: the "have nots", lack of face to face interaction, need for usability and support, managing stress and resistance to change, providing trust, security, confidentiality and policy monitoring, and need for multidisciplinary research.

A basic limitation that is rarely mentioned is the *"have nots"* problem; many people will either have no mobile device to access the services provided, or would find the experience too 'technical' and lacks the human touch i.e. the *face to face interaction* with a human (Brunett & Buerkle, 2006; Rheingold, 2001). Besides, the interaction via the different devices (e.g. mobile phone, PDA, computers) will be a challenge for patients, especially for elderly and people with disabilities, as well as for healthcare professionals; hence, the need for user centered design; indeed, *usability* is of major importance for the success of any information system in healthcare and other sectors (Preece, 2000) and its lack can lead to disastrous consequences (Vicente, 2004), a difficult to use, difficult to learn or remember, user interface impedes the adoption of technology; in this perspective a user centered approach to the interface design would be a must. Since these MVCs are dedicated for patients with chronic diseases, a special attention should be given to situations where the physical capabilities of the member patients does not allow the usual interaction models with a device (e.g. use of buttons, touching a screen). Such situations may arise for people with disabilities (e.g. visual impairment due to diabetes). In such cases, designers need to create new model of interactions using speech recognition to command the devices, or sensors to send an alert in case a patient, such as an elderly, need attention (e.g. falling down, change of some vital parameters) to launch an alert.

Furthermore, healthcare professionals will be managing patients while they are away; therefore, a continuous technical *support* for health professionals is a must to insure a successful experience with their use of the MVCs. This situation is linked to another challenge as well, that the healthcare professionals stress, one concern resides in the fact that if technology helps the professionals to commute less, and hence to spend more time with patients and less time on the roads, then this will result in the health professionals seeing more patients during their working hours, and therefore experience more *stress* and suffer from a "burn out" already experienced by nurses (Aiken, Clarke, Sloane, Sochalski, & Silber, 2002). A more usable interface and more support can play an important role in helping professionals manage their work without adding stress from technology failure and drawbacks in usability. Besides, usability and support address another concern related to *resistance to change* (Longo, 2007; Romm, Pliskin, & Clarke, 1997), without the former, the latter will increase and will jeopardize a successful implementation of a mobile VC; in this context, managing change and addressing caregivers' concerns are vital needs.

Some of the current limitations of current mobile devices are related to the battery life time and the processing power of the devices. Though, upcoming capabilities of mobile devices, such as in the case of 3G mobile phones and smart phones, promise to overcome these limitations. It would be safe to expect that mobile devices will overcome processing power limitations in the future, and will be more adapted for health MVC applications. Moreover, increased network bandwidth in the future will increase the capability of permit mobile devices offer reliable e-health services such as MVCs.

Nevertheless, *security* is a very delicate matter in the health field (Abdul-Kareem, 1998; Aljareh & Rossiter, 2002; Furnell, et al., 1998) indeed, the data exchanged is very sensitive and any breach in security can have a tremendous impact on one's life (i.e. denial of job or insurance); finding, the right balance between security of the system and the flexibility of the service is a challenge for the success of mobile VCs. Data in MVCs does not only involve user (e.g. patient) data but also the user's location, therefore security related to location and context disclosure in general is an important factor to consider (Consolvo, et al., 2005). Other security issues would relate to the frameworks used for MVCs' implementation, in this regard mobile agents are playing a prominent roles and designing a security model for agent-based community is necessary (Chhetri, Price, Krishnaswamy, & Seng, 2006; Malik, Qureshi, Ali, Ahmad, & Suguri, 2005; O'Sullivan & Studdert, 2005; Page, Zaslavsky, & Indrawan, 2004; Spyrou, Samaras, Pitoura, & Evripidou, 2004).

Nonetheless, implementing security solutions is not enough; indeed, security and privacy *policies* should also be developed in order to clarify the *confidentiality* obligations and responsibilities of those accessing patients' information (nurses, physicians, etc.) (Kokolakis, Gritzalis, & Katsikas, 1998); moreover, in order to make sure that the confidentiality is maintained finding strategies to monitor policies' implementation is imperative. Furthermore, establishing *trust* mechanisms between the different mobile VCs' members should be investigated; indeed, trust is one main aspect in health care service delivery (Carter, 1998; van der Bijl, 1998; Williams, 2008).

Finally, studying the determinants of members' behaviour remains an important factor in health mobile VCs (Smith, Orleans, & Jenkins, 2004), the aim would be to deliver an effective healthcare service; we believe that a healthcare oriented mobile VC research and development (R&D) can only be addressed in a *multidisciplinary* way; but although this adds some complexity to R&D, it provides an opportunity for innovation.

CONCLUSION

In an era where the population is ageing, the number of citizens with chronic disease is increasing and the cost of healthcare delivery is on the rise; minimizing the healthcare cost becomes important endeavor. On the other hand, mobile technologies are becoming widespread and virtual communities are evolving taking advantage of users' mobility; we believe that tapping into these two fairly new domains provides an opportunity to manage chronic disease and alleviates challenges in the healthcare system. Our approach presents many advantages for patients; indeed, it can enable a better quality of life and would have a positive impact on their health; besides, it may decrease healthcare delivery cost, and has a positive impact on patient productivity and on the society in general. Though, several challenges are ahead, especially in terms of health data security, confidentiality, and device and software usability; indeed, a user-centered design approach would be essential for the success of mobile VCs for chronic disease management. Finally, spreading the positive outcomes to the marginalized population is a challenge for researchers, governments and social justice advocates.

REFERENCES

Abdul-Kareem, S. (1998). A preliminary study of security in healthcare systems on the information superhighway: the Malaysian perspective. *Health Informatics Journal, 4*(3-4), 223–226. doi:10.1177/146045829800400314

Aiken, L. H., Clarke, S. P., Sloane, D. M., Sochalski, J., & Silber, J. H. (2002). Hospital Nurse Staffing and Patient Mortality, Nurse Burnout, and Job Dissatisfaction. *Journal of the American Medical Association, 288*(16), 1987–1993. doi:10.1001/jama.288.16.1987

Ali Shaikh, A., & Omer, R. (2005). *Formalising trust for online communities.* Paper presented at the Fourth international joint conference on Autonomous agents and multiagent systems, The Netherlands.

Aljareh, S., & Rossiter, N. (2002). Towards security in multi-agency clinical information services. *Health Informatics Journal, 8*(2), 95–103. doi:10.1177/146045820200800207

Angelmar, R. (2007). *Patient empowerment and efficient health outcomes.*

Arnold, Y., Daum, M., & Krcmar, H. (2004). *Virtual Communities in Health Care: Roles, Requirements and Restrictions.* Paper presented at the Multikonferenz Wirtschaftsinformatik (MKWI) 2004.

Arnold, Y., Leimeister, J. M., & Krcmar, H. (2003). *CoPEP: A Development Process Model for Community Platforms for Cancer Patients.* Paper presented at the The XIth European Conference on Information Systems (ECIS).

Axup, J., Viller, S., & Bidwell, N. J. (2005, 15-20 May). *Usability of a mobile, group communication prototype while rendezvousing.* Paper presented at the The 2005 International Symposium on Collaborative Technologies and Systems, Queensland Univ., Qld., Australia.

Becker, S. A. (2004). A study of web usability for older adults seeking online health resources. [TOCHI]. *ACM Transactions on Computer-Human Interaction, 11*(4), 387–406. doi:10.1145/1035575.1035578

Brendel, R., & Krawczyk, H. (2008). *Detection of Roles of Actors in Social Networks Using the Properties of Actors' Neighborhood Structure.* Paper presented at the Dependability of Computer Systems, 2008. DepCos-RELCOMEX '08. Third International Conference on.

Brown, B., Chalmers, M., Bell, M., Hall, I. M. M., & Rudman, P. (2005). *Sharing the square: collaborative leisure in the city streets.* Paper presented at the 9th European Conference on Computer-Supported Cooperative Work (ECSCW'05).

Brunett, G., & Buerkle, H. (2006). Information Exchange in Virtual Communities: A Comparative Study. *Journal of Computer-Mediated Communication, 9*(2).

Canadian Institute for Health Information. (2007). *Health Care in Canada.* Ottawa, Ontario: Canadian Institute for Health Information.

Carter, M. (1998). From security to trust. *Health Informatics Journal, 4*(3-4), 167–173. doi:10.1177/146045829800400306

Cheng, E. Y., & Arthur, D. (2002). *Constructing A Virtual Behavior Change Support System: A Mobile Internet Healthcare Solution For Problem Drinkers.* Paper presented at the European Conference on Information Systems.

Chhetri, M. B., Price, R., Krishnaswamy, S., & Seng, W. L. (2006). *Ontology-Based Agent Mobility Modelling.* Paper presented at the 39th Annual Hawaii International Conference on System Sciences (HICSS '06).

Clark, H. (1998). *Formal Knowledge Networks: A Study of Canadian Experiences Helping Knowledge Networks Work.* Winnipeg: International Institute for Sustainable Development.

Cleland, J. G. F. (2006). The Trans-European Network - Home-Care Management System (TEN-HMS) Study: An Investigation of the Effect of Telemedicine on Outcomes in Europe. *Disease Management & Health Outcomes, 14*(1), 23–28. doi:10.2165/00115677-200614001-00007

Cleland, J. G. F., Louis, A. A., Rigby, A. S., Janssens, U., & Balk, A. H. M. M. (2005). Noninvasive Home Telemonitoring for Patients With Heart Failure at High Risk of Recurrent Admission and Death. *Journal of the American College of Cardiology, 45*(10). doi:10.1016/j.jacc.2005.01.050

Consolvo, S., Smith, I. E., Matthews, T., LaMarca, A., Tabert, J., & Powledge, P. (2005). *Location disclosure to social relations: why, when, & what people want to share.* Paper presented at the SIGCHI conference on Human factors in computing systems, Portland, Oregon, USA.

Cornelia, M. R., Thomas, W., Marguerite, S., Gilbert, F., & Samir, M. K. (2003). Effects of a computerized system to support shared decision making in symptom management of cancer patients: Preliminary results. *Journal of the American Medical Informatics Association, 10*(6), 573. doi:10.1197/jamia.M1365

Davies, J., Duke, A., & Sure, Y. (2003). *OntoShare: a knowledge management environment for virtual communities of practice.* Paper presented at the Proceedings of the 2nd international conference on Knowledge capture.

Demiris, G. (2005). Virtual Communities in Health Care. In B. Silverman, A. Jain, I. A. & L. Jain (Eds.), Intelligent Paradigms for Healthcare Enterprises (Vol. 184, pp. 121-137). Springer.

Demiris, G., Parker Oliver, D. R., Porock, D., & Courtney, K. L. (2004). The Missouri telehospice project: background and next steps. *Home Health Care Technology Report, 1*(4), 55–57.

Denis, A. (2002). The Internet and Health Communication. *Nurse Researcher, 9*(3), 89–91.

Ebner, W., Leimeister, J. M., & Krcmar, H. (2004). *Trust in Virtual Healthcare Communities: Design and Implementation of Trust-Enabling Functionalities.* Paper presented at the Proceedings of the Proceedings of the 37th Annual Hawaii International Conference on System Sciences (HICSS'04) - Track 7 - Volume 7.

El Morr, C. (2007). *Mobile Virtual Communities in Healthcare: Managed Self Care on the move.* Paper presented at the International Association of Science and Technology for Development (IASTED) - Telehealth (2007), Montreal, Canada.

El Morr, C., Subercaze, J., Maret, P., & Rioux, M. (2008). *A Virtual Knowledge Community for Human Rights Monitoring for People with Disabilities*. Paper presented at the IADIS International Conference on Web Based Communities.

Eysenbach, G., Powell, J., Englesakis, M., Rizo, C., & Stern, A. (2004). Health related virtual communities and electronic support groups: systematic review of the effects of online peer to peer interactions. *BMJ (Clinical Research Ed.)*, *328*(7449), 1166. doi:10.1136/bmj.328.7449.1166

Furnell, S. M., Davey, J., Gaunt, P. N., Louwerse, C. P., Mavroudakis, K., & Treacher, A. H. (1998). The ISHTAR guidelines for healthcare security. *Health Informatics Journal*, *4*(3-4), 179–183. doi:10.1177/146045829800400308

Glissmann, S., Smolnik, S., Schierholz, R., Kolbe, L., & Brenner, W. (2005). *Proposition of an m-business procedure model for the development of mobile user interfaces*.

Gustafson, D. H., Hawkins, R. P., Boberg, E. W., McTavish, F., Owens, B., Wise, M., et al. (2001, September 2-5). *CHESS: 10 years of research and development in consumer health informatics for broad populations, including the underserved*. Paper presented at the The 10th World Congress on Medical Informatics (Medinfo 2001), London,UK.

Gustafson, D. H., Hawkins, R. P., Boberg, E. W., McTavish, F., Owens, B., & Wise, M. (2002). CHESS: 10 years of research and development in consumer health informatics for broad populations, including the underserved. *International Journal of Medical Informatics*, *65*(3), 169–177. doi:10.1016/S1386-5056(02)00048-5

Häkkilä, J., & Chatfield, C. (2005). *'It's like if you opened someone else's letter': user perceived privacy and social practices with SMS communication*. Paper presented at the 7th international conference on Human computer interaction with mobile devices & services, Salzburg, Austria.

Halpert, B. J. (2005). *Authentication interface evaluation and design for mobile devices*. Paper presented at the 2nd annual conference on Information security curriculum development, Kennesaw, Georgia.

Hubert, R. (2006). Accessibility and usability guidelines for mobile devices in home health monitoring. *SIGACCESS Accessibility and Computing*(84), 26-29.

Institute of Aging-University of British Columbia. (2007). *The Future is AGING: Institute of Aging Strategic Plan 2007 – 2012*. Canadian Institutes of Health Research.

International Study of Asthma and Allergies in Children (ISAAC) Steering Committee. (1998). Worldwide variations in the prevalence of asthma symptoms: The International Study of Asthma and Allergies in Children. *The European Respiratory Journal*, *12*(2), 315–335. doi:10.1183/09031936.98.12020315

Karin, S. C., Mary Kay, M., Tessa, K.-M., Timothy, M. B., Ronald, K., & Matthew, D. P. (2004). The impact of diabetic retinopathy: perspectives from patient focus groups. *Family Practice*, *21*, 447–453. doi:10.1093/fampra/cmh417

Kawash, J., El Morr, C., & Itani, M. (2007). A Novel Collaboration Model for Mobile Virtual Communities. *International Journal for Web Based Communities*, *3*(1).

Kokolakis, S., Gritzalis, D., & Katsikas, S. (1998). Generic security policies for healthcare information systems. *Health Informatics Journal*, *4*(3-4), 184–195. doi:10.1177/146045829800400309

Krcmar, H., Arnold, Y., Daum, M., & Leimeister, J. M. (2002). Virtual communities in health care: the case of "krebsgemeinschaft.de". *SIGGROUP Bull.*, *23*(3), 18–23.

Leimeister, J. M., Daum, M., & Krcmar, H. (2002). *Mobile Communication and Computing in Healthcare: Designing and Implementing Mobile Virtual Communities for Cancer Patients*. Paper presented at the Tokyo Mobile Business Roundtable.

Leimeister, J. M., Daum, M., & Krcmar, H. (2003). *Towards m-communities: the case of COSMOS healthcare*. Paper presented at the The 36th Annual Hawaii International Conference on System Sciences.

Longo, F. (2007). Implementing managerial innovations in primary care: Can we rank change drivers in complex adaptive organizations? *Health Care Management Review, 32*(3), 213–225.

Luiz Olavo Bonino da Silva, S., Renata, S. S. G., & Marten van, S. (2005). *Agent-oriented context-aware platforms supporting communities of practice in health care*. Paper presented at the The fourth international joint conference on Autonomous agents and multiagent systems, The Netherlands.

Malik, S. S., Qureshi, N. A., Ali, A., Ahmad, H. F., & Suguri, H. (2005). *Inter platform agent mobility in FIPA compliant multi-agent systems*. Paper presented at the 2005 International Conference on Active Media Technology (AMT 2005).

Maloney-Krichmar, D. (2002). *An ethnographic study of an online, mutual-aid health community: group dynamics, roles, and relationships*. Paper presented at the CHI '02 extended abstracts on Human factors in computing systems, Minneapolis, Minnesota, USA.

Maloney-Krichmar, D., & Preece, J. (2005). A multilevel analysis of sociability, usability, and community dynamics in an online health community. *ACM Transactions on Computer-Human Interaction, 12*(2), 201–232. doi:10.1145/1067860.1067864

Mannino, D. M., Homa, D. M., Akinbami, L. J., Moorman, J. E., Gwynn, C., & Redd, S. C. (2002). Surveillance for asthma, United States, 1980-1999.

Maret, P., Hammoud, M., & Calmet, J. (2004). *Muti Agent Based Virtual Knowledge Communities for Distributed Knowledge Management*. Paper presented at the International Workshop on Engineering Societies in the Agents World (ESAW), Toulouse, France.

Marks, J. S. (2008). *Targeting Arthritis: Improving Quality of Life for More Than 46 Million Americans. Centers for Disease Control and Prevention*. CDC.

Menezes, A. M. B., Perez-Padilla, R., Jardim, J. R. B., Muino, A., Lopez, M. V., Valdivia, G., et al. (2005). Chronic obstructive pulmonary disease in five Latin American cities (the PLATINO study): a prevalence study. *The Lancet, 366*(9500), 1875(1877).

Merali, Y., & Davies, J. (2001). *Knowledge capture and utilization in virtual communities*. Paper presented at the Proceedings of the 1st international conference on Knowledge capture.

Meuser, J., Bean, T., Goldman, J., & Reeves, S. (2006). Family health teams: A new Canadian interprofessional initiative. *Journal of Interprofessional Care, 20*(4), 436–428. doi:10.1080/13561820600874726

Moreno, A., & Isern, D. (2002). *A first step towards providing health-care agent-based services to mobile users*. Paper presented at the first international joint conference on Autonomous agents and multiagent systems: part 2, Bologna, Italy.

Narayan, K. M. V., Boyle, J. P., Thompson, T. J., Sorensen, S. W., & Williamson, D. F. (2003). [JAMA]. *Lifetime Risk for Diabetes Mellitus in the United States The Journal of the American Medical Association, 290*, 1884–1890.

@neWorld (2008). A Virtual Community for Kids with Cancer Retrieved October 15, 2008, from http://1worldonline.org/

O'Sullivan, T., & Studdert, R. (2005). *Agent technology and reconfigurable computing for mobile devices.* Paper presented at the 2005 ACM symposium on Applied computing, Santa Fe, New Mexico.

Page, J., Zaslavsky, A., & Indrawan, M. (2004). *A buddy model of security for mobile agent communities operating in pervasive scenarios.* Paper presented at the second workshop on Australasian information security, Data Mining and Web Intelligence, and Software Internationalisation - Volume 32, Dunedin, New Zealand.

Pitsillides, A., Pitsillides, B., Samaras, G., Dikaiakos, M., Christodoulou, E., & Andreou, P. (2004). DITIS: A collaborative virtual medical team for home healthcare of cancer patients. In Istepanian, R. H., Laxminarayan, S., & Pattichis, C. S. (Eds.), *M-Health: Emerging Mobile Health Systems* (pp. 247–266). Springer.

Preece, J. (2000). *Online Communities: Designing Usability supporting Sociability.* John Wiley & Sons Ltd.

Public Health Agency of Canada. (1999). Measuring Up: A Health Surveillance Update on Canadian Children and Youth (No. 0-662-27888-7): Ottawa: Minister of Public Works and Government Services Canada.

Public Health Agency of Canada. (2002). Canadian Paediatric Society, College of Family Physicians and Canadian Teachers' Federation Call for Urgent Action to Boost Physical Activity Levels in Children and Youth Retrieved June 10, 2008, from http://www.phac-aspc.gc.ca/pau-uap/paguide/child_youth/media/realease.html

Reddy, K. S., Shah, B., Varghese, C., & Ramadoss, A. (2005). Responding to the threat of chronic diseases in India.(Author abstract)(Report). *The Lancet, 366*(9498), 1744(1746).

Rheingold, H. (2001, July). Face-to-Face with Virtual Communities. *Campus Technology, 14,* 8–12.

Romm, C., Pliskin, N., & Clarke, R. (1997). Virtual Communities and Society: Toward an Integrative Three Phase Model. *International Journal of Information Management, 17*(4), 261–270. doi:10.1016/S0268-4012(97)00004-2

Santos, L. O. B. S., Guizzardi, R. S. S., & Sinderen, M. v. (2005). *Agent-oriented context-aware platforms supporting communities of practice in health care.* Paper presented at the Proceedings of the fourth international joint conference on Autonomous agents and multiagent systems, The Netherlands.

Schubert, P., & Hampe, J. F. (2005). *Business Models for Mobile Communities.* Paper presented at the 38th Annual Hawaii International Conference on System Sciences(HICSS '05).

Secretariat of the Commission for Environmental Cooperation (CEC). (2006). *Toxic Chemicals and Children's Health in North America.* Montreal: Commission for Environmental Cooperation.

Siau, K., & Shen, Z. (2006). Mobile healthcare informatics. *Informatics for Health & Social Care, 31*(2), 89–99. doi:10.1080/14639230500095651

Smith, T., Orleans, C., & Jenkins, C. (2004). Prevention and Health Promotion: Decades of Progress, New Challenges, and an Emerging Agenda. *Health Psychology, 23*(2), 126–131. doi:10.1037/0278-6133.23.2.126

Spyrou, C., Samaras, G., Pitoura, E., & Evripidou, P. (2004). Mobile agents for wireless computing: the convergence of wireless computational models with mobile-agent technologies. *Mobile Networks and Applications, 9*(5), 517–528. doi:10.1023/B:MONE.0000034705.10830.b7

Temesgen, Z., Knappe-Langworthy, J. E., Marie, M. M. S., Smith, B. A., & Dierkhising, R. A. (2006). Comprehensive Health Enhancement Support System (CHESS) for People with HIV Infection. *AIDS and Behavior*, *10*(1), 35–40. doi:10.1007/s10461-005-9026-x

The Center for Health Enhancement Systems Studies. (2008). Comprehensive Health Enhancement Support System. Retrieved October 15, 2008, from https://chess.wisc.edu/chess/home/home.aspx

Tompa, E. (2002). The Impact of Health on Productivity: Empirical Evidence and Policy Implications. In Banting, K., Sharpe, A., & St-Hilaire, F. (Eds.), *Review of Economic Performance and Social Progress* (*Vol. 2*, pp. 181–202). Centre for the Study of Living Standards and the Institute for Research on Public Policy.

Uauy, R., Albala, C., & Kain, J. (2001). Obesity Trends in Latin America: Transiting from Under- to Overweight. *The Journal of Nutrition*, *131*(3), 893S–899.

United Nations. (2005). *Information Economy Report*. Paper presented at the United Nations Conference on trade and Development.

van der Bijl, N. (1998). Security of information in trusts. *Health Informatics Journal*, *4*(3-4), 210–215. doi:10.1177/146045829800400312

Vicente, K. (2004). *The Human Factor*. Toronto: Vintage Canada.

Wang, S. S., Green, M., & Malkawi, M. (2002). *Mobile positioning technologies and location services*.

Willard, T. (2001). *Helping Knowledge Networks Work*. Winnipeg: International Institute for Sustainable Development.

Williams, P. A. H. (2008). When trust defies common security sense. *Health Informatics Journal*, *14*(3), 211–221. doi:10.1177/1081180X08092831

Winkelman, W. J., & Choo, C. W. (2003). Provider-sponsored virtual communities for chronic patients: improving health outcomes through organizational patient-centred knowledge management. *Health Expectations*, *6*(4), 352–358. doi:10.1046/j.1369-7625.2003.00237.x

Women's Health Matters Network. (2008). Retrieved October 15, 2008, from http://www.womenshealthmatters.ca/

World Health Organization. (2003). The World Health Report 2003—Shaping the Future. Geneva, Switzerland: World Health Organization (WHO).

World Health Organization. (2005). Preventing Chronic Disease: A Vital Investment. Geneva, Switzerland: World Health Organization (WHO).

Xiao, Y., & Chen, H. (Eds.). (2008). *Mobile telemedicine: a computing and networking perspective*. Boca Raton: CRC Press.

Yach, D., Hawkes, C., Gould, C. L., & Hofman, K. J. (2004). The Global Burden of Chronic Diseases: Overcoming Impediments to Prevention and Control. *Journal of the American Medical Association*, *291*(21), 2616–2622. doi:10.1001/jama.291.21.2616

Yusuf, S., Reddy, S., Ounpuu, S., & Anand, S. (2001). Global Burden of Cardiovascular Diseases: Part I: General Considerations, the Epidemiologic Transition, Risk Factors, and Impact of Urbanization. *Circulation*, *104*(22), 2746–2753. doi:10.1161/hc4601.099487

Chapter 14
Privacy Enhancing Technologies in Electronic Health Records

Christian Stingl
Carinthia University of Applied Sciences, Austria

Daniel Slamanig
Carinthia University of Applied Sciences, Austria

ABSTRACT

In recent years, demographic change and increasing treatment costs in North American and European countries demand the adoption of more cost efficient, highly qualitative and integrated health care processes. The rapid growth and availability of the Internet facilitate the development of eHealth services and especially of electronic health records (EHRs) which are promising solutions to meet the aforementioned requirements. The EHR integrates all relevant medical information of a person and represents a lifelong documentation of the medical history. Considering implementations of EHRs, one of the most critical factors of success is the protection of the patient's privacy, which is clearly reflected in surveys concerning such systems. This chapter will provide a security analysis of EHR systems, discuss basic and enhanced security methods and finally introduce levels of security to classify EHR systems.

INTRODUCTION

An electronic health record (EHR) is the integration of relevant medical information of a person and represents a lifelong documentation of the medical history of this person. EHRs improve the availability of medical data and consequently help to improve the quality and efficiency of medical treatment processes. One interesting aspect of EHRs is the moderation of health data. This can

either be realized by authorized medical staff and/or the patients. The second group is especially of high importance in context of Personal Health Records (PHRs). Moderation comprises not only the management of medical data but also the task of granting access to medical data to other parties. Moreover, it is also possible to nominate trustworthy delegates for the moderation of the medical data, e.g. a general practitioner or a relative.

The focus of this chapter is a discussion of security issues regarding EHR systems, where we assume that these systems provide a time and loca-

DOI: 10.4018/978-1-61520-777-0.ch014

Copyright © 2010, IGI Global. Copying or distributing in print or electronic forms without written permission of IGI Global is prohibited.

tion independent access via the Internet. This is, of course, a central aspect in most of the currently available and deployed systems.

As mentioned above, one important aspect of EHR systems is the management of highly sensitive medical data. It must be emphasized that medical data are much more sensitive than data from the banking or telecommunication sectors. Consequently, a high level of security and especially the protection of the patient's privacy are essential for EHR systems. Hence, we claim that this is a critical success factor for the public acceptance of these systems.

The two main issues that will be discussed in this chapter are the security analysis of EHR systems and security concepts that can be applied to encounter the identified threats and thus to achieve a very high level of security.

The security analysis firstly classifies potential attackers, namely external adversaries, internal adversaries and so called curious persons. Secondly, we are focusing on components of an EHR system that can be attacked, i.e. the EHR system itself, the communication channel and the user's client. Thirdly, we will identify data that are vulnerable to attacks and consequences which result from attacks against these data. We want to point out, that the analysis primarily focuses on aspects regarding the patients in order to enhance their privacy.

After this analysis we will introduce methods to realize a security concept for EHR systems. These methods are divided into basic and enhanced ones, whereas the enhanced methods can be used to significantly improve the patient's privacy. Furthermore, we define five security levels which consist of subsets of the above mentioned methods. These levels can be applied for the implementation of security concepts for EHR systems to prevent security threats discussed in the security analysis. Moreover, we will give some characteristic real-world examples as well as some virtual scenarios of attacks against medical data that are in our opinion highly realistic and analyze them with respect to the security levels.

Before we start with the security analysis we will give some background information on electronic health records, health data, legal requirements and cryptography.

BACKGROUND

Health Records

In this section we are going to discuss the basic terminology und characteristics regarding digital health records. In context of these records two main classifications can be found in the literature. The first classification uses the terms electronic medical records (EMRs) and electronic health records (EHRs). Thereby, an EMR includes medical records of patients which are managed by clinicians as well as health care institutions. An EHR additionally includes health information of individuals and furthermore can be managed by individuals themselves (NAHIT, 2008). The second classification uses the terms EMR, EHR and personal health records (PHRs) whereas PHRs are intended to be moderated by the Patients (Tang et al., 2006). Throughout the remainder of this chapter we are using the term EHR to address EHRs and PHRs and patients are able to access their medical data (see Figure 1).

Figure 1 shows the actors involved in a EHR which are relevant to the content of this chapter. However, it must be noted that EHRs may additionally integrate other parties like insurances, pharmacies and other healthcare providers like laboratories, general practitioners, etc.

First of all it must be stated, that EHR applications are ranging from stand-alone applications, e.g. USB-tokens (Wright and Sittig, 2007), to web-based applications (Eichelberg et al., 2005). The latter approach usually integrates different EMRs and consequently holds all relevant medical information regarding individuals. Moreover, individuals are able to access and manage their health information via the Internet. Additionally,

Figure 1. Overview of an electronic health record (EHR) system and involved parties

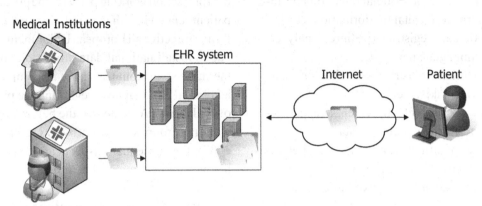

they are able to share these data with other parties and can access data of other parties for whom they are authorized.

Especially, the time and location independent access to patient related data, offers the most promising possibility to improve the quality and efficiency of medical treatment processes. Besides this primary use of medical data one additional feature of EHRs is the so called secondary use of data. It is related to non-direct care use of personal health information including but not limited to analysis, research, quality and safety measurement, public health, payment, provider certification or accreditation, marketing and other business including strictly commercial activities. Nevertheless, in our opinion EHRs should mainly focus on the primary use of medical data to achieve the best possible benefits for the patients.

In contrast to the aforementioned advantages of EHRs, these systems are not free of dangers. This is due to the fact that the central availability of health related data results in an increased potential for the misuse of these data. This problem is often addressed by data protection officers as well as representatives of medical institutions. Major concerns are the so called transparent patient and the transparent physician. The former means that the state of health of a person is fully transparent to parties who are able to obtain access to the EHR. The latter one denotes the transparency

of all actions conducted by a specific physician. Especially, this transparency will be topic of this chapter and we will discuss this aspect in detail. Moreover, we will also provide several approaches to encounter and prevent these problems.

Health Data

According to the U.S. Health Insurance Portability and Accountability Act (HIPAA) health data are any data whether oral or recorded in any form or medium, that is created or received by a health care provider, health plan, public health authority, employer, life insurer, school or university, or health care clearinghouse and relates to the past, present, or future physical or mental health or condition of an individual, the provision of health care to an individual, or the past, present, or future payment for the provision of health care to an individual. Subsequently, we present categories of health data that are of relevance to EHRs (Lowrance, 1997).

- Primary medical, hospital, and clinic data (including various managed-care data)
- Prescribing, pharmacy, clinical laboratory, and imaging data (x-ray, magnetic resonance, sonogram, etc.)
- Administrative and financial data (billing, payment, insurance, audit, etc.)

- Disease registries (melanoma, tuberculosis, burn, congenital malformation, etc.)
- Genetic data registries (pedigree analyses, screening, gene maps, etc.)
- Intervention registries (vaccination, cardiac pacemaker, etc.)
- Tissue samples (blood, semen, ova, pathology, etc.) with associated data
- Surveys of attitudes and practices (diet, alcohol consumption, dental hygiene, etc.)
- Clinical-trial and other experimental data

It is widely agreed upon that medical, hospital and clinic data are very sensitive, since they reflect the state of health of an individual, which is also reflected in laws and regulations. However, this also holds for administrative and financial data which may allow indirect conclusions on the state of health. Consequently, all health data must be considered as sensitive and need to be protected equally in an adequate fashion.

Legal Framework

The necessity for the protection of health data in the emerging field of electronic health care has resulted in national laws and regulations. In the United States these aspects are covered by the HIPAA of 1996 and especially the privacy and the security rule. HIPAA addresses among others the subsequent aspects:

- Identification and authentication of involved parties
- Authorization
- Audits
- Etc.

In the European Union there are at least two major sources that need to be considered in context of data protection. Firstly, the directive 95/46/EC on the protection of individuals with regard to the processing of personal data and on the free movement of such data and secondly the results of the

data protection working party for the processing of patient related health data in EHRs. Based on the former directive all European Union member states had to install national data protection laws. Furthermore some countries have also implemented additional national laws regarding the protection of health data. As stated by the before mentioned working group in a recent working paper (EU, 2007), the subsequent aspects are considered to be relevant in context of health data:

- Identification and authentication of involved parties
- Transmission and content encryption
- Enhanced data protection for highly sensitive health data
- Logging and documentation of processes
- Data protection audits
- Modular access rights (authorization)
- Involuntary (and illegal) disclosure of health data

It is worth mentioning that the legal framework defines the minimum requirements that must be established to realize a secure EHR system. However, we want to point out that methods which are used to realize the legal requirements of course differ in their security level. This will be discussed in detail in this chapter. Furthermore we will identify and discuss additional aspects regarding the privacy of health data that are not at all or not adequately covered by the aforementioned legal frameworks.

Cryptographic Preliminaries

In this section we will discuss the basic requirements for the technical methods that will be discussed in this chapter. In particular, these requirements are cryptographic methods like symmetric and public key encryption, public key infrastructures (PKIs), cryptographic hash functions, digital signatures and the management of cryptographic keys. Subsequently, we will discuss the aforementioned methods at a very abstract level and details can be found in standard textbooks on cryptography (Menezes et al., 1996; Mao, 2003).

Encryption

Encryption is the concept which realizes confidential transmission and storage of electronic data. Symmetric key encryption algorithms like the advanced encryption standard (AES) require a secret encryption key to encrypt and decrypt messages. Consequently, this approach requires that secret keys need to be distributed in a confidential manner between communicating parties. Hence, if the number of communicating parties increases then the effort to manage the key infrastructure will grow enormously. In contrast to symmetric key encryption, public key encryption is based on a completely different paradigm. The main idea is that every party is in possession of a related pair of keys, namely the public encryption key (public key) and the secret decryption key (private key). The point is that the public key can be published and used by any other party to encrypt messages for the owner. However, the corresponding private key is solely known to the owner of the public key and can be used to decrypt messages. Consequently, the holder of the secret key is the only party who is able to decrypt messages which were encrypted using the corresponding public key.

Public Key Infrastructure

For the establishment of an authentic link between public keys and the holders of the corresponding private keys certificates are used. A certificate contains identifying information of the holder together with his public key which is digitally signed by a trusted certification authority. The issuing and management of certificates is in general realized by means of public key infrastructures (PKIs). In context of eHealth so called health cards (smart cards) are increasingly used for identification and authentication purposes and moreover these cards store the above mentioned private keys in a secure manner.

Cryptographic Hash Functions and Digital Signatures

Besides encryption and decryption another important aspect in electronic communication is the authenticity and integrity of data. This means that the originator of the message can uniquely be identified and additionally the receiver is able to recognize if data manipulation took place. In general this will be accomplished by means of digitally signing messages. In order to improve the efficiency of signature generation, in practice one does not sign the entire message, but a fingerprint of the message which is created by means of a cryptographic hash function. A cryptographic hash function is a map from messages of arbitrary size to bit strings of fixed small length (e.g. 160 bit). Clearly, this implies that there are distinct messages which map to the same hash value. This is called a collision. In the practical use it should not be possible to efficiently find collisions of a hash function. Exactly this property is of high relevance regarding the security of digital signatures.

Key Management

Another aspect is the backup of cryptographic keys, which is of enormous importance in context of data encryption. If health data are stored in an encrypted fashion, the availability of these data depends on the availability of the respective cryptographic keys. This means, that the loss of a cryptographic key implies that the health data cannot be decrypted and thus used anymore. Especially in context of medical treatment processes this is a major problem and therefore methods to improve the availability of cryptographic keys need to be realized. However, it must be emphasized that the higher the availability the lower the security of the encrypted data. A suitable compromise between the availability and security is to establish key backup by means of secret sharing. This is a method to split up a secret into shares, e.g. a cryptographic key, and distribute these shares among a set of users. The point is that there are predefined subsets of users such that only these subsets are able to reconstruct the secret by combining their shares.

SECURITY THREATS IN ELECTRONIC HEALTH RECORDS

As mentioned above, health data are very sensitive and need to be protected against misuse by unauthorized persons. Additionally, services which provide online access to health data are even more attractive to attackers, mainly due to the following facts:

- Time and location independent availability of the services
- Access via the Internet
- Central access to a high amount of sensitive and consequently valuable information
- Many parties which can access the system

For these reasons it is in our opinion absolutely necessary to carefully analyze potential attacks when designing and implementing an EHR system. First of all, these attacks can be divided into attacks against the availability of the systems and attacks against medical content data and metadata. The former attacks comprise amongst others denial of service (DoS) and injection of malicious code (malware). The latter ones will be discussed in more detail in this section.

Attacks against content and metadata are in general conducted to acquire (medical) information about specific persons. Subsequently, we will present some examples why people may perform these attacks:

- To sell medical information for financial purposes, e.g. to newspapers, or to use these data for marketing activities, e.g. pharmaceutical companies.
- To compromise other persons by making their health data publicly available.
- To benefit from information about other persons, e.g. about candidates for a job.
- Unauthorized analyses of health data to obtain valuable information and draw potential conclusions.

These reasons illustrate that the misuse of medical data may have enormous negative consequences for individuals and may even threaten their existence. In order to prevent the disclosure of medical data, it is necessary to analyze the following aspects.

- **Target**: which component of the system could be attacked?
- **Adversary**: which group of people conducts these attacks?
- **Attack**: which kind of attacks exist?

Potential Adversaries and Attacks

First of all we will discuss the components of the system that can be attacked, namely the EHR system, the communication channel and the patient's client (see Figure 2).

Depending on the target we distinguish between three different classes of attackers, whereas it must be mentioned that these classes are not necessarily disjoint.

Firstly, internal attackers, e.g. employees of the system or medical staff, conduct attacks mainly against the EHR system. For instance, an operator may steal medical data. It is reflected in current studies that more than 50% of attacks against information systems are conducted by insiders (CSI 2007). But surprisingly enough, insiders are often not considered as potential adversaries

Figure 2. Overview of classes of attackers against EHR systems

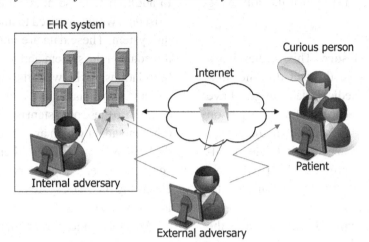

when designing security concepts of systems, or these attacks are solely prevented by means of organizational measures such as security policies and/or non disclosure-agreements.

Secondly, external adversaries can be identified and they are usually considered when discussing security in context of EHR system. These adversaries can either behave active, i.e. hackers, or passive, i.e. eavesdroppers. In contrast to passive adversaries, who are only wiretapping the communication channel, active adversaries also manipulate transferred and stored data. It must be pointed out that, in general, it is easier for an insider to get unauthorized access to medical data than for an external adversary. Consequently, in order to establish a reliable security concept for an EHR system, insider attacks need to be taken into consideration as carefully as external attacks.

Finally, we will introduce a third kind of adversaries which are not taken into consideration in architectures for EHR systems as of now. These attackers will be denoted as "curious persons" here. A curious person is an "attacker" who tries to obtain medical information about persons by influencing this person to present the medical data on their own. This can be achieved by means of more or less sophisticated methods. The former methods mainly comprise methods from social

engineering, e.g. a curious person may convince a patient to hand out login credentials to him. These attacks can only be prevented by raising awareness during security trainings. It must be noted that technical measures cannot be used to counter these attacks, since the attacked person may not perceive the situation as an attack.

In the following we will discuss the above mentioned less sophisticated methods, which have not been considered at all so far, but can be conducted very easily without any know-how regarding the security concept of the EHR system. A concrete scenario can be briefly described as follows: a curious person motivates or even forces another person (the patient) to present the contents of his EHR. This means that the patient logs into the EHR system as usual and gives the curious person an insight into his medical data. In order to make this attack, which we call a "disclosure attack" (Stingl and Slamanig, 2008), more understandable, we will present two illustrative examples.

Consider a person who was suffering a depression applies for a job. It should be noted that up to 18% of people suffer at least once in their lives from depression (Both et al. 2009). We are absolutely sure that this information will negatively affect the chances to get this job if known to the recruiter. Regarding the disclosure of medical data, we are going to distinguish the following two cases.

- **Motivated disclosure**: This means that a person is aware of the fact that the non-disclosure of medical data might have negative consequences. Thus, the person is "motivated" to present the medical data. For instance, another job candidate has already voluntarily presented his EHR in order to demonstrate his "excellent" mental and physical fitness.

- **Enforced disclosure**: In this scenario the recruiter forces the job candidates to open their EHRs in order to determine their "qualifications" for the job. Clearly, this enforcement is in many countries illegal, but nevertheless in our opinion possible. Additionally, this attack cannot be detected during subsequent security audits, since it cannot be distinguished from a standard login by the patient.

A possible alternative in this scenario would be to deny access to the EHR, which however might also result in negative consequences for the candidate. Therefore, it is absolutely necessary to provide a possibility to avoid these consequences in the two above mentioned scenarios. At this point it seems to be paradox to find a satisfiable technical solution to this problem. We will show that there already exists a solution to this problem.

CONTENT DATA AND METADATA IN CONTEXT OF EHR SYSTEMS

The main idea of an EHR system is to represent a life-long documentation of all relevant medical data of a person. This life-long character of an EHR is essential, since many treatment processes require a complete overview of the medical history of a person. Consequently, it is not favorable to remove any (relevant) information from the EHR.

In addition to these medical content data, there exist data which are used to manage the EHRs by the system. These data are in general denoted as metadata of the system and represent for instance the relationships between the involved parties (e.g. patients, physicians) and medical documents. In addition to these persistent metadata, there are also other metadata which are not explicitly stored in the EHR system, but may either be logged by other components, e.g. a web server, or determined by observing the EHR system, e.g. the frequency of logins of a patient.

As already mentioned medical data are generally classified as sensitive. Moreover, a part of these data can be considered as highly sensitive because the unwarranted knowledge of this information can massively violate the patient's privacy and furthermore negatively influence the well-being of the patient. Subsequently, we will briefly present characteristic examples for the three above discussed examples of data.

- Medical content data
- Addictive disorders: drugs, alcohol, pharmaceuticals, etc.
- Mental diseases: depression, etc.
- Psychosomatic diseases
- Venereal diseases
- Infectious diseases, etc.
- EHR metadata provided by the system
- Relationships between patients and specific physicians, e.g. oncologist, psychiatrist.
- Relationships between patients and specific medical documents, e.g. finding of an oncologist or psychiatrist.
- Typical pattern of appointments for treatments, e.g. pregnancy, chemotherapy.
- EHR metadata derived by observing the system
- Number of logins within a specific time period.
- Number of medical documents transferred into the EHR system.

Before we discuss the relevance for protecting these data, we will give some illustrative examples regarding the frequency of some of the above mentioned diseases. As stated above, the number of people that suffer from a depression at least once in their lives is up to 18%. Moreover, there are studies from Germany which say that the number of alcohol and pharmaceutical addicted people is actually each about 2% of people (DHS, 2008). It must be emphasized that the latter numbers only represent the year 2008, but in context of a lifelong EHR the number of concerned patients will actually be considerable higher. However, it must not be ignored that there is no exact information about the number of people who are involved in a treatment concerning their addiction. Nevertheless, considering solely the above mentioned diseases, the number of people whose EHR contains this potentially compromising information is from our point of view relevant. From our point of view it is inevitable that medical content data need to be protected against unauthorized people. But it is natural to ask whether metadata need to be equally protected. This question cannot be answered generally, but we are convinced that protection of the patient's privacy must be a central issue in EHR systems. This is motivated by the fact that people who may enormously profit from an EHR are exactly those who are involved in many different treatment processes and thus have extensive EHRs. But, unfortunately an extensive EHR implies a high amount of metadata so that analyses of these metadata are more likely to disclose compromising information. Hence, we conclude that a reliable architecture for EHR systems needs to consider the protection of medical content data as well as metadata to prevent any possibility of misuse.

MISUSE AND CONSEQUENCES

In this section we will discuss the misuse of medical data regarding the involved parties as well as the consequences for them. Therefore, we need to introduce involved parties:

- **Parties involved in treatment processes**: patients, physicians, etc.
- **EHR provider**: third parties which host the EHR system.
- **EHR initiator**: governments, major software vendors, etc.

Of course, the compromisation of an EHR system will result in a massive loss of confidence for the provider and initiator of the system. Furthermore, this may entail negative economic effects to the threatening of the EHR system's existence. This loss of confidence also applies to the medical parties involved in the treatment process, but the most serious consequences will affect the patients and may massively influence their future. Subsequently, we will present selected areas and consequences for the patient that may result from "public" disclosure of their medical data. In general, immediate consequences are discrimination, stigmatization and uncertainty of the patient respectively.

- **Working environment**: loss of job, reduced chances for jobs, bullying at work, reduced occupational advancements, etc.
- **Social environment**: social exclusion
- **State of health**: mental and/or psychosomatic diseases

These examples underpin the argument that the protection of the patient's privacy and their medical data are essential aspects for the design of EHR systems.

PRIVACY ENHANCING TECHNOLOGIES IN EHR SYSTEMS

Considering information systems, there are measures on different levels which are used to realize a security concept. The security rule of the HIPAA distinguishes between administrative, physical and technical safeguards, whereas the former two are often denoted as organizational safeguards and measures respectively. Subsequently, we will provide some examples from HIPAA and additionally issues that are important when realizing an EHR system.

Administrative, Physical and Technical Safeguards

Administrative safeguards cover policies and procedures which are designed to clearly demonstrate how health care institutions realize security and privacy measures.

- Creation of policies and procedures to document the security aims and define responsibilities
- Non-disclosure agreements for employees
- Schedules for internal and external audits
- Emergency plans
- Training programs regarding IT security
- Etc.

Physical safeguards are used to control physical access to protect against inappropriate access to data.

- The introduction and removal of hardware and software components of the system needs to be managed carefully
- Access to equipment containing health information should be carefully controlled and monitored
- Access to hardware and software must be limited to properly authorized individuals
- Required access controls consist of facility security plans, maintenance records, and visitor sign-in and escorts
- Etc.

Technical safeguards are concerned with controlling access to information systems and protecting stored and transmitted health information.

- Establishment of mechanisms for intrusion detection and prevention
- Confidentiality measures to avoid unauthorized access to health data
- Data integrity methods to detect unauthorized data manipulation and erroneous transmission and storage of data
- Authentication of subjects and objects that are involved in treatment processes

It must be emphasized that security aims may be implemented by means of administrative, physical and/or technical safeguards. For instance, the non-disclosure of health data regarding employees can be achieved among others by non-disclosure agreements and content encryption respectively. In the former case it is obviously necessary to trust employees that they will behave according to the non-disclosure agreement. Clearly, a violation against the agreement implies the disclosure of all health data that can be accessed by this employee. Hence, the trustworthiness of employees is absolutely necessary. On the other hand, proper data encryption mechanisms guarantee that solely authorized parties are able to access health data. Since aforementioned employees are not involved in a treatment process, they will not be given access to health data and are therefore not authorized. Consequently, employees are not able to misuse these data at all. This example shows that in general technical measures are more adequate than administrative or physical measures, since they reduce the necessary trust to the provider and their employees.

Having identified security threats based on the security analysis it is possible to define security properties which counter these threats. Thereby, we distinguish between basic and enhanced security methods. The basic security properties are those which are well known from standard textbooks on information systems and computer security (Menezes et al, 1996; Bishop, 2002). These comprise methods for authentication and authorization, availability, confidentiality and integrity of data and are in our opinion absolutely necessary in context of EHR systems. However, it must be emphasized that these methods mainly protect against external adversaries but marginally against internal adversaries and not at all against curious persons. Therefore, it is inevitable to define enhanced methods to increase the level of security regarding the latter two groups of adversaries. These include anonymity, deniability and unlinkability. In the following we will discuss the basic as well as the enhanced security methods.

Authentication

Entity authentication is the verification of a claimed identity of a person or subject. Typically, this is realized by proving the possession of some secret information to the verifying party, i.e. the EHR system. Subsequently, we will present two basic mechanisms for authentication and an enhanced method. In general authentication mechanisms are classified by means of the number of factors which are used to authenticate a person. Typical factors are knowledge, e.g. a password, personal identification number (PIN), ownership, e.g. smart card, security token, and inherence, e.g. fingerprint, DNA-sequence, voice, etc. **One-factor authentication** is the most widespread technique and is usually based on one of the knowledge factors, e.g. username-password authentication. We want to stress, that one-factor authentication is not adequate in context of sensitive data, since these approaches can be attacked very efficiently, e.g. dictionary or password guessing attacks. If two independent factors are used, this is called a **two-factor authentication**, e.g. smart card and PIN. In European Union countries this type of authentication is the preferred method to get access to health services.

In contrast to conventional authentication, which establishes a unique identification of an authenticating user, **anonymous authentication** enables users to authenticate without disclosing their identity to the verifying party. Especially in context of EHR systems anonymous authentication is very interesting, because these methods enhance the user's privacy by preventing analyses of their behavior. On the other hand it must be noted that methods for anonymous authentication are rarely available today because the implementation effort is either moderate or expensive depending on the prerequisites, e.g. PKI. Furthermore the benefits are not yet presented clear in the current literature.

Another aspect in context of systems which manage user-related data is that anonymous authentication needs to be considered together with data anonymity, which will be discussed later on.

Confidentiality

In order to guarantee that only authorized users are able to access EHR data, confidentiality needs to be realized. In general this will be implemented by means of data encryption techniques. However, data encryption can be applied on three different levels. Firstly, **transmission encryption** can be used in order to protect transmitted data on the communication channel (see Figure 3 a). This encryption technique is in common use and popular representatives are the secure sockets layer (SSL) and its successor transport layer security (TLS) and the Internet protocol security (IPsec) in use with virtual private networks (VPN). These methods focus solely on external adversaries, but do not provide any confidentiality at the client as well as the EHR system. In order to guarantee confidentiality at the EHR system, two different approaches can be applied. The first approach which we call **server-based encryption** uses encryption methods which are provided by the EHR system. For example, database encryption like transparent data

Figure 3. Confidentiality realized by means of transmission encryption (a), transmission encryption in combination with server-based encryption (b) and user-based encryption (c).

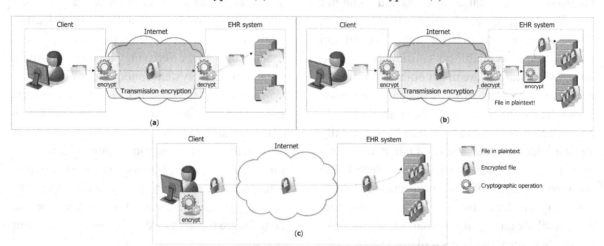

encryption from Oracle 10g, encrypted file systems like EFS from Microsoft, or proprietary content encryption that is performed by the EHR system itself. Even when using server-based encryption in combination with transmission encryption it must be pointed out, that the transmitted data will temporarily be available in plaintext at the EHR system (see Figure 3 b). In particular, this means that the data will be passed in plaintext from the "transmission encryption" to the component of the EHR system which realizes the server-based encryption. Moreover, it must be emphasized that firstly specific employees are able to access data in plaintext and secondly the management of the cryptographic keys that are used for data encryption is realized at the EHR system and consequently is basically vulnerable to attacks.

In contrast to server-based encryption, where the cryptographic keys are solely chosen at the EHR system and all cryptographic operations are performed at the system using the aforementioned keys, **user-based encryption** is based on cryptographic keys that are related to the user. At the user's client these keys can be used to encrypt data and subsequently transmit the encrypted data to the EHR system (see Figure 3 c). In context of user-based encryption this means, that data

are solely in plaintext at the user's clients and consequently stored in the EHR system in an encrypted fashion. Thus, the number of feasible attacks can be reduced significantly. Comparing the two before mentioned approaches, obviously user-based encryption provides a higher level of security, but the infrastructural requirements are higher, e.g. PKI and smart cards, and furthermore the user's client must be able to perform cryptographic operations.

Integrity

Data integrity means that manipulation of transmitted (**transmission integrity**) or stored data (**storage integrity**) can be detected and thus helps to avoid the use of erroneous health data in medical treatment processes. Besides error and manipulation detection codes, there exists also error correction codes to correct errors occurring during transmission or storage of data. Subsequently, we will solely focus on error and manipulation detection codes, which can be realized by means of several techniques such as checksums, message authentication codes or digital signatures. The preferred method to realize data integrity in context of health data are digital signatures.

Because digital signatures additionally provide a property called message authentication. This means that the receiver of a message is able to identify the creator of the message. In context of EHR systems digital signatures should be used to authenticate relevant information that will be integrated into the system. Therefore every creator of health data is required to digitally sign this information and hence the reliability of health data can be increased.

Authorization

Authorization is the concept of providing access to resources only to users who are permitted to do so. Usually the process of authorization takes place after a successful authentication. Mainly, authorization concepts in EHR systems are realized by means of discretionary access control (DAC) strategies, e.g. access control lists (ACLs) or mandatory access control (MAC) strategies, e.g. role based access control (RBAC) (Blobel, 2004; Eyers, 2006; Win, 2005). In the former case, the access policies for objects are specified by their owners, whereas in the latter case access policies are specified by the system. The before mentioned strategies represent only a selection of methods which exists in the literature and in practice today (Bishop, 2002). These methods are typical examples for what we call server-based authorization, since the management, implementation and execution of the authorization is realized solely by the EHR system. To clarify this scenario we will give an example. In server-based authorization, a user may specify access rights to a person for specific health data objects. However, these access rights are stored at the EHR system and an application layer mechanism is responsible to grant or deny access according to these rights. Obviously, specific employees can bypass this barrier to gain unauthorized access to health data. Nevertheless, these methods are used in nearly all systems today.

In order to overcome the before mentioned disadvantages it is possible to either use user-based authorization or anonymous authorization. User-based authorization means that initially solely the creator of health data is able to create access tokens, e.g. a digitally signed data structure, for other parties and solely these authorized parties are able to use these tokens to gain access. Consequently, employees are firstly not able to create another access token and secondly are not able to use such tokens. It must be emphasized that in user-based authorization all cryptographic operations are performed on the user's client. This means, that the creator of health data generates an encrypted access token for every party that should be able to access these health data. These access tokens are stored transparently in the system which means that employees can identify authorized parties, but are not able to use these tokens. In contrast, authorized parties can use their encrypted access token to gain access to the respective health data.

Anonymous authorization has compared with user-based authorization an additional property, namely that access tokens can neither be linked to authorized persons, nor the respective health data. Consequently, unauthorized persons, e.g. employees, are also not able to reveal relationships between authorized persons and health data.

Data Anonymity

In this section we will discuss methods to prevent analyses of EHR metadata. Thereby, anonymous communication provides anonymity for users communicating with the EHR system against eavesdroppers. It must be mentioned, that anonymous communication is a requirement to establish anonymity at the EHR system regarding authentication and authorization. Unlinkability and obfuscation are used to provide anonymity for health data stored in the EHR system.

Anonymous Communication

Mechanisms that provide anonymity and unlinkability of messages sent over a communication channel are denoted as anonymous communication techniques and have been intensively studied in recent years, see (Danezis and Diaz, 2008) for a sound overview. There are several implementations available for low-latency services like Web browsing, e.g. Tor, JAP, as well as high-latency services like E-Mail, e.g. Mixminion. These anonymous communication channels help to improve the privacy of users in context of eavesdroppers and curious communication partners. Especially, regarding the latter one anonymity can be preserved if electronic interaction does not rely on additional identifying information at higher network layers, i.e. the application layer. For example, a user who queries a public web page using an anonymous communication channel may remove all identifying information from higher network layers and thus will stay anonymous.

Unlinkability

Unlinkability of items of interest means that relations between items, which a priori exist, cannot be identified through pure observation of the system (Pfitzmann and Köhntopp, 2000; Steinbrecher and Köpsell, 2003). A system containing n users provides perfect unlinkability, if the relation of an object and a user exists with probability $p = 1/n$ for all objects. Hence, an insider of the system cannot gain any information.

Pseudonymization of person related data is the process of replacing every person identifier for example by a value, a so called pseudonym, which can for instance be the symmetric encryption of the person's identifier. If the used encryption secret is kept secret is practically impossible to invert the pseudonym to obtain the person's identifier. However, a person who is in possession of this key can easily compute the person's identifier given the pseudonym. Based on pseudonymization techniques it is possible to pseudonymize a conceptual model of an EHR system (Slamanig et al., 2007). Basically, this means that every person is assigned one or more pseudonyms that are used to uniquely relate health data to this person. The resulting pseudonymized conceptual model provides unlinkability and can be implemented highly efficient.

Obfuscation

Considering the above mentioned pseudonyms, there exists an injective mapping between users and pseudonyms. Consequently, pseudonyms can be used to analyze the structure of an EHR system. This means that health data that are connected to the same pseudonym are related to the same person. If the authentication method does not provide anonymity, an attacker can easily link the pseudonym to the holder of the pseudonym. However, even if anonymous authentication is used, an attacker who uses so called intersection attacks (Kesdogan et al., 2003), i.e. intersecting the sets of queried health data, may also be able to determine the holder of the pseudonym. In order to prevent these analyses it is possible to break the injectiveness of the mapping between identities and pseudonyms (Damiani et al., 2003; Stingl and Slamanig, 2008). Hence, this complicates the above mentioned attack, but it must be pointed out that when users access their EHR the system will provide health data to them which are not related to them. However, they will not be able to view the content of these data, when health data are encrypted.

Information Hiding

Information hiding means that users are able to hide specific information depending on the situation. To clarify this property we will discuss two scenarios.

- A patient presents his EHR during a treatment process, but wants to hide some information which is not relevant or even compromising from the patient's point of view, e.g. a cured drug addiction or a second opinion.
- A person is forced to present the entire EHR for instance during a job interview or an insurance contract conclusion.

When considering an authorization concept, based on explicitly granting access to specific information to other parties, then information hiding in context of the first example can be realized very easily by the patient. However, this does not apply to the second example. Furthermore, if the patient is not explicitly granting access to other persons prior to the treatment, but logs into his EHR during the treatment and presents the entire data, then it is necessary to provide additional measure to realize information hiding. In the following we will present methods to realize information hiding regarding the aforementioned two scenarios. Additionally, we want to emphasize that we are also considering insiders, who are trying to reveal information on hidden health data.

Pseudo-Information Hiding

This property is characterized by providing methods to hide information without the possibility to plausibly deny the existence of this information. Plausible deniability means, that external parties as well as insiders have no possibility to determine the existence of hidden information and even less their content. Typical examples are classifying health data as hidden in analogy to hidden files, whereas the EHR system does not show health data that is characterized as hidden. Another method is to use encrypted envelopes to store health data in the EHR system, which need to be opened explicitly by additional information solely known to the user. It is easy to comprehend from the aforementioned examples that these methods provide some level of protection, but do not provide a satisfiable solution regarding plausible deniability.

Information Hiding with Plausible Deniability

Therefore we need a measure to provide plausible deniability in a cryptographically provable sense. As countermeasure so called multiple identities (Slamanig and Stingl, 2008b) can be used. In this context multiple identities can be described by means of dividing the EHR of a person into so called sub-identities (see Figure 4). A user can assign a subset of her EHR to each of these sub-identities. Thereby, these subsets do not need to be disjoint. Subject to the person, the medical data are presented to, the user is able to choose one of her sub-identities (e.g. a special prepared, non compromising one) and consequently opens the assigned subset of medical data. Hence, a user can hide sensitive data in a special sub-identity in order to prevent disclosure of medical data. However, one drawback of this approach is that passwords which are used to derive the cryptographic keys for the respective identities need to be chosen independently of each other. More precisely, there must not be any relationship between passwords which clearly could be computed by an adversary too. However, we assume that in practice the number of identities and passwords respectively will be moderate. Furthermore, this concept additionally provides the possibility to create so called super-identities which can hold several sub-identities. Thus, super-identities can be used to comfortably manage the respective sub-identities.

To summarize, we provide an overview of the discussed techniques, a classification regarding the security and privacy and evaluate the effort for implementing these methods. Furthermore, one should keep in mind that the effort may heavily depend on prerequisites, for instance a two-factor authentication may be based on a

Figure 4. Simplified presentation of the aspects unlinkability and plausible deniability. If the user authenticates against the super identity, he can access all health data. But by authenticating against the non-compromising identity (NC) only non-compromising information will be presented (highlighted area). The right hand side of the figure shows that it is not possible to determine any relationship between health data and participating parties.

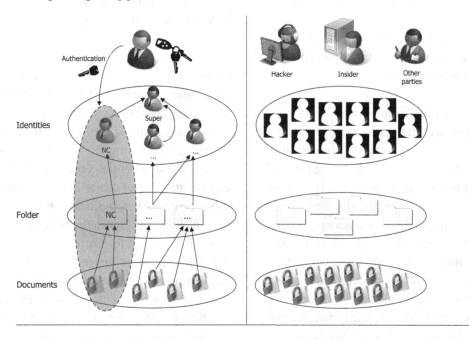

public key infrastructure (PKI). Additionally, we give an estimation for the computational cost considering client and server computations. But, we want to emphasize that the effective costs may massively depend on the chosen protocols to realize the methods and the desired degree of security and privacy. Communication costs are solely relevant when using anonymous communication. However, as above the effective costs depend on the chosen protocols, but need to be considered as expensive.

SOLUTIONS AND RECOMMENDATIONS

In this section we will discuss security levels for EHRs based on the methods introduced in the last section. Thereby, the degree of privacy

provided by an EHR increases with the security level. However, it must not be unmentioned that the effort for implementation increases with the security level too. After introducing the security levels, we will give some characteristic real-world examples as well as some virtual examples that are in our opinion highly realistic. The latter ones did not occur as far as we know, maybe since EHR systems with a high number of users are not available currently. Finally, we will show which level of security will be required to prevent the attacks in the aforementioned examples.

Analyzing the first three examples from table 3, one can conclude that level 2 providing server-based confidentiality is sufficient to avoid these attacks and to prevent misuse of stolen data respectively. Nevertheless, it must be pointed out, that it may be possible to draw potential conclusions based on the analysis of metadata, even though the

Table 1. Overview of the discussed techniques and methods and the implementation effort

Technologies	Methods	Classification	Implementation Effort	Computational Cost
Authentication	One-factor authentication	Basic	Few	Few
	Two-factor	Basic	Few/moderate	Few
	Anonymous	Enhanced	Moderate/expensive	Moderate/expensive
Authorization	Server-based	Basic	Few	Few
	User-based	Enhanced	Moderate	Moderate
	Anonymous	Enhanced	Expensive	Moderate
Confidentiality	Transmission	Basic	Few	Moderate
	Server-based	Basic	Few	Few
	User-based	Enhanced	Moderate	Moderate
Integrity	Transmission	Basic	Few	Few
	Storage	Basic	Moderate	Few
Data anonymity	Anonymous communication	Enhanced	Few	Moderate/expensive
	Obfuscation	Enhanced	Moderate	Moderate
	Unlinkability	Enhanced	Expensive	Moderate
Information hiding	Pseudo-information hiding	Basic	Few	Few
	Information hiding with plausible deniability	Enhanced	Expensive	Few

health data are encrypted. The same argumentation holds for the last example, but in this case it could be possible that server-based confidentiality is not sufficient. This depends on the privileges of the current user of the hijacked computer. Clearly, if the person has access to the EHR system and is consequently able to access health data, then these data are theoretical "available" to the attacker. To avoid this scenario, user-based confidentiality and authorization (level 3) should be applied.

To avoid the attack of the first scenario anonymous authentication and anonymous authorization are required and thus at least level 4 is necessary. In the second scenario the knowledge of one health information of a user enables an attacker to reveal further information of health data of this user. This

Table 2. Definition of security levels for EHRs

Level	Authentication	Authorization	Confidentiality	Integrity	Data anonymity	Information hiding
1	One-factor	Server-based	Transmission	Transmission		
2	Two-factor	Server-based	Transmission Server-based	Transmission Storage		
3	Two-factor	User-based	Transmission User-based	Transmission Storage		
4	Anonymous	Anonymous	Transmission User-based	Transmission Storage		Pseudo-information hiding
5	Anonymous	Anonymous	Transmission User-based	Transmission Storage	Unlinkability Obfuscation	Plausible deniability

Table 3. Some recent examples of attacks against health data

Country	Description	Level
U.S.A	**Laptop with data on 28,000 home care patients stolen in Detroit:** Laptop containing home care information on 28,000 patients has been stolen from the car of a nurse (Computerworld, 2006).	2
U.S.A	**Hackers Break into Virginia Health Professions Database:** Hackers broke into a Virginia state Web site used by pharmacists to track prescription drug abuse and deleted records on more than 8 million patients. (Washington Post, 2009).	2
U.S.A	**Hackers sell health data:** 500 MB of sensitive data in plaintext of hospitals in the U.S.A has been collected by malware which was injected into the respective IT systems (Finjan, 2009).	2
Spain	**Health data on the Internet:** Hacker hijacks a hospital computer to steal health data (El Pais, 2008).	3

Table 4. Virtual scenarios which show potential attacks against EHR systems

Virtual scenario	Level
An EHR system was developed according to level 3. Hence, user-based confidentiality and authorization is used. However, a hacker or an insider has analyzed the behavior of users and the relationships between users and medical institutions or physicians respectively. Consequently, it was possible to determine a detailed list of all parties involved in treatment processes for every user, although having no information about the content of medical data.	4
An EHR system was developed according to level 4. This means that the relationships between parties and health data are anonymized, but not relationships between health data. However, anonymous authentication in combination with user related health data provides information to significantly improve the chances to identify single users and consequently their health data.	5
A job candidate is illegally forced to present the EHR during a job interview.	5

is due to the fact that actually every EHR system is based on a structured concept, e.g. a relational database model. In order to prevent the analysis of the structure, it is recommended to use methods which provide unlinkability. Further improvements can be achieved by means of obfuscation techniques.

To avoid the precarious situation of the third scenario it is necessary that a user can present a part of the EHR containing no compromising information. Consequently, the job recruiter has no possibility to obtain any information whether the entire EHR or a selected part of the EHR is presented.

FUTURE RESEARCH DIRECTIONS

One aspect that was treated rudimentary in this chapter is the vulnerability of the user's client. This issue cannot solely be covered by techni-

cal safeguards which are enforced by the EHR system, since it is very hard to establish uniform administrative measures, e.g. policies, for EHR users. For instance, if the operating system at the user's client is prone to security exploits due to missing security patches, malware could be installed unnoticeably on the client. This malware could steal health data independent of the security level of the EHR system. One approach to counter the client vulnerability is trusted computing (TCG, 2009), which helps to reduce the number of attacks against user's clients. This is mainly due to the fact that software as well as hardware components are authenticated to the client by means of cryptographic operations. A very interesting aspect in this context is the use of direct anonymous attestation (Brickell et al., 2004) which enables the EHR system to enforce that user's client complies with software specifications defined by the EHR system. Furthermore, this approach enables the client to anonymously conduct the aforementioned protocol. This means that the anonymity discussed in this chapter will not be compromised at all.

CONCLUSION

In this chapter we have provided a security analysis of EHR systems and discussed two additional groups of adversaries, namely internal adversaries and "curious persons", which are from our point of view not taken into consideration adequately in many existing EHR approaches. Furthermore we have shown that the consequences for all involved parties in case of disclosure of medical data are serious. Especially, considering the patient this may result in massive disadvantages regarding his working and social environment. In order to prevent attacks conducted by the aforementioned adversaries we have introduced enhanced security properties for EHR systems and discussed methods to realize them. In our opinion these enhanced properties are of enormous relevance when realizing a reliable EHR system. Furthermore we have introduced security levels to firstly classify EHR systems and secondly show that recent attacks against EHR systems can be prevented by applying a certain level of security.

REFERENCES

Article, E. U. 29 Data Protection Working Party (2007). *Working Document on the processing of personal data relating to health in electronic health records (EHR)*. Retrieved February 2009, http://ec.europa.eu/justice_home/fsj/privacy/workinggroup/wpdocs/

Bishop, M. (2002). *Computer Security: Art and Science*. Addison-Wesley.

Blobel, B. (2004). Authorisation and access control for electronic health record systems. *International Journal of Medical Informatics*, 73(3), 251–257. doi:10.1016/j.ijmedinf.2003.11.018

Both, F., Hoogendoorn, M., Klein, M. C. A., & Treur, J. (2009). Design and Analysis of an Ambient Intelligent System Supporting Depression Therapy. In L. Azevedo & A.R. Londral (Eds.), *Proceedings of the Second International Conference on Health Informatics, HEALTHINF 2009* (pp. 142-148). INSTICC Press.

Brickell, E., Camenisch, J., & Chen, L. (2004). Direct anonymous attestation. In *Proceedings of the 11th ACM Conference on Computer and Communications Security, CCS'04* (pp. 132-145). New York: ACM.

Computer Security Institute. CSI (2007). Computer *Crime and Security Survey 2007*. Retrieved February 2009, http://www.gocsi.com/forms/csi survey.jhtml

Computerworld (2009). Laptop with data on 28,000 home care patients stolen in Detroit. Retrieved May 2009 from http://www.computerworld.com/action/article.do?command=view ArticleBasic&articleId=9002685

Damiani, E., Vimercati, S. D., Jajodia, S., Paraboschi, S., & Samarati, P. (2003). Balancing confidentiality and efficiency in untrusted relational DBMSs. In *Proceedings of the 10th ACM Conference on Computer and Communications Security*, CCS '03 (pp. 93-102). New York: ACM.

Danezis, G., & Diaz, C. (2008). *A Survey of Anonymous Communication Channels* (Tech Rep MSRTR-2008-35). Microsoft Research.

Eichelberg, M., Aden, T., Riesmeier, J., Dogac, A., & Laleci, G. B. (2005). A survey and analysis of Electronic Healthcare Record standards. *ACM Computing Surveys*, 37(4), 277–315. doi:10.1145/1118890.1118891

El Pais. (2009). 4.000 historias clínicas de abortos se filtran en la Red a través de eMule. Retrieved May 2009 from http://www.elpais.com/articulo/socie-dad/4000/historias/clinicas/abortos/filtran/Red/traves/eMule/elpepusoc/20080425elpepisoc_3/Tes

Eyers, D. M., Bacon, J., & Moody, K. (2006). OASIS role-based access control for electronic health records. *IEEE Proceedings on Software,* *153*(1), 16–23. doi:10.1049/ip-sen:20045038

Finjan Malicious Code Research Center. (2008). *Malicious Page of the Month.* Retrieved May 2009 from http://www.finjan.com

German Centre for Addiction Issues. DHS (2008). Retrieved February 2009 from http://www.dhs.de/

Kesdogan, D., Agrawal, D., & Penz, S. (2003). Limits of Anonymity in Open Environments. In *Revised Papers From the 5th international Workshop on information Hiding* (pp. 53-69). Springer-Verlag.

Lowrance, W. W. (1997). *Privacy and Health Research. A Report to the U.S. Secretary of Health and Human Services.* Retrieved February 2009 from http://aspe.os.dhhs.gov/datacncl/PHR.htm

Mao, W. (2003). *Modern Cryptography: Theory and Practice.* Prentice Hall.

Menezes, A. J., Vanstone, S. A., & Oorschot, P. C. (1996). *Handbook of Applied Cryptography.* CRC Press, Inc.

National Alliance for Health Information Technology. NAHIT (2008). *Defining Key Health Information Technology Terms.* Retrieved February 2009, http://www.nahit.org/

Pfitzmann, A., & Köhntopp, M. (2000). Anonymity, Unobservability and Pseudonymity - A Proposal for Terminology. In *Proceedings International Workshop on Design Issues in Anonymity and Unobservability* (pp. 1-9). Springer-Verlag.

Slamanig, D., Stingl, C., Lackner, G., & Payer, U. (2007). Preserving Privacy in a Web-based Multiuser-System (German). In P. Horster (Ed.), *Proceedings of DACH-Security 2007* (pp. 98-110). IT-Verlag.

Steinbrecher, S., & Köpsell, S. (2003). Modelling Unlinkability. In [Springer-Verlag.]. *Proceedings of Privacy Enhancing Technologies Workshop, PET, 2003,* 32–47.

Stingl, C., & Slamanig, D. (2008). Privacy-enhancing methods for e-health applications: how to prevent statistical analyses and attacks. *Int. J. Bus. Intell. Data Min.*, *3*(3), 236–254. doi:10.1504/IJBIDM.2008.022135

Trusted Computing Group. TCG (2009). Retrieved February 2009, http://www.trustedcomputing-group.org

Washington Post. (2009). Hackers Break Into Virginia Health Professions Database, Demand Ransom. Retrieved May 2009 from http://voices.washingtonpost.com/securityfix/2009/05/hackers_break_into_virginia_he.html

Win, K. T. (2005). A review of security of electronic health records. *Health Information Management Journal, 34*(1), 13–18.

Wright, A., & Sittig, D. F. (2007). Encryption Characteristics of Two USB-based Personal Health Record Devices. *Journal of the American Medical Informatics Association, 14,* 397–399. doi:10.1197/jamia.M2352

ADDITIONAL READING

Agrawal, R., & Johnson, C. (2006). Securing electronic health records without impeding the flow of information. *International Journal of Medical Informatics, 76,* 471–479. doi:10.1016/j.ijmedinf.2006.09.015

Demuynck, L., & De Decker, B. (2005). Privacy-Preserving Electronic Health Records. In *Proceedings of 9th IFIP TC-6 TC-11 International Conference on Communications and Multimedia Security, CMS 2005* (pp. 150-159). Springer-Verlag.

Gritzalis, S. (2004). Enhancing Privacy and Data Protection in Electronic Medical Environments. *Journal of Medical Systems*, *28*(6), 535–547. doi:10.1023/B:JOMS.0000044956.55209.75

Liu, V., Caelli, W., May, L., Croll, P., & Henricksen, M. (2007). Current approaches to secure health information systems are not sustainable: an analysis. In *Proceedings of the 12th World Congress on Health (Medical) Informatics. Medinfo, 2007*, 2430–2432.

Predd, J., Pfleeger, S. L., Hunker, J., & Bulford, C. (2008). Insiders Behaving Badly. *IEEE Security and Privacy*, *6*(4), 66–70. doi:10.1109/MSP.2008.87

Slamanig, D., & Stingl, C. (2009). How to Preserve Patient's Privacy and Anonymity in Web-based Electronic Health Records. In L. Azevedo & A.R. Londral (Eds.) *Proceedings of the Second International Conference on Health Informatics, HEALTHINF 2009* (pp. 257-264). INSTICC Press.

Tang, P. C., Ash, J. S., Bates, D. W., Overhage, J. M., & Sands, D. Z. (2007). Personal Health Records: Definitions, Benefits, and Strategies for Overcoming Barriers to Adoption. *Journal of the American Medical Informatics Association*, *13*, 121–126. doi:10.1197/jamia.M2025

Win, K. T., Croll, P., Cooper, J., & Alcock, C. (2002). Issues of Privacy, Confidentiality and Access in Electronic Health Record. *Journal of Law and Information Science*, *12*(1), 4–25.

Win, K. T., Susilo, W., & Mu, Y. (2006). Personal Health Record Systems and Their Security Protection. *Journal of Medical Systems*, *30*(4), 309–315. doi:10.1007/s10916-006-9019-y

Chapter 15
Privacy–Based Multiagent Brokering Architecture for Ubiquitous Healthcare Systems

AbdulMutalib Masaud-Wahaishi
United Arab Emirates University, UAE

Hamada Ghenniwa
University of Western Ontario, Canada

ABSTRACT

Ubiquitous healthcare is an emerging technology that promises increases in efficiency, accuracy and availability of medical treatment; however it also introduces the potential for serious abuses including major privacy violations. Brokering is a capability-based coordination approach for ubiquitous healthcare systems (UHS). A major challenge of brokering in open environments is to support privacy. Within the context of brokering, the authors model privacy in terms of the entities' ability to hide or reveal information related to its identities, requests, and/or capabilities. This work presents a privacy-based multi-agent brokering architecture that supports different privacy degrees. Unlike traditional approaches, the brokering is viewed as a set of services in which the brokering role is further classified into several sub-roles each with a specific architecture and interaction protocol that is appropriate to support a required privacy degree. To put the formulation in practice, a prototype of the proposed architecture has been implemented to support information-gathering capabilities in healthcare environments using FIPA-complaint platform (JADE).

INTRODUCTION

Nowadays in modern and ubiquitous computing environments, it is imperative more than ever that the delivery of healthcare quality is clearly crucial in any society. Healthcare workers are expected to continuously improve the quality, timeliness, and cost of their services to the community. An important feature of the various ubiquitous healthcare systems is that they share similar problems and are faced with common challenges for decentralized systems in open environments. In this chapter we focus on the following challenges:

- In open ubiquitous healthcare environments, it is no longer practical to expect healthcare

DOI: 10.4018/978-1-61520-777-0.ch015

Copyright © 2010, IGI Global. Copying or distributing in print or electronic forms without written permission of IGI Global is prohibited.

clinicians, staff, care providers and patients to determine and keep track of the information and services relevant to his/her requests and demands. For example a patient shall be ubiquitously able to access his/her medical record, i.e., from anywhere at any time through any means.

- The distributed nature of data, information, knowledge and services among multiple healthcare locations may require effective coordination and collaboration amongst the participants. The provision of care to hospitalized patients involves various procedures and requires the coordinated interaction amongst various staff and medical members.

- Open healthcare environments usually characterized by multiple participants that may require different degrees of access authorities on data, information, knowledge and services. In such environments, ubiquitous healthcare systems must satisfy different levels of security and privacy requirements.

The proactive health systems have the potential to improve healthcare access and management which significantly decrease the incurred costs through efficient coordinated information flow between various physicians, patients and medical personnel, yet the privacy concerns are key barriers to the growth of health based systems in. Legislations to protect personal medical information were proposed and put in effect to help building a mutual confidence between various participants in the healthcare domain. All these suggest that healthcare needs a major shift towards building cost-effective privacy-based solutions for pervasive and ubiquitous embedded e-Health environments, given that limited financial and human resources will be committed. Without broad trust in medical privacy, patients, professionals, and service providers may diminish the value

and resist the adoption of ubiquitous healthcare services.

The high degree of collaborative work needed in healthcare environments implies that developers and researchers should think of other alternatives to manage and automate this collaboration efficiently. The main goal of this chapter is to provide a thorough analysis, investigation and to develop a privacy-based coordination solution for decentralized systems in open environments that is applicable to ubiquitous healthcare domain. In this chapter we focus on one aspect of coordination that deals with capability-interdependency problem, i.e. to achieve a goal by a group of participants that may go beyond the capability of the individuals. To this end, the chapter presents an in-depth analysis of the capability-based coordination and proposes a novel privacy-based brokering framework and interaction protocols that support different privacy degrees that are applicable to ubiquitous healthcare systems.

BROKERING – CAPABILITY BASED COORDINATION

In developing ubiquitous healthcare environments, coordination is a major challenge. Entities need to locate and interact with others who possess the capabilities to achieve a particular goal. For distributed systems, fulfilling a request may go beyond the capability of the individual entities, this is known as the *capability-interdependency problem* (Ghenniwa and Huhns, 2004)

In the conventional point-to-point interaction configuration, entities interact directly with each other to provide controlled and directed coordination. However, this configuration is both inflexible and computationally expensive. For instance, there is no separation of concerns between computation and coordination. The absence of a separate medium that deals exclusively with the coordination aspects in the system means that the entities, in addition to other computational activities, have to carry out the "interaction work" themselves to satisfy common or local tasks.

As an alternative, the capability-based coordination approach can be a very effective medium for interaction. In this approach, the entities need not to be concerned with how the interaction is performed or done. The essential objectives of capability-based coordination solutions are to facilitate the interaction of various entities who continue to operate in open distributed environment and compete to deliver value-rich services.

Brokering is a capability-based coordination which is viewed as an abstraction level at which a distributed system environment can be viewed collectively as a coherent universe. Furthermore, such coordination gives a *ubiquitous* level of interaction at which the involved entities are not required to be known to each other, nor exist in the same place at the same time in order to work together.

Within this context we define brokering for ubiquitous healthcare as: "*A capability-based coordination solution that enables variety of participants to work together ubiquitously in open distributed environments*".

In capability-based coordination, participants can be distinguished by the role they play (for example, a service requester or a provider). Providers specify services they provide in capabilities. For example, a service that provides weather forecasting is an example of a capability. Capabilities are often accompanied by services parameters, which specify the conditions under which services are offered such as cost and quality. Requesters specify services they need in requests. Requests can be accompanied by preferences, which are counterparts of service parameters.

PRIVACY

A major challenge of brokering in open ubiquitous healthcare environments is to support privacy. In collecting the massive amounts of health information gathered by ubiquitous healthcare systems, close attention needs to be paid to who controls what is gathered, who has access to it, and where/how/whether that information is stored.

Privacy and the confidentiality of medical data, information, knowledge and services have to be especially safeguarded. Healthcare professionals and care-providers prefer to have the ability of controlling the collection, retention and distribution of information about themselves. A recent survey (The Association of American Physicians and Surgeons, 2008) shows that 67% of the American national respondents are concerned about the privacy of their personal medical records, 52% fear that their health insurance information might be used by employers to limit job opportunities while only 30% are willing to share their personal health information with health professionals not directly involved in their case. As few as 27% respondents are willing to share their medical records with various drug companies.

The modern communication infrastructures, networks and technologies, provide extraordinary high data rates, thus allowing cost and time efficient remote delivering of medical data that have been collected from the portable, embedded devices that reside onto the end-users (monitored patients) towards remote distributed Medical Servers, for further processing.

Furthermore, the pervasiveness and ubiquitous characteristics of modern user-centric nomadic environments, in which the user is the central point surrounded by different types of embedded computing devices and sensors, like for example ElectroCardioGraph (ECG) and pulse, oxygen saturation and blood pressure devices, has exemplified the need for essential and vital requirements concerning security and privacy aspects such as the protection of sensitive medical data and measurements, confidentiality, and protection of patients privacy.

With this growing concern about privacy in ubiquitous healthcare environments, considerable research has been conducted focusing on various aspects. Solutions and models put forth by this research address specific challenges of the problem. However, within the context of brokering for ubiquitous healthcare we view Privacy as *"the ability of healthcare entities to decide upon revealing or hiding information related to their identities, requests and capabilities in open distributed environments"*.

BACKGROUND

Many researchers have worked on privacy in ubiquitous healthcare domain and have addressed the privacy issues from various perspectives. Some approaches had proposed criteria for privacy design patterns and identified protection solutions for pseudonymous and anonymity emails by providing guidelines for users to send and exchange emails without revealing their online identity (Chung E. et 2004; Langheinrich, 2001; Schumacher, 2002). The dependability and the perception of privacy based on the case study of a sensor-rich, eldercare facility issue in U-Healthcare was analyzed in and discussed in (Felix & Harald, 2004) [8]. A recent survey has been conducted with focus on the security solutions for pervasive healthcare environments with a special attention on securing data collected by sensors as well as the communication between the sensors. Also, it provides an investigation of mechanisms for controlling the access to medical data using cryptographic primitives (Venkatasubramanian & Gupta, 2007).

Other approaches proposed the use of privacy policies along with physical access means (such as smartcards), in which the access of private information is granted through the presence of another trusted authority that mediate between information requesters and information providers (Clarke, 2007; Yee, Korba, & Song, 2006). A European IST project (Camarinha-Matos & Afsarmanesh, 2001), TelemediaCare, developed

agent-based framework to support patient focused distant care and assistance, in the architecture composes tow different types of agents, namely stationary "static" and mobile agents. Web-service based tools were developed to enable patients to remotely schedule appointments, doctor visits and to access medical data (Silver, Andonyadis & Morales. 1998).

Another approach provides access control mechanisms and tools for protecting requesters' personal privacy (Langheinrich, 2002). Service requesters joining an environment are prompted for the required privacy policies of each service in the environment. A dedicated requester's proxy checks these policies against the user's predefined privacy preferences and accordingly decides upon using or declining the services. Brox (2005) proposes the usage of MPEG-21 standard as a mechanism to access control to medical. However the approach does not provide an architecture or guidelines for utilizing the standards and hence the author considers it as open future research issue.

Gialelis et al (2008) propose a pervasive healthcare architecture into which a wearable health monitoring system is integrated into a broad tele-medical infrastructure allowing high – risk cardiovascular patients to monitor critical changes and get experts feedback. However; the proposed architecture does not address any privacy considerations, which may lead to serious breaches.

Many industrial and government initiatives and programs attempted to develop healthcare systems and networks at domestic and global scales (Health Insurance Portability and Accountability; Initiative for Privacy Standardization in Europe, 2008). A major objective of these networks is to improve the "quality" of healthcare services and make them ubiquitously available and cost-effective. For example, in many cases sharing a complete electronic medical patient case file, between specialists, hospitals and GPs is crucial in diagnosing diseases correctly, avoiding duplicative risky and expensive tests, and developing effective treatment plans. However, medical patient case files may contain some sensitive information about critical and vital topics such as abortions, emotional and psychiatric care, and genetic predisposition to diseases.

However; many of the proposed solutions have the assumption that the computations take place with the existence of a completely trusted third party. Additionally, and to the extent of our knowledge there has not yet been any proposals that have treated privacy as an architectural element within the coordination services for ubiquitous healthcare systems.

THE BROKERING LAYER

Healthcare entities are usually required to work together to satisfy a request. Moreover, these entities should be able to select an appropriate privacy level and play different roles to achieve their goals and get results to their requests regardless of whether the request can be satisfied at a local or remote location. A healthcare entity's role can be categorized as either a service-requester or a service-provider. A service-provider is the role of a domain entity with the capability to meet the needs of another domain entity. A service-requester is the role of a domain entity that attempts to achieve a goal beyond its own capability.

Brokering entities need to interact (on behalf of requesters) with various providers to fulfill a request. The interaction protocols specify the set of allowed message types, message contents and the correct order of messages during any brokering scenario. To facilitate the interaction, entities in uubiquitous healthcare environments need to depend heavily on interact with each other not only to perform requests, but also to advertise their capabilities.

The concern of this chapter is to view privacy in terms of three attributes: the entity's identities (*Id*), capabilities (*Cap*) and requests (*Req*). The brokering enables the entities to participate in the environment with different roles and hence

be capable of automating their privacy concerns and select a particular privacy degree. An entity is able to choose whether to reveal or hide a particular privacy attribute. Each role is represented as a special brokering entity (each has a distinguished name) with a specific architecture and interaction protocol that is appropriate to a required privacy degree.

Responsibilities are separated and defined according to the roles played and the required privacy degree. Within the layer, two sets of brokering entities are available to service requesters and providers. The first set handles interactions with requesters according to the desired privacy degree that is appropriate to their preferences. The other set supports privacy degrees required by service providers. Figure 1 shows a logical view of the brokering layer. Each brokering scenario is accomplished by the combination of the requester role, brokering entity role and the provider role. Note that in the figure, a specific privacy attribute variable $\bar{x}$, $x \in \left\{ Id, Req, Cap \right\}$ represents that the corresponding privacy attribute is not revealed.

The following tables summarize the different scenarios that can be played by the brokering layer categorized by the required privacy degrees of both the requester and the provider entities.

Each interaction protocol is described in terms of a combination of the interaction within the brokering layer and the interaction with the domain entities.

BROKERING INTERACTION PROTOCOLS

Each brokering scenario encapsulates a set of conversation and message exchanges amongst the requester-related brokering entities (called ReqBroker henceforth) and the provider-related brokering entities (called ProvBrokers henceforth) as well as the corresponding domain entity which

Figure 1. Logical view of the brokering layer

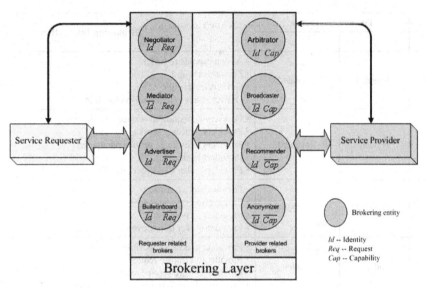

plays a specific role in an interaction protocol. An interaction protocol can be viewed as a set of messages' content and the constraints imposed on the individual roles in different privacy degrees. A role focuses on how the entity in a given state receives a message of a specified type, performs local actions, sends out messages, and switches to another state.

The Requester-Brokering Interaction Patterns

A requester interacts with the environment through sending and receiving messages. In some scenarios (for example, requesters hiding privacy attributes), the ReqBrokers and the domain entities exhibit a proactive behavior to respond to changes in the environment. The following represent the vari-

Table 1. Brokering roles and interaction protocols with requesters

Brokering Role	Privacy Attributes		Brokering Interaction
	Req	*Id*	
Negotiator	Revealed	Revealed	• Receive service request • Forwards request to broker-provider side • Deliver result to requester
Mediator	Hidden	Revealed	• Retrieve service request posted by a requester • Forwards request to broker-provider side • Store result to be retrieved by requester
Advertiser	Revealed	Hidden	• Post service request to service repository • Requester to search repository and request service • Retrieve a service request that was stored by a requester • Forwards request to broker-provider side • Store result to be retrieved by requester
Bulletinboard	Hidden	Hidden	• Requester to store service request • Retrieve service request that was stored by a requester • Forwards request to broker-provider side • Store result to be retrieved by requester

Table 2. Brokering roles and interaction protocols with providers

Brokering Role	Privacy Attributes		Brokering Interaction
	Id	*Cap*	
Arbitrator	Revealed	Revealed	• Assign capable provider • Forwards request • Get service's result • Deliver result to requester-broker side
Broadcaster	Hidden	Revealed	• Post service request to service repository • Providers to access service repository • Providers to evaluate service parameters • Providers to store result • Provider-broker to retrieve stored result
Recommender	Revealed	Hidden	• Forward service request • Provider to evaluate request • Providers to store result • Provider-broker to retrieve stored result
Anonymizer	Hidden	Hidden	• Providers to access repository • Provider to evaluate request • Provider to store service result • Brokering layer to retrieve stored result

ous roles and the associated interaction patterns that can be played by the brokering in supporting requesters with different privacy degrees.

The interaction requires a set of agreed messages, rules for actions based upon reception of various messages and assumptions of the communication channels. These constraints, rules and patterns can be abstracted and formalized as interaction patterns, which are basis for successful capability-based coordination. The interaction protocols range from negotiation schemas to a simple request for a task.

The interaction protocols are viewed as patterns representing both message communication and the corresponding constraints on the content of such messages. In the proposed model, a protocol is modeled as a set of communicating processes executing concurrently. They express the constraints on the relationship between sending and receiving messages which represent the protocol mechanism. This model emphasizes the entities' collaborative behaviors.

In order to define the messages that are needed to support a specific privacy degree, we first identify the required "message-types" that can satisfy the supporting protocol and next, decide on the possible messages that can be assigned to particular role in a given interaction protocols. Note that messages can be accompanied by guard conditions to describe the constraints on the exchanged messages. To summarize the process, the process will be as follows:

1. Define the possible roles that entities can play is a specific protocol.
2. Identify how many types of messages exist in an interaction protocol. Message types are specified as constructors of the actions initiated by the entities.
3. Decide what messages a role can send, check, receive or store.
4. Next, we have to figure out the rules and constraints on these messages.

A message consists of a sender, a set of receivers, "*type*" of message and message "*content*". In all the following interaction protocols, we focus only on message semantics, without caring about its implementation details. For readability purposes, we list the interaction protocols using the message type only.

The Negotiator

Consider the following scenario: a doctor wants to have information about the number of patients who have Hepatitis B in a specific city. The doctor needs to be assessed without exposing its identity and the pertinent request to others.

The above scenarios exemplifies privacy degrees in which revealing sensitive information can lead to catastrophic discrimination outcomes, knowing the scientist's identity might lead to a biased and unfair decision; marketing trends can turn into spamming. Therefore, it might be desirable to not be identified when accessing on-line services. Requester should be able to interact with the corresponding brokering entity to request services, receive service's results, and acknowledge the receipt of service's result.

The proposed protocol protects the requester's identity and requests despite revealing them to the Negotiator. The assumption is that the Negotiator is a trusted entity. Figure 2 depicts the protocol that involves the Negotiator's interaction pattern includes interaction with various ProvBrokers. The Negotiator forwards the request to all the ProvBrokers. The Negotiator issues a Call-For-Proposals (CFP) to ProvBrokers (act as potential contractors) with the request specifications which include:

* **Request abstraction**: a brief description of the request represented by the service name that abstract the required capability.
* **Request specification**: a description and the expected format of the request.
* **Expiration time**: a statement of the time interval during which the announcement is valid.

For example, a doctor might request health information related to the mortality rate amongst the newborns in specific region. Accordingly, a request for service is defined as follows:

$$\langle informationGethering, NewBorn\text{-}Mortality, Region\text{-}Name, PDF, 30 \rangle$$

The request states that an electronic PDF file is required for newborn mortality data in a defined region within a defined time unit.

Figure 2. Interaction pattern for the negotiator

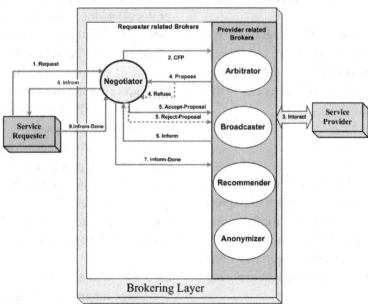

Each ProvBroker submits an offer on behalf of its providers. The interaction protocol represents the message communication and the corresponding content of such messages.

1. **Receive ("Request")**: A service request is received by the Negotiator.
8. **Send ("Inform")**: The Negotiator delivers service's result to the requester.
9. **Receive ("Inform-Done")**: A message is received from the requester indicating the receipt of the service's result.

The interaction within the brokering layer is represented as follows:

2. **Send ("CFP")**: Sending a call for proposal message to ProvBrokers.
4. **Receive ("Propose")**: The Negotiator receives service proposal(s).
4. **Receive ("Refuse")**: A ProvBroker declines to participate in fulfilling a service request.
5. **Send ("Accept-Proposal")**: A message is sent to the wining ProvBroker indicating the acceptance of the proposal.
5. **Send ("Reject-Proposal")**: A rejection message is sent to those ProvBrokers who do not win.
6. **Receive ("Inform")**: The Negotiator receives the service's result1.
7. **Send ("Inform-Done")**: The Negotiator informs the ProvBroker of the receipt of the service's result.

The Mediator

In some cases, such as in healthcare environments, patients with fatal diseases may wish to request services and seek further health related information without the need to reveal their identities.

The requester should have appropriate means that permit requesting services without exposing its identity.

Clearly a direct communication link with the Mediator violates this requirement. Therefore, a requester must convey requests and get results exclusive of related identity information. This can be achieved by providing an access to common storage facilities that are publicly available to post requests and retrieve results. The storage facility can be a dedicated repository, or a database. The Mediator is responsible for granting requesters the right to access these facilities either for a limited number of times or only for a limited-time period (for example during the active involvement of the requester in the interaction protocol).

The requester should have a prior explicit consent to access these storage facilities either to post service's request or to retrieve a result (for example, protection guidelines for Sexual Transmission Disease, STD). Retrieving results implies the ability of requesters to link a particular request to its corresponding result. This can be accomplished by assigning a unique identification key for every posted request. Both the Mediator and the requester use this key during the interaction protocol to identify and link the service request to its relevant result.

It is to be noted that, in order to be authorized for online access to such repositories, the requester might be at the risk of exposing its IP (internet protocol) address and hence the privacy requirement will be violated. To overcome such an issue, requesters will be able to hide their IP through the use of a proxy server utilizing cryptographic techniques in which a dynamic IP address is issued from a pool of IP addresses and therefore making the identity anonymous.

The Mediator checks for available requests that have been posted and accordingly forwards the service request to the ProvBrokers. Figure 3 shows the proposed interaction pattern associated with this privacy degree2. The corresponding protocol will be as follows:

2. The Mediator checks for ("**Request**") message for any available service requests that

Figure 3. The interaction pattern for the mediator

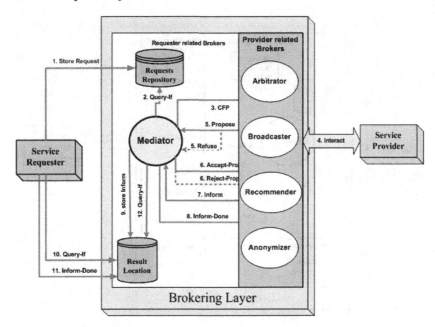

were stored by Requesters and need to be served.

3. **Send ("CFP")**: Sending a call for proposal message to ProvBrokers.

5. **Receive ("Propose")**: The Mediator receives service proposal(s).

5. **Receive ("Refuse")**: A ProvBroker declines to participate in fulfilling a service request.

6. **Send ("Accept-Proposal")**: A message is sent to the wining ProvBroker indicating the acceptance of the proposal.

6. **Send ("Reject-Proposal")**: A rejection message is sent to those ProvBrokers who do not win.

7. **Receive ("Inform")**: The Mediator receives the service's result.

8. **Send ("Inform-Done"):** the Mediator informs the ProvBroker of the receipt of the service's result.

9. The Mediator to store **("Inform")** indicating the availability of a service's result.

12. The Mediator checks for **("Inform-Done")** that has been stored by the Requester (indicating the receipt of the result).

The requester interaction with the relevant Mediator is solely restricted to the following:

1. The requester to store (**"Request"**) into a request repository.

10. The Requester checks for (**"Inform"**), indicating the availability of the result and hence retrieves it.

12. Upon retrieving the service result, the requester stores (**"Inform-Done"**) into the result repository.

The Advertiser

There might be certain situations where requesters prefer to hide their requests. For example, clinicians might benefit from variety of service offerings regarding new medications, tools, medical equipments and health related notifications. The clinicians will be able to check a service's repository for service offerings that have been previously posted and thus decide on choosing an offering that might be of interest.

In order for those clinicians to browse such a repository, an access control should be granted

Figure 4. The interaction pattern for the advertiser

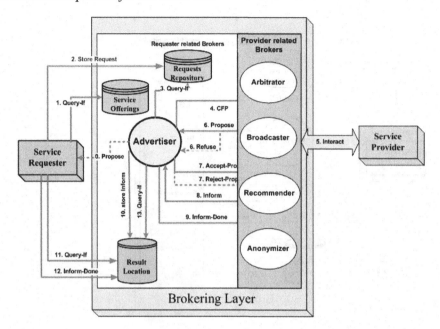

prior to any interaction. The access to this repository provides an appropriate indirect communication channel that allows service requesters to post requests and get results without having to reveal their request to the relevant ReqBroker supporting this privacy degree.

The Advertiser permits requesters to check a service's repository for further information or to search for other service offerings that have been previously posted and accordingly determines services that might be of interest.

Upon selecting a particular offering, the requester informs the Advertiser with the desired a service request as shown in Figure 4. Similarly, the interaction pattern is as follows:

1. The requester to check for (**"Propose"**) for service offerings.
2. The requester to store (**"Request"**) into a request repository.
3. The Advertiser to check for (**"Request"**) which indicates the availability of service requests.

4. **Send ("CFP")**: Sending a call for proposal message to ProvBrokers.
6. **Receive ("Propose")**: The Advertiser receives service proposal(s).
6. **Receive ("Refuse")**: A ProvBroker declines to participate in fulfilling a service request.
7. **Send ("Accept-Proposal")**: A message is sent to the wining ProvBroker indicating the acceptance of the proposal.
7. **Send ("Reject-Proposal")**: A rejection message is sent to those ProvBrokers who do not win.
8. **Receive ("Inform")**: The Advertiser receives the service's result.
9. **Send ("Inform-Done"):** The Advertiser informs the ProvBroker of the receipt of the service's result.
10. The Advertiser to store (**"Inform"**) indicating the availability of a service's result.
11. The requester checks for (**"Inform"**) for the availability of the result and hence retrieves it.

12. Upon retrieving the service result, the requester stores **("Inform-Done")** into the result repository.

13. The Advertiser checks for **("Inform-Done")** that has been stored by the requester (indicating the receipt of the result).

The Bulletinboard

In some cases, requesters desire to hide their identities and requests from the entire environment. For example, patients with narcotic-related problems (such as drug or alcohol addiction) can seek services that provide information about rehabilitation centers, specialized psychiatrists, or programs that will help overcoming a particular critical situation without revealing either their identities nor the desired information.

As shown in Figure 5, requesters will have the ability to either post their requests into physical storage facility (requests repository) or check the service offerings repository for services that might be of interest. In both cases, the requester stores the request in a special storage location (request repository). The Bulletinboard checks and identifies requests that need to be served and accordingly forwards them to the ProvBrokers.

Note that, for this degree of privacy, the requester is responsible to check for the availability of the service's result and hence retrieve it. This implies that the requester should be aware of linking the result to its own request. The protocol is detailed as follows:

3. The Bulletinboard checks for ("**Request**") which indicates the availability of service requests.

4. **Send ("CFP")**: Sending a call for proposal message to ProvBrokers.

6. **Receive ("Propose")**: A Bulletinboard receives service proposal(s).

6. **Receive ("Refuse")**: A ProvBroker declines to participate in fulfilling a service request.

Figure 5. Interaction pattern for the bulletinboard

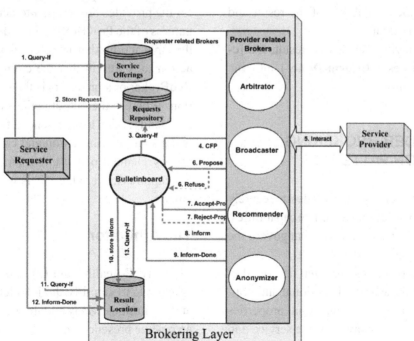

7. **Send ("Accept-Proposal"):** A message is sent to the wining provider indicating the acceptance of the proposal.

7. **Send ("Reject-Proposal"):** A rejection message is sent to those ProvBrokers who do not win.

8. **Receive ("Inform"):** The Bulletinboard receives the service's result.

9. **Send ("Inform-Done"):** the Bulletinboard informs the ProvBroker of the receipt of the service's result.

10. The Bulletinboard to store **("Inform")** indicating the availability of a service's result.

13. The Bulletinboard checks for **("Inform-Done")** that has been stored by the Requester (indicating the receipt of the result).

The requester interaction with the relevant Bulletinboard is restricted to the following:

1. Requester to check for (**"Propose"),** for service offerings that might be of interest.

2. The requester to store (**"Request"**) into a request repository.

11. The Requester checks for ("**Inform**") which indicates the availability of the result and hence retrieves it.

13. Upon retrieving the service result, the requester stores (**"Inform-Done"**) into the result repository.

THE PROVIDER-BROKERING INTERACTION PATTERNS

The interaction patterns allow providers to securely automate their privacy and advertise capabilities; define conditions and constraints that govern the provision of these capabilities.

Providers' capabilities are often described in terms of two main aspects, Functional and non-functional properties. The Functional properties capture the intended behavior of the service and define the input and output parameters.

The input parameters specify the required information that is needed prior to any service provision, while the output parameters specify the result of the service execution (for example, a service provider with information gathering capabilities generate outputs in electronic PDF file). The non-functional properties exhibit the constraints over the functionality of a service and specify additional information about the service capabilities, such as availability, service quality, cost, payment, security, trust and ownership.

However, describing the providers' capabilities is beyond the scope of the work presented here. It is assumed that there are appropriate services and tools (for example, capability description languages) by which providers are able to describe the inherent capabilities.

The following interaction patterns depict the different brokering scenarios categorized by the privacy concerns of service providers. In all the interaction patterns, it is assumed that the Prov-Brokers are able to interpret services' capabilities, match and locate providers who are capable of fulfilling a particular service request.

Note that in representing the different automat for the provider-brokering interaction action signatures of the ProvBrokers include the subsets of the input actions that are referred by the "receive" action to represent that the environment (being ReqBroker or a provider) is the source of the action. Whereas the output actions are referred by the "send" action to represent that the ProvBroker is the source of the action and can be consumed by any element of the environments. The sates are captures as variable labels with instantiation values.

The Arbitrator

In many E-health3 applications, the primary concern is to simplify the interaction with users and institutions. Many countries have established an on-line presence. In most cases, governments need to make decisions related to national security-threatening issues that might involve citizens, institutions and organizations. However, making such decisions might require the collaboration of other parties (for example, intelligence-related services) who need to be protected anonymously from perspectives associated to their identities and capabilities. The Arbitrator provides coordination activities to those providers who can contribute collaboratively to provide services while shielding their identities and capabilities.

To exploit the gain of this collaboration, providers do not have to worry about their privacy from being known by other counterparties. Direct communication with the Arbitrator requires the revealing of the privacy attributes. The protocol must shield and suppress any other entity form coming to know these attributes. In order to satisfy this requirement, it is assumed that the Arbitrator supporting this privacy degree is a trusted entity.

Moreover, the Arbitrator (on behalf of the provider), engages in subsequent interactions with various ReqBrokers without revealing the privacy attributes of the provider. In other words, the identity of the Arbitrator is the only revealed attribute to other entities (ReqBrokers) when sending and receiving messages. Figure 6 depicts the interaction pattern for such a privacy case.

For every received service request (i.e. CFP messages received from various ReqBrokers), the Arbitrator matches the most appropriate providers to fulfill a particular request and accordingly sends the received CFP message to the matched ones. Providers might contribute to fulfill received service requests by submitting proposals to the ProvBroker. On behalf of all potential providers, the Arbitrator sends the received proposals to the relevant pertinent ReqBroker which in turn determines and selects the appropriate service proposal. Once the ReqBroker notifies the Arbitrator about the outcomes of the selection process, the Arbitrator will be able to issue an acceptance message to the corresponding winning provider and a dismiss message for each unselected provider. The proposed interaction pattern that supports this privacy degree will be as follows:

Figure 6. The interaction pattern for the arbitrator

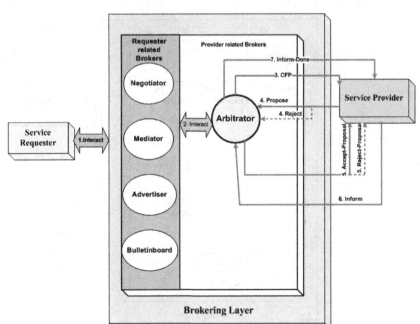

3. **Send** ("**CFP**"), the Arbitrator sends a call for proposals to all providers with known capabilities (this implies that the Arbitrator will be aware of providers who might satisfy a particular service request).

4. **Receive** ("**Propose**"), the Arbitrator receives service proposals from potential providers.

4. **Receive** ("**Reject**"), the Arbitrator receives a decline message from the provider.

5. **Send** ("**Accept-Proposal**"): Upon receiving an acceptance message from the ReqBroker, the Arbitrator in turn notifies the provider (winner) accordingly.

5. **Send** ("**Reject-Proposal**"), a rejection message is sent to non-winning provider.

6. **Receive** ("**Inform**"), the Arbitrator receives the service's result.

7. **Send** ("**Inform-Done**"), the Arbitrator notifies the relevant provider of the receipt of the result.

The interaction pattern assumes that the protocol is initiated upon receipt of CFP message from the ReqBrokers within the brokering layer.

The Broadcaster

Providers avail themselves of more precise and reliable data collected from many sources, to assess their own local performance in comparison to global trends, and to avoid many of the inefficiencies that currently arise because of having less information available for their decision-making.

The protocol permits various to hide their identities and reveal their service offerings to the relevant ProvBroker. The Broadcaster grants providers an access to various repositories (such as request repository, service repository and a result repository) either for a limited number of times or only for a limited-time period (for example during the active involvement of the provider in the corresponding interaction protocol). Service requests are posted to a dedicated repository which can be accessed by providers as shown in Figure 7.

A provider may respond to call-for-proposal request by an offer posted onto a repository. Upon

Figure 7. The interaction pattern for the broadcaster

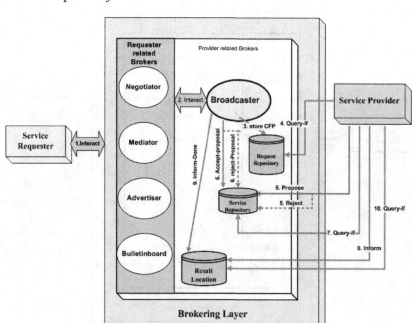

delegating a service request to a provider, the provider post service results to be retrieved by the Broadcaster and delivered to the proper destination. The sequence of events is shown below:

3. The Broadcaster to store ("**CFP**") in request repository.
4. Provider to check for posted services' requests, ("**CFP**").
5. Provider to store ("**Propose**"), indicating a proposed service for a particular request.
5. Provider to store ("**Refuse**"), indicating the refusal for serving a particular request.
6. The Broadcaster to store (**"Accept-Proposal"**): Indicating an acceptance message;
6. The Broadcaster to store (**"Reject-Proposal"**): Indicating a rejection message for a proposed service.
7. Provider to check for services proposal acceptance ("**Propose**").
8. Provider to store (**Inform**) indicating the availability of a service's result.

9. The Broadcaster to store (**Inform-Done**) upon retrieving the service's result.
10. Provider to check for the receipt of the service's result ("**Inform-Done**").

The Recommender

Another setting where hiding provider's capability is a useful situation. Consider a new medical product that has been introduced to the market such that no single (even very large) retailer can accurately predict consumer demand for it. This happens when different retailers target different groups of customers, for which shopping patterns and adaptability to new products vary. Then it is beneficial to all such stores to engage into joint forecasting, while still preserving the privacy of the encapsulated capability.

After receiving a service request, the Recommender sends it to every provider with unknown capabilities. Figure 8 shows the associated interaction pattern.

Once a provider selects a particular service request, it sends a service proposal to the Recom-

Figure 8. Interaction pattern for the recommender

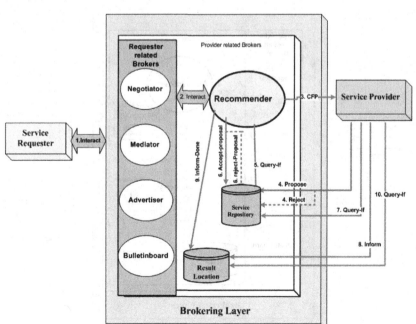

mender who controls the remaining transaction according to the appropriate negotiation mechanisms that are similar to what has been described in former patterns.

3.   **Send** ("**CFP**"), the Recommender sends a call for proposal message to providers.
4.   Provider to store ("**Propose**"), indicating a proposed service for a particular request.
4.   Provider to store ("**Refuse**"), indicating the refusal for serving a particular request.
5.   The Recommender to check for services proposals ("**Propose**").
6.   The Recommender to store (**"Accept-Proposal"**): Indicating an acceptance message;
6.   The Recommender to store (**"Reject-Proposal"**): Indicating a rejection message for a proposed service.
7.   Provider to check for proposal acceptance ("**Accept-Proposal**").
8.   Provider to store **(Inform)** indicating the availability of a service's result.

9.   The Recommender to store **(Inform-Done)** upon retrieving the service's result.
10.   Provider to check for the receipt of the service's result **("Inform-Done").**

The Anonymizer

In many situations, providers would prefer to have secure and safe means that enable them to engage in sharing their capabilities while protecting their privacy attributes. Each provider with this privacy degree will be able to view information relevant to desired requests. A provider contributes to the fulfillment of these requests by proposing services to the designated Anonymizer whose functionality includes the ability to view and send any stored proposals to ReqBrokers. Moreover, it is assumed that the Anonymizer has the ability to match and determine capable providers with the most insight towards fulfilling the service request. Different storage repositories are available to the provider to access as shown Figure 9.

The interaction pattern will be as follows:

Figure 9. The interaction pattern for the anonymizer

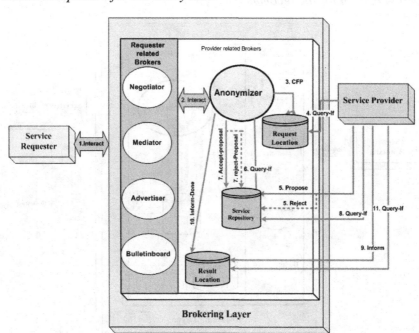

3. The Anonymizer to store ("CFP") message.

4. The provider to check for services requests, ("CFP").

5. Provider to store ("**Propose**") message indicating a proposed service for a particular request.

5. Provider to store ("**Refuse**"), indicating the refusal for serving a particular request.

6. The Anonymizer to for services proposals, ("**Propose**").

7. The Anonymizer to store ("**Accept-Proposal**"): Indicating an acceptance message;

7. The Anonymizer to store ("**Reject-Proposal**"): Indicating a rejection message for a proposed service.

8. Provider to check for ("**Accept-Proposal**") which indicates an acceptance of service's proposal.

9. Provider to store (**Inform**) indicating the availability of a service's result.

10. The Anonymizer to store (**Inform-Done**) upon retrieving the service's result.

11. Provider to check for the receipt of the service's result, (**Inform-Done**).

THE PRIVACY-BASED BROKERING PROTOCOLS

Since brokering protocols can be described as repeatable patterns of a specific interaction, they can be treated as reusable elements. These patterns can be combined and expressed at different levels of abstraction in which the behavior and the functionalities of the entities should be characterized by a succinct and precise description through an interface (Thus, capturing the essence of the behavior of the entity). Therefore, the repeated patterns of the brokering entities can be packaged into various sets of high level protocols. These patterns are arranged into the following protocols:

1. **Service Soliciting Protocol**: this protocol allows domain agents playing the role of requesters to solicit help from the brokering layer. The protocol consists of two sub-protocols that support the following modes:

a. **Direct Soliciting Mode**: in which the brokering agent receives service requests directly from the requester agent. This mode allows the requester to directly solicit help by sending its service request through the message performative REQUEST. The pattern is as follows:

- **Receive** ("**Request**"): The ReqBroker receives a request for service from the requester.

- **Send** ("**Inform**"): The ReqBroker delivers back the service's result

- **Receive** ("**Inform-Done**"): A confirmation message is received from the requester.

b. **Indirect Soliciting Mode:** This mode supports the interaction with requesters hiding one of their privacy attributes. The ReqBroker will be able to retrieve a stored service request, store service's result and query about the receipt of a service's result. The protocol has the following message pattern:

- The ReqBroker checks for ("**Request**") message for any available service requests that were stored by requesters and need to be served.

- The ReqBroker to store ("**Inform**") indicating the availability of a service's result.

- The ReqBroker checks for ("**Inform-Done**") that has been stored by the Requester (indicating the receipt of the result).

2. **Contracting Protocol**: this protocol abstracts all messages exchanged between the brokering agents (ReqBrokers and ProvBrokers) and contains all the behavior relevant to call for proposals, bidding, evaluating proposals and awarding/rejecting service proposal as follows:

   ○ **Send ("CFP")**: Sending a call for proposal message to ProvBrokers.

   ○ **Receive ("Propose")**: A ReqBroker receives service proposal(s).

   ○ **Receive ("Refuse")**: A ProvBroker declines to participate in fulfilling a service request.

   ○ **Send ("Accept-Proposal")**: A message is sent to the wining ProvBroker indicating the acceptance of the proposal.

   ○ **Send ("Reject-Proposal")**: A rejection message is sent to those ProvBrokers who do not win.

   ○ **Receive ("Inform")**: The ReqBroker receives the service's result.

   ○ **Send ("Inform-Done")**: the ReqBroker informs the ProvBroker of the receipt of the service's result.

3. **Service Delivery Protocol**: this protocol abstracts all the messages and the behaviors relevant to provide specific services. The package includes two main sub-protocols, namely:

   a. **Direct Delivery Mode**: This mode allows a provider revealing its privacy attributes to respond directly to a CFP message by proposing a specific service offering to the corresponding ProvBroker. The protocol supports the following pattern:

      ▪ **Send ("CFP")**: Sending a call for proposal message to the provider.

      ▪ **Receive ("Propose")**: A ProvBroker receives service proposal.

   ▪ **Receive ("Refuse")**: A provider declines to participate in fulfilling a service request.

   ▪ **Send ("Accept-Proposal")**: A message is sent to the provider indicating the acceptance of the proposal.

   ▪ **Send ("Reject-Proposal")**: A rejection message is sent to those providers who do not win.

   ▪ **Receive ("Inform")**: The ProvBroker receives the service's result.

   ▪ **Send ("Inform-Done")**: the ProvBroker informs the provider of the receipt of the service's result.

   b. **Indirect Delivery Mode**: in which the service is stored into a repository and to be retrieved by the corresponding entity. This mode entitles the ProvBroker to store responses and to query about replies associated with a specific CFP message. The protocol includes the following:

      ▪ The ProvBroker to store ("CFP") into the request repository.

      ▪ The ProvBroker to store ("Accept-Proposal"): Indicating an acceptance message;

      ▪ The ProvBroker to store ("Reject-Proposal"): Indicating a rejection message for a proposed service.

      ▪ The ProvBroker to check for service's result ("Inform").

      ▪ The ProvBroker to store (Inform-Done) upon retrieving the service's result.

DESIGN AND IMPLEMENTATION

Developing the brokering services comprise the automation of privacy to enhance the overall security of the system and accordingly entities should be able define the desired degree of privacy. In fact the brokering service permits entities to participate in the environment with different roles and hence be capable of automating their privacy concerns and select a particular privacy. The challenge here is how to architect a service that could provide means and mechanisms by which entities would be able to interact with each other and determine any privacy degree that suits a particular satiation. Such interaction is characterized by the non-determinism aspect in addition to the dynamic nature of the environment where these entities exist and operate for which they require to be able to change configurations to participate in different roles. These requirements could not be accomplished using traditional ways of manually configuring software.

We strongly believe that agent-orientation is an appropriate design paradigm for providing coordination services and mechanisms in such settings. Indeed, such a paradigm is essential to modeling open, distributed, and heterogeneous environments in which an agent should be able to operate as a part of a community of cooperative distributed systems environments, including human users. A key aspect of agent-orientation is the ability to design artifacts that are able to perceive, reason, interact and act in a coordinated fashion. Here we view agent-orientation as a metaphorical conceptualization tool at a high level of abstraction (knowledge level) that captures, supports and implements features that are useful for distributed computation in open environments.

These features include cooperation, coordination, interaction, as well as intelligence, adaptability, economic and logical rationality. We define an agent as an individual collection of primitive components that provide a focused and cohesive set of capabilities. We focus on the notion of ag-

enthood as a metaphorical conceptualization tool at a high level of abstraction (knowledge level) that captures supports and implements features that are useful for distributed computation in open environments.

The representative agents of domain and brokering entities within the context of ubiquitous healthcare systems are built on the foundation of CIR-agent architecture (Ghenniwa & Kamel, 2000). The CIR-Agent is an individual collection of primitive components that provide a focused and cohesive set of capabilities. The basic components include problem-solving, interaction, and communication components, as shown in Figure 27(b). A particular arrangement (or interconnection) of components is required to constitute an agent. This arrangement reflects the pattern of the agent's mental state as related to its reasoning about achieving a goal. However, no specific assumptions need to be made on the detailed design of the agent components. Therefore, the internal structure of the components can be designed and implemented using object oriented or another technology, provided that the developer conceptualizes the specified architecture of the agent as described in Figure 10.

Basically, each agent consists of knowledge and capability components. Each of which is tailored according to the agent's specific role. The agent's knowledge contains the information about the environment and the expected world. The knowledge includes the agent self-model, other agents' model, goals that need to be satisfied, possible solutions generated to satisfy each goal, and the local history of the world that consists of all possible local views for an agent at any given time. The agent's knowledge also includes the agent's desires, commitments and intentions toward achieving each goal.

The capability package includes the reasoning component, the domain actions component which contains the possible set of domain actions that when executed, the state of the world will be changed and the communication component

Figure 10. The CIR agent's architecture

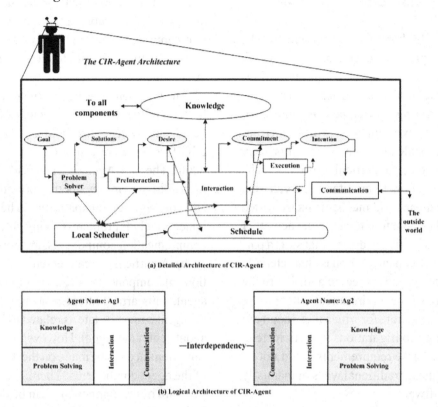

(a) Detailed Architecture of CIR-Agent

(b) Logical Architecture of CIR-Agent

where the agent sends and receives messages to and from other agents and the outside world.

The problem solver component represents the particular role of the agent and provides the agent with the capability of reasoning about its knowledge to generate appropriate solutions directed to satisfy its goal.

During the interaction processes, the agents engage with each other while resolving problems that are related to different types of interdependencies. The coordination mechanisms are meant to reduce and resolve the problems associated with interdependencies. Interdependencies are goal-relevant interrelationships between actions performed by various agents.

The agent's interaction module identifies the type of interdependencies that may exist in a particular domain. Consequently, agents select an appropriate interaction device4 that is suitable

to resolve a particular interdependency. These devices are categorized as follows:

- Contract-based, includes the *assignment* device;
- Negotiation-based, includes *resource scheduling*, *conflict resolution*, *synchronization*, and *redundancy avoidance* devices.

Within the context of brokering, the interdependency problem is classified as *capability interdependency* and the interaction device is the *"assignment"*. The basic characteristics of the assignment device are problem specifications, evaluation parameters, and the sub-processes. The problem specifications might include, for example, the request, the desired-satisfying time, and the expiration time.

A collection of basic components comprises the structure of the agent model and represents its capabilities. The agents' architectures are based on the CIR-Agent model as shown in Figure 11. A brokering session mainly recognizes two types of agents, namely, domain agent (Requester or Provider) and brokering agent (ReqBroker or ProvBroker). The architecture of each agent type is described in details below.

The Domain Agent: Service Providers and Requesters

Service providers and requesters are modeled as domain agents as shown in Figure 29. The requester agent can participate with various privacy degrees and request services from the brokering layer. A requester delegates the service's request(s) to the relevant brokering agent according to the interaction protocol the selected privacy degree. The domain agent possesses knowledge and

capability. The knowledge includes the model of the brokering agents in terms of the supported privacy degree, self model and the local history. The capability is categorized into three components: reasoning that includes problem-solving and coordination, communication and a set of domain actions.

A domain agent playing the role of a service provider can select the appropriate privacy degree and thus participate on providing the capability that meets the needs of another domain entity. The problem solver the domain agent hiding any of the privacy attributes encompasses the accessing of different storage repositories. For example, the problem solver of a requester includes functionalities related to formulating service requests, check for available service offerings and access various storage repositories to store requests or to retrieve service results. On the other hand, the problem solver of a provider hiding its identity and capability attributes consists of modules related

Figure 11. The overall system model

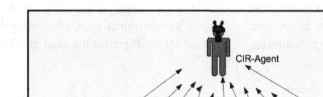

to accessing storage repositories to check for stored service requests that might be fulfilled and hence participating in storing service proposals and service's results.

The coordination component of a requester comprises the interaction device which entails soliciting service from the relevant ReqBroker agent. The interaction device of the provider agent manages the coordination activities which involve proposing services to specific CFP messages and engage in bidding processes.

THE BROKERING AGENTS: REQBROKERS AND PROVBROKERS

A brokering agent is composed of two components namely, the knowledge and capability. The knowledge component contains the information in the agent's memory about the environment and the expected world. As shown in Figure 13, this includes the agent self-model, models of the domain agents in terms of their roles (requester/provider) and/or capabilities and the local history of the world. The knowledge includes all possible local views for an agent at any given time (such as the knowledge of physical repositories

available services requests, services offerings and service results).

The ReqBroker Agent

The ReqBroker's problem solver component includes: accessing various storage repositories, locate and identify services' requests, deliver and store services' results. The interaction component comprises the following activities: (1) Preparing the "CFP" message that formulates the "announcement" to be sent out to the ProvBrokers, (2) Collecting service proposals and (3) evaluating these proposals against certain criteria (for example parameters identified in the service's request).

The ReqBroker Interaction Device: Assignment

The main function of the assignment device is to resolve problems associated with capability and decomposition interdependencies. The basic characteristics of the assignment device are problem specifications and evaluation parameters. With reducing complexity in achieving a goal as the agent's main objective, a solution can be selected based for example on the goal quality.

Figure 12. The domain agent architecture

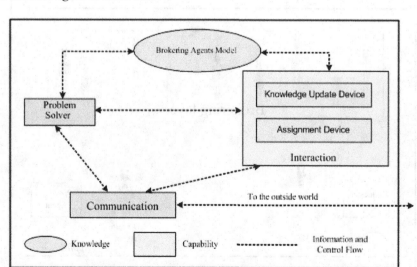

Figure 13. The brokering agent architecture

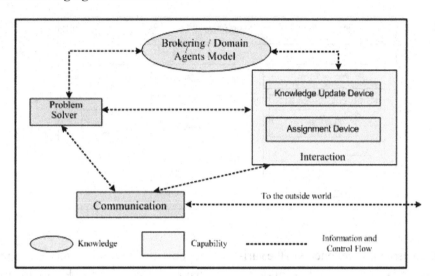

The implementation technique of the assignment device is based on the soliciting approach as in the case of the contract-net approach which depends on (1) the modeling approach for other agent's capabilities, and (2) the solicitation approach for the local schedule and workload of other agents. To achieve a high degree of parallelism in the assignment device, the implementation consists of the following processes:

1. **Call for Proposals:** The initiating ReqBroker agent (or the manager) informs all the other potential ProvBrokers agents (or contractors) of the problem specification by an announcement. The problem specification might include the goal, and the desired satisfying time for example. The ProvBrokers initialize generates a CFP message to the relevant service providers. A focusing strategy might be used by the ProvBrokers to identify the set of potential contractors (service providers) based on their capabilities (in scenarios related to providers revealing their capabilities). At a certain time, ProvBrokers representing their interested relevant providers send "Propose" message to the ReqBroker agent indicating the start of the bidding process.

2. **Evaluate:** At a certain time, ProvBrokers representing their interested relevant providers send "Propose" messages to the ReqBroker agent indicating the start of the bidding process. When the service satisfying deadline reaches, the ReqBroker ceases to accept any new messages related to either request's inquiries or new service offers. Based on the evaluation parameters, the ReqBroker evaluates submitted proposals and accordingly selects the best bid.

3. **Award/Reject:** the process allows the ReqBroker to issue an award/reject message to the potential ProvBrokers. For the selected (winning) ProvBrokers, a contract form is created, an award (Accept-Proposal) message is sent to the corresponding ProvBrokers and a reject (Reject-Proposal) messages is sent to the non-wining.

The reasoning components of the ReqBrokers vary according to the privacy degree they support. Utilizing the privacy-based protocols defined in

Figure 14. Architecture of the negotiator's reasoning component

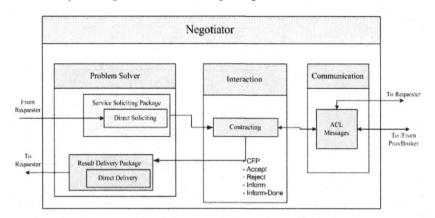

Section 3.5.1 the reasoning components of the various ReqBrokers will be represented as follows:

The Negotiator Design

As shown in Figure 14, the interaction component includes the following protocols: (1) the contracting protocol that exhibits all the interaction with the ProvBrokers and (2) the direct mode of the service soliciting protocol which abstracts all the interaction activities with the service provider.

The Mediator Design

Requestors are permitted to have an access to special repositories by which they would be able to post their required service requests without having to reveal their identity to any other entity in the environment. The Mediator's problem solver functionality is solely to access these repositories to: query about available service requests, store service's result into the result location repository and to check for result's receipt acknowledgments. The interaction component utilizes the contracting protocol as shown in Figure 15.

The Advertiser Design

As shown in Figure 16, the problem solver component includes the service soliciting protocol (indirect mode) while the interaction component includes the contracting protocol.

Figure 15. Architecture of the mediator's reasoning component

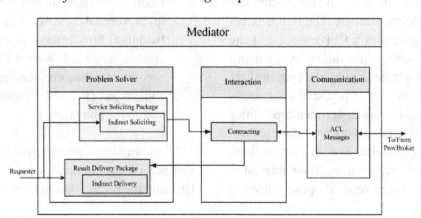

The Bulletinboard Design

The Bulletinboard's problem solver functionalities are limited to accessing the various repositories (either to check for service requests, store service results or to check for receipts acknowledgment). These functionalities are performed by utilizing the indirect mode of the service soliciting protocol as shown in Figure 17.

The ProvBroker Agent

The ReqBroker agent sends (or store) a "CFP" message to service providers. The ProvBroker carries out the interaction with the ReqBrokers and accordingly reports the outcome of the inter-

action to the participating service provider. The ProvBroker's architecture varies according to the supported privacy degrees.

The ProvBroker Interaction Device: Assignment

Similarly, the implementation technique of the assignment device of the ProvBroker is based on the soliciting approach as in the case of the contract-net approach. The implementation consists of the following processes:

1. **Call for Proposals:** The ProvBrokers initialize a CFP message to the relevant service providers. A focusing strategy might be used

Figure 16. Architecture of the advertiser's reasoning component

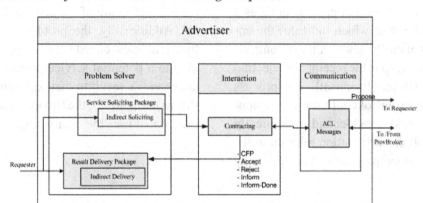

Figure 17. Architecture of the bulletinboard's reasoning component

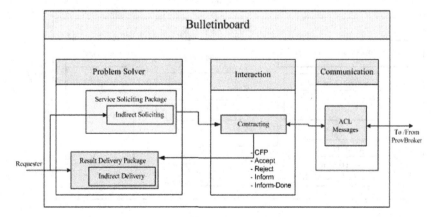

by the ProvBrokers to identify the set of potential contractors (service providers) based on their capabilities (in scenarios related to providers revealing their capabilities).

2. **Propose:** At a certain time, ProvBrokers representing their interested relevant providers send "Propose" messages to the ReqBroker agent indicating the start of the bidding process. A focusing strategy might be used by the ProvBrokers to identify the set of potential contractors (service providers) based on their capabilities (in scenarios related to providers revealing their capabilities).

3. **Winning/Rejection:** By receiving the award message, the ProvBroker creates the winning process and accordingly informs the winning provider (either by sending an acceptance message to the providers or by storing the Accept-Proposal message into a repository). Note that process initiates a commitment state which indicates the engagement of the ProvBroker into a contract. Alternatively, upon the receipt of a rejection message (Reject-Proposal), the process allows the ProvBrokers to notify the non-winning service provider and consequently destroys all the information relevant to the rejected service proposals. The reasoning

components for the ProvBrokers as described in the following sections.

The Arbitrator Design

All interactions with ReqBrokers entail the exposure of only the identity of the engaged Arbitrator. As shown in Figure 18, the interaction component of the Arbitrator includes the contracting protocol and the service delivery protocol (direct mode).

The Broadcaster Design

Providers are allowed to access repositories to check for requests that might be of an interest without having to reveal their identity to any other entity in the environment. All the interaction with provider with this privacy degree is accomplished by the problem solver component which includes the indirect mode of the service delivery protocol. Additionally, the problem solver includes functionalities related to link a specific CFP message to a potential service proposal and to map the service's result to that particular request. As shown in Figure 19, the Broadcaster's interaction component uses the contracting protocol.

Figure 18. Architecture of the arbitrator's reasoning component

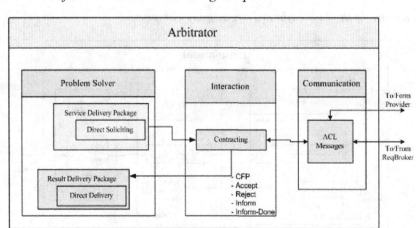

The Recommender Design

The Recommender's interaction enables sending every received CFP service request (from ReqBrokers) to the provider with unknown capabilities. As shown in Figure 20, the interaction component includes the contracting protocol while the problem solver comprises the indirect mode of the service delivery protocol

The Anonymizer Design

All service requests and service offerings and services results are stored into special storage repositories (service request and result locations that are accessed consecutively by both the Anonymizer and the provider). In order to achieve such functionalities, the problem solver component utilizes the indirect mode of the service delivery protocol as shown in Figure 20.

PROTOTYPE IMPLEMENTATION

A prototype of the proposed system has been implemented to support and provide information-gathering capabilities to different participants in healthcare environments where the accessibility

Figure 19. Architecture of the broadcaster's reasoning component

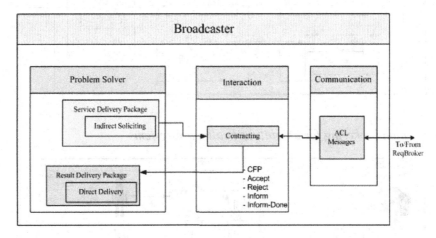

Figure 20. Architecture of the recommender's reasoning component

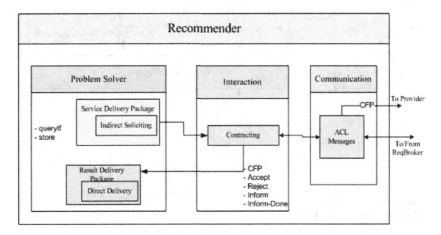

of private information is a desirable feature to various categories of the healthcare personnel, patients, and clinicians.

As shown in Figure 22, three databases represent various medical data for three distributed locations, each being managed by a dedicated agent that can play both roles of an information requester as well as a provider. A web interface is available for healthcare participants to select their desired privacy degree along with any capability they might posses (medical data, patient's diagnosis and treatment reports, Pharmaceutical data reports, etc.). Based on the privacy degree required by both the requester an information provider,

Figure 21. Architecture of the anonymizer reasoning component

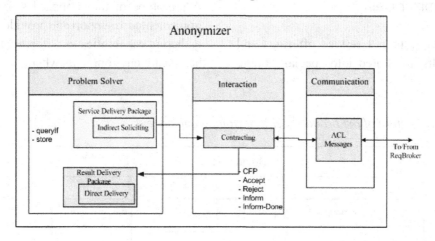

Figure 22. Information brokering for ubiquitous healthcare systems

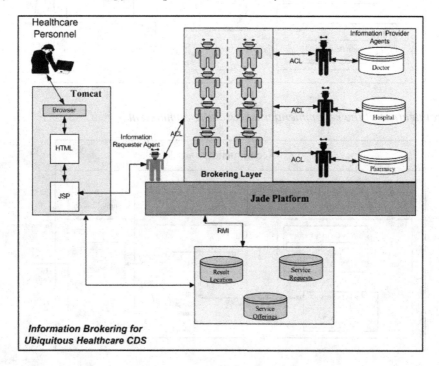

dedicated brokering agents handle the interaction according to the relevant interaction protocols associated to the selected privacy degrees.

The implementation utilizes Java Web Services Development Pack (JWSDP, 2008) and the JADE platform (Jade, 2009), which is a software framework to develop agent applications in compliance with the FIPA specifications for multi-agent systems (FIPA, 2008).

FUTURE RESEARCH DIRECTIONS

A crucial element in addressing privacy concerns is the level of trust between domain entities and the brokering layer. In security, trust relates much to the degree of confidence that an entity has in the ability of other entity to conform to any selected privacy requirements. Entities should be able to generate a quantified trust measure about the brokering layer. Therefore, mapping privacy to trust would provide a mechanism for different participants to determine the relevant privacy degrees. In other words, requesters and service providers would be able to generate trust relationships with the brokering layer prior to any interaction.

To deal with the heterogeneity characteristic of ubiquitous healthcare environments,, the brokering shall have the ability to process requests and description of capabilities by utilizing a formal, adequate and expressiveness representation. Locating relevant services presumes that its capabilities can be named at any instant; this implies the utilization of registration and naming services. However, one direction is to consider the scalability of the proposed brokering model in which brokering entities are to be able to cross register services' capabilities from one society to another

The choice of matching mechanism depends on the structure and semantics of the descriptions to be matched as well as the desired privacy level. One of the important directions for future work

is to expand the proposed model to include the capability of semantic brokering, by introducing new functionality in the layer to resolve common types of structural and semantic heterogeneity.

CONCLUSION

The aim of this chapter is to define a generic brokering architecture that enables cooperation under a desired level of privacy protection in ubiquitous healthcare. The work presents in depth analysis of the capability-based brokering with the ability to support different degrees of privacy and accordingly proposes various interaction protocols and the suitable mechanisms of the coordinated control. Furthermore, we provide a detailed design and implementation guidelines for a privacy-based brokering model in ubiquitous healthcare systems.

Unlike traditional approaches, the brokering is viewed as a capability-based coordination solution in cooperative distributed systems. Architecturally, the proposed model is viewed as a layer of services where different roles can be played by the various entities (requestors, brokers and providers). The brokering role into several sub-roles based on the attributes designated to describe the desired privacy degree of both the service provider and the service requestor. Each role is modeled as an agent with a specific architecture and an interaction protocol that is appropriate to support a required privacy degree.

Within the layer two sets of brokering entities are available to service requesters and providers. The first set handles interactions with requestors according to the desired privacy degree that is appropriate to their preferences, while the other set supports privacy degrees required by service providers. A brokering pattern is realized by the different roles played by the domain entities and their corresponding brokering agent. A complete brokering scenario is accomplished by performing different levels of interaction namely: (1)

Requester-to-Broker Interaction, (2) Broker-to-Broker Interaction and (3) Broker-to-Provider Interaction. Different combinations within the layer can take place to support the Inter-Brokering interactions. The proposed layered-architecture provides an appropriate separation of responsibilities, allowing developers and programmers to focus on modeling solutions and solving their particular application's problems in a manner and semantics most suitable to the local perspective.

Another important innovative aspect of the model is that it treats the privacy as a design issue that has to be taken into consideration in developing brokering services for cooperative distributed systems.

By utilizing the Agent-Oriented paradigm, the privacy-based brokering is modelled at a high level of abstraction, in which the distributed environment is viewed collectively as a coherent universe of interacting and collaborative agents and consequently provides high degree of decentralization of capabilities, which is the key to system scalability and extensibility.

Within the context of brokering, we model privacy in terms of the ability of ubiquitous healthcare entities to reveal or hide its information related to the identities, requests and and/or capabilities. Each privacy degree is supported by a dedicated brokering entity (agent) with a specific architecture and interaction protocol. Requesters and providers are able to conceal their privacy concerns from the whole environment including the brokering layer itself.

The brokering layer incorporates a means of *virtual pseudonymity* (protecting identities) and *anonymity* techniques (hiding the goals and capabilities) since the brokering agents within the layer act as proxies to both service requestors and providers. Clearly, in every protocol, the interactions within the layer are constrained to sending service requests and receiving service offerings and results without having to reveal who is actually requesting or providing the service.

REFERENCES

Beckwith, R. (2003). Designing for Ubiquity: The Perception of Privacy. *IEEE Pervasive Computing / IEEE Computer Society [and] IEEE Communications Society, 2*(2), 40–46. doi:10.1109/MPRV.2003.1203752

Brox, G. A. (2005). MPEG-21 as an access control tool for the National Health Service Care Records Service. *Journal of Telemedicine and Telecare, 11*, 23–25. doi:10.1258/1357633054461868

Camarinha-Matos, L., & Afsarmanesh, H. (2001). Virtual Communities and Elderly Support. In *Advances in Automation, Multimedia and Video Systems, and Modern Computer Science* (pp. 279–284). WSES.

Chung, E., et al. (2004). Development and Evaluation of Emerging Design Patterns for Ubiquitous Computing. *Patterns C1-C15, DIS2004*. Clarke, R. (n.d.). *Identification, Anonymity and Pseudonymity in Consumer Transactions: A Vital System Design and Public Policy Issue*. Retrieved from http://www.anu.edu.au/people/Roger.Clarke/DV/AnonPsPol.html

FIPA. (n.d.). *Foundation of Intelligent Physical Agent*. Retrieved from http://ww.fipa.org/

Ghenniwa, H., & Huhns, M. (2004). Intelligent Enterprise Integration: eMarketplace Model. In Gupta, J., & Sharma, S. (Eds.), *Creating Knowledge Based Organizations* (pp. 46–79). Hershey, PA: Idea Group Publishing.

Ghenniwa H., & Kamel M. (2000). Interaction Devices for Coordinating Cooperative Distributed Systems. *Journal of Intelligent Automation and Soft Computing*.

Gialelis, J., Foundas, P., Kalogeras, A., Georgoudakis, M., Kinalis, A., & Koubias, S. (2008). Wireless Wearable Body Area Network Supporting Person Centric Health Monitoring. In *Proceedings of the 7th IEEE International Workshop on Factory Communication Systems (WFCS 2008), May 20-23, 2008.*

Health Insurance Portability and Accountability Act (HIPAA). Retrieved from http://www.intellimark-it.com/privacysecurity/hipaa.asp

Initiative for Privacy Standardization in Europe (IPSE). Retrieved from http://www.hi-europe.info/files/2002/9963.htm

JADE. (n.d.). Java Agent Development Framework: Jade. Retrieved from http://www.jade.cselt.it/

Jurgen, B., Felix, G., & Harald, V. (2004). Dependability Issues of Pervasive Computing in a Healthcare Environment". In *Security in Pervasive Computing 2003* (LNCS 2802). Retrieved from http://www.vs.inf.ethz.ch/res/papers/bohn_pervasivehospital_spc_2003_final.pdf

Korhonen, I., Parkk, J., & Van Gils, M. (2003). Health Monitoring in the Home of the Future. *IEEE Engineering in Medicine and Biology Magazine, 22*(3), 66–73. doi:10.1109/MEMB.2003.1213628

Langheinrich, M. (2001). Privacy by Design: Principles of Privacy-Aware Ubiquitous Systems. In *Ubicomp 2001*. Retrieved from http://www.vs.inf.ethz.ch/publ/papers/privacy-principles.pdf.

Langheinrich, M. (2002). A Privacy Awareness System for Ubiquitous Computing Environments. *Ubicomp (. LNCS, 2498,* 237–245.

Romanosky, S., et al. (2005). *Privacy Patterns for Online Interactions*. Paper presented at Plop 2005, Monticello, Illinois, Sept. 7-10, 2005.

Schumacher, M. (2002). *Security Patterns and Security Standards - With Selected Security Patterns for Anonymity and Privacy*. Paper presented at European Conference on Pattern Languages of Programs, (EuroPLoP), 2002

Silver, B. G., Andonyadis, C., & Morales, A. (1998). Web-based healthcare agents; the case of reminders and to-dos. *Artificial Intelligence in Medicine, 14*(3), 295–316. doi:10.1016/S0933-3657(98)00039-6

The Association of American Physicians and Surgeons. (n.d.). Doctors Lie to Protect Patient Privacy–Poll Survey. Retrieved from http://www.aapsonline.org/press/nrnewpoll.html

Venkatasubramanian, K., & Gupta, S. (2007). Security Solutions for Pervasive Healthcare. In Security in Distributed, Grid, Mobile, and Pervasive Computing (pp.349-366).

Yee, G., Korba, L., & Song, R. (2006). Ensuring Privacy for E-Health Service. In *Proceedings of the First International Conference on Availability, Reliability and Security (ARES 2006)*. Vienna, Austria. April, 2006

ENDNOTES

[1] A result is the required format depicted in the service's request, (for example, the patient's diagnosis information in PDF as per the patient's service request specification).

[2] Note that in all the interaction diagrams, the Query-If action permits the brokering entity to access the storage repositories and to check stored messages for message types.

[3] E-health refers to the electronic delivery of healthcare services to users

[4] Interaction device is an agent's component by which it interacts with the other elements

of the environment through a communication device. A device is a piece or a component with software characteristics that is designed to service a special purpose or perform a special function.

Chapter 16
Managing E-Health in the Age of Web 2.0:
The Impact on E-Health Evaluation

Benjamin Hughes
ESADE, Spain

ABSTRACT

The use of Web 2.0 internet tools for healthcare is noted for its great potential to address a wide range of healthcare issues or improve overall delivery. However, there have been various criticisms of Web 2.0, including in its application to healthcare where it has been described as more marketing and hype than a real departure from previous medical internet or eHealth trends. Authors have noted that there is scant evidence demonstrating it as a cost efficient mechanism to improve outcomes for patients. Moreover, the investments in Web 2.0 for health, or the wider concept of eHealth, are becoming increasingly significant. Hence given the uncertainty surrounding its value, this chapter aims to critically examine the issues associated with emerging use of Web 2.0 for health. The authors look at how it not only distinguishes itself from previous eHealth trends but also how it enhances them, examining the impact on eHealth investment and management from a policy perspective, and how research can aid this management.

INTRODUCTION

Many authors are excited by the potential impact of Health or Medicine 2.0® (e.g., Guistini, 2006: Sandars & Schroter, 2007; Boulos & Wheeler, 2007; McLean, Richards & Wardman, 2007). The terms denote the use of Web 2.0 tools in healthcare and medicine, and is part of a wider eHealth trend that is becoming increasingly important in health

decisions. As more people go online, they rely on the Internet for important health information. Reports estimate that 80% of Internet American users have searched online for health information at some point in their lives (Fox, 2006; Ferguson, 2007), and a large percentage of "health seekers" indicate the web has a direct effect on the decisions they make and on their interactions with doctors (Madden & Fox, 2005). However there have been major criticisms of Medicine or Health 2.0, and policy makers need to understand how its distinct

DOI: 10.4018/978-1-61520-777-0.ch016

Copyright © 2010, IGI Global. Copying or distributing in print or electronic forms without written permission of IGI Global is prohibited.

features allow improvement in patient outcomes. They are also very new concepts that are hard to define and delineate, both from eHealth in general and between the two terms themselves (Hughes, Joshi, Wareham 2008). For this reason this chapter principally uses the term Medicine 2.0 to denote both terms (Health 2.0 and Medicine 2.0), and examines it through its critical issues. Scholars note that an issues focus can potentially address the gap between research and actual practice in eHealth (Potts, 2006), and that it allows an effective common agenda between researchers, practitioners or policy makers (Amabile et al., 2001).

Although distinct in their reach and pace of change, many of the key issues associated with Web 2.0 in Medicine 2.0® are similar to that of eHealth (Hughes, Joshi, Wareham, 2008). Four such major tensions are identified with the emergence of Web 2.0 tools in healthcare (Hughes, Joshi, Wareham, 2008): 1) Doctors' concerns with patients' use of Web 2.0 in Medicine, even if the information is accurate; 2) Information inaccuracy and potential risks associated with inaccurate Web 2.0 generated information; 3) The consequences of the new methods of creating eHealth, such as privacy and ownership issues with Web 2.0–generated information, or the alternative paths to achieve them and; 4) the delineation of what makes Medicine 2.0, that is not a policy instrument separate to that of eHealth, where Web 2.0's participatory nature may imply that previous outcome measures may become misleading. While this chapter examines all four of these issues, mechanisms for dealing with the first two have already begun to emerge within the wider eHealth domain.

However, elements of the final two issues still pose a concern, not in clarifying the vagueness of the definition of Medicine 2.0, but in understanding: 1) the alternative investment pathways for Web 2.0 within eHealth, and 2) if and how it actually improves patient outcomes. In the first case, Medicine 2.0 opens up alternative pathways for eHealth investment through user contribution

or Web 2.0 business models. This is demonstrated by a wide range of free resources online which perform similar functions to traditional ICT in health. A number of both Web 2.0 investment paths are highlighted in this chapter (such as Facebook, Linux, Patientslikeme.com or similar, eMedicine. com or Medical wikis, Wikipedia.com®, Google Health® or Microsoft HealthVault®), challenging the current orthodoxy on eHealth implementation. They introduce new complexities in eHealth investment decisions, where determining overall eHealth financing is already a key question (European commission, 2008).

In the second case, many authors note Web 2.0's potential through engaging users for creating encyclopedic medical resources, improving medical education or clinical collaboration or providing health information to all types of stakeholders in varying contexts (Guistini, 2006; McLean, Richards & Wardman, 2007; Sandars & Schroter, 2007; Boulos & Wheeler, 2007; Sandars & Haythornthwaite, 2007). While it is understood that eHealth and Web 2.0 tools are used extensively by healthcare companies (Hughes & Wareham, 2008), patients (Ferguson, 2007) and doctors (Manhattan Research, 2008; Sandars & Schroter, 2007; Hughes, Joshi & Lemonde, 2008), Web 2.0 has also been associated with hype rather than a real opportunity to improve health (Skiba, 2006; Hughes, Joshi, Wareham, 2008; Versel, 2008), and in eHealth in general there have been mixed reports of its impact, itself being associated with "hope and hype" (Curry, 2007). For instance, previous research has suggested a great potential in using eHealth to address specific healthcare issues, such as enhanced patient-provider communication (Smedley & Stith, 2003), and applications that are tailored to the individual (Neuhauser & Kreps, 2003) that can tackle socio-economic and health inequalities (Dutta et al., 2008; Wangberg et al., 2008). However, other authors have made contrary suggestions, that eHealth is ineffective (Cashen, Dykes & Gerber, 2004; Korp, 2004), and that it leads to a double divide driven by disparities in internet use (Renahy Parizot & Chauvin, 2008; Lintonen, Konu & Seedhouse, 2007).

In this context of inconsistent reporting of the impact of eHealth, and new methods for developing eHealth interventions with Web 2.0, the chapter examines the various healthcare ICT evaluation frameworks in the practitioner and research domain. No particular framework is consistently applied across ICT evaluations. Moreover, for eHealth evaluation in particular, there is no established framework distinct to healthcare ICT in general (Glasgow, 2007). However, many ICT evaluation frameworks consider impact through user uptake and satisfaction, amongst other outcome measures, which do not automatically imply changes in behavior or patient outcomes. In addition, we previously noted the participatory nature of Web 2.0, which has developed new methods for engaging users, even though the effectiveness of this improved engagement in terms of outcomes is yet to be proven. This development is a cause for concern if use or satisfaction is taken as principal success measure, and suggests that a re-think of eHealth evaluation is required. Moreover, even if this measure is appropriate for certain outcomes, this must be paired with classic issues in economic analysis as defining alternatives, and combining different indicators into an overall evaluation when considering any intervention as a whole (Vimarlund & Olve, 2005). Given that new alternatives exist, it implies a new basis for comparison and eHealth evaluation in the age of Web 2.0, itself unsurprising as technological surges tend to leave research and evaluation techniques far behind (Potts, 2006; Atienza, Hesse, Baker, Abrams, Rimer, Croyl & Volckmann, 2007).

The chapter concludes with a proposal to frame eHealth evaluation in the context of Medicine 2.0, including: 1) following existing good practice frameworks, such as Re-AIM, that focus on ensuring good research and adequate explanation of outcomes; 2) examining the cost-effectiveness of eHealth interventions versus other possible alternatives, including the use of interventions not related to eHealth, or alternative pathways to ICT implementation via Web 2.0; 3) demonstrating the evolution of different eHealth interventions over time, and; 4) investigating the effectiveness of eHealth at a Health care system level by intranational and international comparisons of eHealth effectiveness. In conclusion, the chapter details the role of research in achieving these goals, by extending studies beyond the single intervention, examining issues of transferability and scalability and, creating common frameworks for comparisons of eHealth effectiveness.

BACKGROUND

Healthcare is one of the fastest-growing sectors in all economies, and eHealth is emerging when the challenge for developed countries is meeting ever increasing patient expectation for health care services with limited resources (Cabrera, Burgelman, Boden, da Costa, & Rodriguez, 2004). The objectives of eHealth programs are to improve health outcomes while reducing cost in the clinical system, through diverse capabilities such as online prescription refills, appointment scheduling, online billing, online medical records, improved patient-provider communications, or the proliferation of content-only health gateways, physician directories, physician-only sites, and online pharmacies (Wen & Tan, 2005). Hence eHealth has a wide scope, and is most commonly delineated via Eysenbach's (2005) definition (Oh, Rizo, Enkin & Jadad, 2005) as:

An emerging field in the intersection of medical informatics, public health and business, referring to health services and information delivered or enhanced through the Internet and related technologies. In a broader sense, the term characterizes not only a technical development, but also a state-of-mind, a way of thinking, an attitude, and a commitment for networked, global thinking, to improve health care locally, regionally, and worldwide by using information and communication technology.

This goes beyond simply Internet-based applications. For instance, the EU includes many aspects in its eHealth program, such as health information networks, Electronic Health Records, telemedicine services, personal wearable and portable communicable systems, health portals, and many other information and communication technology-based tools assisting prevention, diagnosis, treatment, health monitoring, and lifestyle management (Commission of the European Communities – COM, 2004). However, this does not include many ICT applications in healthcare or medical informatics, as many systems including the aforementioned Electronic Health Records are implemented without the use of the internet.

Despite this large scope, eHealth has yet to reach its full potential in many developed countries (Wickramasinghe et al., 2005). Encouraging early evidence suggests that behavior change efforts that include eHealth technologies can improve outcomes, and applications that are individually tailored, participatory, personally relevant, and contextually situated are more likely to promote behavior change (Neuhauser & Kreps, 2002). They can play a role in bridging the divide between socio-economic status and health, health inequalities or disparities due to race (Wangber et al., 2008; Dutta, Bodie & Basu, 2008). This has led eHealth to be recognized as a major pathway to address health disparities (Smedley, Stith & Nelson, 2003), via programs that enhance patient-provider communication, trust, and cultural appropriateness of delivered care (Starfield, 2007). Nonetheless, while research to date has identified certain beneficial cost savings, through virtual networking effects, electronic medical records, or physician-patient relationships (Mukherjee & McGinnis, 2007), a number of authors criticize the eHealth initiatives. For instance, authors cite lack of impact due to poor strategy (Wiklund &

Lindh, 2005), its current inability to deliver content that is dynamically tailored to meet the cultural, language, or literacy needs of the individual user (Cashen, Dykes & Gerber, 2004; Korp, 2006), and eHealth has been implicated in the causation or persistence of disparities because of the relative lack of access of some groups. This is coined the double divide (Renahy, Parizot & Chauvin 2008), as high income groups are almost three times as likely to have household internet access as low income groups (Curry, 2007). This has led to calls for more systematic investigation into the role of information and communication technology within health promotion (Lintonen, Konu & Seedhouse, 2007).

While eHealth is relatively new itself, an even newer trend, Medicine 2.0, has emerged in the last couple of years. Medicine 2.0 relies on a new generation of internet tools, which O'Reilly (2005) coined as "Web 2.0". These tools offer new possibilities through their collaborative nature, relying on the "Wisdom of Crowds" and a new participative mindset which is typified by examples such as Wikipedia.com, MySpace. com or Facebook.com (Boulos & Wheeler, 2007; Beer & Burrows, 2008). However, describing the phenomena through the tools, while a good initial sanitizing device, has a severe limitation in delineating its scope and describing its true nature. Hence, scholars consider Web 2.0 more as a philosophy that can be defined as (Hughes. Joshi, Wareham, 2008):

The use of a specific set of Web tools (blogs, Podcasts, tagging, search, wikis, etc) by actors in health care including doctors, patients, and scientists, using principles of open source and generation of content by users, and the power of networks in order to personalize health care, collaborate, and promote health education.

As such, Medicine 2.0 is a trend clearly subsumed by eHealth, and while Web 2.0 focuses on user participation less prominent in eHealth, there is a large overlap and gray boundary between the two (Hughes. Joshi, Wareham, 2008). Moreover, it overlaps with the term Health 2.0, though analysis of the two terms has shown there to be little difference in these concepts (Hughes. Joshi, Wareham, 2008). Gunter Eysenbach, who launched the Medicine 2.0 conference, noted that the main differences are that Health 2.0 is business and U.S. focused, while Medicine 2.0 is targeted at an international and academic audience (Eysenbach, 2008). Given this narrow separation, no major distinction is made between them in this chapter, since each is subsumed by eHealth, and the participatory nature of both is certain to create new possibilities, but also new issues, which we go on to describe in the next section.

HOW WEB 2.0 IMPACTS E-HEALTH EVALUATION AND INVESTMENT DESCISIONS

Looking Beyond Web 2.0's Potential: Emerging Issues with Medicine 2.0

We take an issues based view to examine Web 2.0's impact on eHealth policy, as scholars suggest this can enable the current gap between research and practice to be addressed, promoting a common agenda between researchers and practitioners (Potts, 2006; Amabile et al., 2001). In a recent systematic review of Medicine 2.0 literature, four such major tensions were identified with the emergence of Web 2.0 tools in healthcare (Hughes, Joshi, Wareham, 2008): 1) Doctors' concerns with patients' use of Web 2.0, even if the information is accurate; 2) Information inaccuracy and potential risks associated with inaccurate Web 2.0 information; 3) The consequences of the new methods of creating eHealth, such as privacy and ownership issues with Web 2.0–generated information, or the alternative paths to achieve them and; 4) the delineation of what makes Medicine 2.0, that is not a policy instrument separate to that

of eHealth, where Web 2.0's participatory nature may imply that previous outcome measure may become misleading.

Firstly, doctors' concerns arise from Web 2.0 causing unwanted patient behaviors, such as consulting a physician late or making wrong conclusions about disease management, even if the online information is accurate. The issue is not new and arose with eHealth, where concerns partly arise from what Ferguson (2007) "e-Patient resistant clinicians", due to a sense of loss of control, paternalism, or lack of training driving these doctors' behaviors. In Medicine 2.0 there are amplifying effects to this behavior are identified by certain authors, such as lack of training for doctors (Sandars & Schroter, 2007), or the difficulty of advising patients on use of Web 2.0 tools (Goh, 2006). Overall, doctors are now required to consider roles as advisors to patients and gatekeepers of resources, rather than previous roles as the gatekeeper of medical knowledge. Encouraging early evidence shows that doctors are adapting to this role (Ferguson, 2007; Hughes, Joshi, Lemonde, 2008), and research has begun to provide insights for doctors to adapt to these changes (see Goh, 2006).

Secondly, user-generated information via Web 2.0 has a potential for misinformation, also an adaptation to a hazard long identified with eHealth. This applies to both medical professionals and patients, and scholars have urged all types of uses to seek evidence based decisions, leading to strong criticisms of the use of Web 2.0 tools for decision making in health (Lacovara, 2008). This is demonstrated by responses to articles on Medicine 2.0's potential, such as "the consequences could be disastrous for any inexperienced trainee following the advice" (Giustini, 2006; Tang H, Ng, 2006). However, Esquivel (2006) notes the error and correction rate on an Internet-based cancer support group, examining user generated information that underpins Web 2.0 methods, and found that most information was accurate and most false or misleading statements were rapidly corrected. Eysenbach (2008) also examined the impact of information accuracy and credibility in relation to eHealth in general and noted that that patients will tend to use both intermediated (experts, authorities) and distributed (i.e., Web 2.0) information to make their health decisions, thereby reducing any risk from inaccurate online information. However, despite early evidence of low risk, many practitioners and researchers remain to be convinced. This applies not only to doctors, but to health professionals (Hughes, Joshi, Lemonde, 2008).

Thirdly, scholars have noted other issues relating to the user-generated information via Web 2.0 methods. These include privacy, ethical, legal, and ownership issues (Karkalis & Koutsouris, 2006; Boulos & Burden, 2007) not only for patients, but also doctors who may use social networking sites for medical education and debate (Sandars, Homer, Pell & Croker, 2008). They suggest that potential models of identity management and authorization schemes should also be investigated in the context of Medicine 2.0 research. Once again, this tends to accentuate eHealth trends such as noted by Ferguson (2007), who also highlights that those patient groups who run specific sites claim ownership over this data and are increasingly using it to influence the research agenda. However, Web 2.0 methods of generating eHealth services or platforms also create a new set of possibilities for eHealth development. If Web 2.0 now offers increases in effectiveness for eHealth delivery, and alternative routes for ICT development, this challenges the orthodoxy on eHealth investment, and we go on to describe this issue more in the next section.

Lastly, while new sources of health information are emerging via Web 2.0 methods, many of the issues seem inseparable eHealth issues in general. Scholars therefore ask if Medicine 2.0 or Web 2.0 applied to the medical domain is just hype (Skiba, 2006), and the concept is dogged by continued speculation that terms such as Health 2.0 may be a fake "gold rush" (Versel, 2008).

This final issue is of great concern for two reasons. Firstly, it is impossible for policy makers to judge Web 2.0's contribution to patient health outcomes separately to eHealth. Secondly, Web 2.0's participatory nature will mean misleading outcome measures, such as the depth of a patient's involvement in an internet based intervention, will make these eHealth interventions appear more successful on a number of the typical measures used. If interactivity and clean usable interfaces become ubiquitous in the age of Web 2.0, more caution is require in using them as measure of eHealth success.

Web 2.0 Alternatives to Existing Orthodoxy on E-Health Program Investment

Investments on health care ICT can be immense, an illustrative being the Electronic Health Record (EHR) system for the UK's National Health Services (NHS), a vision to build one online system, accessible everywhere, with individual patient's medical record in digital format. Heavily criticized for 12 billion pounds sterling spent, being four years late, and lacking full implementation, it is one of the most high profile ICT investments in health in recent years (Collins, 2009). While cost estimates of a similar system of the United States as a whole stand at $28 billion investment, and a $16 billion a year operating cost, the benefits are potentially $81 billion a year. (Walker, Pan, Johnston, Adler-Milstein, Bates & Middleton, 2005; Hillestad, Bigelow, Bower, et al., 2005). However, the case of the UK's NHS shows the inherent risks of such a project, and that despite the many benefits large scale ICT projects, progress into developing affordable systems has been slow (Curry, 2007).

What alternatives has the emergence of Web 2.0 presented? The principle of Web 2.0 design is that it is user driven (O'Reilly, 2005), with effective applications arising out of a series of user designed alternatives are selected by large online communities. Developers offer free technology for many reasons, but are often rewarded for successful applications, with reduced costs and risks such as user acquisition (Krohn, Yip, Brodsky, Morris, & Walfish, 2007). A high profile example of this is Facebook, which conformed it own development to Web 2.0 principles by embracing Open Source in May 2007, allowing users to submit applications themselves. One year later, the number of user generated applications had grown to a staggering 33,000, with 400,000 registered developers (Ustinova, 2008; Facebook, 2008). This illustrates the power of Web 2.0 for application development, an approach that created a number of small scale health applications like EHRs within the Facebook platform. However, this type of collaboration need not be small scale, as open source developments such as Linux (Raymond, 1999) have shown the impact that the collaborative philosophies associated with Web 2.0 can bring even to large organizations. Hence, Web 2.0 provides an entirely different approach to development from centrally mandated and designed systems.

When translated into Medicine 2.0, two different approaches are seen. Some alternatives arise from patient adoption, such as patientslikeme.com, a site where members add their own individual-level health experience to a repository of structured outcome data. This site has already attracted over 30,000 patients over a fairly narrow set of conditions, developing an unprecedented data set that informs medical conversation, not only within the patient community but also within the scientific one (Eysenbach, 2008). There are numerous similar efforts, including sites such as Curetogether (http://www.curetogether.com/), DailyStrength (http://www.dailystrength.org/) or RevolutionHealth (http://www.revolutionhealth.com/) to name but a few.

Others are driven by large businesses seeking to profit from the potential in eHealth through Web 2.0 business models. Companies such as Google and Microsoft have entered the field in the past

three years. Like its email and search, Google offers this service for free, though the current functionality is limited and there are concerns over data ownership (Tanne, 2007). However, the success of Google Office®, which faced the same initial criticism (Conner, 2008), means it would be unwise to bet against the success of Google's health services. Its ability to integrate patient records from different health partners, like CVS or Quest Diagnostics, means that Google Health® now has 100s of million of records (Arora, 2009) and is already one of the largest patient record systems worldwide.

Finally, while the focus is on Medicine 2.0 initiatives involving patients directly, major contributions to the working practices of health professional are also observed. For instance, the contributions of thousands of doctors has propelled eMedicine® to an important source of clinical knowledge, and more generic user generated content sources such as Wikipedia are heavily used by certain doctors (Hughes, Joshi, Lemonde, Wareham, 2009). Moreover, there are numerous specialist wikis (of which selected lists can be found at http://hlwiki.slais.ubc.ca/index.php/Medical_wikis). Overall these examples show the tremendous impact Web 2.0 can have on approaches to implementing various types of healthcare ICT. Table 1 summarizes these different examples of Web 2.0 development paths, and its potential for eHealth programs.

EXAMPLES OF ICT EVALUATION FRAMEWORKS IN HEALTH

In respect to the goals of eHealth programs, to reduce cost and improve health outcomes (Cabrera, Burgelman, Boden, da Costa, & Rodriguez, 2004), the measurement of eHealth impact has been limited. On the cost side, economic evaluations of ICT applications in healthcare have been rare (Vimarlund & Olve, 2005). On the outcomes side, scholars note an absence of good evidence

Table 1. Examples of how Web 2.0 can impact eHealth program development

Example	Example type	Description	Impact on eHealth
Facebook	Web 2.0 systems development	Opening of platform to external users for application development – 33,000 applications developed over a year (Ustinova, 2008; Facebook, 2008).	Customized application development
Linux	Web 2.0/Open source development	Development of the world's most popular operating system via open standards	Large scale application development
Patientslikeme.com or similar	Health 2.0 data generation	30,000 patients entering detailed information on symptom control and treatment effectiveness (Eysenbach, 2008).	Patient driven data capture and design
eMedicine.com or Medical wikis	Web 2.0 data generation	Clinical reference tool maintained by 10,000 physician contributors (Hughes et al. 2009).	User generated medical reference
Wikipedia.com	Web 2.0 data generation	Reference tool of choice for junior doctors (Hughes, et al., 2009).	User generated medical and general reference
Google Health® (or Microsoft HealthVault®)	Web 2.0 business models	Assembling of 100s of millions of health records in a couple of years in pursuit of Web 2.0 business models	Use of beta applications, mash-up or data integration, and Web 2.0 business models

on the effects of delivering health promotion online (Duffy, Wimbush, Reece & Eadie, 2003), even though scholars make the case for eHealth through secondary measures, such as satisfaction and acceptance in telemedicine (Arnaert & Delesie, 2001), improving communication (Baldwin, Clarke, Eldabi & Jones, 2002) and in patient empowerment (Bauer, 2002). To address these and other concerns, various frameworks have emerged for ICT evaluation on both the practitioner and academic domains.

In the practitioner domain, an example is Canada Health Infoway, the primary lead in Canada for eHealth-related activities. Their mission is to foster and accelerate the development and adoption of electronic health information systems on a pan-Canadian basis. Infoway's goal is to have an interoperable Electronic Health Record in place for 50 percent of Canada's population by the end of 2009. "Measure Benefits and Adjust" is one of Infoway's business strategies, requiring a process for continual measurement of realized versus planned benefits and needed adjustment (Canada Health Infoway, 2006; Scott & Saeed, 2008). Specifically the following elements are elaborated on the framework:

1. System dimensions, including functionality, performance and security
2. Informational dimensions, including content quality and availability
3. Usage dimensions, including use patterns, self-reported use and intention to use
4. Satisfaction dimensions such as user satisfaction or ease of use
5. Net benefits including, quality (such as patient outcomes), access and productivity. Within productivity there are sub-dimensions that include resource allocation and monetary outcomes.

While a fairly extensive list of prerequisites for successful eHealth intervention, the relation of actual outcome measures to eHealth investments is not entirely clear. Furthermore, Web 2.0 contorts any such evaluation system in two ways: 1) common criteria such as usage and satisfactions will rise, even though patient outcomes may not, and; 2) the investment paths in eHealth more complex, with more alternatives, requiring clearer measures of outcomes per unit of investment (which may be monetary investment or other, depending on the nature on the intervention).

In the research domain, much work has been done in specifying good practice healthcare ICT evaluation, such as the RE-AIM framework, UMIT's inventory of ICT evaluations studies in healthcare and the STARE-HI framework, or CHEATS. These can be briefly described as:

- **RE-AIM (Glasgow, Vogt & Boles 1999;Glasgow, 2002)**: is an acronym that stands for Reach (participation rate and representativeness of participants); Effectiveness (on both primary outcomes and quality of-life/negative consequences); Adoption (participation rate and representativeness among settings and staff implementing a program); Implementation or consistency of program delivery, and Maintenance or sustainability at both patient and setting levels (www. re-aim.org). Within this framework, multiple indices are suggested for tackling issues such as the representativeness of the sample, though their application has not seen much eHealth research.

- **UMIT (University for Health Sciences, Medical Informatics and Technology)**: have cataloged a vast inventory of evaluation studies from 1982 to 2005. Here scholars have observed that ICT evaluation studies suffer many weaknesses, though many findings relate to basic research quality such as adequate explanation of the context or appropriateness of the research questions in their support of the conclusions (de Keizer, 2008). Work in this area has resulted in STARE-HI (Talmon, Ammenwerth, Brender, de Keizer, Nykänen, Rigby, 2008), or Statement on Reporting of Evaluation Studies in Health Informatics, which attempts to raise the quality of evaluation studies in health informatics through standard guidelines on reporting of studies. Specific recommendations include appropriate standardized sections for research,

reporting of the sample, or clear explanation of outcome measures

- **CHEATS (Shaw, 2002)**: is a generic framework for addressing clinical, human and organizational, educational, administrative, ethnical and social explanatory factors in an ICT intervention. As such the CHEATS framework provides a wider range of potential explanatory factors, though fit and moderating factors still need to be determined.

However an issue in applying most of these frameworks is that their focus is to improve the quality of research into ICT use in healthcare. This does not entirely address eHealth evaluation needs, as the objectives of discrete pieces of research are not necessarily aimed at taking the wider view of a programs relative effectiveness. Rather, given common limits on the length or scope of a research articles, focus is often on one aspect of the intervention (such as usability, adoption, satisfaction, etc.). However, any full evaluation requires defining alternatives, the basis for comparison, and combining different indicators into an overall evaluation (Vimarlund & Olve, 2005). As such, while many frameworks exist for ICT evaluation in healthcare, they are often not designed to address full evaluation or the challenges of Web 2.0 (as outlined in table 2).

BEYOND FRAMEWORKS: EXAMPLE E-HEALTH EVALUATION STUDIES IN RESEARCH

To demonstrate this issue more precisely in scholarly work we examine three recent papers *specific* to eHealth. These papers naturally use summary measures of a population's health, allowing comparison of one population to another described as an essential input into evaluations of the performance of different health systems (Murray & Frenk, 2000). However, these should

Table 2. Examples of evaluation frameworks or studies for eHealth and the impact of Web 2.0

Example	Example type	Description	Impact of Web 2.0
Canada Infoway	Practitioner eHealth frame-work	System, satisfaction, Informational, Usage, Net benefits (including, quality, patient outcomes, access and productivity).	• Participation and adoption may rise without change in outcomes • Alternative Web 2.0 investment paths not considered • Weak link between outcomes and invested resources
RE-AIM	Research based eHealth/ICT evaluation framework	Reach, Effectiveness (on both primary outcomes and quality of-life/negative consequences); Adoption, Implementation, and Maintenance or sustainability	• Participation and adoption may rise without change in outcomes • Alternative Web 2.0 investment paths not considered
STARE-HI	Research based ICT evaluation framework	Specific recommendations for every section of a research study (reporting of the sample, explanation of outcome measures, etc.)	• Not a framework specifically positioned for eHealth (unlike RE-AIM) • Recommendations do not specifically address potential issues of misinterpretation of increased use usability or satisfaction due to Web 2.0
CHEATs		Clinical, human and organizational, educational, administrative, ethnical and social explanatory factors in an ICT intervention	

also be considered alongside health financing and inequalities (Murray, Salomon & Mathers 2000; Wilkinson, 1997; 2007). When applied to eHealth evaluations, examples such as Dutta et al. (2008) use a 3 step model where race and socio economic status effect 3 factors including health information orientation, health information efficacy and technological efficacy. These in turn effect health information seeking, and finally, real health outcomes. Similarly, in their study of internet use and health outcomes in the Paris Metropolitan area, Renahy et al. (2008) also use socio-economic status, technological efficacy (home internet access, experience of use) and health information seeking. However they also test a number of other measures such as social integration in relation to subjective health. Other examples include Wangberg et al. (2007), who also use socio economic status, internet use and health information seeking, and social support. The common elements of these models are shown in figure 1.

This approach demonstrates "value" in the realm of evaluation, as defined by Ovretveit (1998), and generally conforms with the factors that should be considered when examining any health intervention (e.g., Murray & Frenk, 2000; Murray, Salomon, Mathers 2000; Wilkinson, 1997; 2007). However, three types of issues arise with the approach as implemented by these studies. Firstly, the influences of the aforementioned factors, such as absolute income or income disparities, are often dulled by grouping in quartiles. Secondly, different outcome measures are used that add to the picture of mixed reports regarding the impact of eHealth, such as the use of subjective health versus other health outcomes. And ultimately, eHealth needs to tackle the thorny issue of the repetitiveness of the sample (Glasgow, 2007), as the different treatments of the most important factors driving health, absolute and relative income (Wilkison, 1997; Wilkinson 2007), are strongly correlated to internet use, meaning that factors such as specifying denominators and the representativeness of samples needed to be addressed.

However this is not a judgment on the value of these specific studies, but rather shows the importance of the aforementioned frameworks in ensuring high quality research. However it also demonstrates that the scope of typical studies is

Figure 1. Common elements in models examining e-health summary outcomes

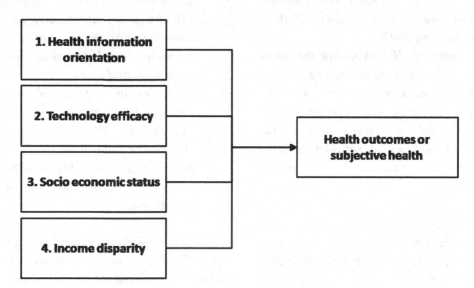

not sufficient to inform policy makers in eHealth investment decisions. The authors may have demonstrated that a particular use of or intervention via eHealth impacts outcomes, perhaps complying with the many of the guidelines set out in the above frameworks, but provides only a narrow view on the value of the intervention. While this is valuable research, a full assessment has to be very specific about such classic issues in economic analysis as defining alternatives (Vimarlund & Olve, 2005). In addition, these example studies do not provide insights to other important evaluation factors, such as the how such eHealth evolves over time or the limits to its scalability (Glasgow, 2007).

Solutions for Addressing Evaluation Techniques in the Age of Web 2.0

The previous sections have outlined the major limitations in the way we examine eHealth initiatives and the inherent risks in applying these techniques with the emergence of Web 2.0. Good evaluations of eHealth have been rare (Vimarlund & Olve, 2005; Duffy, Wimbush, Reece & Eadie, 2003), and while making such assessments is difficult, the use of extensive mixed methods is essential for identifying eHealth programs best practices, and to allow improved management. To address this in the age of Web 2.0, ICT evaluation frameworks also needs to consider: 1) following existing good practice frameworks, such as Re-AIM, that focus on ensuring good research and adequate explanation of outcomes; 2) examine the cost-effectiveness of eHealth interventions versus other possible alternatives, including the use of interventions not related to eHealth; 3) Investigate these factors in terms of their possible evolution over time, and; 4) demonstrate the effectiveness of eHealth at a Health care system level by intra-national comparisons of eHealth effectiveness.

The first becomes even more critical due to the emergence of Medicine 2.0. Web 2.0 applications by their nature potentially increase user's participation, satisfaction or involvement in a particular eHealth-based intervention. As such, successful eHealth evaluation needs to use combined measures by:

- *The outcomes relevant to the specific intervention: By following appropriate frameworks such as RE-AIM (seeMurray & Frenk, 2000;Murray, Salomon, Mathers 2000;Glasgow, 2007)*

- **The impact of eHealth within the intervention:** *Determining the role of eHealth where frameworks such as those used by-Canada Health Infoway (2006)are useful where the link between outcomes and the role of eHealth (usage, satisfaction, influence on behavior change, etc.) are explicitly linked*

In the second instance, the emergence of Web 2.0 has introduced new methods for developing user centric applications. Given the considerable cost of ICT development, the alternative use of the sources of funding for eHealth must be considered in two ways:

- **Alternative pathways within eHealth:** *Using Web 2.0 principles for system development must be considered, which may reduce short or long term benefits and control, but with significantly lower development costs may deliver better value alternative scenarios*
- **Alternative pathways without eHealth:** *eHealth must be compared to the cost of traditional interventions, including a counselor's ability to tailor or personalize motivational messages, goals or feedback to the individual in question.*

In addition these assessments must be made over time using return on investment analysis (Chinn, 2002). Investments in eHealth need significant time periods to provide benefits, however the subsequent value can be much greater than alternatives without ICT. Hence the above evaluations must be made over time, considering the sustained impacts and cost of interventions covering two aspects:

- **Evolution of effect:** *The effectiveness of eHealth interventions can decline over time, however impact can also increase with operational improvements and changes in scale and reach*
- **Evolution of cost:** *Initial cost of traditional ICT investments can be high, though may decline with operation improvements. Alternative maintenance and evolution approaches are available through Web 2.0, with different development and operational cost profiles.*

Finally, it will clearly be challenging to complete the above rigorous analysis in all cases of spending decisions. Some investments are too small to warrant such efforts, however many different small eHealth investments can add up to a significant financial burden for any given Healthcare system. For this reason, the success of eHealth use should also be examined at the macro-level, considering intra- and inter-country comparisons of different overall health systems and their eHealth effectiveness.

- **Intra-system comparisons:** *Regions have specific population and health systems that make inter-regional comparisons difficult, though not impossible. However, given the increase in eHealth use, comparisons between eHealth interventions with similar environmental conditions can be made*
- **Inter-national comparisons:** *With eHealth now a priority for many developed countries, and coordinated and promoted at the European level (European commission. DG INFSO, 2008), the use of standardized metrics will allow best practices to be identified between different health systems*

There are many possible explanations for summary measures of health, such as the specifics of the population (e.g., absolute income, income disparities, cultural factors, etc.) and the nature of the health system (absolute health spending, public vs. private systems, etc.). However, if the use of eHealth *is* having a major impact on healthcare delivery effectiveness, given the varying application of eHealth between countries, the effects of these interventions and inter-systems comparisons must be possible.

While these proposals require significant effort, the value at stake in both eHealth spending and potential benefits is staggering. Researchers have noted that it is possible to follow most evaluation recommendations by simply keeping systematic records, and that there is little impact on patients (Glasgow, 2007). Moreover, Web 2.0 may help policy makers or practitioners share eHealth data and set common comparison measures. Many specialist medical wikis have achieved this is in specific domains, but this is in no way a silver bullet for eHealth evaluation.

FUTURE RESEARCH DIRECTIONS

This chapter has set out both the huge value at stake in eHealth investment, the limitations of current research and evaluation techniques that examine these investments, and highlighted that the emergence of Web 2.0 not only makes typical measurements more misleading (such as use or user satisfaction), but also opens new alternative pathways to eHealth implementation that must be taken into account in these evaluations. As such, an acceleration of research into eHealth evaluation, taking a more holistic approach, is required. These span three axis of examining the macro impact of eHealth, the translational and scalable impact over time, and the relative impact via benchmarks:

Macro impact of eHealth:

- Researchers need to venture outside the research "silos" and the unit of analysis of the single intervention. Much evidence

supporting eHealth effectiveness is case based, demonstrating that that the intervention in question had an effect on a specific disease group, and by focusing on internal validity (Glasgow, 2007). Most health organizations need eHealth programs to produce benefits on multiple variables, and research needs to examine more than one isolated problem in order to demonstrate value.

- Research should examine the impact of eHealth use at the system level. This involves comparing health systems at the national level, isolating confounding factors related to the population and the health system in question, and comparing the effectiveness of eHealth between systems. This is a significant task, however the increase systematic collection of standardized eHealth data will allow this, such as the EU's tracking of eHealth use across member states (see European Commission i2010, 2009).

Longitudinal, translational and scalable impact of eHealth:

- Research needs to consider a wider scope of designs to examine the longitudinal view of eHealth programs. Costs of eHealth systems vary over time, as does the effectiveness of different interventions. For instance, keeping users engaged over time is a common challenge across intervention areas (Glasgow, McKay, Piette & Reynolds, 2001). As such research needs to examine options such as interrupted time series designs that capture how eHealth interventions evolve over time (Shadish, Cook & Campbell, 2002; Rotheram-Borus & Flannery, 2004; Glasgow, 2007), including how this varies in terms of cost effectiveness.

- Examine the transferability and scalability of the intervention via principles of the

Technology Acceptance Model (TAM – Venkatesh, Morris, Davis & Davis, 2003) or diffusion of innovations (Rogers, 2003). A large proportion of research is carried out on the effectiveness of pilot interventions. In order to understand the value of these when scaled to a larger population appropriate frameworks such as the PRECEDE-PROCEED or CURRES models should be used (Glasgow, 2007)

E-Health Benchmarking:

- In order to facilitate the above measurements benchmarks or frameworks for comparability need to be developed. As a minimum a basis for comparison between studies needs to be established by a clear but concise description of 4 elements in studies, outcomes, the role of eHealth the outcome, the resources applied to achieve that outcome, and how these may change over time. It is difficult for reviewers or editors to insist on these elements, but doing so provides a minimum of information for comparisons of intervention effectiveness.

CONCLUSION

Overall the emergence of Medicine 2.0 provides great potential for eHealth effectiveness. Although Medicine 2.0 is clearly distinct in its reach and pace of change, it is important to understand it through its contribution to eHealth as a whole. It can address previous eHealth limitations versus traditional interventions by allowing the further customization and personalization of interventions over the internet. It also provides new alternatives for eHealth investment, using open source and user-contributions as a means to develop ICT applications for healthcare. Despite this improvement, it raises key questions for overall eHealth financing, as evaluation techniques are behind

actual practice and not prepared for its emergence. For instance, simply adding Web 2.0 features to traditional eHealth work may improve indicators of use and satisfaction, without delivering real improvements in patient outcomes. Moreover, even though Web 2.0 opens alternative implementation routes for eHealth projects, such as open source collaborations, many of these are new to the health sector and the organizations that operate within it and may not be considered in assessment of alternative scenarios for ICT implementation.

Given this importance, this chapter detailed how Medicine 2.0 emergence should be viewed for effective management of eHealth, and outlined four dimensions required for thorough evaluations, including: 1) following existing good practice frameworks, such as Re-AIM, that focus on ensuring good research and adequate explanation of outcomes; 2) examining the cost-effectiveness of eHealth interventions versus other possible alternatives, including the use of interventions not related to eHealth, an alternative implementation routes using online collaborations; 3) demonstrating different eHealth interventions evolution over time, and; 4) investigating the effectiveness of eHealth at a Health care system level by intra-national and international comparisons of eHealth effectiveness. In order to achieve these goals scholarly research will also need to play a key role, with longitudinal views, and by developing common frameworks or benchmarks for comparisons of eHealth effectiveness.

REFERENCES

Amabile, T., Patterson, C., Mueller, J., Wokocik, T., Odomirok, P. W., Marsh, M., & Kramer, S. (2001). Academic-practitioner collaboration in management research: A case of cross-profession collaboration. *Academy of Management Journal, 44*(2), 418–432. doi:10.2307/3069464

Arnaert, A., & Delesie, L. (2001). Telenursing for the elderly: The case for care via video-telephony. *Journal of Telemedicine and Telecare, 7*, 311–316. doi:10.1258/1357633011936912

Arora, M. (2009). CVS joins Google Health Rx network: millions can access medication records online. *Official blog from the Product Manager, Google Health.* Retrieved March 6, 2009, from http://www.socresonline.org.uk/12/5/17.html

Atienza, A., Hesse, B., Baker, T., Abrams, D., Rimer, B., Croyle, R., & Volckmann, L. (2007). Critical issues in eHealth research. *American Journal of Preventive Medicine, 32*(5Suppl), S71–S74. doi:10.1016/j.amepre.2007.02.013

Baldwin, L., Clarke, M., Eldabi, T., & Jones, R. (2002). Telemedicine and its role in improving communication in healthcare. *Logistics Information Management, 15*(4), 309–319. doi:10.1108/09576050210436147

Bauer, K.A. (2002). Using the Internet to Empower Patients and to Develop Partnerships with Clinicians. *World Hospital Health Services, 38*(2), 2-10 9.

Beer, D., & Burrows, R. (2007). Sociology and, of and in Web 2.0: Some Initial Considerations. *Sociological Research Online, 12*(5). Retrieved March 6, 2009, from http://www.socresonline.org.uk/12/5/17.html

Boulos, M. N. K., & Burden, D. (2007). Web GIS in practice V: 3-D interactive and real-time mapping in Second Life. *International Journal of Health Geographics, 27*(6), 51. doi:10.1186/1476-072X-6-51

Boulos, M. N. K., & Wheeler, S. (2007). The emerging Web 2.0 social software: an enabling suite of sociable technologies in health and health care education. *Health Information and Libraries Journal, 24*, 2–23. doi:10.1111/j.1471-1842.2007.00701.x

Cabrera, M., Burgelman, J.C., Boden, M., da Costa, O., & Rodriguez, C. (2004*). eHealth in 2010: Realizing a Knowledge-based Approach to Healthcare in the EU – Challenges for the Ambient Care System.* (Report on eHealth related activities by IPTS). European Commission, Directorate-General, Joint Research Centre.

Canada Health Infoway. (2006). *Benefits Evaluation Indicators, Technical Report.* (Version 1.0. September 2006). Retrieved March 6, 2009, from http://www2.infoway-inforoute.ca/Documents/BE%20Techical%20Report%20(EN).pdf

Cashen, M. S., Dykes, P., & Gerber, B. (2004). eHealth technology and Internet resources: barriers for vulnerable populations. *The Journal of Cardiovascular Nursing, 19*(3), 209–214.

Chinn, S. (2002). E-health engineering economics. *International Journal of Healthcare Technology and Management, 4*, 451–455. doi:10.1504/IJHTM.2002.002423

Collins, T. (2009). Minutes of Blair meeting which sparked £13bn NHS IT scheme. Retrieved March 7, 2009, from http://www.computerweekly.com/Articles/2009/02/11/234758/minutes-of-blair-meeting-which-sparked-13bn-nhs-it.html

Commission of the European Communities. (2004). e-Health - making health care better for European citizens: An action plan for a European e-Health Area. (COM 356). Communication from the Commission to the Council, the European Parliament, the European Economic and Social Committee and the Committee of the Regions, Brussels.

Conner, N. (2008). Google Apps: The Missing Manual. Sebastopol, CA: O'Reilly/Pogue Press.

Curry, S. J. (2007). eHealth research and healthcare delivery beyond intervention effectiveness. *American Journal of Preventive Medicine, 32*(5Suppl), S127–S130. doi:10.1016/j.amepre.2007.01.026

de Keizer, N. (2008). The quality of evidence in health informatics: How did the quality of healthcare IT evaluation publications develop from 1982 to 2005? *International Journal of Medical Informatics, 77*(1), 41–49. doi:10.1016/j.ijmedinf.2006.11.009

Duffy, M., Wimbush, E., Reece, J., & Eadie, D. (2003). Net profits? Web site development and health improvement. *Health Education, 103*(5), 278–285. doi:10.1108/09654280310499055

Dutta, M., Bodie, G., & Basu, A. (2008). Health Disparity and the Racial Divide among the Nation's Youth: Internet as a Site for Change? In Everett, A. (Ed.), *Learning Race and Ethnicity: Youth and Digital Media. The John D. and Catherine T. MacArthur. Foundation Series on Digital Media and Learning* (pp. 175–198). Cambridge, MA: The MIT Press.

Esquivel, A., Meric-Bernstam, F., & Bernstam, E.V. (2006). Accuracy and self correction of information received from an internet breast cancer list: content analysis. *British Medical Journal, 22;332*(7547), 939-942.

European commission. DG INFSO (2008). *Sources of financing and policy recommendations to Member States and the European Commission on boosting eHealth investment.* Brussels. Retrieved March 7, 2009, from http://www.financing-eHealth.eu/downloads/documents/FeH_D5_3_final_study_report.pdf

European Commission. i2010 (2009). *Benchmarking.* Brussels. Retrieved March 7, 2009, from http://ec.europa.eu/information_society/eeurope/i2010/benchmarking/index_en.htm

Eysenbach, G. (2001). What is e-health? *Journal of Medical Internet Research, 3*(2), e20. Retrieved March 6, 2009, from http://www.jmir.org/2001/2/e20/

Eysenbach, G. (2008). Credibility of health information and digital media: new perspectives and implications for youth. In Metzger, M. J., & Flanagin, A. J. (Eds.), *Digital Media, Youth, and Credibility. The John D and Catherine T MacArthur Foundation Series on Digital Media and Learning.* Cambridge, MA: MIT Press.

Eysenbach, G. (2008). Medicine 2.0: Social Networking, Collaboration, Participation, Apomediation, and Openness. *Journal of Medical Internet Research, 10,* 3:(e23).Retrieved March 6, 2009, from www.jmir.org/2008/3/e22

Facebook. (2008). Facebook Expands Power of Platform Across the Web and Around the World. Retrieved March 7, 2009, from http://www.facebook.com/press/releases.php?p=48242

Ferguson, T. (2007). ePatients white paper. www.e-patients.net. Retrieved March 6, 2009, from http://www.e-patients.net/e-Patients_White_Paper.pdf on 22/1/08

Fox, S. (2006). Online health search 2006. Pew Internet and American Life Project 2005. Retrieved March 6, 2009, from www.pewinternet.org/PPF/r/190/report_display.asp.

Giustini, D. (2006). How Web 2.0 is changing medicine. *British Medical Journal, 23;333*(7582), 1283-1284.

Glasgow, R. E. (2002). Evaluation of theory-based interventions: the RE-AIM model. Glanz, K., Lewis, F.M., & Rimer, B.K. (Ed.), Health behavior and health education (3rd ed., pp. 531-544). San Francisco CA: John Wiley & Sons.

Glasgow, R. E. (2007). C evaluation and dissemination research. *American Journal of Preventive Medicine, 32*(5Suppl), S119–S126. doi:10.1016/j.amepre.2007.01.023

Glasgow, R. E., McKay, H. G., Piette, J. D., & Reynolds, K. D. (2001). The RE-AIM framework for evaluating interventions: what can it tell us about approaches to chronic illness management? *Patient Education and Counseling, 44*, 119–127. doi:10.1016/S0738-3991(00)00186-5

Glasgow, R. E., Vogt, T. M., & Boles, S. M. (1999). Evaluating the public health impact of health promotion interventions: the RE-AIM framework. *American Journal of Public Health, 89*, 1322–1327. doi:10.2105/AJPH.89.9.1322

Goh, S. H. (2006). The internet as a health education tool: sieving the wheat from the chaff. *Singapore Medical Journal, 47*(1), 3–5.

Hillestad, R., Bigelow, J., Bower, A., Girosi, R., Meili, R., Scoville, R., & Taylor, R. (2005). Can electronic medical record systems transform health care: potential health benefits, savings, and costs? *Health Affairs, 24*, 1103–1117. doi:10.1377/hlthaff.24.5.1103

Hughes, B., Joshi, I., & Lemonde, H. (2008). To 2.0 or not to 2.0? Young doctors have already answered the question. In G. Eysenbach (Ed.), *Proceedings of the Medicine 2.0 congress, 4-5th September 2008, Toronto* (p. 39).

Hughes, B., Joshi, I., Lemonde, H., & Wareham, J. (2009). Junior physician's use of Web 2.0 for information seeking and medical education: a qualitative study. *International Journal of Medical Informatics.*

Hughes, B., Joshi, I., & Wareham, J. (2008). Medicine 2.0: Tensions and controversies in the field. *Journal of Medical Internet Research, 6;10*(3), e23. Retrieved March 7, 2009, from http://www.jmir.org/2008/3/e23/

Hughes, B., & Wareham, J. (2008). Democratized Collaboration in Big Pharma. In G. Soloman (Ed.), *Proceedings of the Academy of Management Conference, 13th August 2008, Anaheim, CA.*

Karkalis, G. I., & Koutsouris, D. D. (October 2006). *E-health and the Web 2.0.* Paper presented at The International Special Topic Conference on Information Technology in Biomedicine, Greece 2006.

Korp, P. (2006). Health on the Internet: implications for health promotion. *Health Education Research, 21*(1), 78–86. doi:10.1093/her/cyh043

Krohn. M., Yip, A., Brodsky, M., Morris, R., & Walfish, M. (November 2007). *A world wide web without walls.* ACM Workshop on Hot Topics in Networks presentated at HotNets-VI, Atlanta, GA.

Lacovara, J. E. (2008). When searching for the evidence, stop using Wikipedia! *Medsurg Nursing, 17*(3), 153.

Lintonen, T. P., Konu, A. I., & Seedhouse, D. (2008). Information technology in health promotion. *Health Education Research, 23*(3), 560–566. doi:10.1093/her/cym001

Madden, M., & Fox, S. (2005). *Finding answers online in sickness and in health.* Washington, DC: Pew Internet and American Life Project.

Manhattan Research Group. (2007). White Paper: Physicians and Web 2.0: 5 Things You Should Know about the Evolving Online Landscape for Physicians. Retrieved March 6, 2009, from http://www.manhattanresearch.com/TTPWhitePaper.aspx

McLean, R., Richards, B., & Wardman, J. (2007). The effect of Web 2.0 on the future of medical practice and education: Darwikinian evolution or folksonomic revolution? *The Medical Journal of Australia, 187*(3), 174–177.

Mukherjee, A., & McGinnis, J. (2007). E-healthcare: an analysis of key themes in research. *International Journal of Pharmaceutical and Healthcare Marketing, 1*(4), 349–363. doi:10.1108/17506120710840170

Murray, C. J. L., & Frenk, J. (2000). A framework for assessing the performance of health systems. *Bulletin of the World Health Organization, 78*(6), 717–731.

Murray, C. J. L., Salomon, J. A., & Mathers, C. D. (2000). A critical examination of summary measures of population health. *Bulletin of the World Health Organization, 78*(8), 981–994.

Neuhauser, L., & Kreps, G. L. (2003). Rethinking communication in the e-health era. *Journal of Health Psychology, 8*(1), 7–22. doi:10.1177/1359105303008001426

Oh, H., Rizo, C., Enkin, M., & Jadad, A. (2005). What Is eHealth (3): A Systematic Review of Published Definitions. *Journal of Medical Internet Research, 7*(1), e1. Retrieved March 7, 2009, from http://www.jmir.org/2005/1/e1/

Øvretveit, J. (1998). *Evaluating health interventions*. London: Open University Press.

Potts, H. W. (2006). Is e-health progressing faster than e-health researchers? *Journal of Medical Internet Research, 8*(3), e23. Retrieved March 7, 2009, from http://www.jmir.org/2006/3/e23/

Raymond, E. (1999). *The Cathedral and the Bazaar*. Sebastapol, CA: O'Reilly Media.

Renahy, E., Parizot, I., & Chauvin, P. (2008). Health information seeking on the Internet: a double divide? Results from a representative survey in the Paris metropolitan area, France, 2005-2006. *BMC Public Health, Feb 21, 8*(1), 69.

Rogers, E. M. (2003). *Diffusion of innovations* (5th ed.). New York: Free Press.

Rotheram-Borus, M. J., & Flannery, N. D. (2004). Interventions that are CURRES: costeffective, useful, realistic, robust, evolving, and sustainable. In Rehmschmidt, H., Belfer, M., & Goodyer, I. M. (Eds.), *Facilitating pathways: care, treatment, and prevention in child and adolescent health*. New York: Springer.

Sandars, J., & Haythornthwaite, C. (2007). New horizons for e-learning in medical education: ecological and Web 2.0 perspectives. *Medical Teacher, 29*(4), 307–310. doi:10.1080/01421590601176406

Sandars, J., & Schroter, S. (2007). Web 2.0 technologies for undergraduate and postgraduate medical education: an online survey. *Postgraduate Medical Journal, 83*, 759–762. doi:10.1136/pgmj.2007.063123

Scott, R. E., & Saeed, A. (2008). Global eHealth–Measuring Outcomes: Why, What, and How. Report commissioned by WHO's Global Observatory for eHealth. Retrieved March 6, 2009, from http://www.eHealth-connection.org/files/conf-materials/Global%20eHealth%20-%20Measuring%20Outcomes_0.pdf

Shadish, W. R., Cook, T. D., & Campbell, D. T. (2002). *Experimental and quasiexperimental design for generalized causal inference*. Boston, MA: Houghton Mifflin.

Shaw, N. T. (2002, May). 'CHEATS': a generic information communication technology (ICT) evaluation framework. [PMID: 11922936]. *Computers in Biology and Medicine, 32*(3), 209–220. doi:10.1016/S0010-4825(02)00016-1

Skiba, D. J. (2006). Web 2.0: next great thing or just marketing hype? *Nursing Education Perspectives, 27*(4), 212–214.

Smedley, B. D., Stith, A. Y., & Nelson, A. R. (2003). *Unequal Treatment; Confronting Racial and Ethnic Disparities in Healthcare*. Washington, DC: National Academies Press.

Starfield, B. (2007). Pathways of influence on equity in health. *Social Science & Medicine, 64*(7), 1355–1362. doi:10.1016/j.socscimed.2006.11.027

Talmon, J., Ammenwerth, E., Brender, J., de Keizer, N., Nykänen, P., & Rigby, M. (2008). STARE-HI—Statement on reporting of evaluation studies in Health Informatics. *International Journal of Medical Informatics, 78*(1), 1. doi:10.1016/j.ijmedinf.2008.09.002

Tang, H., & Ng, J.H.K. (2006). Googling for a diagnosis – use of Google as a diagnostic aid: internet based study. *British Medical Journal, 2;333*(7579), 1143-1145.

Tanne, J. (2007). Google launches free Electronic Health Records service for patients. *British Medical Journal, 336*, 1207. doi:10.1136/bmj.a208

Ustinova, A. (2008). Developers compete at Facebook conference. San Francisco Chronicle. Retrieved March 7, 2009, from http://www.sfgate.com/cgi-bin/article.cgi?f=/c/a/2008/07/23/BU7C11TAES.DTL

Venkatesh, V., Morris, M. G., Davis, G. B., & Davis, F. D. (2003). User Acceptance of Information Technology: Toward a Unified View. *Management Information Systems Quarterly, 27*(3), 425–478.

Versel, N. (2008). Health 2.0. Will its promise be realized? *Managed Care (Langhorne, Pa.), 17*(3), 49–52.

Vimarlund, V., & Olve, N. G. (2005). Economic analyses for ICT in elderly healthcare: questions and challenges. *Health Informatics Journal, 11*(4), 309–321. doi:10.1177/1460458205058758

Walker, J., Pan, E., Johnston, D., Adler-Milstein, J., Bates, D. W., & Middleton, B. (2005). *The value of health care information exchange and interoperability. Health Affairs* (pp. W5-10–W5-18). Millwood: Web Exclusives.

Wangberg, S. C., Andreassen, H. K., Prokosch, H. U., Santana, S. M., Sørensen, T., & Chronaki, C. E. (2008). Relations between Internet use, socio-economic status (SES), social support and subjective health. *Health Promotion International, 23*(1), 70–77. doi:10.1093/heapro/dam039

Wen, J., & Tan, J. (2005). Mapping e-health strategies: thinking outside the traditional healthcare box. *International Journal of Electronic Healthcare, 1*(3), 261–276. doi:10.1504/IJEH.2005.006474

Wickramasinghe, N. S., & Fadlalla, A. M. A. (2005). A framework for assessing e-health preparedness. *International Journal of Electronic Healthcare, 1*(3), 316–334. doi:10.1504/IJEH.2005.006478

Wiklund, H., & Lindh, J. (2005). Development Without Strategy – the case of web-based health care services in Swedish city councils. *International Journal of Public Information Systems, 1*, 71–80.

Wilkinson, R.G. (1997). Socioeconomic determinants of health. Health inequalities: relative or absolute material standards? *British Medical Journal, 22;314*(7080), 591-5.

Wilkinson, R. G. (2007). Comment on: The changing relation between mortality and income. *International Journal of Epidemiology, 36*(3), 484–490. doi:10.1093/ije/dym077

ADDITIONAL READING

Andreassen, H., Bujnowska-Fedak, M., Chronaki, C., Dumitru, R., Pudule, I., & Santana, S. (2007). European citizens' use of E-health services: a study of seven countries. *BMC Public Health, 7*(1), 53. doi:10.1186/1471-2458-7-53

Atkinson, N., & Gold, R. (2002). The promise and challenge of eHealth interventions. *American Journal of Health Behavior*, *26*(6), 494–503.

Boulos, M. N. K., & Wheeler, S. (2007). The emerging Web 2.0 social software: an enabling suite of sociable technologies in health and health care education. *Health Information and Libraries Journal*, *24*, 2–23. doi:10.1111/j.1471-1842.2007.00701.x

Cabrera, M., Burgelman, J.C., Boden, M., da Costa, O., & Rodriguez, C. (2004*). eHealth in 2010: Realizing a Knowledge-based Approach to Healthcare in the EU – Challenges for the Ambient Care System. (*Report on eHealth related activities by IPTS). European Commission, Directorate-General, Joint Research Centre.

Curry, S. J. (2007). eHealth research and healthcare delivery beyond intervention effectiveness. *American Journal of Preventive Medicine*, *32*(5Suppl), S127–S130. doi:10.1016/j.amepre.2007.01.026

Economist, The. (2007). Health 2.0: Technology and society: Is the outbreak of cancer videos, bulimia blogs and other forms of "user generated" medical information a healthy trend? *The Economist*, September 6, 73-74

Eng, T. (2001). *The eHealth Landscape: A Terrain Map of Emerging Information and Communication Technologies in Health and Health Care*. Princeton, NJ: The Robert Wood Johnson Foundation.

European Commission Information Society and Media DG. Study on Economic Impact of e-Health. Retrieved from www.eHealth-impact.org

Eysenbach, G. (2001). What is e-health? *Journal of Medical Internet Research*, *3*(2), e20. doi:10.2196/jmir.3.2.e20

Ferguson, T. (2007). ePatients white paper. www.e-patients.net. Retrieved March 6, 2009, from http://www.e-patients.net/e-Patients_White_Paper.pdf on 22/1/08

Giustini, D. (2006). How Web 2.0 is changing medicine. *British Medical Journal, 23;333*(7582), 1283-1284.

Glasgow, R. E. (2007). eHealth evaluation and dissemination research. *American Journal of Preventive Medicine*, *32*(5Suppl), S119–S126. doi:10.1016/j.amepre.2007.01.023

Gustafson, D., & Wyatt, J. (2004). Evaluation of eHealth systems and services. *British Medical Journal*, *328*(7449), 1150. doi:10.1136/bmj.328.7449.1150

Hughes, B., Joshi, I., & Wareham, J. (2008). Medicine 2.0: Tensions and controversies in the field. *Journal of Medical Internet Research, 6;10*(3), e23.

McLean, R., Richards, B., & Wardman, J. (2007). The effect of Web 2.0 on the future of medical practice and education: Darwikinian evolution or folksonomic revolution? *The Medical Journal of Australia*, *187*(3), 174–177.

Parente, S. (•••). (200). Beyond the hype: A taxonomy of e-Health business models. *Health Affairs*, *19*(6), 89–102. doi:10.1377/hlthaff.19.6.89

Potts, H. W. (2006). Is e-health progressing faster than e-health researchers? *Journal of Medical Internet Research*, *8*(3), e23. doi:10.2196/jmir.8.3.e24

Skiba, D. J. (2006). Web 2.0: next great thing or just marketing hype? *Nursing Education Perspectives*, *27*(4), 212–214.

Versel, N. (2008). Health 2.0. Will its promise be realized? *Managed Care (Langhorne, Pa.)*, *17*(3), 49–52.

Wyatt, J., & Sullivan, F. (2005). eHealth and the future: promise or peril? *British Medical Journal, 331*(7529), 1391–1393. doi:10.1136/bmj.331.7529.1391

KEY TERMS AND DEFINITIONS

eHealth: The intersection of medical informatics, public health and business, referring to health services and information delivered or enhanced through the Internet and related technologies

eMedicine®: A point-of-care clinical reference features up-to-date, searchable, peer-reviewed medical articles organized in specialty-focused textbooks. eMedicine® is a rgistered trademark of theWebMD Health Corporation

Google Health®: A service for users to store and manage all your health information in one place. Google Health® is a trademark of Google Inc.

Health 2.0: As Medicine 2.0, but with a focus on the U.S. and commercial activity

ICT: Information and communications technology

Medicine 2.0: The use of a specific set of Web tools (blogs, Podcasts, tagging, search, wikis, etc) using principles of open source, generation of content by users, and the power of networks in order to personalize health care, collaborate, and promote health education. Medicine 2.0 is a registered trandemark of Gunther Eysenbach, MD, MPH.

Microsoft HealthVault®: A platform from to store and maintain health and fitness information Microsoft HealthVault® is a registered trademark of Microsoft Corporation.

Web 2.0: a second generation of web development and design, that aims to facilitate communication, secure information sharing, interoperability, and collaboration on the World Wide Web.

Wikipedia®: A free encyclopedia that anyone can edit. Wikipedia® is a registered trademark of the Wikimedia Foundation, Inc.

Chapter 17

Academic Family Health Teams:
Collaborative Lessons from the Far Flung North

David Topps
Northern Ontario School of Medicine, Canada

ABSTRACT

Working collaboratively, in widely distributed settings, poses unique challenges. The Academic Family Health Team, affiliated with the Northern Ontario School of Medicine, has had to adopt a wide variety of information sharing practices and collaborative software tools, in order to function effectively in such roles as clinicians, educators and researchers. Based on an ongoing action research model, this chapter describes approaches taken and lessons learned while developing the informatics infrastructure to support interprofessional practice. The author describes how common procedures and software tools can benefit from a Web 2.0 approach, comparing commercial and open-source aspects of possible solutions. Ubiquitous data access for point of care decision making is supported by integrating web services, mobile devices and multi-stream communications. Resource discovery is enabled by integrating information streams into the medical record, into wireless device interfaces and via clinical dashboards. Effective team collaboration is highly enhanced through such infrastructure support.

INTRODUCTION

Coming from a practice environment and an educational environment that has some unique features of Northern Ontario, our Academic Family Health Team is faced with the challenges of providing health care, teaching and learning in a highly distributed fashion. Because these activities are inherently spread across many locations and with many different groups, there is an even greater need than usual to work in a collaborative fashion, with a strong emphasis on effective and open information sharing. Prior to Web 2.0, this would have been extremely difficult, if not impossible. The author shares some of his team's experiences with such information systems and collaborative workflow tools, both from a practical and an action research perspective.

DOI: 10.4018/978-1-61520-777-0.ch017

Copyright © 2010, IGI Global. Copying or distributing in print or electronic forms without written permission of IGI Global is prohibited.

As primary health care and medical education both become more complex, it is likely that the majority of practitioners in this field will face these increasing challenges and the necessity of working effectively and collaboratively, both online and in person, with access to information at the point of care wherever it may be – ubiquitous health care. This chapter will lay out why such collaborative activities have been so important to the success of the team and provide examples of tools and approaches that we have found useful. While specific tools are mentioned as examples, it is more important for readers to look at the underlying principles and apply them to the rapidly changing world that they will encounter.

BACKGROUND

The importance of teamwork and collaboration in primary health care in today's increasingly complex health care systems cannot be over emphasized. The days of the solo general practitioner are dwindling. Many factors are driving this trend: the current fee structures and payment mechanisms are making solo practice increasingly less financially attractive; but the biggest driver is the overall increase in complexity in the health care system as a whole. Patients themselves are more complex – with an aging demographic and the increasing predominance of chronic disease and cancer care, each patient on average poses an increased range of problems to the practitioner. While it is wonderful that modern medicine provides a much broader and more sophisticated armamentarium of diagnostic and therapeutic tools from which the practitioner can select, the interplay of information and clinical choices again presents the practitioner with an increasingly complex scenario of options. Overriding all of this, spiraling healthcare costs and increasing fiscal pressures on the health care system as a whole drive a philosophy of "do more with less". There is less capacity within the system at any given time. As is distressingly evident from the long wait times encountered by any unfortunate who has visited a hospital emergency room, the system is being driven closer to the point of breakdown, and beyond, much of the time.

Governments in many jurisdictions are increasingly turning towards integrated health services with a strong emphasis on interprofessional teams. This is seen across Canada, with some interesting initiatives in the provinces of Alberta and Ontario. The province of Québec has already engaged with the concept of multidisciplinary health teams – their long experience with community health centers represents similar attempts at such health service rationalization. Other governments around the world have also generated some groundbreaking initiatives in the area of primary health care reform. In particular the United Kingdom, with several reforms and iterations of change in how the National Health Service is structured, has attempted to integrate and rationalize the provision of care by various bodies and organizations within the healthcare system. (Mohan, 1995)

In Ontario, the provincial government has also been through several iterations of primary health care teams with the formation of Family Health Networks, Family Health Groups, Family Health Teams, and latterly Family Health Organizations. The distinctions between these are mostly subtle to outsiders but the underlying payment and organizational structure of each arrangement can have profound effects on the overall nature of team collaboration. The fact that there have been so many iterations in such a short time suggests that the solution to finding an optimum collaborative team structure is not a simple one.

What is increasingly clear is that any effective solution is highly dependent on the development of efficient, effective and practical means of information exchange between teams, groups and individuals at all levels within the system (Bellamy & Connelly, 2009). Much has been written on this need for effective informatics support (Reid & Wagner, 2008). This chapter will focus on the emerging tools and technologies that provide opportunities for primary health care teams to function effectively, and on the factors that affect their adoption and uptake within the busy working lives of team members.

COLLABORATIVE CARE AND LEARNING WITH HEALTH 2.0 TOOLS

Issues, Controversies, Problems

To help provide you, the reader, with some sense of context upon which the findings and recommendations of this chapter are based, it might be helpful to briefly relate some of the author's experience in this area. Beginning with remote rural practice in a small isolated community in southern Alberta, the author experienced tight collaborative teamwork at its most quintessential. But two decades ago, with a small team that was entirely collocated, and with relatively simple information needs and resources, this was an essentially simple and feasible exercise. In the days before the Internet, when fax was still a novelty, there were few choices on how to gather and disseminate information. In moving through a variety of suburban and urban-based practice settings, and from there into full-time practice in an academic health science center, it was interesting to see how these various groups dealt with information exchange, delegation, coordination and teamwork. As could be guessed, generally as the group size increased, the ability to effectively manage information flow decreased.

The academic health science center in particular, with the parallel operation of 12 separate teaching pods across three separate teaching sites, became increasingly disconnected and prone to errors of information transfer. With multiple levels of trainees at any one time, differing practice styles, a constant turnover in staff and locums, and differing local administrative structures, there was little to be seen that could be called common practice.

This was recognized at the time – one particular measure that was implemented back then in an attempt to improve coordination of patient care information, and data for education and research purposes, was setting up an electronic medical record across the main family medicine teaching sites associated with the department. This was moderately successful in terms of local patient care within any one teaching site. One simple but glaringly obvious piece of evidence for this improvement was exemplified by the dramatic decrease in the number of daily phone calls from pharmacies about prescribing errors – this dropped from an average of 22 per day to less than five per day for the entire unit. (Topps, 2005)

On moving to Ontario, the author as part of his new portfolio became much more intimately involved with informatics both in the provision of primary health care and of medical education. This dovetailed with the government of Ontario's initiatives in primary health care reform and in particular with the formation of a local Family Health Team. Much of the following commentary on the potential tools and approaches for information sharing within a collaborative team environment in primary health care is based on the author's experiences with establishing education informatics at the Northern Ontario School of Medicine, and with establishing the informatics support for Academic Family Health Teams across Northern Ontario.

The Northern Ontario School of Medicine is the first new medical school in Canada in 35 years. Based in two main locations in Sudbury and Thunder Bay, with two host universities, Laurentian University and Lakehead University, the school's infrastructure has a broad geographic base. The school embraces a model of distributed medical education, and places its learners, both undergraduate and postgraduate, in community-based settings throughout the curriculum. The effective campus covers an area that is the size of France and Germany combined. All medical students are provided with laptops and the curriculum is entirely based on electronic media and web communications. It is important to note that e-learning is not an adjunct, as it is in most medical schools, but the primary means of information distribution at the school.

NOSM has a strong social accountability mandate, which is inherently laced into all the school's activities. Curricular themes have moved beyond the traditional biomedical aspects and encompass strong elements of northern rural and remote healthcare, professionalism and population health. NOSM's social mandate also recognizes the importance of introducing its learners to collaborative practice and interprofessional education and care. Two new initiatives at the school, the formation of Academic Family Health Teams, and the Interprofessional Education unit, emphasize NOSM's attention to this priority.

Looking at the educational needs of our learners, it is interesting to see the first signs of a generational change in study and learning styles. We are starting to see indications of more collaborative activity on learning, as predicted in Millennials Rising by Howe and Strauss (Howe & Strauss, 2000). Our students are much more concerned about success of the group, with a strong emphasis on mutual enhancement of overall performance, compared to their colleagues of yesteryear who regarded medical education as a highly competitive environment. This is a fortunate fit for NOSM's educational style which has much small group work and online activity.

Factors Affecting Collaborative Activity

There has been substantial work on the factors affecting team performance and individual performance in a team environment. O'Connor (2006) has described the extrinsic factors, such as reward structures, collective efficacy, social dilemmata, social identity, interdependence; and also intrinsic factors such as team size, individuals' identity, social status, commitment and desire to achieve,

as being key to overall team performance. Quinlan (2000) has described how team leadership, team structure and team goals significantly affect performance and collaboration. The social culture with respect to scholarly collaboration, work patterns and external activities plays an influential role. D'Amour et al (2005) have described the importance of interprofessional collaboration when trying to establish effective primary health care delivery and highlighted how little work has been done on how such collaborative activity is being facilitated.

San Martin-Rodriquez et al (2005) have described some of the elements found in successful health care teams but point out that there is little support for these positive determinants so far. Reid and Wagner (2008) in particular have highlighted how traditional information transfer methods are inadequate to support coordinated care. While data interoperability of electronic medical record systems will help in this regard, and is long overdue, this in itself will not be sufficient. Information systems and processes that support team work amongst primary health care workers are an essential factor but have had little study or support to date.

Solutions and Recommendations

In this section, we shall discuss how we have used various software applications and web services to support collaborative care and educational activities within our Academic Family Health Teams. The emphasis in this section is on how the group has used and benefited from such applications, with a series of small use case examples. It is not intended to be a generic review of current applications – in a rapidly changing field such as this, publishing timelines would make such a review quickly obsolete. When we do mention specific software examples, this is not intended to be an endorsement. Indeed, the reader will note that many of the applications mentioned are heavily Microsoft centric. This reflects our current working environment and the need for our back-end systems to connect to large Microsoft-based systems. However, in principle we espouse and pursue the philosophy of adopting the use of free and open-source software whenever possible.

It is not the intent of this chapter to delve into the debate of the merits of open-source software, compared to commercial off-the-shelf applications. We will note at this point that widespread collaboration does require that information systems from many organizations and areas can intercourse effectively. This is more readily achieved by adopting open standards and avoiding proprietary data formats. However, during our work so far in establishing software infrastructure to support our collaborative activities, we have generally found that many open-source software applications are not yet sufficiently mature to support our needs – hence the trend has been towards using commercial off-the-shelf applications. We are, however, finding that as these collaborative tools increasingly develop the ability to share data and services with each other, openness becomes essential and that these activities are becoming dominated by open source software – we anticipate that we will move more and more in this direction.

In supporting collaboration, the essential point of Web 2.0 is that software and web services support a greater degree of user to machine interactivity and also application to application interactivity. The importance of easy data interchange between disparate and somewhat autonomous systems cannot be over emphasized. A clear expression of such application to application interactivity is best seen in software mashups – these will be explored later in this chapter.

Groupware

Both teams and groups, when looking to improve teamwork and group collaboration, naturally look to an area of software called groupware. Commonly, this refers to personal information manager software that is designed specifically

to support group activities (although the term is now also used more widely to apply to any software that supports collaborative group activities). This includes group calendaring, shared contact management and to-do lists. Such applications are frequently tied into and use modified e-mail messaging as a means to communicate groupware items between group members. The most sophisticated of these support a very close integration of these components, with easy-to-use features that facilitate connecting actions with events so that meeting coordinators can link attendees, action items and deadlines. This item linking is seen in most personal information managers but the benefits are correspondingly greater when used consistently by the group as a whole.

This leads to the concept of the benefits of networking effects. It has been suggested, as in Metcalfe's law, (Gilder, 1993) that the value of the communications network is proportional to the square of the size of the network. Others have even suggested that, as in Reed's law, (Reed, 2009) the value of a network grows exponentially. However, the work of Odlyzko and Tilly (2005) shows that this is a significant overestimate and that the general value of communication network of size n grows like $n\ log(n)$ – this growth rate is still faster than linear growth but is much slower than the quadratic growth of Metcalfe's law. This common misconception may help explain some of the overestimates in the recent past of the benefits of the Web in general.

To turn now to a more specific use case that demonstrates how the use of groupware has significantly affected the effectiveness of our team, we will highlight the case of the confusion and miscommunication that surrounded introducing new members to complex and overlapping hospital call rotas. Prior to the introduction of a group calendar, call group members had simply been faxing updates to each other as to who is absent, who was following whose patients, and general availability updates. This had worked well, and was simple and convenient, at a time when the call group was small and all members worked full-time. However the introduction of new part-time and highly itinerant physicians to the call group created a situation where dissemination of the information was breaking down on multiple occasions. Changing to a common group calendar relieved much of this problem but still created issues of access to the information. Moreover, it was not reasonable to expect group members to frequently consult the calendar for recent changes.

XML and RSS feeds derived from calendar data, highlighting updates and new changes, provided the means to distribute this information to a variety of endpoints including e-mail, the team blog, and individual messaging systems. This suited the group of physicians much better, as they were able to customize the information flows according to their own personal workflows. Providing the calendar data in the open standard iCal format meant that users could access their calendar information from a variety of software clients including open-source applications and freeware such as Google Calendar™.

Team Site

The next measure that was introduced to improve team collaboration for the Academic Family Health Team was the establishment of an intranet website. After evaluating a number of excellent options, the team chose Microsoft SharePoint™ as a platform for its team sites. As mentioned above, this reflected a standing need to connect to other Microsoft systems, rather than the overall quality of the Microsoft product. The dominant feature in the selection of the software was ease-of-use for the end-user. Previous work at the medical school with other products that showed much greater sophistication and power demonstrated to us that such power was pointless – busy users, in the chaotic environment of a fully functioning medical clinic, do not take the time to study and learn the intricacies of a sophisticated system.

The SharePoint team site provided built-in options for the development of wikis, blogs, discussion boards and folders for file sharing. What turned out to be particularly attractive to our users in this particular team site interface was that actions were easy to perform and easy to find on the presentation page. This was noted not only by members of our Academic Family Health Team but also by several other teams which used the same team site server for their collaborative educational and research projects. There are currently 17 different team sites on this particular server, many of which are in very active use. Many participant groups have commented favorably on their preference for having a central repository for information, rather than having items serially distributed as e-mail attachments.

Shared Folders

The team site feature which most user groups use first when taking advantage of the collaborative tools is the shared folder. Shared network folders are not new and have been available to most units at NOSM for quite some time. However this particular variety of shared folder allows better descriptions of the folder contents but, more importantly, has a sophisticated internal version control system, with rollback to previous copies. This is all automatic and internal to the infrastructure and requires no user intervention, except when users wish to go back to previous versions of a document.

The folder capacity allows much bigger file sizes than are typically allowed as e-mail attachments. This has been a great boon to participants in our Pocketsnips project, who have been developing short educational videos. The ability to send around large multimedia files is essential to this group. Images that are centrally stored can be displayed as small thumbnails so that users do not have to download the large files in order to see the contents.

Figure 1. SharePoint team site for family health team

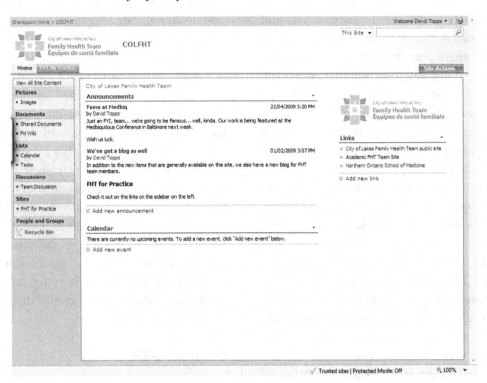

As Web 2.0 tools and services develop, we see increasing availability of vast cloud-based services with enormous storage capacities, trivial costs and ubiquitous accessibility. Amazon, Google and Microsoft now all provide access to such huge storage areas, along with many other providers. These have moved beyond simple storage and are now quite sophisticated in their ability to provide data concurrency, merging of offline changes and multi-site propagation of data. Some of these are particularly health related – Microsoft and Google both provide secure repositories attuned to individuals' needs. These Personal Health Records may be quite disruptive in their effects, and may have arisen out of the public's frustration with the inability of large organizations to provide integrated data sharing mechanisms for essential health care data.

But at a more local level, the interfaces to such file sharing mechanisms are becoming increasingly user friendly. Obscure network resource locators are often hidden from users. Immediate, real-time sharing of notes in a truly seamless manner is now available in such educational tools as Microsoft OneNote™. Open-source tools, based on open standards such as RSS and Atom feeds are also freely available but, so far, our Team has found that these are lacking in ease and utility compared to their commercial equivalents. In a hectic clinical environment, there is little tolerance for software quirkiness.

Wikis

The team site also has a very easy to use wiki. This has been particularly useful for our teams when they are constructing documents that have a very dynamic nature and where formal tracking of changes is not required. As with most wiki engines, rollback of changes to previous edits and versions is easily achieved. This particular factor encourages new users to get in and get their hands dirty, actively participating in collaborative editing because the team can reassure them that any unintended foul-ups are easily remedied and repaired.

Most participants particularly commented that it was reassuring to know that one was always working on the latest version of the draft and that they did not have to go back and search for competing changes or questions. For documentation that is rapidly changing and is largely for internal use, this is particularly attractive. Making use of the ability to notify users of changes with the use of RSS feeds or e-mail notification has also facilitated this process. The document owner no longer feels compelled to constantly go back to her website to see if changes have been posted. This simple convenience again makes integration of wiki activity into the workflows of busy group members much more feasible than with previous sharing mechanisms.

In collaborative healthcare, the ability to rapidly construct simple documentation in a lightweight and highly collaborative manner is a huge advantage. Our Academic Family Health Team has been using this for collective editing of internal recommendations and modifications to care pathways and clinical practice guidelines. The ability to link out to reference documentation from any point within the wiki text is particularly attractive and is very easy to achieve. Easy access to the central documentation from any clinic terminal, Web terminal or even mobile device has also been attractive and helps to encourage team members to make frequent use of this documentation.

One of the big challenges with implementation of clinical practice guidelines has related to the issues surrounding knowledge translation in general. Evidence-based practice has been shown in many fields and disciplines to have the potential to produce major improvements in the quality of healthcare and in the reduction of medical error (Amalberti & Leape, 2002; Bates et al., 2001). However, despite this commonly accepted premise, healthcare practitioners make little actual

use of clinical practice guidelines in their daily workflow (Bonetti et al., 2005; Ely, Burch, & Vinson, 1992). Our academic family Health team is actively exploring some of the communications and information transfer factors in play. It is anticipated that greater integration with the electronic medical record and with other information sources typically accessed during clinic workflows will help to streamline this process.

Blogs

Blogs have not been nearly as successful as a Web 2.0 tool to facilitate our collaboration activities in health care or in education. The reasons for this have not been clear and continue to be studied. After the initial enthusiasm at NOSM for blogging as a simple means of information distribution, there has been significant falloff in interest. Some of this may be due to local technical factors. A common issue appears to be that users are expecting to have to access the contents of the blog via its own originating website. The idea that RSS feeds can be incorporated into the viewing end point that is most convenient for the user has been slow to take off. A few NOSM users have grasped the idea that RSS feeds can be incorporated into their e-mail clients but this is not widely adopted.

In the wider world of continuing medical education, a few attempts have been made to initiate blogging activities. Again, the interest in this has been lukewarm. Informal conversations with experts in the field suggest that this premise may be a victim to the Gartner hype cycle (Fenn, 2009). Much emphasis has been placed in the recent past on the power and potential success of web portals. Much effort and money has been put into the development of web portals, particularly in the area of medicine. There are now many, many examples, with varied and rich content contained within each. However, this also exemplifies one of the pitfalls of the traditional Web 1.0 approach and the need for the user to separately visit each website, searching for these pearls of wisdom.

The Web 2.0 approach where information can be systematically, selectively and simply distilled into a variety of simple RSS feeds which can then be collected into a common viewing point has not yet been appreciated widely in the medical education community.

In order to ease adoption and acceptance of such Web 2.0 approaches, we are instituting local dashboards and customizable personal web pages that are similar in style to the approach taken by iGoogle™ and other customizable services. The ability to customize one's home page or other centralized service in a trivially easy manner provides great potential in helping users move towards simple integration of these information resources into their daily workflows. Furthermore, integration of RSS feeds and simple Web links such as these will also be easier for electronic medical record vendors to incorporate into their proprietary offerings. Such workflow integration is absolutely crucial in furthering the adoption of these information resources in busy clinical practice. A time interval as short as 30 seconds appears to be the limit of tolerance for busy clinicians when searching for patient related information. (Dawes & Sampson, 2003). Not only does there need to be one-stop shopping, there also needs to be one-click shopping, with that one click tied to the current patient and to the current presenting clinical condition.

There are a number of areas that we are investigating in our Academic Family Health Team weblogs, looking at the ability to provide a simple and easy publication mechanism for educational information. Firstly, we are looking at these as a simple means of patient education. Web-based patient education is not a new concept and has been generally very popular in the broader concept of generalized websites. However, apart from sites that are specifically advertising a particular commercial benefit or service, individual clinic websites are rare and tend to be poorly maintained after an initial burst of enthusiasm. This is a common phenomenon in the Web 1.0 world and is seen in most personal websites, not just in medical ones. It is difficult to keep up a steady flow of interesting information and small organizations do not have the resources or manpower to update their sites frequently enough to maintain the interest of their potential visitors. This is where blogging has several benefits.

The biggest overall advantage of blogging, as a distribution mechanism for small teams, offices and organizations, is that the information to be distributed does not have to be updated or refreshed on a frequent basis. If potential users are educated to the idea of incorporating feeds into their other activities, so that information in the form of blog posts are delivered automatically to their viewing end point without user intervention, this relieves the end-user of the need to actively seek out the information by visiting the portal or website that originated the information. Because of this, it matters far less as to whether information is distributed hourly, daily or even monthly. This simple premise may be obvious to those who actively and widely participate in the blogging world. However it has escaped the ken of most end-users – if this could be addressed, blogging as a means of publication of infrequently updated information could become much more popular and effective.

This is as much the case for patient education information from an individual clinic website. Our Academic Family Health Team has set up a blog feed that provides information such as local health news, public health and safety alerts, and local recommendations on activities that are specific to the local environs and to educational programs being conducted by the health team. The blog has been set up such that it allows easy contributions by any team member. There is no need for this information to be filtered through the bottleneck of an individual webmaster. By providing simple one-click "Publish This" access to the blog, team members can post items of interest within seconds, and importantly, can see the results of such a post immediately. This immediate feedback and confirmation should significantly reinforce such behaviors in a very positive manner.

In a similar manner, blogging has also been useful for staff education activities, both within the Academic Family Health Team, and within small user groups at NOSM. For Academic Family Health Team members, the accessibility of such a blog feed within their local workplace dashboard has been effective. We have been using this to publish current alerts such as infectious disease outbreak warnings; local updates on health programs; hospital and laboratory notifications. At NOSM, for general small-group educational use, we have linked our blogs to discussion feeds. This has the positive benefit that blog items can prompt further discussion, especially if they allude to a particularly current or hot topic. Such a connection has been popular with the medical students at NOSM.

Both for these discussion boards and for the blog streams themselves, users can view an RSS feed to see if there are any new posts or additional information. Again, this has the advantage that users do not need to repeatedly visit the initiating website but can rely on this automatic notification. User control over the degree and extent of notification is one of the factors that distinguish the Web 2.0 approach from earlier attempts at push delivery of Web information. "Active push" delivery was originally seen as being a great solution for information publication but the deluge of data produced quickly swamped most users. This is particularly true in health care, where the amount of new information available on daily basis is enormous, both for patients and for health care providers. Highly selective control over which feeds or which particular items of information are actively sent to the recipient's end point is an essential feature of Web 2.0 and helps to ameliorate the information overload suffered by most users.

Messaging

At NOSM and in our Academic Family Health Team, we have explored a number of methods to improve immediate communications within teams and groups. There are many situations within a busy clinic environment where the two commonest forms of rapid communication, e-mail and telephone, are inappropriate and do not work well. It is significantly disruptive to the client-caregiver interaction and relationship to be disturbed by telephone or pager interruptions. E-mail is neither sufficiently selective nor immediate for urgent and emergent issues. Of course, a simple knock on the clinic room door is quick and simple. However, as we have studied interprofessional interactions amongst team members, we have noted many examples of the need for communications where the balance between immediacy and intrusiveness is important but difficult to find. For example, a simple request to fetch additional items of equipment or easily accessible information is a very common occurrence during the workday.

There is a subtle distinction here regarding the intrusiveness of various forms of interruption and this is worth touching upon at this point, as we have seen this to be a key factor in facilitating interprofessional collaboration amongst busy team members. The form or method of interruptions that seems to work best, and is most appealing to both initiators and recipients of such interruptions, has the following features. The interruption needs to be sufficiently intrusive, but only just so, to be noticed by the recipient during conversation with the patient. Telephone ring tones and intercom buzzers demand immediate attention – this seems to be hardwired into our psyches. If the recipient does choose to ignore such an interruption, the effect is still mildly baffling and disruptive to the patient, who wonders why the caregiver is not answering the call. More subtle mechanisms such as screen pop-ups, where the user can control their placement, size, intrusiveness as well as the volume, tone and intrusiveness of any accompanying audio signal, provide the user with a much finer degree of control over factors that they find helpful or annoying.

Secondly, it is enormously helpful if the messaging system can quietly convey in a nonintrusive manner the scope or urgency of the topic at hand. In this way the recipient can choose between directing their attention to the message or to their patient. This choice, which is more satisfying to the recipient, is also very useful to the initiator of the message – they can "test the waters" to see if the caregiver is easily interruptible without fear of being annoying or intrusive.

There are now several communication mechanisms that provide such a degree of fine control over presence and intrusiveness. Instant Messaging (IM) is globally useful in this regard; the convenience features, touched on above, help explain some of the rising popularity of IM accounts. With particular regard to how such messaging mechanisms can be used within a clinical context, we have been analyzing three main mechanisms: public instant messaging (such as MSN messenger), secure instant messaging such as Windows Live Communications Server™, and the instant messaging systems that are built into the electronic medical record.

Public instant messaging systems have the advantage of being free, easy to access, and widely available. Given that our activities at NOSM and in our Academic Family Health Team are distributed across multiple nodes and sites, this simple means of communication has been popular amongst team members. However such systems are, by their nature, not at all secure. They are not suitable for discussing a topic that relates to specific patient information – we have been careful to advise and educate team members on such usage.

A more secure instant messaging service, such as Windows Live Communications Server, can provide the needed protection to facilitate patient specific discussions. However, the most common use of such patient related discussion also needs to be tied to information that is held in the electronic medical record. Because of this, it is usually easiest to then simply use the instant messaging system that is inbuilt within the electronic medical record. The latter also has the advantage that there is automatic logging and audit trails of the information flows, a feature that is required in some jurisdictions. Finding the balance in how these various instant messaging systems should be optimally used is not straightforward; moreover, it is consequent to individual preferences and local circumstances. We have found that it is generally more sensible to provide overall guidelines as to use rather than rigid restrictions – these latter are only applied where patient confidentiality is a concern.

One other feature that is inherent to some instant messaging systems is the mere indicator of Presence. This is of greater use when teams are geographically separated. However some of our team members have found that the user controls inherent to such systems are also an easy means of simply indicating whether they can be disturbed in any particular patient interaction – a simple electronic do-not-disturb sign. This notification of Presence can be automatically tied into other information flows. For example, Live Communications Server can automatically modify the user's Presence indicator according to categories within that user's calendar. So, if the user indicates on the calendar that they are engaged in an important meeting or consultation, this can in turn be disseminated automatically to various forms of Presence indicator. This is a proprietary feature within Microsoft Live Communications Server; however, there are also third-party tools which allow adaptation to a more open standards-based Web 2.0 approach. Our Academic Family Health Team is currently investigating the feasibility of connecting our patient scheduling system with business rules and an automatic indicator of general availability and Presence.

Mobile Devices

As access to the Internet becomes more and more widespread, even ubiquitous, healthcare providers are increasingly looking to have access to their most important information at the point of care. It has been demonstrated that the quick easy access to key data provided by mobile devices is a significant factor in their adoption, and despite some initial reticence about the impact that they might have on the client-caregiver interaction, concerns about intrusiveness were rapidly allayed (Topps, Thomas, & Crutcher, 2003; Topps, Evans, Khan, & Hays, 2004). Early mobile devices provided minimal Web connectivity and the few examples of this were fraught with problems. However, today's smart phones, which combine cell phone-based digital data services with the abilities of the personal digital assistants, are seeing broad acceptance in the health care provider community (Spyglass Group, 2006; Crounse, 2009).

Early concerns about the potential interference of radio frequencies with the function of certain medical devices have largely been refuted (Gilfor, 2004; Myerson & Mitchell, 2003). While such radiofrequency interference has been demonstrated technically, the actual degree of clinical significance has been greatly exaggerated. There remain a few critical clinical environments where the use of generic wireless devices is restricted, but most hospitals are now unconcerned about their use in general traffic areas. Many of the studies which did raise initial concerns did not pay attention to simple physical factors such as the inverse square law and transmission distance, or even whether the degree of interference had an actual impact on the clinical function of telemetry devices.

Mobile devices have been used extensively as data gathering tools in clinical practice. For educational purposes, their use remains quite common but there are extant concerns about the security of storing clinical data on devices that are very prone to being stolen or lost. Although on-device encryption would help with such security concerns, this is generally not considered adequate protection. Because of this, more organizations are looking for means of providing secure communications between the peripheral data-gathering device and the central data server. With database servers that are behind firewalls in a secure clinical environment, there are additional security concerns that such wireless access may open holes in such firewalls. Moreover, in the distributed medical education environment of NOSM, we have had to establish data communications for our wireless mobile devices in a wide variety of hospital settings, both small and large. Small community hospitals are more likely to have atypical firewall configurations and this can create configuration problems for learners and clinicians who are trying to connect to a central data service.

Data Synchronization

Initially we had some success in developing a reliable data synchronization service that was relatively immune to the vicissitudes of such firewalls. This success was based on our ability to utilize the common port 80 access for data transfer, along with a data replication system that minimized the amount of data transfer by simply synchronizing the deltas, or small chunks of actually changed data. Latterly, increasing security restrictions for wireless communications, and the widening variety of common operating systems seen in wireless mobile devices, have pressured us into adopting an entirely different approach. Proprietary data replication services, that are restricted in their availability of choice for operating system and platform, are no longer tenable in this changing environment. Accordingly, we have moved towards exploring a much more platform agnostic approach with XML-based web services at the core.

Adopting a web services approach has several advantages: using a common open standards-based communications format means that we are much less dependent on any particular software tool, database backend, or hardware device platform. It is important to remember that devices come and go but data is persistent. This also makes a better fit with our overall general philosophy regarding data interchange between disparate systems – web services provide us with a mechanism that is much less dependent on the underlying device or system at all levels of complexity. By changing the focus of our mobile device development to be consistent with web services, we will be able to take advantage of new developments in web services in larger systems and in other areas. Web services may be marginally less efficient in terms of the quantity of bits sent during any one transmission, but with falling costs for such communications, this is no longer of great concern.

Ubiquitous access to data has a number of advantages in healthcare education and in a collaborative team environment, such as our Academic Family Health Team. By encouraging our learners to "look it up" rather than memorize facts, and by providing them the means to simply access this information at the point of care, we have been more effective at moving them away from the philosophy of trivia addiction that seems to arise from an environment where educational assessment places more emphasis on fact retention than problem-solving. The half-life of medical knowledge is frequently stated at below five years (Emanuel, 1975) so that, by the time learners enter clinical practice, 50% or more of what they memorized is supposedly obsolete. Additionally, it is well known that our memories are notoriously unreliable for fine detail. It is important to move our learners towards the paradigm where it is better to be reminded or assisted with matters like drug dosing or intravenous infusion rates. Small numerical errors can produce catastrophic results and therefore constructing a culture of skepticism in one's ability to memorize becomes increasingly important.

Paging Doctor Smith

In today's fast-paced and complex clinical environment, especially where teamwork is concerned, ubiquitous access to personnel becomes almost as important as ubiquitous access to data. The increasing sophistication of our wireless mobile devices provides a greater degree of flexibility and control in how they are accessed. Firstly, many clinicians and are becoming tired of the "Batman Belt Syndrome" where they are festooned with multiple devices such as cell phone, pager, PDA and security dongle. These capabilities can now all be rolled into a single device, which produces less clutter, but also interesting capabilities in terms of integration of services. For example, rather than simple pager services which merely transmit a phone number but no indication of urgency or context, many sites are now making use of text messaging or other means of instant bidirectional messaging, thereby eliminating unnecessary steps in the communication process and providing more timely access to the appropriate provider or unit.

Improved integration of services means that a layer of sophistication can now be incorporated into the communications process. This ties into some of our earlier discussions about desktop-based instant messaging, intrusiveness and the effects of Presence. Many wireless communication devices now provide Profiles: preset groups of settings which affect the user's configuration of the device. Their use is widespread – we all expect our fellow patrons to use the "silent" Profile for our cell phones when enjoying a theater performance. In our development work at NOSM, we have been able to combine central calendaring, group communications, and these on-device Profiles. As a result, if a team member is engaged in a delicate surgical procedure, this is now reflected in the calendar booking. The group calendar conveys this information to the mobile device which then modifies its Profile so that calls are forwarded, or at least the ringer is turned off. We've also been able to modify the same mechanism for our team members who travel frequently in covering our distributed medical education environment. When flight bookings are recorded in the group calendar, with accurate start and finish times, this information is transmitted to the device which then in turn automatically modifies its Profile for flight operations so that wireless transmissions are turned on and off at the appropriate times without any user intervention required.

Location Based Services

Our unit has also been exploring the utility of location-based services with wireless mobile devices. The initial commercial excitement over this paradigm has thankfully waned and we are not, at present, overwhelmed with free offers from local coffee vendors. Moving beyond this somewhat limited concept, we have been exploring how Bluetooth proximity sensing, along with assisted GPS, can be used to provide a degree of accurate location awareness, even in an interior environment beyond clear line-of-sight to satellites. Many devices now provide such location awareness, even down to a micro level, detecting whether they are holstered or not, and can now modify their Profiles accordingly. Such location-based services are of great potential interest in a clinical environment: areas where wireless transmissions are of concern can now be protected by automatic turnoff of devices. At a less draconian level, devices can now modify their Profiles and Presence settings according to their location. This is easily modifiable on a user to user, case to case, or location to location basis – this is particularly important because of the concerns of most users when operating with devices that provide central awareness of location – that awkward, almost paranoid, feeling of Big Brother watching you. If the user can control the degree of location awareness and the degree of device response, there is likely to be greater acceptance.

Integration of such services provides different kinds of mashup. By pulling together disparate features, data, and information flows, new emergent properties and functions arise. By focusing on making these properties and data formats as exchangeable and nonproprietary as possible, similar interesting emergent functions will arise from the imaginations of "group think". Christo El Morr, in Chapter 13 of this book, on Mobile Virtual Communities deals with this issue in greater detail.

Education and Research in Primary Health Care

The newly emerging emphasis on teamwork in primary health care, with a move away from volume driven fee-for-service arrangements, has important implications for interprofessional education, care and quality assurance. Governments faced with rising fiscal costs for healthcare provision are increasingly turning to such measures. Redundancy of information gathering and inefficiencies in information transfer are rife in the healthcare industry. In a collaborative team environment, where team members are increasingly interdependent, such information flows are correspondingly of increasing importance. While much faith has been placed on the expected positive benefits of teamwork, little research or evaluation has been conducted on how such information flows help or hinder team collaboration. Our Academic Family Health Team, along with other such groups, has been very active in exploring such opportunities.

Medical education in particular requires much work in this area. Physicians typically receive very little training about team dynamics, group coordination, or effective teamwork; traditionally, they do not spend much time in group study. So, if we do not educate them in group activities, is it not unreasonable then to expect them to naturally indulge in group activities in the workplace? At NOSM, our undergraduate curriculum places much emphasis on small group work, professionalism and interprofessional care. With our focus on training physicians who will be able to effectively work in small communities, where teamwork is essential, this emphasis is of paramount importance. It is germane at this point to emphasize the difference between interprofessional and multidisciplinary care. In today's parlance, "interprofessional" places as much emphasis on how team members from different backgrounds and disciplines actually work together, respect each other's skills and contributions, and communicate effectively.

Communication within the group is of great importance but it is important not to forget the effects of excellent communication between groups, or the benefits of establishing communities of practice that have no relation to geography. Etienne Wenger's communities of practice (Wenger, 2002)(Wenger, 2002 ref_num1766) emphasize the importance of groups of individuals with a common interest or scope of practice. In his report, he discusses a number of tools that facilitate collaboration but these are largely Web 1.0 style (Wenger, 2001). In rural and remote clinical practice, this is particularly important – in our environs of northern Ontario, where geographic communities are widely separated, it can also be difficult for groups with common interests to become effectively established. Over the last 15 years, the availability of the Web and the improved communications that arise therefrom, have been hugely powerful and allowing groups, organizations and widely distributed teams to become established.

Web availability and the deluge of information have tended to create an overall worsening in the signal-to-noise ratio, such that the ability of such groups to form and collaborate has been lessened. The Web 2.0 approach to selective, collaborative, active data interchange between systems and groups provides an improved mechanism where group members retain greater control over their degree of participation and with whom they are

collaborating. The availability of cheap or even free web-based collaboration tools, desktop conferencing and data exchange services will help to renew activity within communities of practice that are spread thinly across the continent.

YouTube™ and PocketSnips

Ubiquitous access to data also applies to educational tools and resources. The use of multimedia in education is not a new concept but has previously been expensive to implement and difficult to distribute. Many an educational CD-ROM, after its enthusiastic initial reception, has been laying gathering dust on the clinic bookshelf. Even for those enthusiastic clinicians who are keen on such innovations, the actual use of such resources has been low, simply because the five minutes required to find said CD-ROM and play it on the relevant display screen has been beyond the workflow tolerance of the typical clinic set up. The explosion in popularity of concise, amusing videos on services like YouTube has led many groups to develop short digital videos of clinical procedures. Much of this activity has been driven by the easy availability of an effective distribution mechanism, with easy-to-use metadata tagging.

Our PocketSnips project has been highly successful in creating a library of such short educational videos. In the creation and production process, our team has made great use of many of the collaborative and communication tools discussed so far. Our SharePoint team site greatly accelerated the collaborative process of creating learning objectives, storyboards, video scripts and adjunct material. The quality of the subject matter was greatly strengthened by a strong peer review process which would not have been possible without these collaborative tools. Easy access to live collaborative editing in the wiki and in the shared folders was a significant factor in the rapid turnaround of high-quality content. The efficiencies afforded by this improved process significantly reduced our production costs:

Figure 2. PocketSnips site for short teaching videos

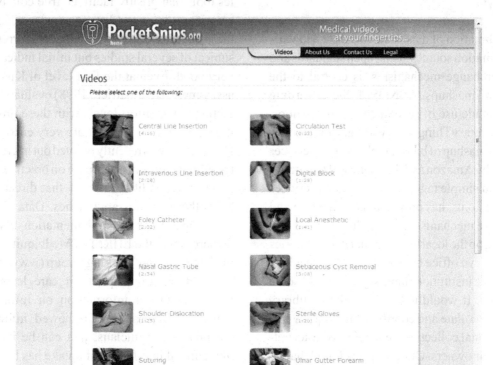

traditionally, high-quality video content had cost around $10,000 per finished minute; our process reduced this by a factor of 10.

Even with such greatly reduced costs, it is still expensive for any one school or organization to produce an extensive library that will meet all their educational needs. Because of this, our project team actively sought collaborative partnerships with other medical schools that were involved in similar projects. Such collaborative activity was further enhanced by the adoption of Creative Commons licensing (http://creativecommons. org/). Our collaborating groups have found this mechanism to be simple to implement and easy for content authors to understand. In particular, we have encouraged our authors to allow "share alike" permissions that greatly facilitate the repurposing of content. Such repurposing is an important factor in content sharing: just as it is unusual for colleagues to share complete and un-modified lectures or PowerPoints™, it is similarly

more helpful for groups to simply extract selected pieces from multimedia presentations rather than mindlessly copying the original whole.

In order to keep the videos short and the file size down, our PocketSnips team placed strong emphasis on the premise that not all content that is relevant to a procedure needs to be included in the video itself. Our distribution mechanism places relevant adjunct material in close proximity to each video, thereby cutting more than 50% on average from each video length. Placing such material outside the video frame also enabled us to easily internationalize the content – it is much cheaper to translate plain text than it is to re-record embedded narration. Furthermore, by avoiding head shots in our videos, it was much easier to synchronize narration with the underlying video frames which further reduces costs. It also allows easy internationalization because there is no need to synchronize moving lips with a different language.

Mashups

The combination of data from disparate and various information sources, using open standards and data interchange mechanisms, is central to the concept of mashups. At NOSM, the e-learning unit has made use of several common mashups. Firstly, LibraryThing (www.librarything.com), which is a mashup of bibliographic search services provided by Amazon and the Library of Congress, along with simple tagging and metadata services from del.icio.us, has provided us with a free and easy-to-use mechanism for coordinating and collaborating on the local holdings, not in our libraries but in our own office bookshelves. Most teachers in academic institutions have significant personal collections. It would not be feasible for library services to collate and coordinate the holdings in these personal collections, even if it were acceptable to their owners. Our group has found that by simply using this mashup service, we have been able to better share our collections, and to trace errant books when they are not returned.

Other interesting services that have been used by colleagues within our group include PubMed Faceoff (www.postgenomic.com/faces/index.php), SciFOAF (www.urbigene.com/foaf/), and various forms of location-based image sharing. It is particularly poignant to note that even companies like Adobe that have traditionally been highly proprietary in their approach to software development have explored the concept of mashups: their development laboratories have been experimenting with Notetaker™ which is a mashup of three open source tools. It will be interesting to see where this progresses over the coming years.

FUTURE RESEARCH DIRECTIONS

At a practical level, our Academic Family Health Team, and a number of our group projects, have benefited considerably from the new informat-ics tools that greatly facilitate true collaborative practice, even over a distance. Just to what extent these benefits have had an impact is currently the subject of several studies but initial indicators are very good. Even at the first level of Kirkpatrick assessment, (Kirkpatrick, 1998) evaluating satisfaction and comfort levels with these processes, the results received so far are very encouraging. However, as was recently pointed out in a review of the effectiveness of e-learning on practice, (Cook, 2009), there is little research that directly compares these various approaches. Data standards may help to improve implementation of Web 2.0 resources into the EHR. The Medbiquitous Point of Care Learning Working Group (www.medbiq.org/working_groups/point_of_care_learning) has some useful information on InfoButtons, a method of providing reviewed information resources for clinicians, that can be integrated into clinical interfaces but uptake has been slow. It will ultimately be ideal if we can demonstrate direct positive health outcomes from some of the approaches described above.

CONCLUSION

We have described our explorations of many of the Web 2.0 based services and tools that we have found useful in supporting collaborative care and teaching in our Academic Family Health Team environment. An essential factor in promoting the daily use of these tools has been the resource discovery and surfacing of the information sources. The focus has to be on making things easier and faster to achieve. The benefits of collaborative care are well documented but such collaboration cannot come with too many layers of organizational overhead or else all will be left aside. The complexity of the information exchange must reside somewhere in the overall system but is clearly most effective when hidden from the team participants themselves.

REFERENCES

Amalberti, R., & Leape, L. L. (2002). *How Hazardous is Healthcare*. Paper presented at the 5th Joint Quality in Health Care Symposium.

Bates, D. W., Cohen, M., Leape, L. L., Overhage, J. M., Shabot, M. M., & Sheridan, T. (2001). Reducing the frequency of errors in medicine using information technology. *Journal of the American Medical Informatics Association*, *8*(4), 299–308.

Bellamy, M., & Connelly, C. (2009). *NHS Connecting for Health*. Retrieved 11/02/09, from http://www.connectingforhealth.nhs.uk/.

Bonetti, D., Eccles, M., Johnston, M., Steen, N., Grimshaw, J., & Baker, R. (2005). Guiding the design and selection of interventions to influence the implementation of evidence-based practice: an experimental simulation of a complex intervention trial. *Social Science & Medicine*, *60*(9), 2135–2147. doi:10.1016/j.socscimed.2004.08.072

Cook, D. A. (2009). The failure of e-learning research to inform educational practice, and what we can do about it. *Medical Teacher*, *31*(2), 158–162. doi:10.1080/01421590802691393

Crounse, W. (2009, 2009/01/27). *The View on Mobile Solutions in Health*. Retrieved 11/2/09, from http://blogs.msdn.com/healthblog/archive/2009/01/27/the-view-on-mobile-solutions-in-health.aspx.

D'Amour, D., Ferrada-Videla, M., San Martin, R. L., & Beaulieu, M. D. (2005). The conceptual basis for interprofessional collaboration: core concepts and theoretical frameworks. *Journal of Interprofessional Care*, *19*(Suppl 1), 116–131. doi:10.1080/13561820500082529

Dawes, M., & Sampson, U. (2003). Knowledge management in clinical practice: a systematic review of information seeking behavior in physicians. *International Journal of Medical Informatics*, *71*(1), 9–15. doi:10.1016/S1386-5056(03)00023-6

Ely, J. W., Burch, R. J., & Vinson, D. C. (1992). The information needs of family physicians: case-specific clinical questions. *The Journal of Family Practice*, *35*(3), 265–269.

Emanuel, E. (1975). A half-life of 5 years. *Canadian Medical Association Journal*, *112*(5), 572.

Fenn, J. (2009, 2009/02/04). *Hype cycle - Wikipedia, the free encyclopedia*. Retrieved 11/02/09, from http://en.wikipedia.org/w/index.php?title=Hype_cycle&oldid=268502613.

Gilder, G. (1993, 2008/10/30). *Metcalfe's law - Wikipedia, the free encyclopedia*. Retrieved 11/02/09, from http://en.wikipedia.org/wiki/Metcalfe%http://en.wikipedia.org/w/index.php?title=Metcalfe%27s_law&oldid=248687837.

Gilfor, J. (2004). *Report on Electromagnetic Interference in Hospitals*, from http://www.pdacortex.com/EMI.htm.

Spyglass Consulting (2006). *Spyglass Studies the Current State of Mobile Communications Adoption by Clinicians*. Marietta, GA: Spyglass Consulting Group.

Howe, N., & Strauss, W. (2000). *Millennials Rising: The Next Great Generation*.

Kirkpatrick, D. (1998). *Evaluating Training Programs: The Four Levels*. San Francisco, CA: Berrett-Koehler.

Mohan, J. (1995). *A National Health Service?: The Restructuring of Health Care in Britain Since 1979*. St. Martin's Press.

Myerson, S. G., & Mitchell, A. R. (2003). Mobile phones in hospitals. *BMJ (Clinical Research Ed.)*, *326*(7387), 460–461. doi:10.1136/bmj.326.7387.460

O'Connor, M. (2006). A review of factors affecting individual performance in team environments. *Library Management*, *27*(3), 135–143. doi:10.1108/01435120610652888

Odlyzko, A., & Tilly, B. (2005). *A refutation of Metcalfe's Lawand a better estimate for the valueof networks and network interconnections*. Minneapolis, Minnesota, USA: University of Minnesota.

Quinlan, K. M., & Ã...kerlind, G. S. (2000). Factors affecting departmental peer collaboration for faculty development: Two cases in context. *Higher Education*, *40*(1), 23–52. doi:10.1023/A:1004096306094

Reed, D. (2009, 2009/01/27). *Reed's law - Wikipedia, the free encyclopedia*. Retrieved 11/02/09, from http://en.wikipedia.org/w/index.php?title=Reed%27s_law&oldid=266758174.

Reid, R. J., & Wagner, E. H. (2008). Strengthening primary care with better transfer of information. *Canadian Medical Association Journal*, *179*(10), 987–988. doi:10.1503/cmaj.081483

San Martin-Rodriguez, L., Beaulieu, M. D., D'Amour, D., & Ferrada-Videla, M. (2005). The determinants of successful collaboration: a review of theoretical and empirical studies. *J Interprof Care, 19*(Suppl 1)\, 132-147.

Topps, D. (2005). *Implementing an EMR across multiple academic family medicine teaching sites*. Calgary: University of Calgary.

Topps, D., Evans, R., Khan, L., & Hays, R. B. (2004). *Personal Digital Assistants in Vocational Training (Adobe PDF)*. Townsville, Queensland: James Cook University.

Topps, D., Thomas, R., & Crutcher, R. (2003). Introducing personal digital assistants to family physician teachers. *Family Medicine*, *35*(1), 55–59.

Wenger, E. (2001). *Etienne Wenger's 2001 study of technology for communities of practice*. Retrieved 11/2/09, from http://www.ewenger.com/tech/.

ADDITIONAL READING

Wenger, E., White, N., & Smith, J. (2009). *Digital Habitats: stewarding technology for communities*.

Section 4
Applications

Chapter 18
The K4Care Platform:
Design and Implementation

David Isern
Universitat Rovira i Virgili, Spain

David Sánchez
Universitat Rovira i Virgili, Spain

Albert Solé-Ribalta
Universitat Rovira i Virgili, Spain

Antonio Moreno
Universitat Rovira i Virgili, Spain

László Z. Varga
Hungarian Academy of Sciences, Hungary

ABSTRACT

This chapter describes the technological challenges faced during the design and implementation of the K4Care system, an agent-based Web-accessible platform that helps medical practitioners to deliver Home Care services in an efficient way. The system incorporates a Knowledge Layer, with an explicit representation of the required medico-organizational knowledge. The administrative and care actions are performed by the coordinated operation of intelligent agents, that represent the human users of the system. Users can access the platform by means of a Web interface. Several Web 2.0 technologies have been used in order to provide a rich interaction, putting an especial care on connecting the Web browser with the multi-agent system in an efficient manner. An intermediate Data Abstraction Layer has been incorporated in order to allow agents to transparently retrieve the appropriate knowledge when needed. The separation of the knowledge from its actual use has allowed the development of a very dynamic, flexible and adaptable system. The platform also includes several techniques to personalize the interaction with the user both from the visual and functional points of view.

DOI: 10.4018/978-1-61520-777-0.ch018

Copyright © 2010, IGI Global. Copying or distributing in print or electronic forms without written permission of IGI Global is prohibited.

INTRODUCTION

Health care usually involves complex and lengthy procedures, in which a large quantity of professionals with a wide range of expertise, knowledge, skills and abilities (from family doctors to medical specialists, nurses, laboratory technicians or social workers) have to co-ordinate efficiently their activities to provide the best possible care to patients. It has been argued that the standard properties of *multi-agent systems* (Wooldridge, 2002) (distributed nature, autonomous behaviour, dynamic problem solving and coordination techniques) fit with the usual characteristics of the problems in health care (Nealon & Moreno, 2003). A natural solution is to represent each of the human actors involved in the health care process with an *agent* that is responsible of the human's knowledge, the actions he/she is allowed to perform, the communication with other actors, and the access to the personal and medical data stored in an Electronic Healthcare Record.

The economic cost of institutionalised health care is one of the heaviest burdens in the budget of most developed countries. A possible way of reducing this cost is the improvement of *Home Care* (HC) services (Jones, *et al.*, 1999), the reason being that these services delay the arrival of patients to health care institutions, which are very resource-consuming. Studies like (Jones, *et al.*, 1999), (Landi, *et al.*, 2001), (Scuvee-Moreau, *et al.*, 2002) and (Kavanagh & Knapp, 2002) show the great difference between the cost of home care and the cost of hospital care. The typical home care patient (HCP) is an elderly patient, with co-morbid conditions and diseases, cognitive and/or physical impairment, functional loss from multiple disabilities, and impaired self-dependency (Campana, *et al.*, 2008). These patients require a continuous monitoring of their medical and social status, and a periodic follow-up and re-planning of personalised treatments. The use of ICT, as illustrated in the Web-based system described in this chapter, eases the access to the appropriate

knowledge by all the involved actors, and facilitates the co-ordination between them.

One of the main problems of the applications in health care is that they are usually designed ad-hoc for a very particular purpose in a specific health care organization, and that makes them rigid, inflexible and not easily extendible or re-usable. The aim of our work has been to make a Web-based platform that facilitates the management and delivery of Home Care services and that is designed in such a way that it can be easily adapted or tailored to accommodate the specific circumstances, resources and working methods of a particular home care centre. This requirement led to the strict separation of the medical and organizational knowledge, explicitly represented in different knowledge structures, from the way in which it is actually used to deliver the care services. Any change in the knowledge repositories automatically triggers the appropriate changes in the behaviours of the actors of the system. Therefore, the code of the system does not have to be changed at all in different instantiations of the platform.

This chapter presents a detailed description of the design, architecture, principal components and main technological challenges faced during the development of the *K4Care platform*, which has been developed within the European K4Care project. The system models a complex environment in a fully decentralized way, eases the management of Home Care services and is remotely accessible via a rich Web interface (based on several Web 2.0 technologies) by any of the users. All the different kinds of professionals involved in HC are considered in the K4Care model (Campana, *et al.*, 2008). The system adapts automatically to the personal profile of each user, allowing only the performance of actions related to the user's role. Moreover, the medical model (defined by means of a series of knowledge structures) is totally separated from the execution environment, defining a very flexible, modular and dynamic system that could be easily re-used in other health care assistance models. The basic pillar of the system's flexibility is the use of ontologies and agent technology (Wooldridge, 2002).

The rest of the chapter is organized as follows. First of all, a review of projects related to K4Care is presented. Then, the general three-layered architecture of the K4Care system is presented. After that, all the knowledge repositories included in the Knowledge Layer are described. The next section describes the upper layer of the system, the K4Care platform, and covers the multi-agent system and the Web interface, describing their interoperation. Then, the intermediate layer introduced to provide a transparent access to knowledge bases is presented. The following section explains the mechanisms that have been used to personalize the use of the system. Next, the security issues concerning the developed system and the implemented solutions are presented. Finally, the last section provides some conclusions and summarises the main contributions of the work.

RELATED WORK

The goals of clinical decision support systems are to deliver appropriate information and to integrate smoothly within a healthcare organization dynamics (Peleg & Tu, 2006). They require a formal knowledge representation and the integration of electronic health records, standard terminologies and messaging standards for exchanging clinical data. As proposed in K4Care, decentralising different elements in the careflow management is a point of view followed in related frameworks such as Arezzo (Sutton & Fox, 2003), DeGeL (Shahar, *et al.*, 2004) and NewGuide (Ciccarese, *et al.*, 2004).

Arezzo™ is a framework composed by several engines: a composer, a tester and a performer. The composer is used to create guidelines using PROforma as representation language (Peleg, *et al.*, 2003). The tester is used to test the guideline logic before deployment. The performer inference

engine can then run the guideline, taking into account data related to patients stored in an electronic medical record. Arezzo™ uses the Domino autonomous agent model (Fox, *et al.*, 2003). The model deals with a large class of medical problems and establishes a relationship between decision making and plan enactment procedures. The main goal of this model is to identify the main resources required in any language to represent clinical guidelines that can be used for both decision making and plan management.

DeGeL is a Web-based, modular and distributed architecture, which facilitates the gradual conversion of clinical guidelines from text to a formal representation in Asbru (Peleg, *et al.*, 2003). DeGeL contains a set of tools that support guideline classification, semantic mark-up, content-sensitive search, browsing, run-time application, and retrospective quality assessment. The system maintains a repository of guidelines, and it allows the user to search, browse, retrieve and visualise all available guidelines. The system uses different standards to represent the clinical information: LOINC-3 for observations and laboratory tests, ICD-9-CM for diagnosis codes, and CPT-4 for procedure codes (Lau & Shakib, 2005). The authors have designed some tools to solve different issues. A tool called Uruz allows practitioners or medical experts to create new medical guidelines. Another tool called IndexiGuide facilitates guideline retrieval. VisiGuide allows browsing and visualising guidelines. The run-time application, called Spock, incorporates an inference engine that can retrieve data stored in an EHR (Young & Shahar, 2005).

NewGuide is a framework for modelling and executing clinical practice guidelines that proposes the use of the Unified Medical Language System (UMLS (Lau & Shakib, 2005)) as a standard for terminology and a Medical Text Mark-up language called Guideline text mark-up for describing tasks within a guideline (Kumar, *et al.*, 2002). Guidelines are represented using a representation language called GUIDE, which is

Figure 1. K4Care platform architecture

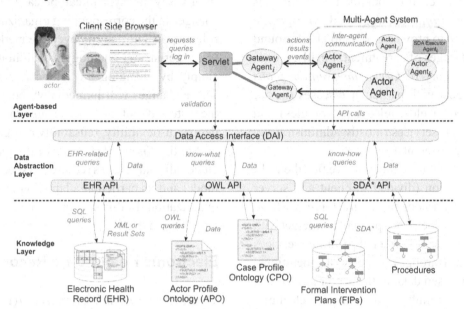

based on Petri Nets. It allows to model complex concurrent processes as well as temporal, data and hierarchical issues. GUIDE is integrated into a workflow management system which proposes an infrastructure that enables inter- and intra-organisational communication through a *Careflow Management System* that, on the basis of the available best practice medical knowledge, is able to coordinate the care provider's activities. The final goal of this architecture is to provide health care organizations with technical solutions which should enable them to improve process efficiency, outcomes and quality of care.

Summarising, the presented systems propose some kind of interfaces to separate the knowledge required during the enactment of a careflow procedure from its storage. However, these systems are designed as a decision support system that proposes some recommendations when some values are out of a particular range, whereas the K4Care platform goes a step forward and proposes an integrated system that reacts to some daily tasks performed by the users (practitioners), but also is acting autonomously in the background according to general rules of behaviour. The knowledge-

driven approach followed by K4Care also offers an added value over previous approaches, allowing to immediately adapt the system behaviour to changes on the medical organization.

GENERAL OVERVIEW OF THE K4CARE ARCHITECTURE

The K4Care platform offers a distributed implementation of the K4Care Home Care (HC) model (Campana, *et al.*, 2008). Its design is focused on decoupling the system's implementation from the knowledge structures which represent the HC model of a concrete organization. The architecture of the K4Care platform (shown in Figure 1) is divided in three main modules: the *Knowledge Layer*, the *Data Abstraction Layer*, and the *K4Care agent-based platform*.

At the bottom of the architecture we find the *Knowledge Layer* that includes all the data and knowledge sources required by the platform. It contains an *Electronic Health Record* subsystem that stores patient records with personal information, results of medical visits and ongoing treatments. This layer also contains two ontologies called *actor profile ontology* and *case profile ontology* used to provide a semantic background in different stages of a treatment. Finally, it contains a repository of *formal intervention plans* created to deal with particular diseases (in our case, centred in elder-related pathologies) and a collection of services (mostly administrative) delivered by different actors.

At the top of the architecture, we find the web-based application (divided in client and server sides). The client side permits an actor (*e.g.,* a head nurse, a family doctor or a patient) to interact with the platform executing a set of permitted services and accessing (through read and write operations) his/her authorised data. In the server side of this layer we find the multi-agent system which implements the system's execution logic. It contains a set of autonomous agents that represent all actors involved in healthcare activities and their associated behaviours. Representing human users, actor agents may have different roles through which they can execute different services.

Between the upper layer (that exploits medical knowledge and data) and the knowledge layer (that stores them), a set of middleware facilities called *Data Abstraction Layer* (DAL) provide independence between the knowledge representation and its use.

In the following sections all these elements will be described in detail, paying special attention to the technologies used to implement them.

KNOWLEDGE BASES

The K4Care platform presents a knowledge-driven design, which implies that its execution behaviour is guided by the knowledge available in several knowledge bases (Campana, *et al.*, 2008). Those sources model heterogeneous information about patient data, actor's skills and interactions, clinical guidelines, medical knowledge, and the procedural and organizational model of a particular centre.

In this way, the system can be easily adapted to changes in the corresponding organization, actor role responsibilities and even the medical scope (*e.g.,* geriatrics, oncology, rehabilitation, etc.) simply by changing the knowledge structures. Those changes will immediately be adopted by the system at runtime. This design provides a high degree of flexibility, reusability and generality.

So, the *Knowledge Layer* of the platform includes all data sources required to specify the HC model and its particular adaptation to a concrete organization. In this section, its components are described in detail.

Electronic Health-Care Record

The *Electronic Health-Care Record* (EHR) stores two kinds of data (Aubrecht, *et al.*, 2008). On the one hand, information related to actors registered in the system, like their personal data and persistent information such as ongoing treatments. These data are used by the platform during the initialization process in order to create and set the different agents associated to real health-care actors. This is stored in a standard SQL relational database incorporating a Java-based hibernate layer. With this approach, the EHR offers an efficient access to data and a minimization of the number of remote accesses to the physical database. On the other hand, it stores the medical record of concrete patients (*i.e.,* the results of tests, health-care processes, analysis, etc) in the form of XML documents. The use of XML representation eases the visualization, transformation and retrieval of -potentially complex- medical data (introduced by means of web formularies) using XLS transformations.

Medico-Organizational Ontologies

Services available in the K4Care platform describe what should be done in a particular point of a procedure. However, those structures require extra information in order to explain how they should be executed under the context (*i.e.*, geriatric, oncology, rehabilitation departments) defined by a healthcare organization. All this knowledge is modelled using the ontologies.

Ontologies are one of the most flexible and powerful models to express knowledge. They are defined as a formal and explicit specification of a shared conceptualization (Studer, *et al.*, 1998). In our case, they will be vehicles to both personalise the access to the K4Care platform and also describe the healthcare case to attend. Two ontologies have been designed: and application ontology called *Actor Profile Ontology*, and a domain ontology called *Case Profile Ontology*.

The *Actor Profile Ontology* (APO) represents the organizational knowledge of a healthcare centre (Casals, *et al.*, 2007). It models the relationships among services (such as patient admission, physical examination, etc), actions (such as a blood transfusion) and documents that store the

results of the tests, treatments or examinations (see the general class structure in Figure 2). Generic entities (actors such as Physician in Charge and groups of them, such as Evaluation Units) are also represented, specifying their skills and permissions. The APO is consulted in execution time in order to adapt the system's behaviour according to the profile of a particular actor which is logged in (*i.e.,* which services an actor may start, which actions he/she may execute, which documents he/she may read) and guide how a treatment should be executed (*i.e.*, who would be able to execute a delegated action, which document should be filled-out, etc.). In this manner, the user's interaction with the system and the healthcare workflow is transparently guided by the knowledge stored in the APO.

The *Case Profile Ontology* (CPO) models the knowledge of a medical sub domain in which the healthcare of an organization or care unit is framed

Figure 2. Actor profile ontology general design

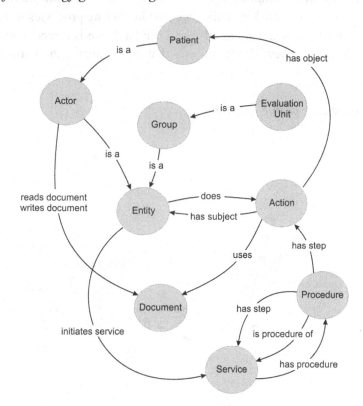

(Riaño, *et al.*, 2009). In the K4Care project, the context is defined by syndromes of cognitive impairment and immobility in the home care service. The CPO, as shown in Figure 3, includes medical terms (syndromes, symptoms, diseases, assessment tests, clinical interventions, laboratory analysis, and social issues) and the relationships among them (*e.g.*, the diseases included in a certain syndrome, the symptoms of a disease, the interventions for a disease or syndrome or the assessment of a set of symptoms). Medical data of this ontology are used to pre-fill or assist the composition of documents associated to a healthcare procedure. They are also used to detect interactions between syndromes, diseases and treatments that a patient may suffer. This information is proactively presented to the practitioner in order to provide assistance during the healthcare process.

Since the advantage of the ontological representation is to be machine readable, the contents of both ontologies are encoded in a standard ontological language: Ontology Web Language (OWL) (W3C, 2004). The definition of both ontologies is the result of the collaboration of a panel of medical and social experts in the field of geriatrics and Home Care, from both old and new European countries, and knowledge engineers. In this manner we ensure the adherence of the modelled HC to the European healthcare model and its logical coherence from the ontological point of view. The Ontological Engineering process (Gómez-Pérez, *et al.*, 2004) was based on the guidelines proposed by the On-To-Knowledge methodology (Staab, *et al.*, 2001). It is focused in the creation of ontologies to improve knowledge management in large and distributed organizations. Through an iterative process composed by five steps (feasibility study, kick-off, refinement, evaluation and maintenance), it allowed to identify hidden and non-trivial inconsistencies or redundancies or incomplete definitions. This helped the experts to elicit as much implicit knowledge as possible and to correct deficiencies in the model.

Intervention Plans and Procedures

The K4Care knowledge layer incorporates two databases with procedural knowledge. They indicate the main steps to be followed during administrative and healthcare processes in a structured way.

First, there is a repository of the *procedures* that implement administrative services (*e.g.*,

Figure 3. Overview of the case profile ontology

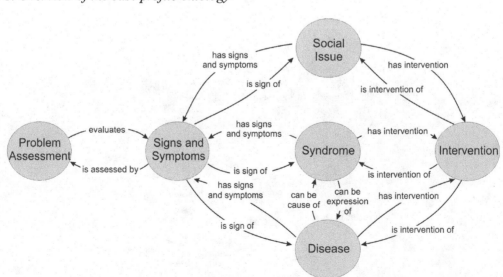

patient admission, discharge, actor assignment, etc.). Next, there is a store of *Formal Intervention Plans* (FIPs) which are general descriptions, usually defined by international care organizations, of the way in which a particular pathology should be treated (*e.g.,* hypertension, anaemia, etc.). FIPs may be related to a *syndrome* (*e.g.,* cognitive impairment), a *symptom* (*e.g.,* abdominal pain) or a *disease* (*e.g.,* dementia). However, a patient may suffer from several of these conditions; thus, the recommendations made by several FIPs must be taken into account to construct an *Individual Intervention Plan* (IIP). The IIP indicates the personalised care actions to be applied on a specific patient (Isern, *et al.*, 2008).

Both structures, which are very similar to clinical guidelines (Fox & Das, 2000), are expressed in a formal notation called *States-Decisions-Actions* (SDA*). SDA* is a flowchart-based representation of clinical guidelines. It is especially suitable to represent the procedural knowledge defined in the K4Care model and it provides several advantages over other languages, such as its intuitiveness and support for temporal constraints (Riaño, 2007). As shown in Figure 4, an SDA* stores three types of variables:

- *States:* determine the condition of the patient at a certain stage (*e.g.,* a patient with chronic kidney disease).

Figure 4. SDA* flowchart for the treatment of hypertension

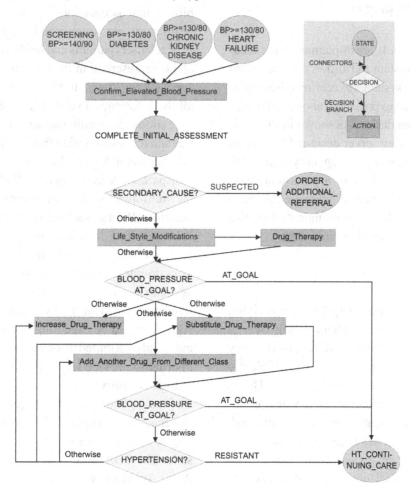

- *Decisions*: are required by medical experts to choose among alternative medical, surgical, clinical or management actions within a treatment. A decision contains a set of logical conditions that should be evaluated before proceeding. Some of the values required can be retrieved from the patient's record (*e.g.,* the last value of the patient's blood pressure), but others should be entered by the practitioner during the medical visit (*e.g.,* consider a secondary cause of hypertension).
- *Actions:* represent the medical, surgical, clinical or management actions that may appear within a treatment (*e.g.,* define or change a drug therapy).

K4CARE PLATFORM

The upper layer of K4Care implements the execution logic of the system and allows the interaction with the user. The system's execution relies on the knowledge structures presented above, offering a knowledge-driven design. As shown in Figure 1, it incorporates a Web server designed to interact with the final user and a multi-agent system which models real world actors in a persistent manner. A specially designed middleware has been implemented in order to communicate the Web side with the agent-based environment.

Multi-Agent System

Agents are active entities capable of perceiving their external environment and acting over it (Wooldridge, 2002). In the K4Care project, they exchange knowledge and co-ordinate efficiently their activities to deliver the HC services. This is a core idea in modern computing, where cooperation and communication are heavily stressed. The agent paradigm advances the modelling of technological systems, as agents embody a stronger and more natural notion of autonomy and control than objects. More generally, Multi-Agent Systems (MAS) (Wooldridge, 2002) provide several advantages in comparison to classical software paradigms when dealing with complex distributed environments like healthcare, such as modularity, flexibility and decentralization (Isern, *et al.,* 2010b).

The main goal of the K4Care MAS is to co-ordinate the activities enclosed in administrative procedures and Individual Intervention Plans between all involved actors. Agents act semi-autonomously, in the sense that several actions, such as exchange of information, collection of heterogeneous data concerning a patient (results, current treatment, next recommended step, past history), or the management of pending actions, are performed by agents without supervision, but others that may have some degree of responsibility (such as decisions taken in the process of healthcare), are supervised by users.

Each user (patients and healthcare professionals) is represented in the system by a permanent agent (*Actor Agents* in Figure 1). Each one owns all the information related to its current service executions and pending actions and manages queries and requests coming from the associated user or other Actor Agents. In order to provide access transparency to end users, the Web interface and the multi-agent system are connected by a bridge constituted by a servlet and a *Gateway Agent* (GA). When an actor logs into the system, the servlet creates a Gateway Agent whose mission is to keep a one-to-one connectivity with the corresponding agent. In this manner, the Actor Agent's execution is independent of the user's location. Ideally, Actor Agents should be executing in a secure environment and distributed through a computer network in order to provide load balancing in conditions of high concurrency.

Finally, *SDA* Executor Agents* (SDA-Es) allow enacting a care plan by recommending the next step to follow according to the patient's current state. The SDA-E is dynamically created by an Actor Agent in order to enact a SDA* structure corresponding to a healthcare process (like an Individual Intervention Plan) or to a management procedure. The SDA-E agent, after loading a SDA* from the repository, is ready to receive queries about its execution. Those queries are performed by the Actor Agent in order to know the next step to follow; meanwhile, the SDA-E stores the current state of the SDA* and the results (documents) of the finished tasks.

In any transition, the SDA-E can send to the Actor Agent the information related to an *action*, a *decision*, or a *state*. In the case of an action, the Actor Agent should contact the role responsible for performing the action. The responsible role (a type of actor which is able to perform the action) is retrieved from the APO. Then, the Actor Agent looks for an Actor Agent which matches the required role. Usually, the final assignment of an action to a concrete user requires his/her acceptance. All the requested tasks are queued to the user's pending tasks, stored in his/her Actor Agent and shown to the user when he/she logs into the system. If the SDA-E informs that the next stage contains a *decision*, all branches and their embedded logical conditions are presented to the user, who selects the most appropriate one (according the previous actions or the patient's EHR). Finally, the last possibility is the existence of *states* that play the role of check points during the whole plan. The interested reader may find a more detailed explanation of how the agents coordinate their activities to execute an Individual Intervention Plan in (Isern, *et al.*, 2008).

All agent functionalities are implemented over communication protocols and share a common knowledge representation (modelled by ontologies). Mainly, agents use two well-known protocols: FIPA-Request and FIPA-Contract Net, and also have an internal ontology to represent all exchanged data (FIPA, 2002). The MAS has been implemented with the JADE tool, which is compliant with the FIPA specification for agent development (Bellifemine, *et al.*, 2007).

Web Server and User Front-End

The final component of the K4Care upper layer is a Web interface which allows the interaction of the final users with the system. Considering the requirements of mobility, home care and remote access of the target users (both patients and practitioners) of the K4Care front end, its design should fulfil the following conditions: simple installation, simple configuration, fast access and, finally, an intuitive interaction.

The Web interface has been designed to provide to the user the same level of functionality of a usual desktop application, without software or hardware requirements, but with the intuitiveness, simplicity and smooth learning curve of Web applications; to this end, *Rich Internet Applications* (RIA) concepts have been applied (Holdener III, 2008). The RIA Web interface architecture is Web-efficient: the application is fully loaded at the client side when a user accesses the Web interface for the first time, and the same application/page persists until the user leaves the page. Therefore, just dynamic information is queried to the server and, moreover, this information is just requested when needed or required by the user. This behaviour improves the performance and response time of the system because the information that is not needed is never transmitted.

One of the most powerful technologies to implement RIA applications, using a standard Web browser, is the use of the *XMLHttpRequest* JavaScript object (commonly known as AJAX - *Asynchronous JavaScript and XML*-). This object provides the ability to perform asynchronous calls to the server, what allows the browser to continue executing code while the query is processed and avoiding interruptions of other running tasks. The K4Care front-end is updated (*e.g.,* pop-up windows, menu bars, visualization of documents, etc.) in real time using this object, without doing continuous requests for new information. This avoids the waste of network resources and improves the performance of the system.

In addition to those technologies, the K4Care client side, embedded into a standard Web browser, has been fully developed using *JavaScript*. K4Care also offers a mechanism to add new functionalities, programmed over browser plug-ins (*e.g.,* Java applets or Flash interfaces), when *JavaScript* is not rich enough to provide them. An example of those components is the *IIP Editor*, an applet (shown in Figure 5) which allows actors to graphically construct/edit/modify/join FIP/IIP SDA*-compliant diagrams when needed. In this way, the K4Care system represents a complete and integrated framework where the user can work without other applications.

In addition, due to the heterogeneous nature of the K4Care users, the Web interface supports the personalizing the look and feel. In this manner, the kind of information and the way in which it is presented can be tailored according to the expected skills and knowledge of the current user. This is based on the use of *CSS style sheets*.

So, it can be adapted to elder people, who often have some kind of disability and it can be used to show only the actions associated to the role of the logged user.

K4Care defines three different CSSs for patients, head nurses and the rest of practitioners. As the typical patients of K4Care are elderly and disabled citizens, the interface presented in this case gives a very simple and reduced view of the information, employing easily readable characters, big sizes and easily understandable terminology. In the case of head nurses, the interface is focused on allowing an easy access to administrative functions related with the supervision of medical services and acknowledgments of actors to pending tasks. Finally, in the case of practitioners, the interface offers particular shortcuts to medical services regarding the creation of individual intervention plans and the inclusion of the results of medical visits into the patient's health record.

Figure 5. Web-based visual editor of individual intervention plans

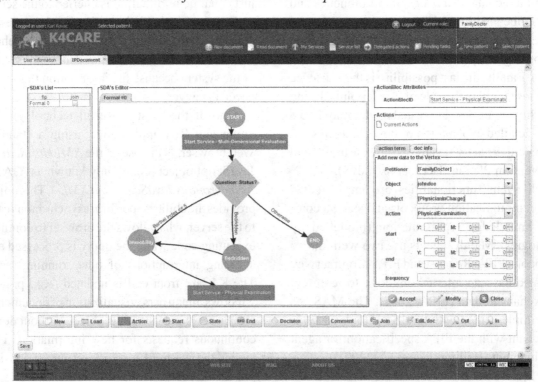

Considering that one of the aims of K4Care project is to present an infrastructure that can be adapted to communities and countries all around Europe, different languages and character sets are also supported by the Web interface. All the information visualized is stored as keys in dictionary files which provide translations to several languages. So, before logging-in, the user may select between the languages which are currently supported: English, Spanish, Catalan, Italian and Hungarian.

The last aspect of the interface adaptation regards the way in which EHR related information is visualized. As different organizations may use different formats for storing clinical data, we opted, as introduced before for storing all this information by means of standard XML documents. In this manner, the interaction format of those documents (both for visualization and data introduction) may be decoupled from the data storage. Therefore, it is possible to configure the rendering of documents for concrete organizations or a type of users by using XSL style sheets which define *how* and *which* data are visualised.

Data Flow between the User and His/Her Actor Agent

Actor Agents represent real users in the platform. So, as the user interacts with the system by means of a Web application, a communication channel should be established between the Web context and the Multi-Agent System. As those are completely independent environments (running on different Java Virtual Machines, one for the Web server and another one for the JADE framework), we have introduced an intermediate layer which acts as a gateway.

In more detail, the data flow between the user and the MAS passes through three layers (see Figure 6): Client layer (*i.e.*, Web browser or front end), Servlet layer (*i.e.*, Web server), and a Gateway layer (special agent embedded in the MAS). This process defines two different and parallel channels of communication: the first one for synchronous messages and second one for asynchronous messages, both shown on Figure 6.

The interaction between the Servlet layer and the Gateway Agent layer is one of the cores of the architecture, since it is able to adapt the protocols between the client side (HTTPS requests) and the MAS (FIPA-compliant messages).

Client Layer

As mentioned above, the client layer consists on a Web browser from which the user interacts with the system. K4Care exploits Web 2.0 possibilities using use of the latest technologies like AJAX, CSS and *JavaScript*.

Servlet Layer

The Servlet layer, based on an HTTP server (in our case Apache Tomcat 6.0), is responsible for receiving secured HTTPS requests in both synchronous

Figure 6. Front-end, multi-agent system workflow architecture

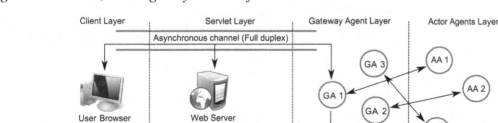

and asynchronous ways (more on this later). The Servlet reads and interprets the HTTPS requests (Get or Post) which are sent to the Gateway Agent (GA). It also deals with the answer returned by the GA. The response for the HTTPS request is always returned to the front end in XML format. This standard codification allows other systems (different from a Web browser) to connect and work together with the K4Care core. Therefore, the system can easily incorporate add-ons using XML as message codification.

Gateway Agent Layer

The Gateway Agent layer consists of a group of agents which are used as a bridge between the Servlet Layer and the Actor Agents Layer (see Figure 7). The GA must be used in order to gener-ate FIPA-compliant messages because the Servlet layer is not embedded inside the multi-agent ex-ecution runtime (JADE-based framework).

In this architecture, the GA has two main responsibilities. The first one is to codify and send FIPA compliant messages. These messages are constructed using the information that lower layers provide, and a given Agent communication ontology. The second responsibility is to receive, interpret and forward FIPA messages from Actor Agents to the Servlet.

In our system, each Actor Agent is associated with a unique Gateway Agent. However, this GA is only alive when the user is logged in. Till disconnection, the GA acts as a bridge between the Servlet and the Actor Agent. When the user logs off, the GA is useless; therefore, in order to free resources, it is removed from the MAS. A

Figure 7. Brower-agents message protocol

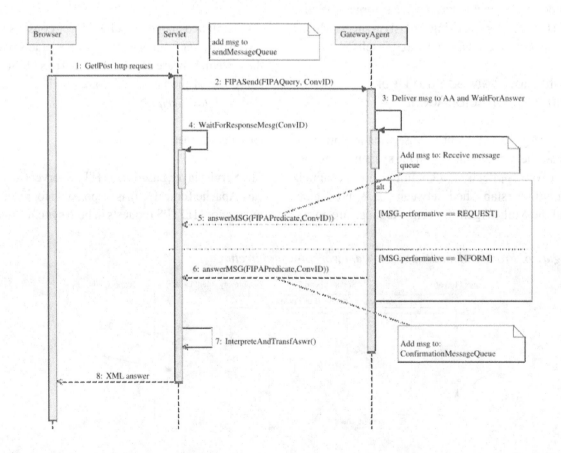

new GA will be created the next time the user logs into the system.

All the messages that the GA sends/receives to/from the MAS are defined in the communication *ontology*, giving a well detailed communication interface between both layers.

Traffic Workflow Adaptation

Each of the layers that compose the K4Care front-end architecture has a different communication protocol; therefore an adaptation of messages that travel from the Web browser to the MAS is needed.

In order to achieve a standard communication among browser and Servlet layers, XML has been chosen as the data codification for the transmitted information. Each message is encoded using a previously defined format that indicates to the server the operation to be made and the result that must be returned. Those messages can be distinguished depending on their purpose, in two types: *synchronous* and *asynchronous*. *Synchronous* messages are defined as standard query messages, that is, the front-end queries information to the server and the server returns a response. On the other hand, with *asynchronous* messages, the server informs the Web browser that has new information for the user. Synchronous traffic is addressed to messages that don't need much time to be processed, and asynchronous traffic is addressed to messages that will take a long time to be responded or processed. This second type of traffic is used to update the Web interface in real time (*i.e.,* inform about new messages or pending actions to be executed).

Both channels follow the same workflow until the GA, as shown in Figure 7. At first, the browser calls an HTTP request to the servlet, providing some parameters which indicate the operation to do (step 1). The servlet interprets these parameters and "conceptually" initiates a new FIPA compliant communicative act (identified using an ID). After the Servlet Layer has processed and sent

the message to the GA (step 2), the GA forwards it to the AAs (step 3).

Then, for the synchronous channel (being full-duplex), the browser sends information to the AAs, and those return a response to the browser. In this case, step 4 from Figure 7 will be quickly generated leaving, in this way, one browser communication call always available to use.

For the asynchronous channel (being half-duplex), the information just travels from the AAs to the browser. In this case, step 4 from Figure 7 will take a while to be responded; specifically, as long as the actors don't have any real time information to transmit to the browser.

It is worth to say that steps 3 and 4 from Figure 7 are designed and developed to be blocking calls, therefore they are just blocked while waiting for new messages to arrive. These blocking processes do not consume CPU time, only memory.

For the last intra-layer interaction, from the Gateway Agent to the MAS, the communication is defined using FIPA messages, the standard agent communication protocol.

This entire communication framework is designed to allow the Web browser to send messages to a multi-agent system and backwards in an efficient way, where neither continuous requests are made to the Web server to request new information nor the network performance is degraded because of the great amount of transmitted information.

DATA ABSTRACTION LAYER

The K4Care knowledge bases guide the execution behaviour of the multi-agent system. So, agents have to access the different data sources at runtime in order to retrieve medical and organizational knowledge, patient's EHR or clinical guidelines. These data are distributed in several sources and encoded in different formats (XML documents, SQL data base, OWL ontologies, SDA* FIPs). This multiple language representation makes the accessing, retrieval and interpretation of the data a difficult process.

In order to tackle this problem, a last component is introduced in the K4Care platform: the *Data Abstraction Layer* (DAL) (Batet, *et al.*, 2007). Its main functions are: *1)* to understand the different languages used to represent the data and *2)* to know where the knowledge is located. It provides a set of Java methods that allow the K4Care agents to retrieve the data and knowledge they need to perform their duties in a transparent manner. It is composed by different *Application Programming Interfaces* (APIs) and a general framework called *Data Access Interface* (DAI), which works as a bridge between the knowledge stored in a particular place and the rest of the system. It incorporates functions to translate data of different knowledge sources into Java objects required by the multi-agent system. It also has an active role, as it is in charge of controlling the access to the different data sources according to the user's role, it prepares the forms for the data to be displayed into the Web browser and it combines information from different sources to give a unique answer to high-level queries.

The different APIs which compose the DAL are the following: the EHR API allows accessing the actors' administrative data and the clinical record by means of SQL queries and XML document retrieval; the SDA API is able to interpret the knowledge stored in FIPs and procedures, expressed in the SDA* notation; and the APO and CPO APIs are able to consult the knowledge contained in the ontologies by means of an OWL wrapper.

PERSONALIZATION

Due to the heterogeneous nature of the K4Care user (from an elderly patient to several types of doctors and practitioners from different organizations), an important aspect of the K4Care platform design is the personalization of the user's interaction. This covers commented aspects regarding the interface, document data visualization and also the system's functionality and behaviour, both for administrative procedures and the enactment of healthcare processes. This last aspect is tackled by the definition and execution of Individual Intervention Plans (as presented previously). This is a very complex matter which is beyond the scope of this chapter (more details can be found in (Campana, *et al.*, 2008) and (Isern, *et al.*, 2010a)).

In this section, we cover the details of the personalization, covering the system's adaptation to a particular organization and the tailoring of the skills and duties associated to the profile of a professional actor.

As previously introduced, K4Care agents incorporate the knowledge contained in the APO to guide their execution and simulate the behaviour of a real institution. With this approach, the APO makes the system scalable and adaptable even to evaluation of healthcare management policies that the APO may capture in the future. This knowledge can be continuously updated and the system will automatically and seamlessly adapt to new laws, norms or ways of doing with a null re-programming effort. New care units or actors (with their corresponding interrelations) can be incorporated into the APO in order to adapt K4Care to concrete healthcare organizations.

Going even further, adaptability may support personalization capabilities at an individual level. In our case, personalization of the system interaction at a user or profile level can take advantage of the APO. From a technical point of view, the personalization can be done by tailoring the APO (Batet, *et al.*, 2008). This consists in creating a local copy of the ontology with a partial view of the APO especially adapted to the user's requirements. Then, the personal agent will use this modified ontology instead of the general one to act according to the individually modelled user's profile. This is a transparent process which can be executed at runtime and results in immediate changes in the system's behaviour.

For example, Doctor Smith, as a Family Doctor, may decide to delegate the execution of some administrative activities or to request permissions for accessing some documents. Those changes are stored in his local APO and the Physician in Charge of the Home Care unit is requested to validate them. After the validation, the local APO is immediately associated to his profile and used by his agent in place of the general ontology in order to readapt its overall execution.

The APO tailoring implemented in K4Care covers the requests for access permissions to forbidden documents, the delegation of actions and the incorporation of additional care units.

SECURITY

One critical aspect in the design and implementation of any health care system is related with security and privacy preserving, inherent with the management of sensitive and confidential data such as medical histories. During the development of the K4Care platform, the following issues were considered (Lhotská, *et al.*, 2008):

- The system must be protected against external attacks and non-authorized accesses. This has been implemented on the server side by the classical approach of *identification, authentication* and *user's failure mechanisms*. Each of the K4Care users may log in by providing a username and password. In addition, the distributed system design allows physically locating critical parts (such as the EHCR or the MAS) in a controlled and secured environment.
- In HC systems, different users play different roles and, thus, they must have different access rights. Thus the system must guarantee, from a technical point of view, that every user is allowed to do the activities for which he/she is competent. K4Care

uses an *authorization* mechanism based on the definition of *user profiles* modeled in the APO ontology. A physical user may have several profiles (*e.g.* the same person may be, at the same time, a physician in charge of the HC unit and a family doctor). In consequence, he/she may be linked to several Actor Agents (each one implementing one of his/her profiles) by means of a Gateway Agent which acts as a bridge. The system gives the possibility of changing the active role of a certain user at each moment, resulting in changes both in the interface and in the system's behaviour.

- Another issue to be taken into account is related to the kind of information that is accessible to every user when several professionals with different types coexist. K4Care implements it by defining personal *information access rights* associated to user profiles which are also included in the APO.
- When a system is distributed and remotely accessible via a Web interface, the security problems inherent to transactions in public networks arise. Since most of the transactions will involve private medical information, it is critical to implement mechanisms to guarantee the preservation of privacy. The K4Care Web server incorporates secured communications via the HTTPS protocol.
- Finally, one of the biggest problems in any computer system is *internal security leaks*. Technical staff may have physical access to the data storage (*i.e.* the EHR) and the possibility to steal such data together with its high price and with the anonymity of such act can be too tempting. The K4Care EHR has been secured by splitting it into two independent parts which decouple sensible medical data from its owner. Those are linked by a cryptographic algorithm to

prevent unauthorized accesses to confidential data. All data are also encrypted and signed to be safely transmitted.

CONCLUSION

This chapter described the design and implementation of the K4Care platform, a system devoted to the provision of healthcare services in a remote and intuitive way, allowing an easy adaptation of its behaviour (with respect to visualization, data format and functionalities) both for medical organizations and concrete professionals. This flexibility, dynamicity, reusability and tailoring possibilities relies heavily on the explicit separation between the representation of the knowledge required to provide Home Care and the way in which it is used to provide the e-care services. As an example, in K4Care the procedures used in potential instantiations of the system in different countries could be adapted to the methods of work in each place, the Formal Intervention Plans used in each medical centre could take into account only the resources they have available or the ontologies can be adapted and extended to model new care units or new procedural or medical knowledge related to the healthcare party.

In this sense, the explicit formalization of all the required knowledge also opens interesting opportunities for user customization, since it is feasible to create and adapt personal views of certain knowledge structures with the preferences or requirements of each user. As shown in the previous section, in the case of K4Care this aspect has been applied to the personalization of Actor Profile Ontologies.

The use of agent technology certainly seems an interesting option to consider in this kind of distributed systems. Moreover, nowadays, the use of a Web interface to allow physically distributed users to access the system anytime and anywhere with an intuitive interface is becoming almost mandatory. Web 2.0 technologies open the possibility of designing and implementing rich Web interfaces, providing the same degree of interaction of a desktop application but without introducing software or hardware requirements or advanced ICT skills. Personalization and adaptation also covers the data visualization and interface interaction according to specific roles and document formats by using CSS, XSL transformations. Security is also ensured by the use of ciphered HTTPS connections and the decoupling of sensible data from its owner in the EHR.

The developed system is composed by several modules implemented with different state of the art technologies covering aspect of rich, secured and multi-language Web-based interaction (AJAX, JavaScript, Servlets), Distributed Artificial Intelligence based on FIPA agents (implemented in JADE) or data storage and knowledge modelling using OWL ontologies, SDA* procedures and hybrid SQL/XML EHR. As introduced in the text, each one offered several advantages compared to classical approaches (typically based on centralized and standalone ad-hoc application) especially when dealing with highly complex environments like healthcare and ensuring a great degree of adaptability and flexibility. However, from a technical point of view, the interoperation of such heterogeneous technologies was neither direct nor trivial. In consequence, several technological challenges were faced during the development, designing, for each case, a concrete intercommunication or adaptation solution.

The final version of the platform is currently tested with real medical data and it is being deployed for the community of the town of Pollenza (Italy). The test deployment will involve the entire Home Care facility, General Practitioners, the Municipality, social assistants and citizens' representatives. The K4Care platform will be applied in the usual care activity delivered during the period of study.

ACKNOWLEDGMENT

This work has been funded by the European IST project K4Care: Knowledge Based Home Care eServices for an Ageing Europe (IST-2004-026968). The authors would like to acknowledge the work of the other members of the K4Care consortium, especially the medical partners, led by Dr. Fabio Campana, and Dr. David Riaño (project co-ordinator and designer of the SDA* formalism).

REFERENCES

W3C (2004). OWL Web Ontology Language. Retrieved from http://www.w3.org/tr/owl-features

Aubrecht, P., Matousek, K., & Lhotská, L. (2008). On Designing an EHCR Repository. In L. Azevedo & A. R. Londral (Eds.), *Proc. of the International Conference on Health Informatics (HEALTHINF 08)* (pp. 280-285). Funchal, Madeira, Portugal.

Batet, M., Gibert, K., & Valls, A. (2007). The Data Abstraction Layer as Knowledge Provider for a Medical Multi-Agent System. In Riaño, D., & Campana, F. (Eds.), *Proc. of the From Knowledge to Global Care AIME 2007 Workshop K4CARE 2007* (pp. 87–100). Amsterdam, The Netherlands.

Batet, M., Gibert, K., & Valls, A. (2008). Tailoring of the Actor Profile Ontology in the K4Care Project. In D. Riaño (Ed.), *Proc. of the ECAI 2008 Workshop Knowledge Management for Health Care Procedures, K4HelP 2008* (pp. 104-122). Patras, Greece.

Bellifemine, F., Caire, G., & Greenwood, D. (2007). *Developing multi-agent systems with JADE*. Chichester, England: John Wiley and Sons. doi:10.1002/9780470058411

Campana, F., Moreno, A., Riaño, D., & Varga, L. (2008). K4Care: Knowledge-Based Homecare e-Services for an Ageing Europe. In Annicchiarico, R., Cortés, U., & Urdiales, C. (Eds.), *Agent Technology and e-Health* (pp. 95–115). Basel, Switzerland: Birkhäuser Basel. doi:10.1007/978-3-7643-8547-7_6

Casals, J., Gibert, K., & Valls, A. (2007). Enlarging a medical actor profile ontology with new care units. In Riaño, D. (Ed.), *Proc. of the From Knowledge to Global Care AIME 2007 Workshop K4CARE 2007* (pp. 101–116). Amsterdam, The Netherlands.

Ciccarese, P., Caffi, E., Boiocchi, L., Quaglini, S., & Stefanelli, M. (2004). A Guideline Management System. In M. Fieschi, E. Coiera & J. X. Li (Eds.), *Proc. of the 11th World Congress on Medical Informatics, MEDINFO 2004* (pp. 28-32). San Francisco, USA.

FIPA. (2002). FIPA Interaction Protocol Library Specification (Specification No. DC00025F). Geneva, Switzerland: Foundation for Intelligent and Physical Agents (FIPA).

Fox, J., Beveridge, M., & Glasspool, D. (2003). Understanding intelligent agents: analysis and synthesis. *AI Communications*, *16*(3), 139–152.

Fox, J., & Das, S. (2000). *Safe and Sound*. Menlo Park, CA, USA: AAAI and MIT Press.

Gómez-Pérez, A., Fernández-López, M., & Corcho, O. (2004). *Ontological Engineering with examples from the areas of Knowledge Management, e-Commerce and the Semantic Web* (2nd ed.). Berlin, Germany: Springer Verlag.

Holdener, A. T., III. (2008). Ajax: The Definitive Guide. Sebastopol, CA, US: O'Reilly Media, Inc.

Isern, D., Millan, M., Moreno, A., Pedone, G., & Varga, L. Z. (2008). Home Care Individual Intervention Plans in the K4Care Platform. In S. Puuronen, M. Pechenizkiy, A. Tsymbal & D.-J. Lee (Eds.), *Proc. of the 21st IEEE International Symposium on Computer-Based Medical Systems, 2008 IEEE CBMS* (pp. 455-457). Jywaskyla, Finland.

Isern, D., Moreno, A., Sánchez, D., Hajnal, A., Pedone, G., & Varga, L. Z. (2010a). Agent-based execution of personalised home care treatments. *Applied Intelligence.* doi:.doi:10.1007/s10489-009-0187-6

Isern, D., Sánchez, D., & Moreno, A. (2010b). Agents Applied in Health Care: A Review. *International Journal of Medical Informatics, 75*(3), 145–166. doi:10.1016/j.ijmedinf.2010.01.003

Jones, J., Wilson, A., Parker, H., Wynn, A., Jagger, C., Spiers, N., & Parker, G. (1999). Economic evaluation of hospital at home versus hospital care: cost minimisation analysis of data from randomised controlled trial. *British Medical Journal, 319*(7224), 1547–1550.

Kavanagh, S., & Knapp, M. (2002). Costs and cognitive disability: modelling the underlying associations. *The British Journal of Psychiatry, 180*, 120–125. doi:10.1192/bjp.180.2.120

Kumar, A., Quaglini, S., Stefanelli, M., Ciccarese, P., Caffi, E., & Boiocchi, L. (2002). A framework for representing and executing a clinical practice guideline for the management of high blood pressure in pregnancy. *Technology and Health Care, 10*(6), 517–519.

Landi, F., Onder, G., Russo, A., Tabaccanti, S., Rollo, R., & Federici, S. (2001). A new model of integrated home care for the elderly: impact on hospital use. *Journal of Clinical Epidemiology, 54*(9), 968–970. doi:10.1016/S0895-4356(01)00366-3

Lau, L. M., & Shakib, S. (2005). Towards Data Interoperability: Practical Issues in Terminology Implementation and Mappingof the HIC 2005. *Thirteenth National Health Informatics Conference* (pp. 208-213). Melbourne, Australia.

Lhotská, L., Aubrecht, P., Valls, A., & Gibert, K. (2008). Security recommendations for implementation in distributed healthcare systems. In M. Klima (Ed.), *Proc. of the 42th IEEE Int. Carnahan Conference on Security Technology (IEEE ICCST 08)* (pp. 76-83). Prague, Czech Republic.

Nealon, J. L., & Moreno, A. (2003). Agent-Based Applications in Health Care. In Nealon, J. L., & Moreno, A. (Eds.), *Applications of Software Agent Technology in the Health Care Domain* (pp. 3–18). Basel, Switzerland: Birkhäuser Verlag.

Peleg, M., & Tu, S. W. (2006). Decision Support, Knowledge Representation and Management in Medicine. In Haux, R., & Kulikowski, C. (Eds.), *International Medical Informatics Association (IMIA) Yearbook of Medical Informatics 2006. Schattauer GmbH.* Germany: International Medical Informatics Association.

Peleg, M., Tu, S. W., Bury, J., Ciccarese, P., Fox, J., & Greenes, R. A. (2003). Comparing Computer-Interpretable Guideline Models: A Case-Study Approach. *Journal of the American Medical Informatics Association, 10*(1), 52–68. doi:10.1197/jamia.M1135

Riaño, D. (2007). The SDA* Model: A Set Theory Approach In P. Kokol, V. Podgorelec, M. Dušanka, M. Zorman & M. Verlic (Eds.), *Proc. of the 20th IEEE International Symposium on Computer-Based Medical Systems, IEEE CBMS 2007* (pp. 563-568). Maribor, Slovenia.

Riaño, D., Real, F., Campana, F., Ercolani, S., & Annicchiarico, R. (2009). An Ontology for the Care of the Elder at Home In C. Combi, Y. Shahar & A. Abu-Hanna (Eds.), *Proc. of the 12th Conference on Artificial Intelligence in Medicine, AIME 2009* (pp. 235-239). Verona, Italy.

Scuvee-Moreau, J., Kurz, X., & Dresse, A. (2002). National dementia economic study group. The economic impact of dementia in Belgium: results of the National Dementia Economic Study (NADES). *Acta Neurologica Belgica, 102*(3), 104–113.

Shahar, Y., Young, O., Shalom, E., Galperin, M., Mayaffit, A., Moskovitch, R., & Hessing, A. (2004). A Framework for a Distributed, Hybrid, Multiple-Ontology Clinical-Guideline Library and Automated Guideline-Support Tools. *Journal of Biomedical Informatics, 37*(5), 325–344. doi:10.1016/j.jbi.2004.07.001

Staab, S., Schnurr, H., Studer, R., & Sure, Y. (2001). Knowledge process and ontologies. *IEEE Intelligent Systems, 16*(1), 26–34. doi:10.1109/5254.912382

Studer, R., Benjamins, V. R., & Fensel, D. (1998). Knowledge Engineering: Principles and Methods. *IEEE Transactions on Knowledge and Data Engineering, 25*(1-2), 161–197.

Sutton, D. R., & Fox, J. (2003). The syntax and semantics of the PROforma guideline modeling language. *Journal of the American Medical Informatics Association, 10*(5), 433–443. doi:10.1197/jamia.M1264

Wooldridge, M. (2002). *An Introduction to multiagent systems*. West Sussex, England: John Wiley and Sons, Ltd.

Young, O., & Shahar, Y. (2005). The Spock System: Developing a Runtime Application Engine for Hybrid-Asbru Guidelines. In S. Miksch, J. Hunter & E. Keravnou (Eds.), *Proc. of the 10th Conference on Artificial Intelligence in Medicine, AIME 2005* (pp. 166-170). Aberdeen, Scotland. Key Terms Medical Informatics, Ubiquitous Health care, Web 2.0 approaches for clinical practice, design and development of ICT methodologies for health care.

Chapter 19
Electronic Environments for Integrated Care Management:
Case of Depression Treatment

Matic Meglič
UP PINT, Slovenia

Andrej Brodnik
UP PINT, Slovenia

ABSTRACT

This chapter provides a basic overview of care process management and active patient engagement principles. It builds upon these principles to describe in more detail the way information and communication technology can provide support for them. It later discusses their impact on quality and cost-efficiency of care. The authors specify care models suitable for ICT support, specific process support characteristics related to health care, standards and communication devices that are being used. The chapter also provides a description of development and implementation of such an environment to support treatment of patients with depression.

INTRODUCTION

Information and communication technology (ICT) offers to the health care systems a new and ever expanding horizon of possibilities to reshape and transform existing health care services as well as implement new, so called eHealth services that were unthinkable of just 10 years ago. Care process management, active patient involvement (so called patient empowerment) and remote care are some of the components of care benefiting most from innovations in eHealth. These components are important not only in improving long-term healthcare but also in sustaining or decreasing financial burden as long-term care is using increasingly more financial and human resources in health care in developed countries. The goal of this chapter is to offer to the reader an insight into some of the challenges the health care systems are facing and describe the way eHealth is helping to support care process management, active patient engagement and remote care. The technologies we focus on include process support, internet and IP multimedia subsystems (IMS). The objectives of this chapter are: to describe modern approaches to health care organization and active patient engagement; to explain

DOI: 10.4018/978-1-61520-777-0.ch019

Copyright © 2010, IGI Global. Copying or distributing in print or electronic forms without written permission of IGI Global is prohibited.

how these modern approaches can be supported by some of the information and communication technologies of today; to provide a case description of an existing environment to support treatment of patients with depression; and to discuss impact on cost of care, quality, and future trends. In the following section we describe some of the general trends and issues in health care and some specific issues that ICT can solve. The section is followed by a description of different models of health care organization. In section 'ICT support for care management and active patient engagement' we present three components of ICT support for these models and then apply the findings to a specific case of depression treatment. In the case description we focus on depression treatment issues, state of the art in ICT support in depression treatment, methods used in the study, preliminary results and the problems we faced in designing, developing and implementing the depression treatment support environment.

We conclude the chapter with some of the future research directions.

BACKGROUND

Health care in the developed world is facing a combination of changes that forces the health care systems to rethink the principles of care provision and to reinvent themselves especially in terms of cost-efficiency, access to care, and quality of care (Bloom, 2002).

The changes on the horizon are on one side a growing population of elderly combined with an increasingly growing numbers of chronically ill patients and patients with one or more chronic conditions - such as hypertension, diabetes mellitus, depression, obesity, asthma, and chronic obstructive pulmonary disease. On the other side is a powerful drive of the health care and pharmaceutical industry to introduce more advanced treatments and procedures, sell more expensive drugs and lower the threshold of diagnosis and

consequent earlier treatment initiation (as has been seen in hyperlipidemia with lipid-lowering drugs).

Combining the two trends – demographic changes and ever present industry interest – we can foresee a further need and drive for increase in the scope and extent of health services to be provided. The increase in scope is almost invariably combined with an increase in cost. This poses a threat to cost-sustainability of health care systems as the costs are already spiraling upwards (Bodenheimer, 2005a; Bodenheimer, 2005b; Marmor, Oberlander & White, 2009). There are several measures to prevent the uncontrolled increase of system - level health care cost. Most of them are restrictive in nature and are focused on readjusting the extent of services provided within the public health care, introducing co-payments and concomitant new insurance schemes, often reducing the availability of services (Bodenheimer, 2005c; Marmor et al., 2009).

Besides these measures a change of thinking is needed for health care systems to provide accessible and affordable future care to the growing population of patients with long-term conditions (Wilson, Bunn & Morgan, 2009). Some of the aspects of needed changes are described in more detail below.

Looking at the cost we can say that the more specialized and institutionalized the care, the more expensive it is. Emergency hospital care and subsequent rehabilitation and consecutive life-long drug therapy due to a myocardial infarction are much more expensive than primary or secondary preventive activities organized by a general physician (Bennett et al., 2008; Jovicic, Holroyd-Leduc & Straus, 2006). These preemptive (or preventive as they are called) activities usually involve the patient to a greater extent and place a part of the prevention process on patient's shoulders. The costs of the patient performing preventive activities at home to the health care system are second to none besides education and motivation. We can argue that the patient him- or herself is the cheapest provider of own care when properly motivated, empowered and provided the tools to do so. Of course the actual implementation and reach of such activities is another issue as several groups of population are not motivated or capable of performing them.

Looking at access to care, the available technology already enables us to implement new health care services that reduce the extent of resource utilization whilst providing innovative preventive, screening and therapeutic services to support or partly replace existing services that are human resource intensive. Remote access to care using TV sets coupled with set-top boxes (we will refer to them as digital TVs), personal computers and mobile devices using internet access as well as phone and video is moving the so called 'point of care' from surgeries and hospitals to patients' homes, further enabling access to care to elderly and disabled (Clark, Inglis, McAlister, Cleland & Stewart, 2007; Kobb, Chumbler, Brennan & Rabinowitz, 2008).

Another aspect of change is the organizational one. Research shows that the treatment outcome (i.e. the percentage of patients cured of all patients treated) is related to the well planned and organized care process (Geyman, 2007; Gilbody, Bower, Fletcher, Richards & Sutton, 2006). An average patient with an escalation of a chronic condition (i.e. hypertensive crisis in a hypertensive patient) sees at least five health care professionals within at least three different health care institutions – a nurse and general practitioner at local practice, a nurse and a specialist in the hospital, and a pharmacist at the pharmacy. Adequate and timely exchange of information between them and a clear definition of their roles and tasks for the particular patient are necessary. As obvious and simple as this may sound, it is surprising to see how often the activities do not follow the correct sequence and the crucial information is not provided to the professional or patient to perform the right tasks.

To make this simple case more realistic we can imagine a patient having more than one chronic condition – i.e. chronic cardiovascular disease and diabetes. The patient receives different long-term drug therapies for each of the conditions. In case of an escalation of one of the conditions the other condition is often to move from a stable to unstable state and require therapy adjustments and potentially other care.

In United Kingdom a third of planned appointments do not take place due either to patient no-show (10%), patient cancellation (10%) or provider cancellation (12%), costing the health care system 700 Million GBP per year (Wilson, 2006). Another example of inadequate service provisioning is treatment of depression. Just over ten years ago results of the first large pan-European survey of depression (Lepine, Gastpar, Mendlewicz & Tylee, 1997) have shown that less than 8% of patients with depression were prescribed antidepressant drugs. At that same time another study (Lin et al., 1995) has shown that 44% of patients stopped taking the medication before 3rd month of therapy, further reducing the number of properly treated patients to just above 4%. Knowing the cost of lost productivity (measured in thousands of USD a year) of patients with depression at their workplace one can grasp the immense burden of untreated depression on the overall productivity of a country. One could argue that the above examples bear no resemblance. The reason to describe them is to point out that advances in care management (i.e. electronic patient scheduling, drug and schedule reminder service) and active patient engagement (i.e. self-reporting on depression treatment, confirmation of scheduled appointments) are crucial to successfully deliver care and improve quality and outcome (Crosson & Madvig, 2004; Fireman, Bartlett & Selby, 2004).

The methodologies to improve care organization and delivery are not easy to implement (Ludwick & Doucette, 2009; Trivedi et al.,

2009). To improve care management in the past a provider needed to employ one or more additional staff members and equip them with tools to monitor the individual patients within the care process and communicate with care professionals or providers the tasks and timings. In days when in developed countries broadband, computers, laptops, netbooks, palmtops and personal digital assistants (PDAs) are becoming almost as ubiquitous as mobile phones, we can extensively reduce human resources usage for care management and patient empowerment by utilizing: (1) these devices (including palmtops, smart phones, remote monitoring devices, body area networks); (2) knowledge and information processing tools (such as process management, data mining, clinical decision support tools); and (3) contemporary communication and information exchange channels such as internet, mobile (push) mail, SMS (short message service) etc. – in general using unified messaging system. The importance of internet is growing not only as a communication and information retrieval tool but also for developing and implementing new public health interventions as well as various monitoring and prediction tools – from disease surveillance to behavior monitoring (Atkinson & Gold, 2002; Eysenbach, 2008; Eysenbach, 2009). The reasons for using internet as an environment of intervention delivery are: low cost and resource implications; reduction of cost and increase of convenience for users; reduction of health service costs; simplicity of overcoming isolation of users; support for timely information; stigma reduction; and simplicity for increased user and supplier control of the intervention (Griffiths, Lindenmeyer, Powell, Lowe & Thorogood, 2006). Interventions, most of them being prevention focused, are promising but not yet reaching their full potential and thus need to be further improved (Neuhauser & Kreps, 2003; Norman et al., 2007). Further benefits in terms of usability and cost are expected in the near future from increased syntactic interoperability of information solutions already used and

the growing semantic interoperability of clinical tools (Blobel, Engel & Pharow, 2006; Lopez & Blobel, 2009).

The designers of eHealth interventions must constantly avoid the danger of increasing disparity in their access between the technologically privileged and those who have limited access to technology or limited capabilities of using it (Cashen, Dykes & Gerber, 2004; Gilmour, 2007). It is also imperative to evaluate interventions in practical trials and use methodologies for evaluating that are rigorous - including for example measures of participation and representativeness at both patient and healthcare setting levels, consistency of outcomes across different subgroups, tendency of an eHealth program to ameliorate versus exacerbate health disparities, implementation and program adaptation, cost, and quality-of-life outcomes (Glasgow, 2007). An important distinction of eHealth evaluation trials is also a higher dropout rate compared to other clinical trials (i.e. drugs). This can cause underestimations of the impact. Methods exist to account for this (Eysenbach, 2005).

Acknowledging the sheer breadth of use of the internet and mobile technologies in healthcare we decided to focus this chapter on methodologies suitable for care management and patient engagement in the process of care and partly secondary prevention. To avoid oversimplification the chapter does not cover primary prevention focused internet and mobile phone interventions or infomediation. In the following sections we describe the basics of care management and patient empowerment and the means and examples of supporting them with ICT.

MODELS AND ENVIRONMENTS FOR CARE MANAGEMENT AND ACTIVE PATIENT INVOLVEMENT

First we focus on laying out the prerequisites for organizational improvement of the care process.

To do so we describe the care process and models of managing the care process more efficiently. Then we describe means to support these models with modern ICT.

The Health Care Process and Models

Health care process is a set of interrelated activities performed by one or more health care professionals, the patient and other actors with the goal of improving or sustaining a specific component of patient's health. The process incorporates various types of activities. The core activities of the process – the ones that are directly related to the goal of the process – are of clinical nature and can be sorted into the following main categories: screening, prevention, treatment and care. Besides these core activities there are supporting activities that ensure that the process runs efficiently; these activities are mostly administrative and include care coordination, information sharing, reminding and scheduling activities.

We propose a distinction between three perspectives of care process based on the completeness of the process and the extent of involved providers: the correct sequence of individual clinical decisions made by each of the involved professionals; the timely synchronization of several health care professionals within a single

health care provider; and the synchronization of various health care providers.

In clinical terms these three perspectives could be named: clinical decision process, clinical pathway and integrated care process (Figure 1).

To improve the process of care in terms of efficiency, bottlenecks, resource utilization and timing one needs to be able to describe the process in detail and measure the indicators. The description includes the right set of tasks and decisions and their sequence, dedicated profiles to execute these tasks and decisions, rules and input data to support the decisions, timings and interrelations. By measuring indicators like resource usage and time spent on each of the tasks for a particular output one can find spare capacities and spare timing in the process and redesign it to be more efficient.

The mix of care models showing the most promise is a combination of integrated care, care management, disease management, case management, stepped care and active patient engagement including self-care, supported extensively by ICT.

Integrated care is defined as a coherent set of products and services, delivered by collaborating local and regional health care agencies to patients with multiple coexisting conditions (Hardy, Mur-Veemanu, Steenbergen & Wistow, 1999). WHO

Figure 1. Dimensions of care process (hc: health care; cd: clinical decision)

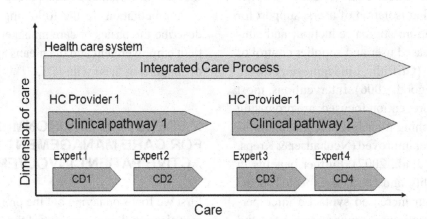

defines it as bringing together inputs, delivery, management and organisation of services related to diagnosis, treatment, care, rehabilitation and health promotion (Grone & Garcia-Barbero, 2001). In relation to process management view it is important that in integrated care we define roles and tasks for specialists and other health care professionals in multidisciplinary teams (Campbell, Hotchkiss, Bradshaw & Porteous, 1998) and aim to provide a bundle of services to cover all necessary health care needs of patients.

Case, disease and care management all focus on efficiently generating, planning, organizing and administering the care and services but differ in scope. Case management focuses on particular cases (relapse of disease), disease management focuses on a particular disease whereas care management includes other services as well (nursing, social etc).

In stepped care needs for interventions are triaged based on clinical or organizational decision criteria that define what type of action is required in a specific situation. This way more expensive resources (i.e. doctors and nurses) can focus on performing difficult clinical tasks whereas other staff performs less complex tasks where rules can be applied with a greater certainty. Administration staff can in this case perform a broader set of organizational tasks related to patient follow-up and scheduling, previously assigned to clinical personnel. The described care models have been shown to improve the quality of care and resource utilization but require additional coordination effort (Geyman, 2007).

Active patient participation means that patients take an active role and engage in the process of care. The final step in patient engagement is patient empowerment (Ash & Bates, 2005), where the patient takes an active role in care process as well as in monitoring of his or her process of care. According to Angelmar (2007) patient empowerment refers to patient's power over a range of decisions (e.g. provider and treatment choice) and to increase of this power by patient

education and legal rights. To it we could also add possibility of reacting to deviations from the planned care process.

We reach that level by providing to the patient relevant disease information, specific localized health care information (e.g. eligible services, scope of insurance coverage) and make available and transparent the information about the specific instance of the care process (s)he takes part in. The benefits of patient empowerment are explained below into further detail.

The patient can perform tasks previously performed in part by professionals (e.g. various self-assessments performed at home instead of the surgery or hospital) and - accordingly - provider resource utilization is reduced. The patient is also able to monitor own care process, exert control and report deviations when necessary – e.g. the patient notifies the care manager of an overdue waiting time for a therapeutic procedure. This way the care quality and efficiency control is enhanced as the control of the services provided is not only controlled by the payer but also by the recipient of care. The perceived quality of care is increased as the patient is more actively involved in the process of care.

ICT Support for Care Management and Active Patient Engagement

Until recently the problem was how to implement these care models without an extensive increase in coordination effort. With the advent of ICT and its use in health, commonly referred to as 'eHealth', an increasing array of electronic information management tools, information exchange and communication technologies are available and being used to support the implementation of modern care model into practice. A survey by Southern California Evidence Based Practice Center shows that health information technology improves quality by increasing adherence to guidelines, enhancing disease surveillance, and decreasing medication errors. Much of the evidence on quality improvement is related to primary and secondary preventive care. The major efficiency benefit was to decrease utilization of care (Chaudhry et al., 2006).

We propose to divide eHealth tools for support of care management and patient engagement broadly into three categories: (1) process support environment, (2) tools for information integration, and (3) user interaction tools. This division is first of all based on the processes we find in health care, the technology supporting these processes as well as their specific added value.

Process Support Environments

In the business world Business Process Management (BPM) is a well known methodology in use for well over a quarter of a century. It is used in several business functions: it helps to monitor and control the core process and support processes; it serves as a means of improvement of the production process (finding and eliminating bottlenecks); it supports efficient enterprise resource planning and just in time inventories; the simulations enable strategic decisions. Several tools using information technology have been developed for use of BPM methodology. In simple terms the basic tools are: a database to store all business process related information, an execution engine to execute particular instances of a defined process, and a designer tool that helps process designer to transform the actual processes into a model that serves as a template for the execution engine. Correspondingly to the broad use of BPM there is a broad market of products and services to support BPM. These range from off the shelf proprietary and open – source software (IBM®, Microsoft®, Eclipse™ based Intalio®, jBOSS® jBPM, TIBCO® or others like Enhydra™ Shark, Bonita) to complete BPM outsourcing services. A limited number of standards to support BPM were developed and some of them are: XML Process Definition Language (XPDL) for exchange of BPM diagrams; Business Process Execution Language (BPEL) for programming web services and specifying interactions between them; Business Process Modeling Notation (BPMN) to model processes using a graphical notation; and Business Process Definition Metamodel (BPDM) to define concepts used in expressing business process models.

In health care the use of process management was predominantly a domain of large health care organizations using them to support non-clinical processes. In the last years they are increasingly being used in hospitals to support clinical processes but in out-of-hospital setting they are only seldomly used.

The reason to increase the adoption of BPM in health care, especially in care or disease process management is the following: in several ways the care process is similar to other processes in manufacturing: the patient has a distinct predefined pathway through the system, there are several tasks to be performed on this patient, alternative processes and sub-processes, decision and quality control points and sets of rules associated with the process. The reader might wonder why the adoption of BPM in care management has not yet occurred to a similar extent as in business. The reasons probably lie in the fact that the general perception of treatment decision-making is part art and part knowledge and to a smaller extent to the specifics of care process which we describe in more detail.

The health care process is not always a single process but for one instance (one patient) several processes might run in parallel. An example would be parallel sub-processes of cognitive behavioral therapy, psychiatric therapy and peer to peer training in depression. Another example would be a reminder sub-process triggered by a missed task, that runs parallel to treatment process. The process can be highly variable due to complex treatment protocols and the decision criteria and rules of decision process can not always be specified. Another problem lies in the two-dimensional variability of clinical information: besides the specific variable value the relative weight of that value might be different in different patients depending on their specific health status. Sometimes a value of a variable can be used as a decision criterion but sometimes the clinical importance of that value is reduced and other values need to be taken into account that might not be important in other patients.

There are efforts to improve the process management methodology to fit better to health care specifics as well as to adapt the care processes to fit better to the process view. The former includes using adapted methodologies like process matrices and the latter includes the fast growing clinical pathways related activities in various countries and an increasing trend of shifting from structural to process organization within health care providers.

In design and specification of processes the use of process matrices is an alternative way of laying out the process as compared to flowcharts. It allows multiple tasks and processes to be run in parallel for a single instance and allows variability of sub-process invocation rules (meaning the conditions on which a specific sub-process is started). Our experience is that the process matrices are (though less graphical and transparent than flowcharts) successfully used to describe and allow complex sub-process relationships. An important guideline when describing or redesigning care processes is also the level of fragmentation of tasks and especially fragmentation of clinical decision making tasks. In our experience the clinical decision making process of different clinicians can be quite different. Consequently the consensus among them can be difficult to reach in the design phase, disagreements also occur once the process management is implemented. In these cases two options remain for the process designer: use of accepted clinical guidelines or an agreement to focus more on the administrative and operational issues of the process, leaving the clinical decision making to the clinicians themselves without coding the rules into the process support

system. Clinical decision support tools and expert systems are in our opinion to be discerned from most process support tools. They also use different methodologies – clinical decision support tools use mostly analytical methods based on statistics whereas expert systems use artificial intelligence and statistical modeling.

To assess the growth of IT support for process management in health care a survey of IT care process management related publications in PUBMED® between 1990 and 2007 was conducted (Figure 2) showing an overall exponential growth of publications with an additional increase from the year 2003 (Meglič, 2007).

Technologies for Information Integration

The care process related information in the clinical setting is often extensive and structured to various extents. Process management environment is dependent on information to steer the process and is of limited value without it. This information is of two types: the information that does not yet exist and needs to be entered into the system and the information that already exists in an electronic format in a different information system. For process management environments

Figure 2. Number of publications on IT & care process management (logarithmic scale)

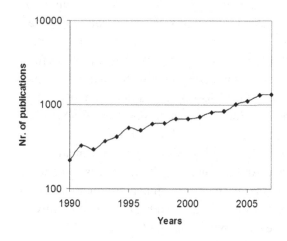

to be unobtrusive and user friendly (1) the user must be able to enter new information in a simple and efficient way and most importantly (2) the information already existing in electronic format must be made available to the care process environment as automatically as possible. Why is this so important? Various information systems and e-business solutions provide crucial information in electronic format to be used as input information for care management, thus avoiding duplication of entry of information, which is one of the major obstacles for adoption of eHealth solutions. To name a few of them, these are electronic healthcare records, hospital-, laboratory- and radiology information systems, personal healthcare records, picture archiving and communication systems.

To successfully exchange information between different information systems there needs to be an agreement on the format of exchange and the format of datasets and information structure. The most often used ones are HL7®, CEN™ 13606, HISA and CCD. The OpenEHR® archetype concept is also gaining popularity in the last years. As the descriptions of the standards are beyond the scope of this chapter, we list them below only to provide a starting point for readers that might be further interested in that topic.

HL7 family of standards is provided by Health Level Seven (www.hl7.org), a not-for-profit organization. Several versions exist, the most commonly used is version 2.x and the latest one is version 3. The European Committee for standardization's (CEN) Health informatics - Electronic Health Record Communication (EN 13606) European Standard family defines information architecture for communicating part or all of the Electronic Health Record of a single patient. The same organization also offers Standard Architecture for Healthcare Information Systems (EN 12967), also called Health Informatics Service Architecture or HISA. This is a standard to support the development of modular open systems to support healthcare. For continuity of care two separate standards exist (HL7 CDA and ASTM® CCR) – perhaps the new Continuity of Care Document (CCD) created by joined efforts of both organizations and approved in 2007 by American National Standards Institute (ANSI®) will take the future role of a single standard in this field. OpenEHR initiative (www.openehr.org) is developing a semantically oriented open source shared platform for health computing.

User Interaction Technologies

Now that we have described the care process support tools which are the core of the environment let us turn to user interaction tools that create the link between the users and the care process management environment. The primary goal of user interaction tools is to enable users to enter information when prompted and access relevant information whenever they need it. This interaction needs to be simple and efficient. To support these requirements from a hardware point of view we can use several types of devices and information exchange and communication technologies. Types of devices commonly used for interaction in clinical and patient home setting are personal computers, laptops, netbooks, palmtops, PDAs, smartphones, ordinary mobile phones, wearable or portable measurement devices and digital TV. Personal computers, laptops, netbooks, palmtops and digital TV offer a wide array of interaction possibilities due to relatively large screens and inbuilt or attachable keyboards. With PDAs and smartphones the ease of entering and presenting information is somewhat reduced whereas ordinary mobile phones and wearable or portable measurement devices offer a very limited scope of interaction.

In the design of user interaction these specifics are taken into account. Suitable combinations of ease of portability and connectivity of the device on one hand and the needed scope of interaction on the other hand are established for a particular user profile. In case that there is not a single combination (i.e. some of the tasks like manipulating a database require using a personal computer or laptop whereas some of the tasks require 24/7 remote access to basic patient information) two or more combinations are set for each of the profiles and different functionalities are assigned to each of them.

For communication purposes we have at hand a wide variety of networks: global WAN or broadband wireless networks (e.g. IEEE® 802.16™; local (LAN) which can also be wireless (WLAN, e.g. IEEE Standard 802.11™ based); on a short distance we can use networks like Bluetooth® (IEEE Standard 802.15.1™ based) or older infrared connections. Furthermore, for communication we can also use telecommunication networks such as GSM, GPRS, UMTS, HSDPA, etc. The choice of specific communication infrastructure depends on the functionalities we need to provide to users when supporting the care process. On top of a communication infrastructure a communication protocol is deployed. A general agreement is that this protocol is IP protocol (IPv4 or IPv6). The advent of an IMS standard enabled us to use the same protocol in the telecommunication networks as well and consequently made IP-based services (i.e. internet services including http and consequently also web services) accessible in telecommunication networks.

For health care simple communication is far from sufficient. We have to provide not only secure communication, but also secure applications and secure storage of data. The data we are dealing with are highly sensitive personal data and for their handling we have to build an access model that clearly defines which individual has access to which piece of information. To implement the model we use various cryptographic protocols and infrastructure which are all supported by an adequate trust model and trust infrastructure.

In the following section we describe an implementation of some of the above concepts (web and mobile based care process management environment) on the case of depression treatment.

CASE DESCRIPTION OF USE OF WEB AND IMS SUPPORTED ENVIRONMENT FOR PROCESS SUPPORT: E-DEPRESSION PROJECT

In this section we try to give the readers an example of how to approach applicative research, development and clinical testing of eHealth environments. The project that we describe is not outstanding in terms of scale or resources involved but shows how specific problems of a particular group of patients (in this case the poor compliance with drug therapy of patients with depression) can be addressed by putting into practice contemporary eHealth concepts.

Before delving into details let us first describe the ICT landscape already in place to support active patient engagement and care management support. In Europe several countries have long ago adopted eHealth strategies that are addressing the above issues, which in 2005 was also a requirement from the European Comission to all EU member states. Most of these strategies involve developing nation level electronic health records (EHR) or at least interoperability of local EHRs within a health care system, enabling paperless practices in hospitals and other care centres, exchanging electronically all relevant documentation (such as prescriptions, insurance claims, referral and discharge letters etc.), establishing environments where users can access own health information and interact online with the health care system. United Kingdom National Health Service's National Programme for IT (NPfIT) that supports the NHS Connecting for Health (www.connectingforhealth.nhs.uk) has in last years implemented in several of the above mentioned services. HealthSpace™ enables users to store personal health data and is in concept similar to US based HealthVault ™ or Google™ Health. Choose&Book enables users to have influence on choice of secondary care provider. This service has caused some stir in the general practitioners' community due to the way it was implemented. NHS Direct is a service offering expert advice and information both online as well as over the phone. GP2GP enables exchange of EHRs between GP practices. In Denmark the national and regional health portal 'sundhed.dk' built on MedCom's infrastructure enables citizens and care providers to access and to manage individual person related health information. The described solutions are all necessary prerequisites for efficient health care in the 21st century and need to be addressed regionally or nationally. In order to reach full potential of eHealth there are several services that can further add value on top of the above mentioned nation-wide services. These are often of lesser value when standing alone or can serve smaller and more specific groups of healthy users, patients as well as health care providers. These include knowledge management solutions (i.e. disease databases, drug interaction databases), decision support systems and expert systems (for clinical and self-help purposes), and of course care management support.

Let us now return to the aim of this section, which is to describe a way to address an issue of poor compliance with drug therapy in depressed patients. The aim of the 3 year applicative project called eDepression, running at Primorska Institute for Natural Sciences and Technology (PINT), University of Primorska, Slovenia was to develop and evaluate an environment to support the treatment process of patients with depression that would incorporate integrated, managed and stepped care concepts on the basis of business process management principles. The initiator of the project was the late psychiatrist prof. Andrej Marušič. The project is financed by Slovene Ministry of Health and Slovene Research Agency. The plan was to develop a web- and internet multimedia subsystem (IMS)- based environment to connect patients, care managers, doctors and psychologists. Together with developing the environment a new health service model was also described to be piloted and evaluated in terms of cost-efficiency. As existing nation-level eHealth

services in Slovenia do not include services similar to NHS Direct or HealthSpace, we needed to add these functionalities (call centre, access to personal health information, exchange of closed circuit electronic messages) to the planned care management solution.

While working on eDepression project at UP PINT in Slovenia we identified the following goals to be achieved in the project:

- Improvement of the care process;
- Reduction in resource utilization;
- Improvement in patient perceived quality of care;
- Improvement in patient satisfaction; and
- Reduction in treatment related risks.

The means of achieving these goals were the following:

- To develop and implement a generic care process support environment (later applicable also to management of other chronic condition);
- To actively engage and empower the patients;
- To enable participation of various types of health care professionals and providers;
- To use care process support or streamlining using BPM principles;
- To store patient information in a way that is accessible to any involved actor that has been granted access to it; and
- To offer easy access to the environment using common devices and communication means.

Considering Figure 1 (dimensions of care process) we focused on supporting the upper two levels of care, namely integrated care and clinical pathways, while leaving out the support for clinical decisions taken by specific care professionals. The integrated care perspective involved defining and monitoring execution of tasks performed over the whole process of care by different care professionals. The clinical pathways perspective involved offering e-education on relevant clinical pathways to involved professionals and building into the system rules of data analysis and task execution that supported the guidelines (i.e. suggestion of therapy adjustment or antidepressant replacement when a specific time parameter and a relative BDI change in time were met).

DEPRESSION TREATMENT ISSUES

Depressive disorders have been identified as the second leading cause of disability worldwide (Kessler et al., 2003). Depression is one of the diseases with increasingly high prevalence among patients with co-morbidities as well as other age and social groups. It is the most common mental disease with prevalence from 16 to 18% during entire life span. In every moment approximately 12% of patients in general practitioners' offices are there because of depression (de Graaf et al., 2008; Siriwardena, Lawson, Vahl, Middleton & de Zeeuv, 2008; Spitzer et al., 1995).

Existing screening, diagnostics and treatment are not optimal due to reasons such as stigmatization, somatisation, delayed response to antidepressant treatment, the lack of motivation etc. Poor screening often results in patients developing advanced disease before being diagnosed. There is room for improvement both in prevention and in the process of treatment (Lin et al., 1995). The most important problem related to pharmaceutical treatment of depression is poor compliance (Pampallona, Bollini, Tibaldi, Kupelnick & Munizza, 2002). Patients often find it hard to comply with the treatment plan because of delayed treatment response and troublesome side effects that precede depression remission by weeks (Lin et al., 1995). Due to complexity of influence of disease on patient's lifestyle there is a need for multidisciplinary approach to treatment including psychologists and peers.

Looking at the effects of new organizational approaches, a review study in the United States of America found managed care to cause significant improvements in quality of depression care at acceptable costs ranging from $9,051 to $49,500 per quality-adjusted life-year (Neumeyer-Gromen, Lampert, Stark & Kallischnigg, 2004).

State of the Art

ICT support for disease management is growing popular in the last years in fields such as COPD, asthma, diabetes and hypertension but its effects are often yet to be proven (Cummings & Turner, 2009; Garcia-Lizana & Sarria-Santamera, 2007). Several interventions were designed in the field of primary and secondary prevention. Examples are weight management (Stevens et al., 2008; Tufano & Karras, 2005) and smoking cessation (Bock, Graham, Whiteley & Stoddard, 2008). In this chapter we focus on those that involve the therapeutic process as well. It is difficult to find existing care process management solutions to handle depressed patients with the exception of work of Robertson et al. (Robertson, Smith & Tannenbaum, 2005; Robertson, Smith, Castle & Tannenbaum, 2006). There have been experiments of handling data, screening tests, therapy and diagnostics of depressed patients with ICT which generally included electronic forms for screening purposes and systems for decision support for diagnostics and treatment (Plant, Murrell & Moreno, 1994; Trivedi, Kern, Grannemann, Altshuler & Sunderajan, 2004) and centralized patients' data (Crowther, Gask, Ives & Jakenfelds, 2001). The IMPACT study (integrated support for specialists treating elderly depressed patients) has shown improved guidelines adherence and improvements in treatment outcome (Hunkeler et al., 2006; Unutzer, Choi, Cook & Oishi, 2002). In contrast to the eDepression project the authors do not describe any interaction between the system and patients. Robertson and colleagues (Robertson et al., 2006) describe implementation of *RecoveryRoad*, an internet application where intervention is organized in monthly sessions. It offers e-consultations, improvement questionnaires, psychoeducation, physician access to results of questionnaires and information on evidence based treatment. Coordination of care is based on automated reminders for consistent adherence and responses of coordinator over email or telephone. Process support is not described except for the later stage where care managers manually monitored patients' depression scores. Preliminary results are promising.

Focusing on patient engagement aspect, several online cognitive behavioural therapy tools aimed at the patient exist, such as Moodgym and eCouch (available at moodgym.anu.edu.au and ecouch. anu.edu.au, respectively) but there is currently still a lack of online tools that offer process support and automated clinical knowledge besides connecting patients to health care professionals (with the above exceptions).

Methods

To address the mentioned issues of poor patient compliance, poor care management and follow-up, we developed the first two of the mentioned components of ICT care support, namely process support environment and user interaction technologies. Technologies for information integration were not used due to the limited duration and scope of the project. In contrast with existing published research the focus of the project was on establishing automated individual (instance specific) case management in an integrated environment.

We created an environment to fit the health care system in Slovenia but to be adaptable enough to replicate it in similar health care systems in other countries. A team of a psychiatrist, three psychologists, an eHealth expert, an ICT expert and a general practitioner have defined the depression care process and related functionalities of the environment for the following profiles: patient, psychologist, care coordinator, general practitioner, psychiatrist, mentor and system administrator.

To define the process in a format suitable for coding, process matrix was successfully employed as it allows multiple sub-processes (e.g. simultaneously running a set of actions reminding a patient who forgot to fill in a questionnaire and reminding the physician about a missing summary of the same patient's visit that already took place) to be instantiated and finished at various decision points in the process without diverting from the core treatment process.

The optimal treatment process and related task sets were defined for specific profiles and a task set to be performed automatically by the system. Clinical knowledge for decisions and rules was added to support the automated tasks and clinical output (i.e. interpretations of patients' questionnaires, task generation) was linked to the rules. Same was done for administrative decisions, rules and output (i.e. reminders of missed questionnaires, administrative task generation). One of the goals we set was how to make the system intelligent enough to analyze basic clinical data. Use of questionnaires such as BDI and questionnaire in which symptoms and signs as a consequence of medication treatment are evaluated were used to interactively acquire data about progression or regression of disease and compliance with medication regime and possible side effects. But just collection of the data would make no sense unless someone would check and evaluate it regularly. That is why a complex clinical evaluation system was designed. Its core is a process matrix that defines clinical and organizational thresholds at which the system is prompted to create tasks. The designed system was coded into a simple process management system running within a content management system that handled the remaining functionalities of the web- and mobile environment (static content, messages, forums etc.).

In October 2008 we started the clinical trial to evaluate the patient care quality and cost-efficiency of the new service. The clinical trial lasted until end of 2009 and aimed to confirm whether the above described approach improves outcome of depression treatment. The methodology used was a quasi-randomized controlled trial comparing treatment as usual to treatment as usual upgraded by improvehealth.eu service. Patients with first diagnosed episode or a relapse of depression or mixed anxiety-depression disorder were invited to participate by the doctors that diagnosed them. Semi-randomization with systematic alternating order was used with the extent that the doctors, patients or eDepression team had no influence on the grouping of particular patients. In the trial each patient was evaluated with a demographic questionnaire and Beck depression inventory® (BDI) (Beck, Ward, Mendelson, Mock & Erbaugh, 1961) at the start of the treatment and after six months and the difference in pre- and post- BDI score was used to measure outcome. Approximately 80 patients enrolled the trial. The outcomes of patients in both groups will be compared and influence of

various factors (e.g. demography, differences in therapy, internet usage) on the outcome will be evaluated. If we confirm a positive connection between the new intervention and the outcome we will extend the study to perform a cost-efficiency study and compare both the classical approach and the combined classical and new approach in terms of outcome related cost.

Preliminary Results

The environment is available online at www.improvehealth.eu or www.boljsezdravje.si (Figure 3). All functionalities are at the moment available in Slovene language only. The main page includes information about depression and depression treatment, links, news, team contact information and help. People in need of urgent help can find contact information on this page and there is a screening questionnaire for depression with automated results analysis available to all visitors to

Figure 3. Sample screenshot of www.improvehealth.eu

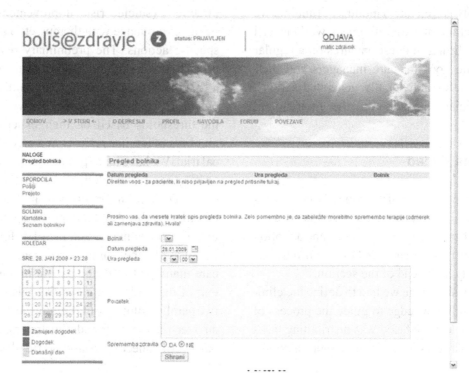

improve depression recognition. Patient specific pages of the environment consist of calendar with important events, personal record with all the data from treatment process, messaging system and a forum. The tasks section enables them to perform self-assessments about depression symptoms and medication side effects. They also provide dates of check-up visits to the doctor. The forum is available for communication between all users of the environment whereas the internal messaging system is used for communication between each patient and individual professionals involved in particular patient's care.

Care professionals' part of the environment has other functions besides the common information, forum and communication modules. General practitioners and psychiatrists see charts of their patients and can write visit summaries whereas the care manager has the most elaborate interface. Care manager can see charts of all the patients he takes care of and can observe patient specific crucial clinical and organizational parameters of care in the default view including pending tasks that were automatically generated by the system. As the study is well into 6 months of running, we observe that automated monitoring is working well with users filling in questionnaires on a regular basis. Same goes for care managers and their performance of individually generated actions. The physicians are adopting the environment very slowly.

Problems Faced

Here we describe some of the issues the project has faced to demonstrate the measures we have taken to deal with them. As usability, trust and adoption are common issues in such studies we will describe them briefly at the end of the section.

In the design stage we had to define the clinical rules and knowledge to guide the process of care. A problem we faced was distributing tasks not previously existing between existing actors in the care process and defining a new type of actor (care manager) and the accompanying roles and responsibilities. Another issue of the design stage was the uppermost complexity of tasks assigned to the patient.

After having developed the environment there were still several parts of the process that were unsupported by the user interfaces such as time tracking of care manager (to measure time spent on particular tasks) and tracking of the patient registration process. For these processes we had to establish additional online forms and additional database. One could argue that these could be planned for and developed in advance but the practical experience is that often several changes are being made during the development process and one can not predict them all in the design stage.

One of the key issues that we were looking at was the quality and setup of threshold levels of computer analysis to provide warnings and automated tasks related to specific patients. By using results of a quantifiable questionnaire the computer could analyze patient status in several directions (suicide risk, improvement of well-being, compliance with therapy etc.) and trigger specific actions. The preliminary results show that the thresholds and actions need to be set on a basis of evidence from experts in the field. In our case the psychologists involved proposed the thresholds based on their experience with numbers of similar patients in a preceding clinical trial. We have had a problem with overflow of tasks generated in relation to patient's exit of the study. The reason for this was the tight timeline of patient follow-up. Example: if a patient forgot to fill a questionnaire and then left for a week's vacation off-line, our protocol would suggest the care manager to call the patient in regard to his exit of the study. For cases like this we suggest two parallel solutions: (1) building into the system an over-run option for administrators, cancelling batches of unnecessary tasks and (2) designing the rule base of the solution and the execution engine in such way that the rules can be edited while the application is running.

A usability study was conducted involving six healthy random users and one usability expert. The design of the study involved tasks to be performed without any help and evaluating the success rate and remarks related to each of the tasks. Users were randomly selected and were from different groups regarding age, computer literacy and internet usage. Usability study results have confirmed that the environment is easy to use as the users finished most of the tasks without external help in their first session. The bottleneck as shown by the usability study was the registration using digital certificates. The bottleneck was solved by an adjustment in the process of patient registration where phone support was made available to the enrolling user.

One of the drawbacks of the study design was also discrimination caused by lack of access to personal computers with internet access. The environment was upgraded to enable access over smart phones but as their use in general population is not widespread the problem persisted. Another problem that we expect to arise when gathering feedback is the need to repetitively fill in the same questionnaire over a longer period of time. The way to solve some of these issues could be by using body sensors (for stress and movement monitoring) and portable devices (for more handy subjective reporting) that are already showing promising results in research and clinical setting (Aziz et al., 2008; Sung, Marci & Pentland, 2005).

One of the limitations of web and mobile environments is lack of physical contact between patients and depression care professionals. To avoid issues of mistrust the service currently runs in parallel to existing care and is not meant to replace the physician-patient relationship but to upgrade it and enable stepped approach to treatment.

On the other hand there are many foreseen benefits that ease the process of depression care. Self evaluation questionnaires are filled out by patients on a weekly basis or even more and the environment is available at all times. If a patient does not fill out the questionnaires regularly enough or there is some other type of inactivity the system warns the patient over email or SMS. If the patient does not respond to SMS a task is automatically spawn for the care manager to call the patient. This way we expect to improve compliance and improve close follow-up. Close follow-up is crucial in the first weeks as modifications of therapy are often needed.

Suicide prevention service would need to be further developed and evaluated as at the moment we can not offer 24 hour telephone contact and for urgent matters the patients are advised to use existing providers of urgent care (contact information is provided on the homepage).

Back-end integration with existing EHRs was not in scope of the project. This was identified as a threat and has caused compliance issues with some physicians that need to retype some of the information into improvehealth.eu. Slow physician adoption can be partly accredited to lack of back-end integration, lack of financial motivation, lack of time during patient visits and lack of IT usage experience.

As the public part of the environment offered a screening tool for depression, we expected feedback from potential new users that received positive screening feedback. The response was slim partly to the fact that we redirected the test users to visit their GPs and because we are holding back information on the site's availability to general public as the clinical trial is not concluded yet.

An issue the case will be facing in near future is sustainability. Existing funding schemes in health care in Slovenia and several other countries do not count on-line communication and services as eligible for reimbursements by health insurance companies. To persuade insurance companies to cover such services on a broader scale we will need to conduct cost-efficiency analyses with results comparable to other interventions.

FUTURE RESEARCH DIRECTIONS

Looking from what we have learned in the description of the case study and from the review of the literature we can draw some conclusions. If we want to provide solutions for integrated health care facility- based and home-based care process support, further research is needed especially in the field of remote automated monitoring, clinical data processing and care model financing. The aim of remote automated monitoring is to acquire important information on patient status regularly, automatically and in a way that is not disturbing for the user. For this purpose portable, wearable and implantable sensors are increasingly being developed. Researchers connect several sensor types into Body Sensor Networks and Body Area Networks to acquire multimodal data (Aziz et al., 2008; Sung et al., 2005) that can be interpreted either in a closed-loop or open-loop approach to provide feedback to the user and when necessary trigger additional interventions on the health care provider side. The data gathered will permit us and later clinicians to gather and analyze relevant

medical data either preemptively (prevention, before a disease state is clinically present) or as a means of therapeutic follow-up.

Additionally with parallel development of electronic health care records, hospital information systems and personal health care records more and more clinical information will be available for process support, diminishing the barriers to adoption of these solutions. Specific analyses focused on Health Technology Assessment aimed at demonstrating the cost-efficiency of the above approaches as compared to other interventions are already underway.

The final goal of all these approaches is to create ubiquitous ICT environments that:

- respects personal dignity and privacy;
- unobtrusively monitors apparently healthy people and provide them with feedback on health related risk behavior (e.g. overeating, lack of recreation, abusive drinking, etc.);
- monitors the treatment process (e.g. blood level of antibiotics or antidepressants, fluctuations in blood sugar levels in diabetic patients);
- predicts relapses of diseases (e.g. changes in behavior patterns in patients with manic depression);

Figure 4. Population pools, disease process (right pointing arrows) and interventions (left pointing arrows and circular arrow)

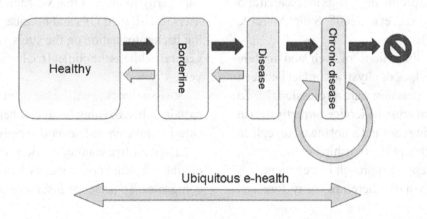

- supports each and every of the profiles of health care professionals involved in the care process with personalized information and task generation; and
- provides automated motivation and reminders to ensure timeliness of the care process.

The future ICT solutions will thus support integrated screening, prevention, treatment and care processes as one and help us streamline healthy people into health improvement programmes, persons at risk into prevention programmes, acute patients into treatment programmes, patients with chronic conditions into treatment and care programmes (as proposed in Figure 4).

This way there will be potential to develop entirely new preventive and screening programmes that will better segment screening, prevention and treatment efforts. To achieve widespread adoption adaptations of existing funding schemes will need to be developed, enabling providers to receive payments based on their population's performance at virtual screenings, individual patients' care process status and clinical improvements of their patients. Health care provision will have the means to become more optimized in terms of human resource utilization and redirection of responsibilities and health related activities to the patients and healthy individuals that will help drive down the disease burden as well as sustain or reduce cost of care.

CONCLUSION

eHealth is already playing an important role in support of health care providers' activities but further improvements in the field of care process support and active patient engagement and empowerment are underway. In view of the rising health care costs due to demographic changes new care models will need to be developed especially in the field of long-term care for the growing population of elderly with one or more chronic conditions. ICT

supported care management and patient empowerment and the resource utilization they enable will play a crucial role in improving health care systems, reducing human resource utilization, improving home care support, patient engagement and consecutive long-term cost-sustainability of these new care models.

ACKNOWLEDGMENT

The authors would like to express their sincere gratitude to late Professor Andrej Marušič MD PhD BSc for setting up eDepression project and for his efforts to invent new methods of treatment for patients with depression.

REFERENCES

Angelmar, R. (2007). Patient empowerment and efficient health outcomes. *Financing sustainable healthcare in Europe: New approaches for better outcomes,* 141. Retrieved February 28, 2009 from http://www.sustainhealthcare.org/cox.php

Ash, J. S., & Bates, D. W. (2005). Factors and forces affecting EHR system adoption: report of a 2004 ACMI discussion. *Journal of the American Medical Informatics Association, 12,* 8–12. doi:10.1197/jamia.M1684

Atkinson, N. L., & Gold, R. S. (2002). The promise and challenge of eHealth interventions. *American Journal of Health Behavior, 26,* 494–503.

Aziz, O., Lo, B., Pansiot, J., Atallah, L., Yang, G. Z., & Darzi, A. (2008). From computers to ubiquitous computing by 2010: health care. *Philos. Transact. A Math. Phys. Eng Sci., 366,* 3805–3811.

Beck, A. T., Ward, C. H., Mendelson, M., Mock, J., & Erbaugh, J. (1961). An inventory for measuring depression. *Archives of General Psychiatry, 4,* 561–571.

Bennett, K., Kabir, Z., Barry, M., Tilson, L., Fidan, D., & Shelley, E. (2008). *Cost-Effectiveness of Treatments Reducing Coronary Heart Disease Mortality in Ireland, 2000 to 2010.* Value. Health.

Blobel, B. G., Engel, K., & Pharow, P. (2006). Semantic interoperability--HL7 Version 3 compared to advanced architecture standards. *Methods of Information in Medicine, 45*, 343–353.

Bloom, B. S. (2002). Crossing the Quality Chasm: A New Health System for the 21st Century. *JAMA: The Journal of the American Medical Association, 287*, 646–64a. doi:10.1001/jama.287.5.646-a

Bock, B. C., Graham, A. L., Whiteley, J. A., & Stoddard, J. L. (2008). A review of web-assisted tobacco interventions (WATIs). *Journal of Medical Internet Research, 10*, e39. doi:10.2196/jmir.989

Bodenheimer, T. (2005a). High and Rising Health Care Costs. Part 1: Seeking an Explanation. *Annals of Internal Medicine, 142*, 847–854.

Bodenheimer, T. (2005b). High and Rising Health Care Costs. Part 2: Technologic Innovation. *Annals of Internal Medicine, 142*, 932–937.

Bodenheimer, T. (2005c). High and Rising Health Care Costs. Part 3: The Role of Health Care Providers. *Annals of Internal Medicine, 142*, 996–1002.

Campbell, H., Hotchkiss, R., Bradshaw, N., & Porteous, M. (1998). Integrated care pathways. *BMJ (Clinical Research Ed.), 316*, 133–137.

Cashen, M. S., Dykes, P., & Gerber, B. (2004). eHealth technology and Internet resources: barriers for vulnerable populations. *The Journal of Cardiovascular Nursing, 19*, 209–214.

Chaudhry, B., Wang, J., Wu, S., Maglione, M., Mojica, W., & Roth, E. (2006). Systematic review: impact of health information technology on quality, efficiency, and costs of medical care. *Annals of Internal Medicine, 144*, 742–752.

Clark, R. A., Inglis, S. C., McAlister, F. A., Cleland, J. G., & Stewart, S. (2007). Telemonitoring or structured telephone support programmes for patients with chronic heart failure: systematic review and meta-analysis. *BMJ (Clinical Research Ed.), 334*, 942. doi:10.1136/bmj.39156.536968.55

Crosson, F. J., & Madvig, P. (2004). Does Population Management Of Chronic Disease Lead To Lower Costs Of Care? *Health Affairs, 23*, 76–78. doi:10.1377/hlthaff.23.6.76

Crowther, R., Gask, L., Ives, R., & Jakenfelds, J. (2001). A program designed to monitor the course and management of depressive illness across the primary/secondary interface. *Medinfo, 10*, 719–723.

Cummings, E., & Turner, P. (2009). Patient self-management and chronic illness: evaluating outcomes and impacts of information technology. *Studies in Health Technology and Informatics, 143*, 229–234.

de Graaf, L. E., Gerhards, S. A., Evers, S. M., Arntz, A., Riper, H., & Severens, J. L. (2008). Clinical and cost-effectiveness of computerised cognitive behavioural therapy for depression in primary care: design of a randomised trial. *BMC Public Health, 8*, 224. doi:10.1186/1471-2458-8-224

Eysenbach, G. (2005). The law of attrition. *Journal of Medical Internet Research, 7*, e11. doi:10.2196/jmir.7.1.e11

Eysenbach, G. (2008). Medicine 2.0: social networking, collaboration, participation, apomediation, and openness. *Journal of Medical Internet Research, 10*, e22. doi:10.2196/jmir.1030

Eysenbach, G. (2009). Infodemiology and info-veillance: framework for an emerging set of public health informatics methods to analyze search, communication and publication behavior on the Internet. *Journal of Medical Internet Research*, *11*, e11. doi:10.2196/jmir.1157

Fireman, B., Bartlett, J., & Selby, J. (2004). Can Disease Management Reduce Health Care Costs By Improving Quality? *Health Affairs*, *23*, 63–75. doi:10.1377/hlthaff.23.6.63

Garcia-Lizana, F., & Sarria-Santamera, A. (2007). New technologies for chronic disease management and control: a systematic review. *Journal of Telemedicine and Telecare*, *13*, 62–68. doi:10.1258/135763307780096140

Geyman, J. P. (2007). Disease management: panacea, another false hope, or something in between? *Annals of Family Medicine*, *5*, 257–260. doi:10.1370/afm.649

Gilbody, S., Bower, P., Fletcher, J., Richards, D., & Sutton, A. J. (2006). Collaborative care for depression: a cumulative meta-analysis and review of longer-term outcomes. *Archives of Internal Medicine*, *166*, 2314–2321. doi:10.1001/archinte.166.21.2314

Gilmour, J. A. (2007). Reducing disparities in the access and use of Internet health information. a discussion paper. *International Journal of Nursing Studies*, *44*, 1270–1278. doi:10.1016/j.ijnurstu.2006.05.007

Glasgow, R. E. (2007). eHealth evaluation and dissemination research. *American Journal of Preventive Medicine*, *32*, S119–S126. doi:10.1016/j.amepre.2007.01.023

Griffiths, F., Lindenmeyer, A., Powell, J., Lowe, P., & Thorogood, M. (2006). Why are health care interventions delivered over the internet? A systematic review of the published literature. *Journal of Medical Internet Research*, *8*, e10. doi:10.2196/jmir.8.2.e10

Grone, O., & Garcia-Barbero, M. (2001). Integrated care: a position paper of the WHO European Office for Integrated Health Care Services. *International Journal of Integrated Care*, *1*, e21.

Hardy, B., Mur-Veemanu, I., Steenbergen, M., & Wistow, G. (1999). Inter-agency services in England and The Netherlands. A comparative study of integrated care development and delivery. *Health Policy (Amsterdam)*, *48*, 87–105. doi:10.1016/S0168-8510(99)00037-8

Hunkeler, E. M., Katon, W., Tang, L., Williams, J. W. Jr, Kroenke, K., & Lin, E. H. (2006). Long term outcomes from the IMPACT randomised trial for depressed elderly patients in primary care. *BMJ (Clinical Research Ed.)*, *332*, 259–263. doi:10.1136/bmj.38683.710255.BE

Jovicic, A., Holroyd-Leduc, J. M., & Straus, S. E. (2006). Effects of self-management intervention on health outcomes of patients with heart failure: a systematic review of randomized controlled trials. *BMC Cardiovascular Disorders*, *6*, 43. doi:10.1186/1471-2261-6-43

Kessler, R. C., Berglund, P., Demler, O., Jin, R., Koretz, D., & Merikangas, K. R. (2003). The epidemiology of major depressive disorder: results from the National Comorbidity Survey Replication (NCS-R). *JAMA. Journal of the American Medical Association*, *289*, 3095–3105. doi:10.1001/jama.289.23.3095

Kobb, R., Chumbler, N. R., Brennan, D. M., & Rabinowitz, T. (2008). Home telehealth: mainstreaming what we do well. *Telemed.J.E. Health*, *14*, 977–981.

Lepine, J. P., Gastpar, M., Mendlewicz, J., & Tylee, A. (1997). Depression in the community: the first pan-European study DEPRES (Depression Research in European Society). *International Clinical Psychopharmacology*, *12*, 19–29.

Lin, E. H., Von, K. M., Katon, W., Bush, T., Simon, G. E., & Walker, E. (1995). The role of the primary care physician in patients' adherence to antidepressant therapy. *Medical Care, 33*, 67–74. doi:10.1097/00005650-199501000-00006

Lopez, D. M., & Blobel, B. (2009). Enhanced semantic interoperability by profiling health informatics standards. *Methods of Information in Medicine, 48*, 170–177.

Ludwick, D. A., & Doucette, J. (2009). Primary Care Physicians' Experience with Electronic Medical Records: Barriers to Implementation in a Fee-for-Service Environment. *Int. J. Telemed. Appl., 2009*, 853524.

Marmor, T., Oberlander, J., & White, J. (2009). The Obama Administration's Options for Health Care Cost Control: Hope Versus Reality. *Annals of Internal Medicine, 150*, 485–489.

Meglič, M. (2007, September). *Care management using BPM: case of depression.* Paper presented at EFMI Special Topic Conference on Open Source in Health care, London, United Kingdom.

Neuhauser, L., & Kreps, G. L. (2003). Rethinking Communication in the E-health Era. *Journal of Health Psychology, 8*, 7–23. doi:10.1177/1359105303008001426

Neumeyer-Gromen, A., Lampert, T., Stark, K., & Kallischnigg, G. (2004). Disease management programs for depression: a systematic review and meta-analysis of randomized controlled trials. *Medical Care, 42*, 1211–1221. doi:10.1097/00005650-200412000-00008

Norman, G. J., Zabinski, M. F., Adams, M. A., Rosenberg, D. E., Yaroch, A. L., & Atienza, A. A. (2007). A review of eHealth interventions for physical activity and dietary behavior change. *American Journal of Preventive Medicine, 33*, 336–345. doi:10.1016/j.amepre.2007.05.007

Pampallona, S., Bollini, P., Tibaldi, G., Kupelnick, B., & Munizza, C. (2002). Patient adherence in the treatment of depression. *The British Journal of Psychiatry, 180*, 104–109. doi:10.1192/bjp.180.2.104

Plant, R. T., Murrell, S., & Moreno, H. R. (1994). Prototype decision support system for a differential diagnosis of psychotic, mood, and organic mental disorders: Part II. *Medical Decision Making, 14*, 273–288. doi:10.1177/0272989X9401400310

Robertson, L., Smith, M., Castle, D., & Tannenbaum, D. (2006). Using the Internet to enhance the treatment of depression. *Australasian Psychiatry, 14*, 413–417.

Robertson, L., Smith, M., & Tannenbaum, D. (2005). Case management and adherence to an online disease management system. *Journal of Telemedicine and Telecare, 11*(Suppl 2), S73–S75. doi:10.1258/135763305775124885

Siriwardena, A. N., Lawson, S., Vahl, M., Middleton, H., & de Zeeuv, G. (2008). Emerging technologies for developing and improving patients' health experience. *Quality in Primary Care, 16*, 1–5.

Spitzer, R. L., Kroenke, K., Linzer, M., Hahn, S. R., Williams, J. B., & deGruy, F. V. III (1995). Health-related quality of life in primary care patients with mental disorders. Results from the PRIME-MD 1000 Study. *JAMA: The Journal of the American Medical Association, 274*, 1511–1517. doi:10.1001/jama.274.19.1511

Stevens, V. J., Funk, K. L., Brantley, P. J., Erlinger, T. P., Myers, V. H., & Champagne, C. M. (2008). Design and implementation of an interactive website to support long-term maintenance of weight loss. *Journal of Medical Internet Research, 10*, e1. doi:10.2196/jmir.931

Sung, M., Marci, C., & Pentland, A. (2005). Wearable feedback systems for rehabilitation. *Journal of Neuroengineering and Rehabilitation, 2*, 17. doi:10.1186/1743-0003-2-17

Trivedi, M. H., Daly, E. J., Kern, J. K., Grannemann, B. D., Sunderajan, P., & Claassen, C. A. (2009). Barriers to implementation of a computerized decision support system for depression: an observational report on lessons learned in "real world" clinical settings. *BMC Medical Informatics and Decision Making, 9*, 6. doi:10.1186/1472-6947-9-6

Trivedi, M. H., Kern, J. K., Grannemann, B. D., Altshuler, K. Z., & Sunderajan, P. (2004). A computerized clinical decision support system as a means of implementing depression guidelines. *Psychiatric Services (Washington, D.C.), 55*, 879–885. doi:10.1176/appi.ps.55.8.879

Tufano, J. T., & Karras, B. T. (2005). Mobile eHealth interventions for obesity: a timely opportunity to leverage convergence trends. *Journal of Medical Internet Research, 7*, e58. doi:10.2196/jmir.7.5.e58

Unutzer, J., Choi, Y., Cook, I. A., & Oishi, S. (2002). A web-based data management system to improve care for depression in a multicenter clinical trial. *Psychiatric Services (Washington, D.C.), 53*, 671–673, 678. doi:10.1176/appi.ps.53.6.671

Wilson, G. (2006) 'No show' hospital patients cost NHS £700m, *Telegraph.co.uk,* retrieved February 23, 2009 from http://www.telegraph.co.uk/news/uknews/1517730/%27No-show%27-hospital-patients-cost-NHS-andpound700m.html

Wilson, P., Bunn, F., & Morgan, J. (2009). A mapping of the evidence on integrated long term condition services. *British Journal of Community Nursing, 14*, 202–206.

Chapter 20
Building Virtual Communities for Health Promotion:
Emerging Best Practices through an Analysis of the International Health Challenge & Related Literature in Second Life

Sameer Siddiqi
University of Houston, USA

Rebecca E. Lee
University of Houston, USA

ABSTRACT

Contemporary Multi-User Virtual Environments (MUVEs) allow health educators, researchers, and practitioners (ERPs) to engage students, participants, and patients through innovative and uniquely rewarding methods. The technology's value lies in its access to non-traditional participant pools, novel forms of social interaction, and cost-effective improvements to existing methods. These benefits are built on key Web 2.0 principles, namely social networking, community synthesis, and collaborative content generation. In light of ongoing dynamic development of virtual platforms, advancements in networking and immersion technology, and sustained consumer interest, the appeal of these environments will likely increase. Linden Lab's Second Life (SL), a widely recognized and heavily populated MUVE, illustrates the technology's broad spectrum of possibilities through the documented efforts of early adopters involved in health promotion, research, and therapy. However, ERPs must be mindful of the medium's complexities, technological and social parameters, and weaknesses before considering development within virtual worlds (in-world). As these environments operate independently of the real world in some aspects, knowledge of gathering and creating relevant in-world and real-world resources, attracting and retaining project interest, and addressing common obstacles is essential. Through an analysis of

DOI: 10.4018/978-1-61520-777-0.ch020

Copyright © 2010, IGI Global. Copying or distributing in print or electronic forms without written permission of IGI Global is prohibited.

the Texas Obesity Research Center at the University of Houston's International Health Challenge in SL and the documented findings of past and existing health-related programs in SL, the authors seek to provide best practices to overcome these challenges and establish realistic parameters for program design and implementation.

INTRODUCTION

The emerging best practices discussed herein are primarily derived from the observations of Texas Obesity Research Center (TORC) research team, through their development and implementation of the International Health Challenge (IHC) in the Multi-User Virtual Environment (MUVE) of Second Life (SL). The innovative intent of the IHC and fundamental lack of relevant literature has allowed TORC's undergraduate and graduate team and faculty co-investigators to test novel solutions based on health promotion and interventions in the real world and recent or on-going in-world projects. Therefore, the best practices we report herein reflect scholarly diversity and comparative study. Additional practices, many of which were tested in the IHC, are provided through a variety of scholarly and informal works, including peer-reviewed articles, in-world and real-world conference proceedings, published discussions of existing or past in-world projects, Linden Lab recommendations, and documentation collected by in-world health and education related organizations. This diverse array of sources provides a means to assess the validity and quality of our own practices in the IHC and those of others. Through these practices we seek to provide best practices for health educators, researchers, and practitioners (ERPs) to overcome these challenges and establish realistic parameters for program design and implementation.

BACKGROUND

Multi-User Virtual Environments (MUVEs) are networked, synchronous, computer-simulated environments which facilitate social interaction among uniquely identified users through rich visual, auditory, or textual interfaces. The technology is rooted in early text-based computer gaming applications known as Multi-User Dungeons (MUDs) (Bartle, 1990). In light of evolving computer processing and connectivity capabilities, these technologically simplistic networks began to incorporate two-dimensional images and audio, and later, animated three-dimensional models and larger numbers of users. Virtual worlds focused on role-playing gaming were informally labeled Massive Multiplayer Online Role Playing Games (MMORPGs), whereas those more interested in social interaction were designated MUVEs (Dieterle and Clarke, 2007). In the last five years, however, MUVEs have come to describe persistent, three-dimensional, mixed media virtual worlds, complete with monetary or commodity based economies and large populations of unique human-controlled characters, or avatars.

Contemporary MUVEs incorporate a number of core Web 2.0 concepts, namely synchronous social networking, organic community synthesis, and collaborative content generation. These principles lay the foundation for the technology's most attractive aspects, including participatory learning (Brown and Adler, 2008) and enhanced social presence (Schroeder, 2002).

Linden Lab's Second Life (SL), the most widely recognized contemporary MUVE, is home to over one million active residents (unique logins per 30 day intervals) and a robust cash-based economy with over $100 million USD in quarterly transactions (Linden Lab, 2009a). SL is mechanically defined as an international multi-user, multi-sensory albeit image-centric, persistent, stigmergic, private ownership based, collaborative and conditional environment built on a publicly accessible wide area network (Robbins, 2007). These central components are manifested through a number of client features and in-world trends, which we will discuss in greater detail later in the chapter.

THE MECHANICS, ECONOMY, AND COMMUNITY OF SECOND LIFE

Before delving into the details of program design and development within SL, there are certain topics worth discussing in brief detail, namely the nature of the client, network, and virtual world. The recently open-sourced end-user client, SL Viewer, runs on sufficiently capable Windows, Mac, and Linux operating systems (refer to Linden Lab's official system requirements for details); performance depends primarily on video processing power and bandwidth (Linden Lab, 2009b). Connections and content processing, storage, and delivery are handled through a collection of networked servers, or grids, operated by Linden Lab (Linden Lab, 2009c). In order to access the virtual world, users are required to login into their unique, near infinitely customizable avatars, via unverified, age-restricted accounts (13 years of age and over). Users are subsequently filtered to one of two grids, Teen (13-17 year olds) or Main (18+ year olds); the Teen grid is far less populated, limited with respect to ownership rights, and includes content censorship among other safety features (Linden Lab). Once in-world, users can associate with one another through organized, miniature social networks, or Groups, which often share contacts, object resources, and land rights. Property within SL, commonly referred to as land, is divided into regions, which in turn are divided into parcels; either can be purchased or leased directly from Linden Lab or through residents, and customized accordingly. Land is populated with objects comprised of geometric and sculpted building blocks known as "prims"; a significant

majority of in-world objects are user-generated, and are made through the Viewer's intuitive object modeling and texturing features and the expansive capabilities of Linden Scripting Language (LSL) (similar to C & Java) (Linden Lab).

As of Q4 2008, Second Life's active population is predominantly male (n=59%), between the ages of 25-44 (n=63%), and resides for the most part in the U.S. (n=39%) and to some extent in other developed Asian and European countries (e.g.: United Kingdom, Germany, Japan, France) (Linden Lab, 2008). Central to SL's speedy adoption is the volume and growth of its currency - based economy (250 Linden ($L) equals approximately 1$USD). Linden Lab reports Q4 2008 user-to-user transactions within the virtual world to be in excess of $100 million $USD, a 54% increase from Q4 2007. Such data supports probable further economic development and resident enrollment in SL or other MUVEs.

This growth is reflected inside SL by the presence of countless special interest groups, which collectively form rich in-world communities focused on a number of loosely related interests. Though most Groups are concerned with in-world entertainment and commercial entities, there are also many focused on creative, instructional, educational, academic, and sociopolitical topics. It is this mixture that best reflects the overall social nature of SL: a network of communities of varied interests with a tilt toward entertainment.

VALUE OF SECOND LIFE TO HEALTH EDUCATORS, RESEARCHERS, AND PRACTITIONERS (ERPs)

SL presents exciting possibilities for (ERPs, as it (a) provides access to a host of valuable demographics, (b) allows for novel forms of interaction not normally feasible in traditional health settings, and (c) improves existing forms of participant / patient / student interaction through more cost effective and beneficial solutions. With regard to demographics, SL is an ideal setting to reach adult members of industrialized societies who may require, but not have practical access to, uncommon health resources (specific health education courses, therapeutic support groups, health interventions, collaboration opportunities, etc.). Participants aside, SL offers radically innovative means of delivering educational content, facilitating therapy, and conducting human subject research, via methods physically or practically impossible to create in the real world, that show positive evidence-based results. In the same vein, SL offers improvements to traditional practices through less costly and time-consuming solutions. This is facilitated by the ability of MUVEs to partially imitate reality; Rheingold (1993) reports that virtual communities show characteristics of love, hate, betrayal, and others common to traditional settings, thereby linking, in some aspects, real world and in-world practices.

In recognition of these benefits, many ERPs, often with the support of large academic, governmental or nonprofit institutions, have begun to explore SL and subsequently document their findings. Early adopters, with specific regard to health research and education, include Indiana University, Ohio University, University of Houston, the National Institutes of Health, FasterCures, and many more; hundreds of similar institutions also have in-world campuses, which often offer virtual classes, meeting and presentation space, and promotional tours. Frequently observed areas of interest include obesity and nutrition, preventive care with regard to chronic illness, support methods for mental and physical disabilities, as well as more procedural issues like cataloging academic and nonprofit resources and compiling databases of research and education techniques and facilitators. Significant health-related contributions are also attributable to groups of individual ERPs unattached to funding institutions. Their efforts have led to the development of grassroots professional Groups within SL, which have in turn

developed valuable land and object resources, contact directories, collaborative opportunities, and more recently, many major real world conferences and workshops.

As is the case with any emerging medium, there are significant challenges that must be addressed before more widespread adoption can occur. Through an analysis of the International Health Challenge (IHC) in SL and dozens of other scholarly works and in-world projects, we intend to contribute to the pressing need for organized evidence-based best practices specific to eHealth endeavors in MUVEs.

THE INTERNATIONAL HEALTH CHALLENGE IN SECOND LIFE

The IHC is an elaborate health promotion study in the virtual world of SL that moves beyond simply improving health knowledge by seeking to positively affect attitudes and behaviors in real life. The purpose of the study is to determine the feasibility of health interventions in MUVEs and role of social cohesion on virtual participation. The program is the result of international collaboration between the Texas Obesity Research Center (TORC) in the Department of Health and Human Performance at the University of Houston and researchers at Wilfrid Laurier University. The IHC is funded by grants from the Network Culture Project of the Annenberg School for Communication at the University of Southern California and the Department of Health and Human Performance at the University of Houston. Evidence based educational content on the topics of physical activity, dietary habits, and behavioral strategies to improve health habits are conveyed through incentivized modes of delivery familiar to virtual world residents. The IHC initially started as a strategy to develop an interactive, multilingual, and multicultural health promotion project in SL as evidenced by a full service build, activities, and participating residents. Using existing resources

Figure 1. Interactive area for surveys, questionnaires, physical activity and dietary habits monitoring logs, and quizzes

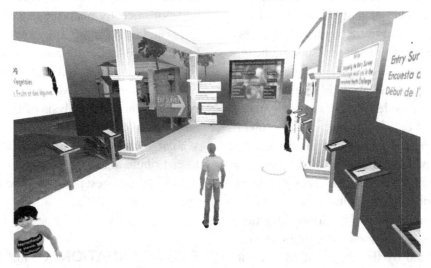

and extensive social networks, together with volunteer assistance, the IHC has flourished into a full scale health intervention with the goals of improving health knowledge, attitudes and behavior among residents.

The IHC project site is located above the University of Houston's Health and Human Performance Island, a virtual property belonging to the Department of Health and Human Performance; such land ownership allows for complete customization of the environment and control over access. The interactive components of the IHC are compartmentalized and arranged in a functional open-air layout. All of these components were modeled and created by in-world and out –of-world TORC staff members, volunteers, and SL-specific contractors. Surveys, questionnaires, physical activity and dietary habits monitoring logs, and quizzes are offered weekly to participants through the site (Figure 1). The adapted educational content referenced earlier is delivered via slide-displays scattered throughout the IHC site; selected topics include:

- Physical Activity Injury Prevention & Safety

- Health Goal Setting
- Social Support and Self Efficacy with regard to Health Goals
- Relapse Prevention

Core measurement instruments are located in specifically designated areas designed to stimulate prolonged participant presence and social interaction. These goals are realized through the use of incentivized interactive objects modeled and scripted to represent real-world physical activity and dietary resources (e.g.: exercise equipment, food items) (Figures 2 & 3). IHC site use and project participation is tracked by scripted sensors and visualized through a scoreboard-like mechanism, which prominently displays the most active members. Access to these features is limited to participants enrolled in the four week program.

Participants are recruited through a number of methods including project promotion at various locations throughout the virtual world by trained staff members following an established protocol, advertisement within special-interest groups, and through unpaid referrals. Such a comprehensive approach minimizes selection bias all while providing the ability to test the efficacy of each

Figure 2. Physical activity pavilion

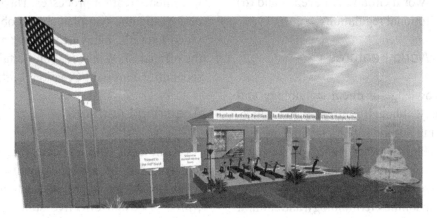

technique. Participant retention is accomplished through a similarly varied system. Trained staff members routinely deliver personalized and universal messages to assigned participants, thereby ensuring regular participant contact. Retention is further enhanced by regular incentivized group activities. We will discuss these techniques and many more in greater detail later in the chapter.

The program is currently concluding active enrollment and participation. Data collection, scoring, and analysis will begin shortly and be made available when appropriate.

MAIN FOCUS OF CHAPTER

Issues, Controversies, Problems & Solutions and Recommendations

Program Design

The inherent complexity and foreignness of virtual environments requires an extraordinary focus on preliminary planning. In this segment, we present techniques with which to become familiar with (a) client features and in-world culture, (b) available sources of literature and collaboration,

Figure 3. Dietary resources pavilion

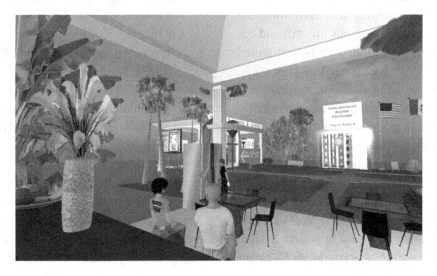

(c) relevant in-world Groups and events, and (d) legal and institutional regulations.

Client & In-World Features

A cursory knowledge of client technology and in-world society, although common to most interested in utilizing Second Life for health purposes (programs), is far from what is needed to develop an effective in-world presence. Program designers should move beyond interface familiarity and examine the capabilities, terminology, and cultural norms of the SL Viewer, in-world economy, and content generation. All of these factors profoundly influence program interactivity, target audience, budget, and scope.

Rather than rely solely on trial and error, EPRs should systematically explore official and user-created documentation. The official Second Life Wiki Help Portal (http://wiki.secondlife.com/wiki/Help_Portal) provides succinct summaries of all of the above topics and links to external text and especially helpful video tutorials. There are also a slew of in-world tutorials, which provide a more interactive learning experience. For those entirely new to SL, in-world and video sessions, both guided and exploratory, should precede any examination of documentation. When working with a larger team, there are many additional considerations. Throughout your own learning process, consider retaining and compiling the most useful guides and tutorials for staff and co-investigators; create a guide that is best suited for the diversity and background of your team. In our experience, interactive video tutorials and in-world orientations, completed individually then discussed as a group, are an effective way to collectively address concerns; document the most common difficulties for future reference.

As mentioned earlier, user-generated content is a definitive feature of SL. Therefore, even a limited understanding of LSL, land use, and object manipulation is helpful in project design, regardless of the level of personal involvement

in content creation processes. Have at least one co-investigator complete basic object creation video tutorials, many of which can be found on the official SL Wiki Creation Portal (http://wiki.secondlife.com/wiki/Creation_Portal).

Acquiring Literature

As is the case with any scientific endeavor, an understanding of prior and existing research and related conclusions provides a foundation from which to design effective studies. Fortunately, there exists a growing body of recent scholarly and informal literature on the topic of virtual worlds, and SL in particular, in the form of journals, conferences, and wiki-based databases.

Novel, peer-reviewed, special interest journals are quickly becoming premier sources of information on virtual environments. Of note are:

- Journal of Virtual Worlds Research (ISSNISSN: 1941-8477)
- CyberPsychology & Behavior (ISSN: 1094-9313)
- Telemedicine and e-Health (ISSN: 1530-5627)
- Journal of Medical Internet Research (ISSN: 1438-8871)
- Studies in Health Technology and Informatics (ISSN: 0926-9630)
- Simulation and Gaming (ISSN: 1046-8781)
- Journal of CyberTherapy & Rehabilitation (ISSN: Not available)
- Annual Review of CyberTherapy and Telemedicine (ISSN: 1554-8716)
- ACM Transactions on Graphics (ISSN: 0730-0301)

The documented proceedings of health or education related, professionally organized, in-world and / or real-world conferences are among the most valuable sources of information on current best practices, findings, and collaborative opportunities. Although proceedings are essential, attendance is strongly encouraged, as doing so provides access to valuable contacts and potential collaborators. Of note are:

- Virtual Worlds Best Practices in Education Conference (http://www.vwbpe.org/)
- Second Life Community Convention (http://www.slconvention.org/)
- New Media Consortium Summer Conference (http://www.nmc.org/)
- Games for Health Annual Conference (http://www.gamesforhealth.org/)
- Medicine Meets Virtual Reality (http://www.nextmed.com/)
- Special Interest Group on Graphics and Interactive Techniques (http://www.sig-graph.org/)
- 3-D Training, Learning, and Collaboration (http://www.3dtlc.com/)

Wiki-based databases of in-world projects also provide valuable documentation of current and past projects and the details and contact information related to each. Of note are:

- RezEd (http://www.rezed.org/)
- University of Oregon's SaLamander Project (http://eduisland.net/salamander-wiki/index.php)
- SimTeach (http://www.simteach.com/wiki/index.php)
- SimTeach Educational Content and Presence Database (http://simteach.com/sled/db/)
- Nonprofit Commons (http://npsl.wikispaces.com/)
- Multimedia Educational Resource for Online Learning and Teaching (http://www.merlot.org/)

Notable In-World Groups

Engaging communities, groups, and projects in SL is as essential to a successful program as is an examination of literature and conference proceedings. Given the significant degree of social-networking in SL, there exist dozens of in-world groups focused on health, research, and education. Regular meetings, group chats, events, resources sharing, and access to members are but a few of the benefits of participating in them. To find groups of interest, use the Community Search function; consider group size and instances of recent activity when selecting groups to engage. Engaging groups on a regular basis is strongly recommended. Of note are:

- Second Life Educators Listserv (https://lists.secondlife.com/cgi-bin/mailman/listinfo/educators)
- Virtual Worlds Research Discussion Group
- Virtual Ability Research Group
- Health Support Coalition
- Health Info Island
- Nonprofit Commons
- Commonwealth Island
- New Media Consortium

Legal & Institutional Considerations

Although virtual, studies involving SL must take human subject interaction, client terms, and property rules into consideration. Projects in SL must be conducted within the confines of Linden Lab's Terms of Service and Community Standards, both of which are readily available online. Health-related ERPs should also consider the regulations of local Institutional Review Boards, as they will likely be required to attain approval before execution. Last, all staff and investigators which will interact with avatars as part of the study should secure Certification for the Protection of Human Subjects or an equivalent document relative to their country; in the United States, certification can be obtained for free from the National Institutes of Health (http://phrp.nihtraining.com/).

Leveraging Real & In-World Resources

ERPs anchored to large educational institutions may have access to faculty colleagues, students, technical support departments, and campus-wide communication channels. Generating faculty interest across various academic and professional disciplines creates a more academically productive, educational, and reputable presence in virtual environments (Liu, 2006). It has been our experience that many faculty are often unwilling to take virtual environments seriously, are unable to operate or setup the software, or simply do not know where to begin once in-world. All of these concerns can be at least partly addressed through regular meetings focused on overcoming technical issues, introductory orientations, and examining the work of in-world peer organizations. These sessions should ultimately lead toward collaboration, which creates a series of benefits. During development, the IHC heavily incorporated fellow faculty members from various departments (Education, Technology, and Health and Human Performance). Such an approach fostered a sense of communal accountability, urgency, motivation, and served as an informative springboard for those considering projects of their own. For campuses with faculty already in-world, organize a central in-world group and create logoed objects to enhance your campus's virtual presence.

As technical difficulties are often a major issue with SL, consider asking your technical support department to provide adequate hardware, perform regular client updates, and troubleshoot, all of which issues will undoubtedly be encountered on a regular basis. Last, we strongly recommend incorporating undergraduate and graduate students in design and testing processes, as they often have strong technical skills, a keen interest in innovative educational, research and health promotion strategies, and an intrinsic understanding of technology and trends within the context of contemporary virtual resources (e.g.: social-networks, virtual worlds).

Third-Party Resources

Linden Lab, the creator and operator of SL, provides a number of resources to ERPs, including but not limited to subsidized and discounted land (for nonprofits), concise setup guides, in-world consultation services, and networking opportunities. Visit their Enterprises and Educators page to access to learn more about these resources (http://secondlife.com/land/privatepricing.php). Many private organizations within SL also offer subsidized regions or parcels; locating such opportunities is a worthwhile challenge. When designing or testing program components, consider using "Sandboxes", areas in SL that are free and open to content creation. In either case, remain mindful of land use and access rights.

Possible Uses of SL for Health Related Educators, Researchers, and Practitioners (ERPs)

SL's emphasis on user-generated content allows for tremendous flexibility in designing and implementing targeted research, education, and health lifestyle related programs. Through an analysis of the IHC and existing and past in-world projects, we present a variety of possible uses and associated benefits.

Research

Researchers at major academic and nonprofit institutions have emerged as early adopters of virtual environments like SL. Although the technology's benefits are too numerous to list, the most prominent include participant access, scalability, design freedom, and cost effectiveness. In the case of the IHC, SL provides access to demographics difficult to target in traditional settings, namely non-local or interspersed populations; such a benefit is essential to studies involving human subject participation. Furthermore, the scalability and design freedom allowed for by the technology's intuitive content generation system permit researchers to create projects spatially impossible in traditional settings. Last, the relatively low-cost nature of the in-world services and goods market allows for programs either too expensive or time-consuming for real world development. However, in its current state, the technology does have a number of weaknesses applicable to research, namely a lack of stringent privacy and confidentiality features, considerable hardware and technical knowledge requirements, inconsistent user access and experience, and sparse foundational research.

Education

SL's immersive, anonymous, lack of serious repercussions, multi-sensory means of social interaction, and collaborative development features support a rich educational experience uncommon to earlier technologies; it's hardly surprising that educators have positioned themselves as the pioneers of virtual world scholarship and professional utilization. Research shows that immersive environments facilitate greater learning independence (Vygotsky, 1978); that social interaction supports more active learning through reflective processes (Wenger, 2000); that anonymity may promote learning behaviors individuals are unlikely to learn independently in real life (Boulos, Hetherington, & Wheeler, 2007); and that collaboration toward an education goal creates communities of learners, which in turn produce a high quality learning experience(Boulos, Hetherington, & Wheeler). In addition to improving quality of instruction, these three components also facilitate uniquely beneficial forms of content delivery. Richter, Anderson-Inman, and Frisbee (2007) define five observed modes of education in SL:

1. **Demonstration**: Facilitates engagement through observation, primarily through textual, visual and auditory in-world objects. By far the most commonly utilized.

2. **Experiential**: Alters the experience of users via immersion for the purpose of conveying educational content. This technique makes the most of the technology's features.

3. **Diagnostic**: Interactive environments that promote self-learning. Most commonly manifested by manipulation-enabled simulations.

4. **Role Play**: Assumption of role or character, so as to experience scenario from first-person perspective.

5. **Constructive**: Use of experimentation, discovery, and construction to convey information. Utilizes collaborative content creation.

The IHC used both Demonstrative and Diagnostic modes of delivery through the use of slide shows, surveys, and modeled interactive physical activity and dietary equipment. As there is little evidence on the effectiveness of each form in virtual environments, programs should attempt to incorporate a variety of aspects with respect to desired outcomes.

Educators must note that SL's primary function is to entertain and so naturally, the client and virtual economy work to that end. Rather than limit SL's inherently playful nature in favor of strict pedagogy, we recommend embracing this aspect by encouraging students and instructors to develop a virtual identity, network with in-world groups outside real world circles, and explore relevant in-world locales. Program designers should also consider the entertainment value of every interactive component.

Also, Bowers, Ragas, and Neely (2009) report that instructors who conduct classes entirely in SL report satisfactions levels greater than those who conduct classes only partially in-world.

Despite SL's immense potential with regard to education, there are noteworthy limitations, the most apparent being technical difficulties and the inconsistencies which result. A student or instructor's educational experience is subject to change based on their technical skills, computer hardware, bandwidth, software incompatibility, and knowledge of SL. For instance, although most participants in the IHC were already familiar with the SL, they had difficulty using the site, and they required step-by-step, written, sometimes live, assistance. Even more, investigators were not clear on the software's capabilities, and could not make effective design changes without consulting third party experts. Steady improvements in hardware and the client will likely address many compatibility and usability issues; later in the chapter, we will propose solutions to overcoming at least some of these difficulties. As is the case with research, a lack of strong confidentiality features, steep learning curve, and limited foundational research are also notable weaknesses.

eHealth

In addition to education and research, SL is becoming increasingly attractive to health practitioners that see virtual environments as a means to deliver care and lifestyle related health information, a process referred herein as eHealth (Wyatt and Liu, 2002). SL offers patients the benefits of social presence, multi-sensory forms of communication, and group cohesion; it also allows care-providers greater control of treatment intensity and experience and the ability to participate in treatment alongside patients (Gorini, Gaggioli, Vigna, and Riva, 2008). Even more, virtual-reality based therapy has been shown to be particularly effective in treating psychological disorders, including but not limited to phobias, eating disorders, social anxiety disorders, sexual disorders, and posttraumatic stress disorders (Riva et al, 2007). Currently, eHealth is primarily manifested in-world through support groups focused on specific disorders; these extensively networked groups are highly active and worth engaging for specific best practices and resources. Researchers do not see eHealth as a replacement; rather, they recommend concurrent real world engagement (Gorini, Gaggioli, Vigna,

and Riva). Limitations include privacy issues (which may be countered via series of passwords & disclosure of insecure systems), a lack of fundamental research on therapeutic effectiveness, lack of built-in clinical features and environments, and the inconsistencies in user experience which result from technical difficulties.

Scaling to Fit Participants

Regardless of intended use, program designers must consider the technical familiarity, learning ability, and hardware accessibility of target participants. Projects ideally should be able to handle participants of varying levels of the aforementioned factors (Joseph, 2007). In the IHC, descriptive written guides were sufficient for many participants, whereas live guided tours were needed for others; in the absence of either, we lost potential participants. Target participant considerations should be derived from focus group surveys and routine beta testing by in-world volunteers, staff, or students.

In-World Staff

The appearance of avatars which represent your team, staff, program site, or program has an effect on participants. Baylor and Rye find students are more likely to remain attentive if the avatars of instructors reflect how they actually appear. Additionally, many private companies in SL make use of complex "appearance codes", policies which prohibit certain forms of clothing, attributes, and other forms of avatar customization (McArthur, 2008). In the IHC, in-world staff is encouraged to wear an item (shirt) that identifies them as members of the program. However, we also find that SL residents are more receptive to customized and unique avatars. Aside from clothing, it is also necessary to conduct training sessions on ethics in SL, acceptable behavior, and the level of avatar autonomy (e.g.: ability to join groups, add friends)

Data Types & Storage

The ultimate objective of any in-world project is to not only benefit participants, but also share conclusive analysis of findings for future efforts. Bell (2007) defines four primary means of quantitative data collection in virtual environments:

- **Experimental**: Controlled, scientific tests that seek to determine cause and effect outcomes. This technique is difficult to practice in virtual worlds given the lack of ultimate control.
- **Survey**: Automated question and response based solution. This technique requires the use of complex data storage and retrieval systems.
- **Textual Analysis**: Participant describes and interprets artifacts. This technique is difficult to practice in virtual worlds given the lack of visual uniformity and varied graphical output (depending on a participant's hardware).
- **Naturalistic Inquiry**: Observing reactions and action of avatars interacting with in-world objects. Obviously, observable reactions are limited in virtual worlds, and so this method requires innovation.

The IHC relies on surveys, which are a mixture of custom and open-source scripts that utilize XML-RPC protocols to rely information between in-world input and web databases. Given the growth of open source communities within SL, we strongly recommend seeking out an open source solution either online or in-world. Regardless of solution choice, pay particular attention to data security, multi-user usability, and retrieval simplicity. When working with human subjects, it is especially important to consider who and how data will be handled; securely collecting and storing data within legal and institutional bounds is imperative.

Program Setup

Upon finalizing an objective, team, mode of content delivery, and system of outcome measurement, you can begin to realize your project, in earnest, in SL. Regardless of whether outside developers will be used, it is necessary to develop a detailed specification document, which outlines in as much detail as possible, all interactive objects and associated mechanisms, site layout, aesthetic principles, estimated costs, projected timeframe, and so on and so forth. As virtual worlds are a novel medium for many ERPs, it is likely that this document will change as the project moves forward; in the case of the IHC, we made many changes during development because of technological discoveries, user recommendations, or unnecessary complexity. At least one version of this document should contain non-technical language, as it may serve as a blueprint for in-world developers unfamiliar with discipline-specific terminology.

Developers

There are two methods to developing a program site: hiring private in-world contractors or utilizing freely available resources and relying on self-instruction for all else. The latter approach is best suited for modest budgets or small teams with a strong interest in developing their knowledge of virtual content creation (3D modeling and scripting), or projects whose interactive components are already widely used and may exist as open source or non-commercial resources elsewhere. Free items, or "freebies," can be readily obtained via appropriate Community Search queries or on the internet. Often, such items have limited modification, duplication, and transfer rights. In such cases, or when an item of script simply cannot be found, there may exist guides or open-source solutions available on the internet; as mentioned earlier, we recommend use of SL specific wikis and video tutorials. For projects with larger budgets, more complex teams, or limited time, in-world contractors are strongly recommended. Developers with various backgrounds and skills can be identified and reached through Linden Lab's "Solution Provider" directory (http://secondlife.com/solution_providers/listings.php). In-world groups and listservs should also be referenced.

There is also considerable in-world interest in volunteer development, especially for nonprofit or research-related projects. However, volunteers must be selected and managed with proper care, so as to avoid lapses in commitment or delays. Settings deadlines, sharing specification sheets, and involving volunteers (time permitting) in team meetings are all methods to maintain consistent and acceptable volunteer performance. In order to attract volunteers, consider reaching out to in-world groups or listservs with backgrounds in education, research, or nonprofit assistance (as listed earlier). Volunteers are most attracted to properly publicized programs with serious potential and real-world backing. With regard to retention, volunteers should be publicly recognized, given credit through objects, and referred to colleagues.

The IHC relied on a variety of development techniques, including hired in-world and in-house developers for complex scripts, a volunteer scripter for common interactive components, self-instruction and use of "freebies" for décor and informational objects.

Land

Although site acquisition and design are matters of personal and creative preference, there are certain considerations specific to health-related educators, researchers, and practitioners. Academic or nonprofit institutions not only receive discount rates and special packages from Linden Lab (see http://secondlifegrid.net/slfe/education-use-virtual-world), but also have the opportunity to lease areas of land belonging to in-world groups focused on nonprofit or academic development (see LIST above) freely or at significantly discounted

rates. The latter option should be considered for projects of limited scope, modest budgets, or experimental interest.

As is the case in real world research and education, interactive spaces should consider participant privacy, functionality, and overall security. In order to facilitate a sense of privacy and security, interactive areas should be separated with dividers, elevation or distance, and parcel restrictions. For instance, the IHC site is elevated thousands of meters in the sky so as to prevent uninterested non-participants from seeing, hearing, or interacting with those on the site. SL's land management settings, which allow thorough access controls, should be considered for especially sensitive programs. Though these settings, avatars can be banned, required to be pre-identified, or diverted to specific areas upon entry.

An aspect of virtual design that is often misunderstood is the use of confined spaces. Although walls and enclosing structures are necessary in real life for privacy, security, and structural purposes, they may create more difficulty than benefit in virtual settings. Camera controls and navigation become significantly more complex when avatars are forced into confined spaces. For this reason, we recommend placing greater emphasis on virtual function than real world simulation; this suggestion applies to all components of the program site.

Program designers are also encouraged to create site rules with consideration of funding sources and Linden Lab Terms of Service and Community Standards. Rules should be posted in an object on the land or distributed as a notecard, and enforced via staff presence.

Real World Integration

Consider using websites and other forms of real-world technology to integrate virtual world participants with other networks. In general, virtual destinations should have, at the very least, a website presence, which can be linked to locations within SL via SLURLs, web addresses that work with the SL client. Many groups also use real world wikis and social networks to organize more effectively.

Testing

Once a site has been designed and populated with scripted and modeled objects, it should be beta tested by individuals of diverse skill-sets, levels of technical knowledge, and hardware / software configurations. For those at academic institutions, we recommend using the insight of undergraduate or graduate students and non-collaborating colleagues, and making changes accordingly. Beta testers should complete all activities and interact with all objects on the site from various computers, software configurations, geographic locations, and client versions (if applicable), and ideally, have varying technical backgrounds. Testing should be continued throughout the course of the program, albeit on a more infrequent basis, so as to ensure a consistent user-experience.

Recruitment & Publicity

Upon completing testing and receiving legal and institutional approval to interact with human subjects, resources should be shifted to promoting the project and thereby attracting academic and professional interest, and where necessary, participants. In-world publicity consists of two major components: networking within special interest groups and commercial advertising. Before approaching either, develop promotional materials which can be viewed and distributed virtually, that is, in the form of "notecards" (brief, non-formatted, in-world txt files) and images. As has been made apparent, interaction with groups of related interests is essential to almost every phase of establishing an in-world program. In promoting the IHC, we attended group meetings at which we spoke about and shared informational materials, asked group leaders to distribute our materials

among members, and requested non-commercial advertising space on their properties. Commercial opportunities include use of the official SL Classifieds Directory, dozens of ad-based affiliate networks, marketing contractors (see Solution Provider Directory), and private ad space available on the most populated sites.

In-world recruitment, however, requires is more complex. Competitive incentives must be combined with either highly targeted advertisements or regular recruitment via designated recruiters. For instance, the IHC developed a detailed training protocol for recruiters, with which we trained in-house staff to not only recruit themselves, but also train virtual residents to recruit. Recruitment entailed regular, brief, and informative dialogues with residents of virtual areas identified to contain receptive populations. Recruiters were also required to submit routine reports summarizing their activities and handle the concerns of assigned groups of participants (usually those they recruited). As in reality, competitive financial incentives in the form of Linden are among the most effective means of recruitment. Recruitment can also be conducted in the real world via SL-related blogs, social networks, listservs, and press. Generally, SL media are interested in novel uses of the virtual world in research and education.

Participant Retention

Sustaining commitments in virtual worlds, in the case of the IHC, can be difficult, as there may not be a perceived personal connection between participants and instructors / researchers. This is especially true in the highly incentivized virtual economy of SL, in which residents are accustomed to competing survey-providers. To address this, we designed a "follow-up" protocol which included impersonal, daily messages and personal, semi-weekly contact along with weekly group activities and regular staff presence on the site. Although time-consuming, preliminary findings show improvement in retention from earlier strategies relying solely on semi-weekly contact. As use of virtual environments expands, we expect this issue to be addressed with greater innovation in best practices.

Incorporating Feedback

In addition to participant recruitment and retention, program operators must be able to maintain technical stability, accessibility, and security within the site. The inherent technical complexities of health-related programs within virtual environments create the need for continuous feedback and subsequent changes. As discussed earlier, significant changes should be avoided, so as to protect scientific fidelity; however, technical and aesthetic issues should be addressed in order to allow for a consistent user experience. Consider creating a bug reporting feature via objects or through individual follow-ups.

Handling Abuse

Unfortunately, like many online networks, virtual environments are plagued with abusive residents that aim to intentionally disrupt site operations and harass avatars. These users are identified in-world as "griefers". Many commercially available in-world scripts provide thorough anti-griefer controls, but ultimately, consistent enforcement of rules via warnings and bans is the most cost effective solution. Refer to Linden Lab's Community Standards to identify disruptive in-world behavior.

Managing Expectations

A handful of issues which afflict most in-world programs, regardless of approach, are: technical delays, the necessity of feedback-based changes, and participant attraction and retention. As has been discussed ad nauseam, technical delays are an inescapable reality of virtual worlds. Project

schedules should allow for extensive beta testing and allocate necessary resources to address discovered errors. Even after testing, difficulties will likely arise when participants begin the program. Although maintaining scientific fidelity is essential to any scientific endeavor, issues related to unintended end-user experiences may require immediate resolutions. For instance, when a number of participants in the IHC reported teleporting difficulties, we were forced to overhaul the site teleport system, which in turn affected all participants. Considerable attention must also be directed toward attracting and retaining participants, particularly if the recruitment pool exists solely in SL. Most programs that do not actively and consistently promote themselves attract very few participants.

FUTURE RESEARCH

The limited breadth of this chapter highlights the need for greater research in a variety of areas, namely foundational research on the value of in-world education, research, and therapy, the means by which to systematically leverage real world resources and develop partnerships, measuring complex qualitative and quantitative data, implications of privacy and security limitations, and more concise guidelines on navigating through available in-world resources. As ERPs continue to migrate toward the medium, and with greater availability of funding and hosting institutions, these topics will likely be addressed in the near future.

CONCLUSION

Developments in computational and connectivity capabilities, and growing interest among ERPs and funding agencies, present a favorable future for virtual environments. Though the technology offers a slew of substantial improvements and innovative solutions to existing approaches and looming questions in health education, research, and therapy, it also presents a number of series challenges. In order to transition from anecdotal successes to consistent models of best practices, early adopters must continue documenting, publishing, and expanding subject literature, just as we intend to do with the IHC.

REFERENCES

Bartle, R. (1999). *Early MUD History*. Retrieved February 28, 2009 from http://www.mud.co.uk/richard/mudhist.htm

Bell, M. (2007, August). *By the Numbers: Quantitative Research Methods in Second Life*. Paper presented at the meeting of the Second Life Educator's Communities Conference, Chicago, IL.

Boulus, M., & Htherington, L., Wheeler&, S. (2007). Second Life: An Overview of the Potential of 3-D Virtual Worlds in Medical and Health Education. *Health Information and Libraries Journal*, *24*(4), 233–245. doi:10.1111/j.1471-1842.2007.00733.x

Bowers, K. W., Ragas, M. W., & Neely, J. C. (2009). Assessing the Value of Virtual Worlds for Post- Secondary Instructors: A Survey of Innovators, Early Adopters and the Early Majority in Second Life. *Intl. Journal of Humanities and Social Sciences*, *3*(1), 40–51.

Brown, J. S., & Adler, R. P. (2008). Minds on Fire: Open Education, the Long Tail, and Learning 2.0. *EDUCAUSE Review*, *43*(1), 16–32.

Dieterle, E., & Clarke, J. (in press). Multi-user virtual environments for teaching and learning. In Pagani, M. (Ed.), *Encyclopedia of multimedia technology and networking* (2nd ed.). Hershey, PA: Idea Group, Inc.

Gorini, A., Gaggioli, A., Vigna, C., & Riva, G. (2008). A second life for ehealth: Prospects for the use of 3-d virtual worlds in clinical psychology. *Journal of Medical Internet Research*, *10*(3). doi:10.2196/jmir.1029

Joseph, B. (2007, August). *Global Kids Inc.'s Best Practices in Using Virtual Worlds for Education*. Paper presented at the meeting of the Second Life Educator's Communities Conference, Chicago, IL.

Linden Lab. (2008). *Second Life – Economy Stats 11/2008*. Retrieved February 28, 2009 from http://static.secondlife.com/economy/stats_200811.xls

Linden Lab. (2009a). *Second Life Economic* Statistics. Retrieved February 28, 2009 from http://secondlife.com/statistics/economy-data.php

Linden Lab. (2009b). *Second Life System Requirements*. Retrieved February 28, 2009 from http://secondlife.com/support/sysreqs.php

Linden Lab. (2009c). *What is Second Life?* Retrieved February 28, 2009 from http://secondlife.com/whatis/

Liu, C. (2006, August). *Second Life Learning Community: A Peer-Based Approach to Involving More Faculty Members in Second Life*. Paper presented at the meeting of the Second Life Educator's Communities Conference, San Fransisco, CA.

McArthur, V. (2008). Real ethics in a virtual world. *Conference on Human Factors in Computing (CHI) Proceedings* (pp. 3315-3320).

Rheingold, H. (1993). *The virtual community: Homesteading on the electronic frontier*. Reading, MA: Addison-Wesley.

Richter, J., Anderson-Inman, L., & Frisbee, M. (August, 2007). *Critical engagement of teachers in second life: Progress in the SaLamander project*. Paper presented at the meeting of the Second Life Educator's Communities Conference, Chicago, IL.

Robbins, S. (2007). *A Futurist's View of Second Life Education: A Developing Taxonomy of Digital Spaces*. Paper presented at the meeting of the Second Life Educator's Communities Conference, Chicago, IL.

Schroeder, R. (2002). *The Social Life of Avatars*. New York: Springer.

Vygotsky, L. S. (1978). *Mind Society: the Development of Higher Mental Processes*. Cambridge, MA: Harvard University Press.

Wenger, E. (2000). Communities of practice social learning systems. *Organization, 7*, 225–256. doi:10.1177/135050840072002

Wyatt, J. C., & Liu, J. L. Y. (2002). Basic concepts in medical informatics. *Journal of Epidemiology and Community Health, 56*(11), 808–812. doi:10.1136/jech.56.11.808

ADDITIONAL READING

Anderson, P., Rothbaum, B., & Hodges, L. (2000). Virtual Reality: Using the virtual world to improve quality of life in the real world. *Menninger Winter Psychiatry Conference, 65*(1), 78-91.

Bell, M. (2007, August). *By the Numbers: Quantitative Research Methods in Second Life*. Paper presented at the meeting of the Second Life Educator's Communities Conference, Chicago, IL.

Boulus, M., Htherington, L., & Wheeler, S. (2007). Second Life: An Overview of the Potential of 3-D Virtual Worlds in Medical and Health Education. *Health Information and Libraries Journal, 24*(4), 233–245. doi:10.1111/j.1471-1842.2007.00733.x

Bowers, K. W., Ragas, M. W., & Neely, J. C. (2009). Assessing the Value of Virtual Worlds for Post- Secondary Instructors: A Survey of Innovators, Early Adopters and the Early Majority in Second Life. *Intl. Journal of Humanities and Social Sciences, 3*(1), 40–51.

Collins, C., & Jennings, N. (2006, August). *Emerging Best Practices for Campus Builds in Second Life*. Paper presented at the meeting of the Second Life Educator's Communities Conference, San Fransisco, CA.

Dieterle, E., & Clarke, J. (in press). Multi-user virtual environments for teaching and learning. In Pagani, M. (Ed.), *Encyclopedia of multimedia technology and networking* (2nd ed.). Hershey, PA: Idea Group, Inc.

Global Kids Inc. (2008, August). Summer 2008 RezEd Report. *Global Kids, 1*(1). Retrieved February 28, 2009 from http://www.rezed.org/.

Gorini, A., Gaggioli, A., Vigna, C., & Riva, G. (2008). A second life for ehealth: Prospects for the use of 3-d virtual worlds in clinical psychology. *Journal of Medical Internet Research, 10*(3). doi:10.2196/jmir.1029

Joseph, B. (2007, August). *Global Kids Inc.'s Best Practices in Using Virtual Worlds for Education*. Paper presented at the meeting of the Second Life Educator's Communities Conference, Chicago, IL.

Linden Lab. (2009c). What is Second Life? Retrieved February 28, 2009 from http://secondlife.com/whatis/

Linden Labs. (2009). *Second Life Economic Statistics*. Retrieved February 28, 2009 from http://secondlife.com/statistics/economy-data.php

Liu, C. (2006, August). *Second Life Learning Community: A Peer-Based Approach to Involving More Faculty Members in Second Life*. Paper presented at the meeting of the Second Life Educator's Communities Conference, San Fransisco, CA.

Mason, H., & Moutahir, M. (2006, August). *Multidisciplinary Experiential Education in Second Life: A Global Approach*. Paper presented at the meeting of the Second Life Educator's Communities Conference, San Francisco, CA.

New Media Consortium. (2008, May). *Spring 2007 Survey Educators in Second Life*. [Online].

Richter, J., Anderson-Inman, L., & Frisbee, M. (August, 2007). *Critical engagement of teachers in second life: Progress in the SaLamander project*. Paper presented at the meeting of the Second Life Educator's Communities Conference, Chicago, IL.

Robbins, S. (2006, August). *"Image Slippage": Navigating the Dichotomies of an Academic Identity in a Non-academic Virtual World*. Paper presented at the meeting of the Second Life Educator's Communities Conference, San Fransisco, CA.

Robbins, S. (2007). *A Futurist's View of Second Life Education: A Developing Taxonomy of Digital Spaces*. Paper presented at the meeting of the Second Life Educator's Communities Conference, Chicago, IL.

Schott, G., & Hodgetts, D. (2006). Health and digital gaming: the benefits of a community of practice. *Journal of Health Psychology, 11*, 309–316. doi:10.1177/1359105306061189

Toro-Troconis, M., Mellström, U., Partridge, M., Meeran, K., Barrett, M., & Higham, J. (2008, July). Designing game-based learning activities for virtual patients in Second Life. *Journal of CyberTherapy & Rehabilitation, 1*(3), 227–239. Retrieved February 28, 2009 from http://www.elearningimperial.com/SL/J-CyberTherapy-Rehab_Toro-Troconis_V04.pdf

Toro-Troconis, M., Partridge, M., Barrett, M., & Mellström, U. (2008, July). Game-based learning for the delivery of virtual patients in Second Life. *The Academy Subject Centre for Medicine, Dentistry and Veterinary Medicine Newsletter, 1*(17). Retrieved February 28, 2009 from http://www.medev.ac.uk/external_files/pdfs/01_newsletter/0117_lo_res.pdf

Toro-Troconis, M., Partridge, M., Mellström, U., Meeran, K., & Higham, J. (2008, July). Technical infrastructure and initial findings in the design and delivery of game-based learning for virtual patients in Second Life. In *Proceedings of Researching Learning in Virtual Environments*. Milton Keynes: The Open University. Retrieved February 28, 2009 from http://www.elearningimperial.com/SL/ReLIVE_paper_Maria_Toro_Troconis_V03.pdf

KEY TERMS AND DEFINITIONS

Multi-User Virtual Environments: Networked, synchronous, computer-simulated environments which facilitate social interaction among uniquely identified users through rich visual, auditory, or textual interfaces.

Second Life: An international multi-user, multi-sensory albeit image-centric, persistent, stigmergic, private ownership based, collaborative and conditional environment built on a publicly accessible wide area network (Robbins, 2007).

Avatar: A dynamic, customizable visual or textual virtual representation controlled by a human user.

Region: An area of premium property (256m x 256m) hosted on a physical server machine; can be either mature or PG; can hold up to 100 avatars and 15,000 prims (Linden Lab, 2009). Subdivided into smaller units of land known as parcels.

LSL: Computer programming language of SL used to script function of in-world object mechanisms. Similar to C and Java.

Prim: Fundamental building blocks of SL, comprise larger structures. Can be geometric or sculpted.

Grid: The term used to describe Linden Lab's network on which SL operates. Though there exist two Grids (Main & Teen), they are actually hosted within the same infrastructure.

Griefer: Abusive residents that aim to intentionally disrupt site operations and harass avatars

Experiential Education: Alters the experience of users via immersion for the purpose of conveying educational content. This technique makes the most of the technology's features.

Group: Hierarchal miniature social networks within SL, often share contacts, object resources, and land. The fundamental social unit of SL.

eHealth: In the context of SL, the term refers to the use of SL as a means to deliver therapy and lifestyle-related health information.

Chapter 21

Dynamic Business Processes and Virtual Communities in Wireless eHealth Environments

Dimosthenis Georgiadis
University of Cyprus, Cyprus

Panagiotis Germanakos
University of Nicosia, Cyprus

Constantinos Mourlas
National & Kapodistrian University of Athens, Greece

George Samaras
University of Cyprus, Cyprus

Eleni Christodoulou
University of Cyprus, Cyprus

ABSTRACT

Computer Supported Collaborative Work (CSCW) related applications tend to be a trend for most successful businesses, organizations and domains nowadays, as is the Healthcare sector. Healthcare specialists often work in remote areas facing many problems and challenges driven mainly from the limitations and constraints of the mobile and wireless technologies in relation to the tasks at hand. Due to the sensitive area of healthcare provision, this chapter discusses that additional features need to be incorporated in current CSCW systems, like the dynamic creation of medical virtual teams, dynamic workflows and the automatic triggered events upon time expiration, in order to be more effective and efficient. In this respect and having in mind the new Web 2.0 characteristics, a set of new features applied in our proposed CSCW system, DITIS, is analyzed in an attempt to encapsulate all the needs of eHealth applications. Furthermore, an extensive evaluation of the system is presented, supporting the need for such enhancements since a significant increase in communication, coordination and collaboration has been shown among the subjects.

DOI: 10.4018/978-1-61520-777-0.ch021

Copyright © 2010, IGI Global. Copying or distributing in print or electronic forms without written permission of IGI Global is prohibited.

INTRODUCTION

Nowadays, many organizations are distributed across sites, in different countries and continents. Within these organizations the nature of working activities is constantly changing due to this geographical expansion and diversification of practices. Employees are now on the move with their notebooks, Personal Digital Assistants (PDAs) and mobile phones. Some have referred to this trend as nomadic working (G Reif et al. 2001). These organizations have to provide an effective IT infrastructure to enable their employees to share information and collaborate efficiently. Therefore, the need of supportive Computer Supported Collaborative Work (CSCW) systems is spawned. Analyzing more thoroughly this nomadic way of working further constrains of the wireless environment/medium arise, like the mobile devices capabilities, the delivery of an effective and efficient collaboration, the lack of dynamic workflows and the need for time driven events. Thus, a big challenge is to deploy a competent CSCW system that will satisfy all the aforementioned conceptualizations and limitations to the benefit of the end user.

CSCW-related applications tend to be a trend for most successful businesses and organizations, and especially for the healthcare sector. Healthcare specialists often work in remote areas where the wireless network is limited with many disconnections, while they are experiencing problems with the devices constrains like the small sizes with inefficient input methods, small screens, limited battery life and are prone to damage and spoilage. In this respect, the need for dynamic workflows development and time driven events came to the surface. Specialists expect substantial help from the system they are using, saving them time and effort, i.e. they should not analyze their requirements all over again, waiting for developers to add the new workflow into the system. Furthermore, particular events may underlie some time constraints according the priority of the medical incident.

In general, eHealth applications are far more demanding than any other systems and the need of approaches that will consider all the above-mentioned problems and constraints should be formulated. Such systems must have:

- **Availability awareness:** The system must be aware on the user status (availability), in order to manage better any critical situations.
- **Flexible messaging methods:** Healthcare specialists are not always computer literate and the system has to adopt to their communication skills. Some specialists prefer the use of emails and other prefer the use of SMS text messages. The system has to provide all means of communication.
- **Confidentiality:** One of the special needs of an eHealth application is the confidentiality of the information. Patient's data are sensitive information and can't be viewed by anyone. Laws were instituted for protecting this kind of data and thus, eHealth applications have to follow these strict guidelines.
- **Security:** In order to support the above characteristic, solid security schemas have to be enforced. Furthermore, we have to provide data restriction access not only table or column level but also row level (database rows and columns). This is due the confidentiality of the data, not only between roles, but also between users. For example, doctors don't share their patient's information with other doctors (row level security).
- **Availability:** An eHealth application has to be available 24/7 from anyplace and by any means. For example, users can access the application even from a mobile phone while they are at the beach.
- **Expandability:** An eHealth application has to be able to expand easily with new features and services. If not, the rapid

changes in the eHealth field will set the application to obsolete.

- **Easy information sharing:** Users must be able to share the information they want with other users, with minimum effort. We have to constantly remember the mobile devices limitations for input and output.

Furthermore, given the sensitive area of healthcare provision and the vast upcoming of the Web 2.0, the conventional CSCW systems need to be enhanced with additional features like the dynamic creation of virtual team, collaboration workflows and the automatic triggered events upon time expiration. An extensive reference and analysis of these concepts, since they figure as the primary components of our proposed CSCW system, namely DITIS, will be presented in this chapter.

Our study is focused on the identification of needs for collaboration in the health care sector and more particularly in the virtual health care teams and the creation of dynamic business processes under the same sector. More specifically, it emphasizes on the collaboration in the health domain, due to the special needs and peculiarities of this sector on collaboration techniques and systems. Unlike other domains, the eHealth domain is more demanding on the integrity of the information, the time constrains, the security (due to the medical record singularity) and the messaging urgency (depending the severity of the case).

The innovation of this work is presented through our system that tries to comprehensively approach most of the given problems in the eHealth sector. We underpin the decision of our selection with regards to the computational model, we describe the system's components namely, (i) User Component, (ii) Message Component, (iii) Questionnaire Component and (iv) Workflow Component, and we illustrate some screenshots of the system.

Using as a case study an established medical organization namely, PASYKAF, we assess the proposed system efficiency and effectiveness through a three-phase evaluation scenarios. We present the evaluation methodology and the evaluation results. The positive impact of the system in the whole process is that users' support has gradually improved over the last years as they have been increasingly interacted with the system capabilities and have recognized the advantages of the system in their daily work for both administrative and consultation purposes. Finally, we describe the findings and we further discuss future trends and opportunities with regards to collaboration in dynamic eHealth environments.

BACKGROUND THEORY

In an attempt to thoroughly approach all the possible dimensions and implications included in the demanding eHealth environment, we conducted an extended research on the aspects of the virtual teams, collaboration and workflow management, presenting the outcome of this research on the basis of the abovementioned concepts (such as definitions, existing systems, standards and technical trends).

Virtual Teams

Collaboration and virtual teams refer to the concept that a team of professionals decide to collaborate over the internet and thus create a virtual team that eliminates the need of physical presence. The collaboration requirements are based on identified scenarios of collaboration analyzed using UML schemas. These scenarios can identify the communication and collaborative requirements a computational model must support in an integrated fashion. Creating virtual collaborative teams for the healthcare environment can further introduce new and more specialized requirements. The collaborative functionality of artifacts may be also enhanced with embedded hybrid intelligence as well.

The usual scenery of a working group in a company contains meetings, encounters in the hallway, getting together for lunch and dropping into one another's offices. People that work together sometimes do not meet one another especially when they are in different places or spread out around the world or even housed in different parts of the same city. Many teams today never meet face-to-face, but work together only online. Face-to-face interactions among people from the same organization are the typical old model of teamwork (Lipnack & Stamps 2000).

In short a virtual team can be described as a group of people who work interdependently with a shared purpose across space, time, and organization boundaries using technology. The main benefit is that in a virtual team you can do what you can't do alone. The challenge of our time is to learn to work in virtual teams and networks while retaining the benefits of earlier forms. In time, virtual teams will become the natural way to work. Since many virtual teams do meet periodically, or a few times, or at least once, they also find themselves in the conventional face-to-face setting. It is generally agreed that a good virtual team is, in a way, a good team.

Four words capture the essence of virtual teams: people, purpose, links, and time. People populate and lead small groups and teams of every kind at every level, from the executive suite to the subcommittees of the local school's parent association. Purpose holds groups together, which for teams mean a focus on tasks that makes work progressing from goals to results. Links are the channels, interactions, and relationships. The greatest difference between in-the-same-place teams and virtual ones lies in the nature and variety of their links. Time is a dimension common to schedules, milestones, calendars, processes, and life cycles (Lipnack & Stamps 2000).

Sometimes virtual teams fail. One major reason why many virtual teams fail is because they overlook the implications of the obvious differences in their working environments. People do not make accommodation for how different it really is when they and their colleagues no longer work face-to-face. Teams fail when they do not adjust to this new reality by closing the virtual gap. So, why put up with the trouble of working across boundaries? Because, when the virtual team is successful, the business performance is improved dramatically. In brief, the cost can be reduced by cutting travel costs and time, the cycle time can be shorten by moving from serial to parallel processes and establishing better communications, the innovation can be increased by permitting more diverse participation, stimulating product and process creativity, and encouraging new business development synergies and finally we can succeed leverage of learning by capturing knowledge in the natural course of doing the work, gaining wider access to expertise, and sharing best practices (Lipnack & Stamps 2000).

Even though interactivity is often presented as a key characteristic of a computer-mediated communication system, the emphasis is often on the computer-human interaction rather than on human-to-human computer-mediated interaction (Panteli & Dibben 2001). The latter is particularly important since virtual teams are effective not only because of the technological advancements but also and most importantly because individuals are able to interact and thus constructively engage in knowledge sharing and creation in the increasingly emergent virtual work environments.

During the last few years there has been an increasing volume of literature on virtual organizations and virtual teams. This body of research generally agrees that virtual teams consist of a collection of geographically dispersed individuals who work on a joint project or common tasks and communicate electronically. For example, Lipnack and Stamps (2000) define a virtual team as "a group of people who interact through interdependent tasks guided by a common purpose" that "works across space, time and organizational boundaries with links strengthened by webs of communication technologies". Indeed, virtual teams have been presented in the popular literature as a communication intensive and a computer-mediated linked type of group. Electronic data interchange, computer-supported cooperative work, group support systems, as well as email, videoconferencing and teleconferencing facilities, to name but a few, enable people based in different locations to communicate and coordinate their actions with great speed and effectiveness.

To this definition then were added 5 new criteria: (1) members work apart more than they do at the same location, (2) they are based on telecommunications technologies as computer networks, email, groupware, and phones, (3) members solve problems and make decisions jointly, (4) members are mutually accountable for results and (5) members in such organizations can be brought together for a finite time to solve specific tasks or problems (Tiwana 2000).

Collaboration through Computer Supported Collaborated Work

Collaboration is a structured, recursive process where two or more people work together toward a common goal - typically an intellectual endeavor that is creative in nature (Simpson & Weiner 1989)

- by sharing knowledge, learning and building consensus. Collaboration does not require leadership and can even bring better results through decentralization and egalitarianism (Muneera 2006). In particular, teams that work collaboratively can obtain greater resources, recognition and reward when facing competition for finite resources (Wagner & Leydesdorff 2005).

The term "Computer-Supported Cooperative Work" (CSCW) was first used by Irene Greif and Paul Cashman back in 1984. It used to describe the topic of an interdisciplinary workshop they were organizing on how to support people in their work arrangements with computers (Schmind & Bannon 1992).

CSCW has emerged as an identifiable research area which focuses on the role of the computer in group work. It is a generic term which combines the understanding of the nature of group working with the enabling technologies of computer networking, systems support and applications.

An essential precursor to the study of collaborative systems is the definition of a mechanism for classifying these systems. Two principal characteristics (see *Figure 1*) are common to all cooperative systems (Rodden 1991).

Figure 1. Time/space CSCW matrix

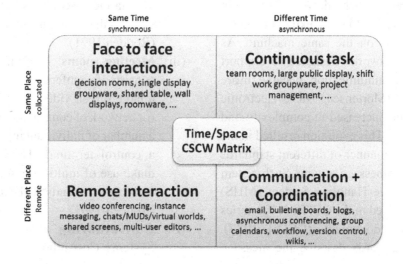

1.   The form of interaction (synchronous versus asynchronous) Some creative problems require group members to collaborate in a synchronous manner since the creative input of each group member is required to generate a strategy for solving a task. In contrast, prescriptive tasks have a previously formulated solution strategy where group members take on particular roles and work in an asynchronous manner often without the presence of other group members. Cooperative systems are therefore either synchronous or asynchronous systems.

2.   The geographical nature of the users (remote versus co-located) Cooperative systems are either remote or co-located. This division is as much logical as physical and is concerned with the accessibility of users to each other rather than their absolute physical proximity. The term co-located is used to emphasis this logical division and to avoid confusion with the distinction between remote and local communication systems.

Collaboration systems can be classified into four major categories:

(i)   **Message systems**: Message systems are the most mature class of system. Over the years, they have evolved from electronic mail programs which allowed a user using a central machine to send textual messages to other users on the same machine. As wide area networks designed to support computer communication became more widespread (Mortensen 1985), electronic mail systems increased in complexity and functionality. This evolution resulted in the creation of a number of different standards for electronic message systems. Such system is the Message Handling System (MHS) model described in the CCITT X400 series of standards documents (CCITT 1987). Message standards describe the message format used to transfer information in message systems. Structured message systems are based on the principle of extending the available amount of machines processing semantic information by adding syntactic structure to the existing message structures (Rodden 1991).

(ii)   **Computer conferencing**: The computer conferencing systems are related to electronic mail programs. However, the principles are different in that structure as in terms of how messages are grouped. A characteristic computer conferencing system consists of a number of groups (called conferences), each of them has a set of members and a sequence of messages. These conferences are often arranged so that they address a single topic and users subscribe to conferences of interest. Usually, the system stores information about the progress of every member in each conference. The needed information is usually held with conference messages within a central database rather than the individual mailbox approach used in messaging systems. Reliable high speed communications has lead to the emergence of new real-time conferencing systems that conference members can communicate in real-time. As computers become more powerful their capability to handle wider classes of data increased. This led to multi-media systems that integrate audio, text and video (Rodden 1991).

(iii)   **Meeting rooms**: Meeting rooms, usually consists of a conference room enhanced with a large screen video projector, a computer (or network of computers), video terminals, a number of individual input terminals, and a control terminal. These systems often make use of multi-user software based on some form of analytical decision technique (Rodden 1991).

(iv)   **Co-Authoring and Argumentation Systems**: Co-Authoring and argumentation systems are systems that aim to support and represent the negotiation and argumentation involved in group working. The collaborative authoring of documents is an example of this class of cooperation where the final generation of the document represents the product of the process of negotiation between authors (Rodden 1991).

Workflow Management

Workflow management (WFM) is a very active field with numerous products and research groups. It is an exciting field since it combines technologies, principles and methodologies from numerous areas of computer science. The landscape is being transformed significantly due to the absorption of emerging technologies like the worldwide web, and due to mergers and partnerships involving numerous companies which produce complementary products. With the appearance of support for workflow management in process modeling and application development tools, WFMSs are becoming a little easier to use. Workflow management has a very significant role to play in disparate organizations' drive to improve their efficiency and customer service (Mohan 1997).

Various definitions have been proposed for concepts relating to WFM. Giga Group (www.gigaweb.com) once gave the following definition: "we call the operational aspects of a business process - the sequence of tasks and who performs them, the information flow to support the tasks, and the tracking and reporting mechanisms that measure and control them - the workflow" (Mohan 1997).

Giga also defined the associated management software as follows: "workflow software is designed to improve business processes by providing the technology enabler for automating these aspects of the workflow: routing work in the proper sequence, providing access to the data and documents required by the individual work

performers, and tracking all aspects of the process execution" (Mohan 1997).

In the last few years, the focus on business process reengineering by enterprises is as a cost saving and service improvement measure has contributed significantly to the recent popularity of Workflow Management Systems (WFMS). WFMSs engage a longer sales cycle, since their adoption requires executive approval and end user commitment. Adopting a WFMS necessitates a cultural change in the way an organization does its business. It requires group consensus and retraining. Typically, implementing a workflow solution involves the hiring of consultants for advice.

Workflow Standards

The Workflow Management Coalition (WFMC - www.aiai.ed.ac.uk/project/wfmc) is the main organization that is involved in workflow management standardization efforts. It was formed in 1993 and it currently has about 200 members (vendors, users, analysts, systems integrators, universities, ...). WFMC defined a reference model for a WFMS's architecture. Version 1.1 of the document (WFMC-TC-1003) describing the model was published in November 1994. This model has 5 interfaces and application program interfaces (APIs) relating to those interfaces are intended to be standardized. The interfaces/APIs are (i) Process definition model and interchange APIs, (ii) Client APIs, (iii) Application invocation interface, (iv) Workflow interoperability, and (v) Administration and monitoring.

While users find it very convenient to define process models using graphical tools, different products provide the graphical support differently. As a result, WFMC decided that it would be too difficult to arrive at a graphical standard for process definitions. Consequently, a language based standard is being worked on for this purpose. Products like FlowMark already support such a language (FlowMark Definition Language, FDL) to allow the convenient export and import of process definitions between different workflow installations.

Technical Trends

WFM, as mentioned above, brings together principles, methodologies and technologies from various areas of computer science and management science: database management, client server computing, programming languages, heterogeneous distributed computing, mobile computing, graphical user interfaces, application (new and legacy) and subsystem (e.g., CICS and MQSeries) integration, messaging, document management, simulation, and business practices and reengineering. Integrating different concepts from these areas poses many challenges. Factors like scalability, high availability, manageability, usability and security also further aggravate the demands on the designs of WFMSs (Mohan 1997).

Many general purpose business application packages have been developed for managing human resources, manufacturing, sales, accounting, etc. by companies like Baan, Oracle, PeopleSoft and SAP. The market for such products has grown tremendously as customer organizations try to avoid producing homegrown solutions. Vendors' generic application packages can be tailored to take into account the special needs of a particular enterprise. Developers of such packages, like SAP (www.sap.com/workflow) and PeopleSoft (www.peoplesoft.com), have incorporated workflow functionality into their products

With the widespread and rapid popularity of the worldwide web, very quickly many WFMS products have been adapted to work in the context of the web. The level of sophistication of web support varies from product to product. Some products permit workflows to be initiated or controlled from a browser. Worklist handling via the web is another form of support that is provided by a few products. In summary, it is the client side

WFMS functionality that has been made available through a web browser. The advantage of web support is that no specialized WFMS-specific client software needs to be installed to invoke workflow functionality at a workflow server. Some of the products with basic web support are: JetForm's InTempo (www.jetform.com/p&s/intempo.html), Mosaix's ViewStar Process@ Work (www2.mosaix.com/ProcessAutomation), Staffware's Staffware Global (www.staffware.com), and Ultimus's Ultimus CyberFlow (www.ultimus1.com).

A PROPOSED EXTENDED MODEL

Having thoroughly considered the notions of virtual team, collaboration and workflow management, we hereafter propose a related extended model, always under the eHealth umbrella. Virtual teams are classified according to eHealth, the Collaboration schema is extended to support cross-organizations structure and workflows became dynamic to support the peculiarity of the medical sector.

Medical Virtual Teams

Medical Virtual Teams (MVTs) are Virtual Teams built around medical objectives and medical specialists (e.g. doctors, nurses, physiotherapists, and psychologists). Medical Virtual Teams can be categorized into three major categories based on the distance between the team members. It is interesting to note that the distance among team members defined the urgency of the collaboration.

Short Distance Medical Virtual Teams (Hospital Medical VTs)

The Short Distance Medical Virtual Teams (SDs) are Medical Virtual Teams (MVTs) that are limited into the boundaries of a building, like a hospital.

On figure 5 we can see the SDs as the number 1 virtual team type. In this case all the team members are collaborating mostly wirelessly (via a wireless LAN). In case of an emergency, the existence of the MVT ceased. The team members after they alerted for the emergency, they meet for the best settlement of the problem. This type of MVT requires a less synchronous model and because of that, the team members are unknown before any action taken (shift based teams).

Long Distance Medical Virtual Teams (Home Care Medical VTs)

The Long Distance Medical Virtual Teams (LDs) are MVTs that their team members works mostly separated and the lifetime of the time is a bit exteneded. On figure 5 we can see the LDs as the number 2 virtual team type. In this case all the team members are collaborating wirelessly (via a wireless WAN). Due to the limitations of the wireless link this MVT model requires an asynchronous model which in essence guarantees the continuous running of the team. For that reason the team members are well known before any homecare visit (subject based teams). If a team member is unavailable, the system will record the request and when the team member will be available, the request will be served. In case of extreme emergency a backup member is usually assign. A good example of a LD is a home care medical virtual team such as DITIS (www.ditis.ucy.ac.cy). DITIS, is the system that hosts our model and supports the activities of PASYKAF (Cypriot Association of Cancer Patients and Friends), who run a national home-based healthcare service for cancer patients living all over Cyprus (Pitsillides et al. 1999).

Variable Distance Medical Virtual Teams (Emergency Medical VTs)

Variable Distance Medical Virtual Teams (VDs) are MVTs that can be change between SDs and LDs depending on the situation that will occur. On figure 5 the VDs can vary between the number 1 & 2 virtual team types. In this case all the team members are collaborating wirelessly apart from few exceptions. An example of a VD is a MVT that handles Emergency medical occurrences, such as the MVTs of the Kardio-T project. In the Kardio-T project, persons having a heart condition, are monitored and for better monitoring of the MVT. This MVT model requires a high synchronous model. As the first model, the team members are unknown before any action taken (shift based teams).

The main problem in all types of the MVTs is that all the properties that we mentioned above, can change dynamically. Every system must be tolerant in every change that may occur.

E-Health Collaboration

As mention before, eHealth applications are very unique with regards the special needs and specifications. Furthermore, the CSCW system that will support the medical virtual teams must be formulated to cover all these needs. Such CSCW system must have:

- **Availability Awareness:** The CSCW system must be aware on the user status (availability), in order to manage better any critical situations.
- **Flexible messaging methods:** Healthcare specialists are not always computer literate and the system has to adopt to their communication skills. Some specialists prefer the use of emails and other prefer the use of SMS text messages. The system has to provide all means of communication.
- **Confidentiality:** Collaboration messages must be confidential and only available to the intended receivers.
- **Security:** All collaboration messages must be secured (at least at a respectable level).

- **Availability:** A CSCW system has to be available 24/7 from anyplace and by any means.
- **Expandability:** A CSCW system has to be able to expand easily with new workflows and collaboration schemas.
- **Easy information sharing:** Users must be able to share the information they want (and nothing more) with other users, with minimum effort.

During our work, a third characteristic was spawned that, to our knowledge, it has never been mentioned so far and it's one of the innovative contributions of this work to this area. This third characteristic is the working organization of the users. The members of a virtual team can emanate from the same or different organizations. These members can also be in the same labor space or in different states. In an attempt to categorize all the virtual team types, we depict below the Time/Space/Organization CSCW matrix (see *Figure 2*).

THE WORKING ORGANIZATION OF THE USERS (SAME VERSUS DIFFERENT)

In the medical sector, we have users for different organizations that are collaborating for the patients' benefit and for providing a better service provision. Users collaborating from hospitals, social worker office, nurses from various organizations, etc for a certain goal.

The above figure presents a clear classification of the various types and forms of virtual teams based on the dimensions of time, place and organization. As a result, eight groups of collaboration were identified. Four cases of groups have their members working in the same organization, four cases of groups sharing same labor space and another four cases of groups working simultaneously (Georgiadis 2002).

E-Health Workflow Management

After an extensive analysis of the Medical Virtual Teams we came to the conclusion that such system must be:

Figure 2. Time/space/organization CSCW matrix

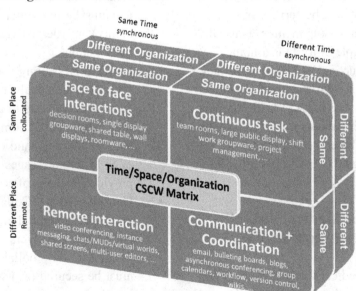

- **Web-based:** Been a web-based application is a newly trend that offers many advantages. Some of them are the ability of accessibility (anytime, anywhere and by any means) and always updated.
- **Ad-hoc (Dynamic):** Workflows supporting Medical Virtual Teams have to be dynamic in order to support the ongoing rapid changes that occur in the medical field. Team members' availability and patients' condition constantly changes providing a dynamic context, thus only dynamic workflows can cope with.
- **Recursive:** Workflows must be able to call other workflows and the second ones call other workflows till a solution to the problem is found. Even recursive workflows can be found.
- **Event driven:** Workflows must be able to be initiated (triggered) by events. Such events can be the change of patient's condition, a message dispatch or even by a medical virtual team member.
- **Time triggered:** Furthermore, workflows must be able to be initiated on time expirations (time triggered). For example, a backup workflow is initiated in case no action is taken for a specific event.

All the above, produce a set of primal specifications of the workflows for Medical Virtual Teams (MVT).

ISSUES, CONTROVERSIES, PROBLEMS

Discussion and Technical Requirements

In the previous section, we mentioned in brief the preferences that categorize the MVTs. In more detail, these preferences that make these categorizations are the collaboration model, the identity of the team members, the type of the network that the MVT will be active on, the distance between the team members and finally the devices that the member will use.

Before the creation of the MVT, it must be clear the needs of collaboration between the team members. This analysis, will determine if the MVT will use a synchronous or asynchronous collaboration model. For instance if we conduct an analysis that will show that the system requires rapid requests and responses then we will use definitely a synchronous collaboration model. Otherwise we prefer the asynchronous collaboration model, if the need for rapid messaging is limited, like the case of DITIS.

Our next concern should be the type of the network and the type of Medical Devices we will use. These two preferences will determine the application model that we will use. As we saw above, all the types of the MVTs are using wireless network. Therefore, as we mentioned in a previous section, it would be better to use an application model that supports an agent to the fixed network that will maintain the user's instance all the time. There are two models for this functionality; the Client/Agent/Server and the Client/Intercept/Server Model. Considering the capabilities of the mobile devices that it will be used, we choose between the two application models. Nowadays, most of the Medical Mobile Devices are small in resources and size. This reason makes the Client/Intercept/Model inappropriate.

Another characteristic is the boundaries that the MVTs will act. This is very important characteristic, because the MVTs types are categorized mainly by the distance between the team members. The distance, between others, determines many things like the cost of supporting the MVT (which is vital to the MVT's existence) and the need for synchronous or asynchronous model.

Finally the identity of the team members affects the type of the MVT. When we say identity of the team member we mean the advantage of knowing the person in the other side. It's better

Table 1. Mobile medical teams' properties

	SD	LD	VD
Collaboration Model	Synchronous	Asynchronous	Synchronous
Medical Mobile Devices	Small-Mid Devices	Small Devices	Med-High Devices
Team Member Identity	Shift Based	Subject Based	Shift Based
Boundaries	Within a Building	None	Vary
Network	Wireless	Wireless	Wireless
Suggested Application Model	Client/Agent/Server	Client/Agent/Server	Client/Agent/Server or Client/Intercept/Server

to know the other users, because the impersonal relationships are proved to be ineffective.

Summarizing the above, we can compare the three models of the MVTs with the following table (see Table 1).

The continuous presence of the collaboration even during members' disconnections should be an indisputable fact in all types of virtual teams.

The Computational Model for Wireless Virtual Medical Teams

In such unpredictable environments, like the wireless ones, it is expected that an appropriate system will be persistent and fault tolerant, even when disconnections occur. The question that rises is: "which is the best combination of technologies for creating collaborative virtual medical teams?" For a more comprehensive approach to the latter question, it could be wise to split the problem into different layers. The first one is the technological layer, in which we examine the technologies that we'll use for the wireless networking and the types of the devices that the team members will use. The second layer is the application architecture layer. In this layer we examine the proper application model that we'll use, depending on the decisions that we'll make in the first layer. Finally, there is a third layer in which we examine the way that the collaborative virtual team will be implemented. This layer is related with the other two layers. Thus, these three layers are dependent to each other, so the procedures of the analysis and de-

ployment start together for all three of the layers (Georgiadis 2002).

The technological layer must be examined after the analysis of the third layer, because we have to understand first the nature of the virtual teams. We can easily exclude the technologies that they depend on being in direct line of sight or technologies that work within few meters (e.g. IrDA, Bluetooth), because when we talk about virtual teams, we assume that a respective distance between the team members, exists. Two of the things that we have to determine are the immediateness of the communication and the real distance between the team members. The distance between the team members reflect on the type of the wireless network that we will choose. If the virtual team moves within the boundaries of a hospital a WLAN may be suitable. If the team members work all over the country, we would use GSM/GPRS/UMTS type of networks. The immediateness of the communication determines the type of the connection that we'll use. For example if we want to send information to the team members all the time we'll choose a connection that the users will be always online (e.g. GPRS or UMTS) (Georgiadis 2002).

In the application architecture layer, appropriate models are the Client/Agent/Server and the Client/Intercept/Server, depending of the resources that the mobile devices will have. If the team members possess mobile devices with many resources, then we can have a Client-side Agent for handling disconnections that may occur.

The certain thing is that we'll have a Server-side Agent. This agent will not only exist for sustaining the user's existence in the network, but also for sustaining the user's existence in the virtual medical team (Georgiadis 2002).

In the final third layer, we have to guarantee that every team member will be equal the other team members in the virtual team anytime. Thus, we can use an agent for each user, representing his in every action. The agent will be always online and connected with the other members of his virtual team. Users can communicate with each other through their agents. The agent receives the message from the senders' agent and forwards it to his user for advising. If the user isn't connected, the agent waits for the user to connect or responds by himself depending on his responsibilities (Georgiadis 2002).

A system that applies successfully the technologies that mentioned above is DITIS (Collaborative Virtual Medical team for home healthcare of cancer patients) (Pitsillides et al. 1999). In DITIS the Client/Agent/Server application model is used. Every user is represented by a mobile agent. Thus the virtual medical team exists anytime. During DITIS deployment, serious stability and steadiness problems were observed due the use of the mobile agent technology. Mobile agent technologies were research platforms running under Java virtual machines, slowing down the process of data and having late responses in data requests due to technology heterogeneity. In order to overcome this problem, we adopted web services and SOA model. All issues that were handled by agents were also managed as well as with web services. The only advantage of the mobile agents was the ability to move between computers, but due to the limited processing of the mobile devices, this feature was disabled. SOA architecture was proven to be more stable and suitable to this type of applications.

Through our system, we assist in the delivery of an enhanced home-care service. This is achieved by offering the health-care team the opportunity to accomplish a seamless continuum of health and health-related services, despite the structural problems of home-care, as compared to facility based care (as for example the geographic proximity and geographic separation between the team members and the patient). We managed to overcome these difficulties by maintaining a dynamic collaborative virtual healthcare team, as well as secure, easy, and timely access to a unified Electronic Medical Record database for the continuous home-treatment of patients. The virtual healthcare team is created explicitly to satisfy the needs of each particular patient at a point in time.

Mobile wireless computing brings about a new paradigm of distributed computing in which communications may be achieved through wireless networks and users can continue computing even as they relocate from one support environment to another. The impact of wireless computing on system design goes beyond the networking level and directly affects data management and data computational paradigms. Infrastructure research on communication and networking is essential for realizing wireless and mobile systems. Equally important, however, is the design and implementation of data management applications for these systems (e.g., wireless virtual teams) a task directly affected by the characteristics of the wireless medium, the limitations of mobile computing devices, and the resulting mobility of resources and computation.

These limitations require a more flexible computational model than the one supporting wireline communications. This is because most of the assumptions that influence the definition and evolution of the traditional client/server model for distributed computing (Gray 1993) are no longer valid. These assumptions include: (a) fast, reliable and cheap communications, (b) robust and resource rich devices, and finally (c) stationary and fixed locations of the participating devices.

Wireless networks, however, are more expensive, offer less bandwidth, and are less reliable than wireline networks. Consequently, network connectivity is weak and often intermittent. Moreover, mobile elements must be light and small to be easily carried around and thus in general have less resources than static elements, including memory, screen size and disk capacity. These result in an asymmetry in mobile computing systems: fixed hosts have sufficient resources, while mobile elements are resource poor. Furthermore, since mobile elements must rely for their operation on the finite energy provided by batteries, energy consumption is a major concern. Mobile elements are also easier to be accidentally damaged, stolen or lost. Finally, having mobile hosts roaming around, changing their location and therefore their point of attachment to the fixed network places new requirements on system design. The center of activity, the system load and the notion of locality changes dynamically. The search cost to locate mobile elements is added to the cost of each communication involving them. Moreover, as mobile elements enter regions in which communication is provided by different means, connectivity becomes highly variable in performance and reliability.

These limitations of mobility and wireless communications result in a form of distributed computing with drastically different connectivity assumptions than in traditional distributed systems. Thus, it is necessary to employ new computational paradigms to achieve a usable system. These new software models must cope with the special characteristics and limitations of the mobile/wireless environment. They should also provide efficient access to both existing and new applications which is a key requirement for the wide acceptance of mobile computing. In summary, the appropriate mobile computing models must efficiently deal with:

- Disconnections, to allow the mobile unit to operate even when disconnected
- Weak connectivity, to alleviate the effect of low bandwidth

- Both light-weight and heavy-weight mobile clients, i.e., clients with different resource capacities
- Dynamic adjustment of the mobile host functionality, i.e., the type and degree of functionality assign to mobile hosts
- The variability of the wireless environment
- Multiple types and application models, including: current, and future TCP/IP applications, and emerging mobile application paradigms.

To this end, a number of models have been introduced recently including the client/agent/server (Badrinath et al. 1993; Fox et al. 1996; Oracle 1997; Zenel & Duchamp 1997; Tennenhouse et al. 1996), the client/intercept (Samaras & Pistillides 1997; Housel et al. 1996), the peer-to-peer (Reiher et al. 1996; Athan & Duchamp 1993), and the mobile agent (Chess et al. 1995; White 1996; IBM Aglets 2001) models.

Through this system, we identified the shortcomings of the wireline client/server model and its inability to support mobile computing. The requirements pertaining to wireless/mobile software models are clearly stated and the positive and negative aspects of the various models are presented in relation to these requirements. Defining a taxonomy of models and providing a methodology for building software for mobile computing is critical, since it provides the framework for the development of future applications and a yardstick to measure their effectiveness in addressing the challenges of mobile/wireless computing.

A PROPOSED CSCW SYSTEM

In our research, several elements were illustrated and choreographed to produce the desired result. The outcome of this research was implemented in the system called, DITIS. In order to better understand the model that DITIS is based upon we introduce in the following sections these features with their definition.

Architecture

The system architecture is basically divided into 5 layers. These layers are the Application/User, the Workflows, the Services, the Sensors and the Database having the last two as parallel (*Figure 3*).

The Application/Users layer is the layer that hosts our GUI that provides all the necessary functionality for a flexible, efficient and effective collaboration, covering all the pre-mentioned requirements. This layer can be altered according to the hosting organization's needs maximizing the added value of the system.

The Workflows layer is the layer that hosts the dynamic workflows as described earlier. It resembles the business processes layer in the SOA architecture, having an orchestration and coordination of the basic system services, but in a more dynamic and ad-hoc manner.

The services layer hosts the basic services that provide all the functionality of the system such as security, messaging, database access, sensors data

access, etc. These services can be called directly from the application or from a workflow, and even more from another workflow.

Finally, the last two layers are the Sensor that hosts all the available sensors of the system (such as: temperature, sound, light, vital signals, etc) and the Database layer that hosts the DBMS of the system. This DBMS can store reading from the sensors for future use by the application, all the data for the user management, collaboration features, virtual teams, dynamic workflows, actions, questionnaires, etc.

Features

The basic features of our system are the management of medical virtual teams, the dynamic questionnaires, the actions, the dynamic workflow management, the responsibilities, the timeouts & triggers, the medical diaries and the proactiveness. Below, we describe these features in more detail.

Medical Virtual Teams

The key elements of our collaboration system are the users, the roles and the virtual teams. By

Figure 3. System architecture

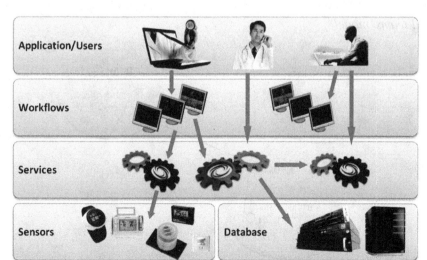

Users we denote the set U of the users that are participating in the system.

Users: $U = \{u_1, u_2, \ldots, u_n\}$

By Roles we denote the set R of all the available roles that a user can participate in the system.

Roles: $R = \{r_1, r_2, \ldots, r_m\}$

Additionally, users have a default role upon their establishment in the collaboration system. This default role is accessed by the function:

$dr(u_i) = r_j$

The notion of a virtual team Ti is denoted by the Cartesian product of the sets U and R. In other words, we have:

$$T_i \subseteq UxR \Rightarrow T_i = \{(u,r) : u \in U, r \in R\} \neq \varnothing, i \in N$$

Through this definition, we can see that the users can participate in a virtual team having a role different than their default one. Furthermore, users can participate in a virtual team having multiple roles and many users participate in a team with the same specific role. The set of all virtual teams VT is defined as:

$$VT = \bigcup_{i=1}^{n} T_i$$

Consequently, the number of all possible virtual team is: $|VT|=2|UxR|$. We can see a graphical representation of the model in Figure 4.

Dynamic Questionnaires (Voting)

Questionnaires can be described as a collection of questions. The questionnaires can be sent to individuals in order to be completed. The results are sent back to the sender and gathered in one place, so we can review the results one by one or just have an overall result (voting). This service allows us to create, view, modify, delete and complete questionnaires.

Another key feature of our system is the questionnaires. In order to give a proper definition of what is a questionnaire, we have to define first all the sub components of a questionnaire. These sub components are the questions and the answers. Similarly to the above we have a set of answers.

Answers: $AN = \{an_1, an_2, \ldots, an_z\}$

A question qi is defined as a set of answers. In other words:

Figure 4. Virtual teams' model

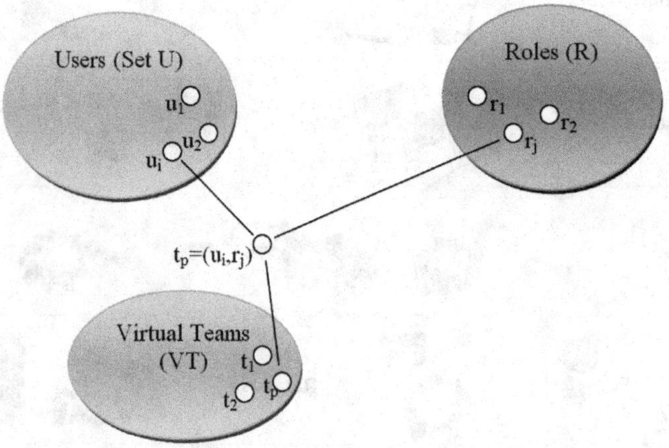

Questions: $Q = \{q_1, q_2, ..., q_z\}$

where $q_i = \{an : an \in AN\}$

Finally, a questionnaire qui is a set of questions.

Questionnaire: $QU = \{qu_1, qu_2, ..., qu_z\}$

where $qu_i = \{q : q \in Q\}$

In Figure 5 we see the graphical representation of the model.

Actions

An action is what a person can do. It could be just sending a message or a more complicated act. These messages are predefined and created by the system administrator. The more complicated act is a calling of a stored procedure. This act can encapsulate information that the administrator and/or the users passes. Additionally, an action can call an existing workflow by sending an interactive message.

Actions: $A = \{a_1, a_2, ..., a_z\}$

Dynamic Workflows (Interactive Message)

Dynamic workflows are sets of actions. They are also called interactive messages because users initiate them by sending a predefined message to another user. These messages are special messages that trigger actions and thus they make the users to interact to each other.

A more complicated notion is the one of the workflows. Workflows are defined as a set of actions connected with users or roles or virtual teams or virtual teams and roles together and with another workflow. For example, we can have the action "Visit Patient" and send it to:

- one user of the system,
- or to every doctor of the system,
- or to the virtual team of the patient,
- or to the doctors of the virtual team.

So, if A is the set of all actions of the system (Actions: $A = \{a_1, a_2, ..., a_z\}$), then:

$$W = \{(x,y) : x \in A, y \in U \cup R \cup T \cup RxT \cup W\}$$

Under the notion of the pre-mentioned timeouts and triggers, the idea of the events is spawned.

Figure 5. Questionnaires model

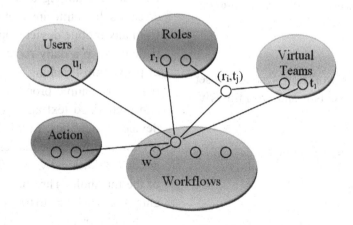

Figure 6. Workflow model

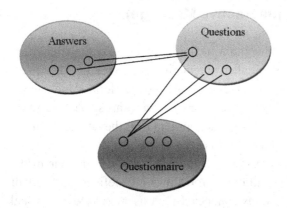

Events are the elements e of the set E that triggers a workflow. Such events are the decision making of a user (complete an action) of it can be a timeout (predefined time expiration of a task). In other words, actions can trigger an event and events can trigger a workflow. So, if the definition of events is:

Events: $E = \{e_1, e_2, ..., e_m\}$,

then there is a function g that given an action a, it returns the generated event.

$$g(a) = \begin{cases} e & \text{if a triggers a new event} \\ NULL & \text{otherwise} \end{cases}$$

Similarly, we have a function f that given an event, it returns the workflow w that it triggers:

$$f(e) = w$$

In other words, the workflow system is a set of ordered pairs of events e and workflows w (e,w).

Dynamic Workflows $= \{(e,w) : e \in E, w \in W\}$

Responsibilities

Some actions are set to be performed by only one user of a certain role. We can notify all users of this role and send them an action to be performed. The first user that will get the action can take the responsibility of completing this task. All other users will be notified that this task is handled by another person. This way we avoid duplication of work. For instance, we can have the scenario that one nurse is asking for a drug prescription from all doctors. We don't want to have more than one doctor to prescribe the same drug. The Responsibility feature solves this problem.

Timeouts & Triggers

Under the scope of the medical virtual teams, we have assignments of roles to patients. There are times though that certain tasks are of vital significance (urgent tasks) and thus the need for the dimension of time is spawned. We can set a timeout on such crucial action. When the time that we set passes, another action or workflow is trigged. For example, we can have a nurse asking for a doctor's help. Nurse will initially ask help from the doctor of the patient's virtual team. After the timeout occurs, another action will be triggered. The new action will be about asking help from any doctor of the system.

Medical Diaries

Web 2.0 concepts include information/experience sharing among users. Medical diaries are an easy self monitoring method, used by patients from any mobile device. During this procedure, patients keep a daily record of their symptoms or pain control ranking the symptom on a scale. It's a very simple procedure, using only clicks and predefined text answers due to the mobile devices limitations. Medical Virtual Team can review anytime these diaries and suggest or take actions. Additionally, we introduced the notion of the threshold. Threshold is a limit on a diary entry that can be set to trigger a workflow or alert the team. For instance, a patient marks a pain of grade 10 in his pain diary. Then, a message can be send to his Medical virtual team, notifying them about this event.

Pro-Activeness

European Committee is focusing on activity motivation services. The activity motivation services include services that will motivate and encourage persons with chronic conditions to undertake physical and mental exercises and activities, change life style, socialize etc. Daily tasks assistance will provide to patients with direction indications, explanations on how to perform some tasks, or even instructions on how to call for human assistance for example through the use of the socialization services. Additionally, the system can assist patients by providing them with a type of memory help (reminders, directions indications to a place, memory assistance etc).

During the following pages, I will present the implementation of the system. For this implementation, we used all the notions and components that are mentioned and presented in the previous chapters. The system was implemented into two different applications. The windows-based application, that it's used from the administrator, in order to setup the collaboration rules and the web-based application

that is customized to work on every mobile device and give the ability to the users of using the system 24/7 everywhere and by any means.

Implementation

For the system's implementation, we used all the notions and components that are mentioned and presented in the previous sections. The system was implemented as two different but also interrelated applications. The windows-based application, that it's used from the administrator, in order to setup the collaboration rules and the dynamic workflows and the web-based application that is customized to work on every mobile device and give the ability to users of using the system 24/7 everywhere and by any means.

Windows-Based Application (Administration)

As mentioned before, this application is designed to be used by the administrator to coordinate the whole system. Following I will present the screens that are implemented in this application.

In Figure 7 we demonstrate the administrators' main menu. The administrator can choose from

Figure 7. Administrator's interface

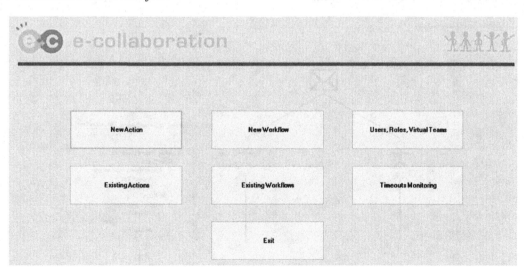

creating new Action, Workflows, Users, Roles and Virtual Teams, or manage the existing ones. Finally, the administrator can manage the workflow timeouts. The administrator can also view the timeouts, in order to start/stop the existing timeouts monitoring process. Additionally, the administrator can populate lists (that will be used by the end users) manually (List of all possible selections – '|' separated or from database query. e.g. Yes | No | Maybe or 'Select Name, Value From Users') or with the use of plain SQL commands.

The workflows are graphically represented and as tree view (*Figure 8*) for better understanding and error prevention for more complicated workflows. In addition there is a circle prevention mechanism that prevents the creation of workflows that may result in dead-end.

Web-Based Application (Users)

Web-based application is used by users in a 24/7 basis through any device (*Figure 9*). Users have access in their data, and can collaborate in innovative ways, using dynamic interactive messages (workflows), questionnaires and virtual teams. In this chapter we present the functionality of the web-based application through the use of a PDA.

Users in the healthcare sector have limited knowledge of mobile devices and ability to use state-of-the-art technologies such as PDAs and smartphones. Thus, we adopted screens that are easy to understand and no need much effort on accessing information by using as much as possible key buttons and minimizing the "clicks" and consequently we speed up the process.

EVALUATION

Methodology and Sampling

Our research site is PASYKAF, a cancer support care organization in Cyprus. PASYKAF was founded in 1986 to provide support to cancer patients and their families during their period of rehabilitation and is manned with highly qualified medical, paramedical and nursing staff. In 1992 it has started a home care service for cancer patients. Specially trained palliative care nurses in close co-operation with doctors (general practitioners and oncologists), physiotherapists and psychologists, attend and care for patients at home, focusing on maintaining the best possible quality of life, including medical care and psychological support.

Figure 8. Workflow graphical representation

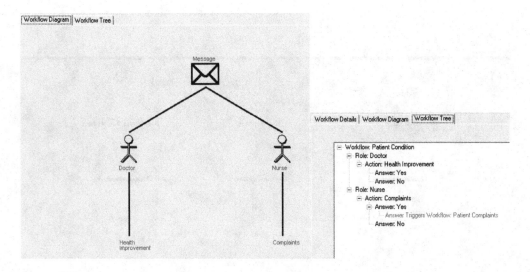

The fieldwork has taken place in various district sites of PASYKAF. Each site is served by palliative care nurses who visit regularly patients at their house offering health care. Data on our system (aka DITIS) implementation were collected on different stages of the implementation process as follows:

- **Phase 1:** The preliminary part of the research has studied the use of mobile telephones by a group of palliative care nurses during a period of 2 months. Interviews with four nurses and two doctors in the Larnaca site have enabled the study of nurses-to-nurses interactions and nurses and doctors/other specialists interactions via the use of mobile telephones whilst also contributed to gathering information on their level of awareness about the system and its potential use in palliative care.
- **Phase 2:** This part of the study took place about 6 months after the 1st phase and involved the use of a structured questionnaire that was sent to the system developers

and potential users. It aimed to explore stakeholders' expectations regarding the system.

- **Phase 3:** The final phase of data collection took place almost 2 years after the completion of the 2nd phase. By this time DITIS has been implemented and deployed in four district sites (Nicosia, Limassol, Larnaca and Paphos). During this phase, current users of the system in three of the district offices of PASYKAF (Larnaca, Limassol and Paphos) were interviewed (psychologists and nurses). The main issues explored during interviews in phase 3 of the study included the following:
  ◦ Participants' actual use of the system.
  ◦ Participants' own explanation of why they use the system, the way they do.
  ◦ Participants' understanding of what users' and others stakeholders' role should be for achieving effective system's use.

Figure 9. User's interface

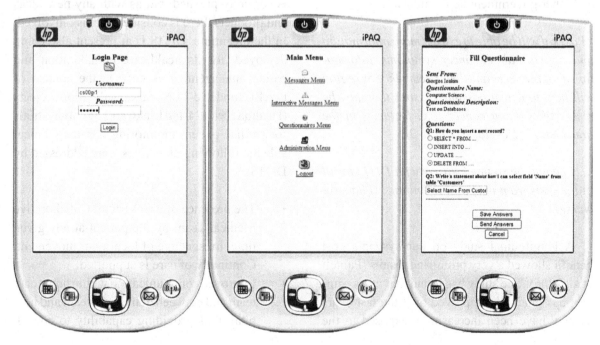

Due to the nature of the system which is patient oriented, there were created more than 200 medical virtual teams assigned to all system users. This sample was used to extract the added value and cost effectiveness of the system.

Results

Overall, the data reveal that the system offers innumerable opportunities for palliative care nurses and other cancer-care practitioners and it's currently widely accepted as an invaluable tool in palliative care (Panteli 2003; Panteli et al. 2006). Nurses, psychologists and doctors acknowledge that the system has numerous advantages and that they are willing to incorporate it in their work activities. Additionally, the system improved the communication, coordination and collaboration among members. Due to the huge amount of data regarding new and old patient records that need to be handled on a daily basis, the system enabled users to access data quickly either from their office or remotely. Furthermore, it was used as a statistical tool, for producing internal reports for the district offices and the head office as well as external reports required by the Ministry of Health and other government departments.

"Pasykaf will be able to extract more information and statistics about cancer symptoms. Information about cancers and their occurrence by region will help to detect possible reasons that may be responsible about cancer (e.g. factories in the areas, etc)" (Developer, Phase 2).

"...Life will be so much easier with DITIS to fill in the gaps from unknown to known" (Limassol Nurse).

A longitudinal study on our system's cost benefit showed a very promising results (Panteli et al. 2006). The study has found that users' support has gradually improved over the last years as they have been increasingly exposed to the

system capabilities and have recognized the advantages of the system in their day to day work for both administrative and consultation purposes. Another reason for this is that the nurses have gained participation in the project team with periodical meetings with the project manager and developers. The study in (Mitchell et al. 1997) had adopted the stakeholders' analysis. It found that there are different relationship characteristics among the key stakeholders showing diversity in interests, expectations and level of involvement in the implementation of the system. DITIS has appeared to act as a useful fuel for improving patient-records and promoting an integrated approach that has a direct impact on the quality of treatment and health care support to home-based cancer patients. However, even though this is a novel application and despite the fact that it has been introduced five years ago, the implementation has remained slow and the system has not yet been able to secure its place and its future in the health sector; though it has been making an impact on the health care support provided by the PASYKAF nurses and medical staff. Speedy commercialization of the system seems to be the solution for its long term survivability, and this is currently pursued, but as with any new ideas and products there is considerable risk involved. In the meantime, DITIS is at present also being deployed, for its healthcare collaboration and patient management aspects, in the context of two EU funded e-TEN market validation projects (HealthService24 and LinkCare), involving trials for cardiac patient monitoring. On the Clinical side the following objectives were addressed by DITIS:

- The presence of the (Virtual) Collaborative Medical Team by the patient at any given time, irrespective of locality or movement. Continuity of care is supported.
- Improved communication within home care team and between home-care team and hospital, thus providing capability to consult

within a team of experts (e.g. home nurse with treating doctor or oncologist), without need to move patient from his home to each one of them. This results in reduction of number of visits to health professionals and reduces burden not only on patient but also his relatives, and makes better use of the scarce and expensive medical professionals and scarce hospital beds.

- Improved and secure, timely access to patient information, in accordance with their authorization levels, through unified information space centred around the patient. As an added benefit, the patient need not provide the same history to multiple professionals.
- Improved and flexible collection of statistical data for further audit and research within the home care setting.
- Improved evaluation through the capability to offer audit and research.
- Improved cost effectiveness through improved communications and better planning of services.
- Improved health practices (shift toward evidence-based) and reduction of bureaucratic overhead.
- Assists in promoting the dependant role of the home-nurse legally binding (for example, in the home setting when interacting with a hospital doctor for the prescription of drugs in the home).

As a consequence of meeting the above clinical objectives the system improves the provision of health care to Cancer patients, thereby achieving better quality of life, in the warmth of their own home.

CONCLUSION

In this chapter we presented the current situation in collaboration and workflow management and more specifically in the eHealth sector. After an extensive research on existing systems and trends, we proposed an extended model for collaboration and dynamic workflow management system within the demanding eHealth context. Additionally, we took under consideration issues like the technical requirements and the most appropriate computational model for this type of application since they are developed to work under wireless environments that many disconnections occur.

The need for new features like medical virtual teams, questionnaires, actions, dynamic workflows, responsibilities, triggers & timeouts, medical diaries and pro-activeness is noted and they were analyzed, modeled and implemented within our system.

The system architecture along with the equivalent layers were presented and described in more detail. Furthermore, the users' graphical interface was presented, both for the administrator and the end users. Through the administrators interface, users can choose from various features like creating new Action, Workflows, Users, Roles and Virtual Teams, or manage the existing ones, among many other features. End-users can access the system anywhere and anytime through any mobile device as long as there is a support of an internet browser and an internet connection. This interface was purposely kept simple by minimizing the need for adding text and minimizing the "clicks", since the users in the eHealth domain aren't so computer and internet cultured.

Eventually, we presented the evaluation of the system, using a real test bed facility (an organization that provides homecare to cancer patients called PASYKAF). The methodology used for this evaluation was consisted of 3 steps and provided the overall evaluation results. The results found that users' support has gradually improved over the last years and the cost effectiveness for the organization was even greater. However, a further experimental evaluation with a larger sample is needed in order to estimate safe conclusions about the effectiveness of this system in the Web 2.0 eHealth context.

Future research directions within the eHealth context are focus in social based VTs, motivation and socialization of the patients. In general, it's a marriage of Ambient Assisted Living (aka AAL) and mobile healthcare. Within this context, systems will have to support an innovative social community model encouraging and supporting active participation, communication, socialization, mutual assistance and self-organization of the elderly, promoting seamless integration and interaction of different people (family members, caretakers, medical professionals, friends etc.) from all ages at any time and any place and providing daily activity monitoring. The model places the patient in the centre of the services, making him both a consumer and producer of assistance.

The use of innovative validated systems will intrinsically have a high positive impact in improving the quality of life of the patient, but also of their families and care personnel, by prolonging the time the person can live independently in a socially integrated community manner thereby reducing the demand for care and the associated care cost.

Furthermore, research has to be done on the effective and efficient integration of Vital Signal Monitoring (VSM) devices and sensors networks. Research will have to be conducted on new algorithms that will be integrated with the VSM devices and sensors for prevention and prediction of possible medical incidents. Due to the critical and importance of the information in eHealth, the margin for errors are prone to null. You have to bear in mind that a mistake here can be result into a loss of a human's life and this is not acceptable by anyone, especially by the medical personnel.

REFERENCES

Aglets Workbench, I. B. M. (2001). IBM Japan Research Group. http://aglets.trl.ibm.co.jp

Athan, A., & Duchamp, D. (1993). *Agent-Mediated Message Passing for Constrained Environments*. In *Proceedings USENIX Symposium on Mobile and Location-Independent Computing* (pp. 103-1070). Cambridge, MA.

Badrinath, B. R., Bakre, A., Imielinski, T., & Marantz, R. (1993). Handling Mobile Clients: A Case for Indirect Interaction. In *Proceedings of the 4th Workshop on Workstation Operating Systems, Aigen, Austria, October.*

CCITT (1987), *Draft Recommendation on Message Handling Systems, X 400, Version 5,* November.

Chess, D., Grosof, B., Harrison, C., Levine, D., Parris, C., & Tsudik, G. (1995). Itinerant Agents for Mobile Computing. *Journal IEEE Personal Communications, 2*(5).

Fox, A., Gribble, S. D., Brewer, E. A., & Amir, E. (1996). *Adapting* to Network and Client Variability via On-Demand Dynamic Distillation. In *Proceedings of the ASPLOS-VII, Cambridge, MA, October*.

Georgiadis, T. D. (2002). *Dynamic Creation of Collaborating System and Database Management, Using Mobile Agents*. Master thesis supervised by George Samaras, Computer Science Department, University of Cyprus, June.

Gray, J., & Reuter, A. (1993). *Transaction Processing: Concepts and Techniques*. Morgan Kaufman Publishers, Inc.

Housel, B. C., Samaras, G., & Lindquist, D. B. (1996). *WebExpress: A Client/Intercept Based System for Optimizing Web Browsing in a Wireless Environment. Journal ACM/Baltzer Mobile Networking and Applications (MONET)*. Special Issue on Mobile Networking on the Internet.

Lipnack, J., & Stamps, J. (2000). *VIRTUAL TEAMS: People Working Across Boundaries with Technology* (2nd ed.). New York: John Wiley & Sons.

Mitchell, R., Agle, B., & Wood, D. (1997). Towards a theory of stakeholder identification and salience. *Academy of Management Review*, *22*(4), 853–887. doi:10.2307/259247

Mohan, C. (1997). *Recent Trends in Workflow Management Products, Standards and Research* (pp. 396–409). Workflow Management Systems and Interoperability.

Mortensen, E. (1985). Trends in electronic Mail and it's role in office automation. *Electronic Publishing Review*, *5*(4), 257–268.

Muneera, S. U. (2006). *Graphic Design: Collaborative Processes = Understanding Self and Others, Art 325: Collaborative Processes*. Corvallis, Oregon: Fairbanks Hall, Oregon State University.

Oracle (1997). *Oracle Mobile Agents Technical Product Summary*. Retrieved from www.oracle.com/products/ networking/mobile/agents/html

Panteli, N. (2003). *DITIS: An eHealth Mobile Application in Cyprus. A user's Perspective*. May, Internal DITIS report. Retrieved from http://www.ditis.ucy.ac.cy/publications/internalreports.htm

Panteli, N., & Dibben, M. R. (2001). Reflections on Mobile communication systems. *Futures*, *33*(5), 379–391. doi:10.1016/S0016-3287(00)00081-1

Panteli, N., Pitsillides, B., Pitsillides, A., & Samaras, G. (2006). An E-healthcare Mobile application: A Stakeholders' analysis. In Al-Hakim, L. (Ed.), *Web Mobile-Based Applications for Healthcare Management*. Hershey, PA: IGI Global.

Pitsillides, A., Samaras, G., Dikaiakos, M., & Christodoulou, E. (1999), *DITIS: Collaborative Virtual Medical team for home healthcare of cancer patients*. Conference on the Information Society and Telematics Applications, Catania, Italy, 16-18 April.

Reif, G., et al. (2001). A Web-based peer-to-peer architecture for collaborative nomadic working. *10th IEEE Workshops on Enabling Technologies: Infrastructures for Collaborative Enterprises (WETICE 2001), Boston, MA, USA* (pp. 334-339).

Reiher, P., Popek, J., Gunter, M., Salomone, J., & Ratner, D. (1996). Peer-to-Peer Reconciliation Based Replication for Mobile Computers. In *Proceedings of the European Conference on Object Oriented Programming 2nd Workshop on Mobility and Replication, June*.

Rodden, T. (1991). A Survey of CSCW Systems. *Interacting with Computers*, *3*(3), 319–353. doi:10.1016/0953-5438(91)90020-3

Samaras, G., & Pitsillides, A. (1997). Client/Intercept: a Computational Model for Wireless Environments. In *Proceedings of the 4th International Conference on Telecommunications (ICT'97), Melbourne, Australia, April*.

Schmidt, K., & Bannon, L. (1992). Taking CSCW seriously. [CSCW]. *Computer Supported Cooperative Work*, *1*(1). doi:10.1007/BF00752449

Simpson, J. A., & Weiner, E. S. C. (1989). *Collaboration. Oxford English Dictionary* (2nd ed.). Oxford University Press.

Tennenhouse, D. L., Smith, J. M., Sincoskie, W. D., & Minden, G. J. (1996). A Survey of Active Network Research. *Journal IEEE Communication Magazine*, *35*(1), 80–86. doi:10.1109/35.568214

Tiwana, A. (2000). From Intuition to Institution: Supporting Collaborative Diagnoses in Telemedicine Teams. In *Proceedings of the 33rd Hawaii International Conference on System Sciences.*

Wagner, C.S. & Leydesdorff, L. (2005). *The diffusion of international collaboration and the formation of a core group.* Globalisation in the network of science in 2005.

White, J. E. (1996). *Mobile Agents* [General Magic White Paper]. Retrieved from http://www.genmagic.com/agents.

Zenel, B., & Duchamp, D. (1997). General Purpose Proxies: Solved and Unsolved Problems. In *Proceedings of the Hot-OS VI.*

Chapter 22
Digital Pathology and Virtual Microscopy Integration in E–Health Records

Marcial García Rojo
Hospital General de Ciudad Real, Spain

Christel Daniel
Université René Descartes, France

ABSTRACT

In anatomic pathology, digital pathology integrates information management systems to manage both digital images and text-based information. Digital pathology allows information sharing for diagnosis, biomedical research and education. Virtual microscopy resulting in digital slides is an outreaching technology in anatomic pathology. Limiting factors in the expansion of virtual microscopy are formidable storage dimension, scanning speed, quality of image and cultural change. Anatomic pathology data and images should be an important part of the patient electronic health records as well as of clinical data-warehouses, epidemiological or biomedical research databases, and platforms dedicated to translational medicine. Integrating anatomic pathology to the "healthcare enterprise" can only be achieved using existing and emerging medical informatics standards like Digital Imaging and Communications in Medicine (DICOM®[1]), Health Level Seven (HL7®), and Systematized Nomenclature of Medicine-Clinical Terms (SNOMED CT®), following the recommendations of Integrating the Healthcare Enterprise (IHE®).

INTRODUCTION: WHAT IS DIGITAL PATHOLOGY?

Several socioeconomic factors have accelerated the dissemination of information technology in anatomic pathology. The spread in the use of Internet, the presence of computers in doctor's offices, and the increasing demand of second opinion from the patient has facilitated the adoption of local, national, and international governmental initiatives to explore and adopt digital pathology and telepathology programmes, and to support the developing of patient electronic health (e-Health) records. Patient electronic health records (EHR) should contain a full range of data set, including the digital images of all types of imaging studies ever performed on the patient.

DOI: 10.4018/978-1-61520-777-0.ch022

Copyright © 2010, IGI Global. Copying or distributing in print or electronic forms without written permission of IGI Global is prohibited.

The concept digital pathology comprises the information technology that allows for the management of information, including data and images, generated in an anatomic pathology department. Anatomic pathology information system and digital imaging modalities are two main components of digital pathology.

Anatomic pathology information systems manage computerized orders of anatomic pathology examination of specimen collected from patients as well as the fulfilment of these orders.

In most anatomic pathology departments, images are more and more being used in a digital format. Photographic images are digitized during specimen macroscopic study and microscopic images during microscopy evaluation and molecular pathology documentation.

Nowadays most of the anatomic pathology departments using digital imaging in microscopy, which is the essential tool of pathologists, are equipped with imaging modalities producing only still images captured from a selected field under the microscope. The use of still microscopic images in the diagnostic process is time consuming and results in frustration for clinicians and pathologists. In the last 5 years, slide scanners have become very popular since they allow a complete digitization of tissue and cytology slides, a process termed whole slides imaging (WSI), to create digital slides. Since this disruptive innovation allows a realistic simulation of the work performed with the conventional optical microscope (figure 1), it is known as virtual microscopy (Ferreira, 1997; Afework, 1998).

Conventional glass slides are fragile, and they are non permanent, since stain will fade over time, especially in immunofluorescence. Also, in cytology, it is not possible to distribute copies of the slides. These disadvantages of conventional slides can be overcome with digital slides, which also have additional advantages, like having lower magnification pictures with extraordinary quality, a dynamic map of the slide, tracking and playing back the path followed by the pathologist during the examination of the slide, images are permanently stored, and it is possible to make annotations that can also be recorded. Additional advantages of digital slides over glass slides are

Figure 1. Using virtual microscopy systems, pathologists can review complete microscopy slides simulating the operation of an optical microscope.

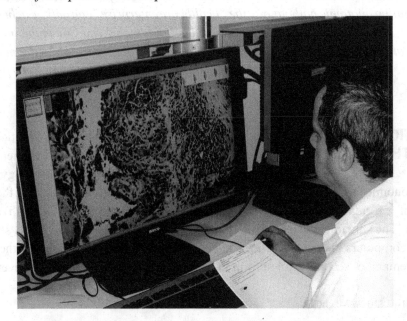

the possibility to distribute multiple copies on a DVD of exactly the same slide, and the high quality always on focus and well illuminated images that decreases eye fatigue, and other ergonomic advantages by reducing back and neck fatigue (Zeineh, 2005).

Virtual microscopy is already being applied in anatomic pathology for primary histopathology diagnosis, primary cytopathology diagnosis, cytological cancer screening. The use of digital images is been validated for diagnostic applications in surgical pathology (Gilbertson, 2006), cytopathology (Dee, 2007), and immunohistochemistry (O'Malley, 2008). There is no statistically significant difference in the diagnostic accuracy either between virtual microscopy and conventional light microscopy. Some automated image analysis algorithms that are being used on digital slides have been U.S. Food and Drug Administration (FDA) 510(k)-cleared for assessing the level or certain immunohistochemical markers. However, there is little experience in the use of virtual microscopy in diagnostic pathology daily practice, and there in no slide scanner that is FDA approved for primary or initial diagnosis.

The consequences of the full digitalization of pathology departments are hard to foresee, but short term issues have arisen that imply interesting challenges for health care standardization bodies.

Digital pathology in an anatomic pathology department also includes biomedical equipments, like laboratory autostainers control software, automated image analysis tools, quality assurance program management systems, etc, that are used during the fulfilment of the orders. These equipments need to be properly interfaced to the anatomic pathology information system.

Digital pathology also addresses information technology used for inter-laboratories exchanges for collaborative diagnostic processes including telepathology for second opinion.

Telepathology is the practice of pathology at a distance using some of the elements that compose digital pathology (still images, digital slides, and less frequently video microscopy). It can be aimed to primary diagnosis or to second opinion teleconsultation (Kayser, 1999).

Telepathology developed in some countries as a response to a shortage of pathologists (Sawai, 2007a). It was classically divided into static telepathology (store and forward, generally sending still images files of representative areas by e-mail or FTP) and dynamic or real time telepathology (video transmission) (Cowan, 2005). Digital or virtual slides can be considered a special type of store and forward telepathology where the whole slide is scanned and saved, to be transmitted under user-demand, with the advantage of sending only requested areas that can be sent using conventional Internet bandwidth. Due to this dynamic interaction between users and the digital slide, some users classify virtual microscopy as digital dynamic telepathology systems (Afework, 1998).

In Japan, since 2000, telepathology is included as an insured healthcare service (Sawai, 2007a).

At last, digital pathology is not only dedicated to patient care and also addresses the use of information systems during research and teaching activities.

Education libraries, biobanks managing systems, or cancer registry databases are part of digital pathology. Virtual microscopy, for example, is already being widely applied in undergraduate teaching, distance learning and continuous medical education, proficiency testing, pathology quality assurance programs, and research (tumour banking).

Digital pathology comprises the use of information technology for all the different activities of the pathologists and should be integrated to the "Healthcare Enterprise" information system for patient care (integration to electronic healthcare record or personal healthcare record) and research activities (integration to biomedical or epidemiological research databases, to cancer registries, to tissue or images banks, to clinical datawarehouses, to translational medicine platforms, etc).

DIGITAL ORDERS AND REPORTS IN ANATOMIC PATHOLOGY

Typical anatomic pathology cases represent the analysis of (all) tissue removed in a single collection procedure (e.g., surgical operation/event, biopsy, scrape, aspiration etc.).

With regards to the diagnostic activities, digital pathology addresses the management of both digital (or computerized) orders for anatomic pathology examination of specimen and digital reports, delivered in fulfilment of these orders.

Like in clinical laboratory, the diagnostic process in anatomic pathology is specimen-driven (figure 2). However, the diagnostic process in anatomic pathology differs from that in the clinical laboratory since it relies on image interpretation. It also differs from that in radiology since, in the current daily practice, digital imaging is not systematically performed.

DIGITAL IMAGING IN ANATOMIC PATHOLOGY

Digital imaging is one major component of digital pathology. Digital imaging solutions include image acquisition modalities, post processing stations, image viewers and picture image and distribution systems (PACS). There are different types of digital image acquisition modalities in anatomic pathology. Scanning speed, quality of image during capture and viewing processes, automated image analysis or computer-aided decisions, adoption of health care standards, and internal organizational issues, are some of the important factors that need to be addressed in the integration of digital slides in EHR.

Figure 2. Overview of anatomic pathology workflow

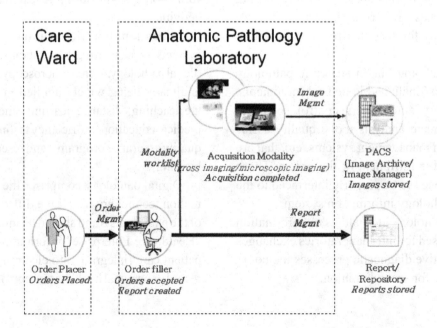

Acquiring Digital Images in Anatomic Pathology

Digital images in anatomic pathology consist in photographic gross images or microscopic images. Photographic gross images capture relevant information about specimen at a macroscopic level (photographs of specimen or derived specimen (e.g. paraffin blocks), etc). The acquisition modality for macroscopic (or gross) imaging is photo camera.

Microscopic images capture relevant information about specimen at a microscopic level. The main objective of virtual microscopy system or whole slide imaging (WSI) devices is building digital slides. They are capable of digitizing slides at high magnifications. Two main groups of acquisition modalities for microscopic images (WSI devices) can be distinguished: modalities using both a motorized microscope and a camera and slide scanners (Rojo, 2006).

Multispectral microscopy is considered an alternative to the red-green-blue (RGB) imaging used by current automated imaging systems, since RGB sensors have shown to be insufficient to distinguish between similar chromogens above all if they overlap spatially. These problems can be solved acquiring a stack of images at multiple wavelengths, and obtaining the determination of precise optical spectra at every pixel location.

Slide scanners are closed systems that include components similar to those used in motorized microscopes (an objective to optically magnify the specimen, digital camera, and motorized stage) but with some modifications, such as absence of eyepieces and absence of position and focus control.

There are many different slide scanning solutions available for pathology slides (table 1) (Rojo, 2006; Yagi, 2007).

A virtual microscopy system has three essential elements: slide scanner, image storage, and viewer (Tofukuji, 2007b). The main barriers to the shift to digital imaging are the storage capacity, the scanning speed and the quality assessment of digital slides in different contexts of use.

Storage Dimension

Digital slides carry a huge amount of data. A single glass slide size is 76 mm x 26 mm and includes a label area and an area of interest with the specimen (tissue or cytology) of about 25 mm x 50 mm. When scanned using a 40x objective, this specimen area can be converted into an up to 220,000 x 90,000 pixels size image, over 55 GB uncompressed data.

A typical specimen of 15 x 15 mm digitized with a 20x objective at a resolution of 0.3 μm/pixel contains 50,000 x 50,000 pixels. For each pixel containing 3 bytes colour information, the total one single slide size is 50,000 x 50,000 x 3 = 7.5 GB of uncompressed data (Tofukuji, 2007b). These figures are related to one single X-Y plane, and they can be increased by several orders of magnitude in those 3D scanning systems capable of saving multiple planes in the Z-axis.

Specimens (tissue slices or cytology smears) usually doesn't occupy the complete specimen area, and since most digital slides are used in compressed format (generally JPEG2000 or JPEG), we can estimate an average of 1 GB per slide (100 times an X-ray film) when scanned at 40x.

A medium-sized anatomic pathology department manages over 100,000 slides per year, which means that a storage capacity of 100 TB is needed every year, only for the microscopic images of the anatomic pathology department.

The price of magneto-optical disks and new storage devices decreases every year. In 1999, the price of 1 TB on magnetic hard disks was 10,000 US dollars (Kayser, 1999); ten years later, the price has dropped to about 100 US dollars.

Scanning Speed

In a slide scanner, specimens are highly magnified optically to obtain desired information. In some

Table 1. Pathology digital slide scanners

System	Vendor	Objective/NA(1)	# slides	Light path	File format
ACIS® III	Dako(2) http://www.dako.com/	Nikon 4x, 10x, 20x, 40x, 60x	100	Halogen lamp	JPEG, TIFF, BMP
Applied Imaging Ariol®	Genetix http://www.genetix.com/	Motorized microscope. 1.25x, 5x, 10x, 20x (0.36 μm/pixel), 40x (0.18 μm/pixel)	50	Fluorescence available	JPEG
dotSlide™	Olympus http://www.olympus.co.uk/microscopy/22_slide.htm	Motorized microscope. 2x plapon, 10x, 20x, 40x uplsapo	1 (50)	Halogen lamp. Fluorescence, polarisation available	Olympus VSI, JPEG, TIFF, JPEG2000
DX40®	Dmetrix http://www.dmetrix.com/	Array of 80 objectives (20X)	40	Bright-field,	DMetrix format. Export to JPEG,TIFF
GoodSpeed®	Alphelys http://www.alphelys.com/	Motorized microscope	4 or 8	Dark field and fluorescence available	JPEG
iSan™	BioImagene http://www.bioimagene.com/	20x/0.50 Plan Fluor 40x/0.75 Plan Fluor	160	Bright-field, integrated LED	JPEG2000, JPEG, TIFF
Leica SCN400	Leica Microsystems http://www.leica-microsystems.com/	x40 (0.25 μm/pixel)	4 (384)	Bright-field,	Leica format, JPG, PNG, MS Silverlight
NanoZoomer® HT	Hamamatsu http://www.hamamatsu.com/	20x/0.7. Modes: x20 (0.46 μm/pixel) x40 (0.23 μm/pixel)	210	Fluorescence available	JPEG, TIFF
NanoZoomer® RS	Hamamatsu http://www.hamamatsu.com/	20x/0.75. Modes: x10 (0.92 μm/pixel) x20 (0.46 μm/pixel) x40 (0.23 μm/pixel)	6	Fluorescence available	JPEG, TIFF
Pannoramic 250®	3D Histech http://www.3dhistech.com/	20x/0.80 (0.23 μm) Plan Apo. 40x/0.95 Plan Apo	250	Fluorescence available	Mirax format, JPEG, TIFF
Panoramic Desk®	3D Histech http://www.3dhistech.com/	20x/0.80 (0.23 μm) Plan Apo. 40x/0.95 Plan Apo	1	Bright-field, halogen lamp	Mirax format, JPEG, TIFF
Panoramic Midi®	3D Histech http://www.3dhistech.com/	20x/0.80 (0.23 μm) Plan Apo. 40x/0.95 Plan Apo	12	Fluorescence available	Mirax format, JPEG, TIFF
Panoramic Scan®	3D Histech http://www.3dhistech.com/	20x/0.80 (0.23 μm) Plan Apo. 40x/0.95 Plan Apo	150	Fluorescence available	Mirax format, JPEG, TIFF
ScanScope® CS	Aperio http://www.aperio.com/	20x/0.75 Plan Apo	5	Bright-field, halogen lamp	TIFF (Aperio SVS), CWS
ScanScope® GL	Aperio http://www.aperio.com/	20x/0.75 Plan Apo	1	Bright-field, halogen lamp	TIFF (Aperio SVS), CWS
ScanScope® GL-E	Aperio http://www.aperio.com/	20x/0.75 Plan Apo	1	Bright-field, halogen lamp	Composite Web-Slide (CWS)
ScanScope® OS	Aperio http://www.aperio.com/	60x/1.35 Plan Apo	1	Oil immersion	TIFF (Aperio SVS), CWS
ScanScope® XT	Aperio http://www.aperio.com/	20x/0.75 Plan Apo	120	Bright-field, halogen lamp	TIFF (Aperio SVS), CWS
Toco™	Claro http://www.claro-inc.jp/	Carl Zeiss Aplan 20x, 40x	1	Bright-field, flat LED	Claro format, JPEG
Vassalo™	Claro http://www.claro-inc.jp/	Carl Zeiss Aplan 20x,40x	80 or 20	Bright-field, flat LED	Claro format, JPEG

(1) NA: Numerical Aperture

(2) In March 2009, Carl Zeiss MicroImaging, Inc. acquired ACIS® and Trestle® Instrument Systems from Clarient, Inc.

cases, digitizing pathology slides using a 20x lens, instead of a 40x one, is enough. This saves time and disk space, but most pathologists feel more confident having their specimens scanned with the highest resolution available, even more if those files are considered for a long-term use.

A 10 mm x 10 mm area can be scanned at 20x magnification in 6 min (Claro Vassalo™), in 2 minutes (Aperio ScanScope® XT) or in less than 50 seconds (DMetrix® DX-40 array-microscope). With these scanning times, it is possible to use digital slide and virtual microscopy systems for quick frozen intra-operative telepathology diagnosis (Tsuchihashi, 2008).

When higher resolutions and quality are needed, for instance using oil immersion with an objective 100x, the same area needs about 20 minutes to be scanned (Aperio ScanScope® OS). In our experience, average scanning time with an objective 40x for each slide is 15 minutes with Aperio ScanScope® XT. However, when using large tissue areas (e.g. cytology smears) that need to be scanned at 40x, with optical quality including multiple focusing points, scanning time of a single slide can be over 1 hour.

At the moment, because of the slowness of current slide scanners a selection of glass slides to be scanned seems necessary. An anatomic pathology department generates about 500 slides per day in the routine workload.

In an integrated environment, where digital slides are sent to a central server, scanning speed may be affected by the network traffic. Image compression time should also be considered when computing slide scanning throughput.

With current technology, a full-digitalization approach would require multiple scanners running in parallel to avoid a significant delay in anatomic pathology service. For that reason, users are currently demanding faster or ultrarapid scanners, integrated with PACS.

Compression

Since digital slide files are large by current standards, it is highly desirable to compress those files. JPEG image compression at ratios less than 20:1 do no compromise diagnostic accuracy. JPEG2000 provides higher image quality than JPEG for the same compression rations (Soenksen, 2005).

The pyramidal image file format, used by some systems, stores the image in several resolutions (e.g. 40x, 10x and 2.5x) simultaneously. This increases the efficiency of viewing, since only the appropriate resolution level is sent to the digital slide viewer. TIFF and JP2 file formats support multiple pyramidal images within one file.

Quality of Digital Slides

The main quality factor in microscopic images is spatial resolution in micrometers per pixel, determined by the numerical aperture (NA) of the objective, and the quality of the lenses. An objective 20x with a 0.70 NA objective is frequently found inside many current slide scanners. It can yield a 0.23 µm/pixel resolution. Higher NA objectives, like 40x (NA 0.95) increases spatial resolution, although it offers less depth of field and correct focusing of thicker sections or cytological smears can become a problem.

The camera used by the scanner is another essential element that limits the quality of obtained images. They can be charge-coupled devices (CCD) or complementary metal oxide semiconductor (CMOS). According to the scanning method, these capturing devices can be area sensors, area transference sensor, linear sensors or array microscope sensors. Digital cameras in scanners have been reviewed elsewhere (Rojo, 2006).

Microscopy specimens are difficult to be scanned because they contain relevant information not only in X and Y axis, but also in Z axis. This is especially true in cytology specimens. For that reason, most manufacturers offer an enhanced focusing mode to digitize multiple Z-axis planes (z-stacks), with the possibility to obtain as a result either a single plane collecting the best focused areas of each of these planes, or a stack of images with the possibility to navigate in the Z-axis, at least in a small portion of the digital slide.

Almost every current digital slide contains at least small out-of-focus areas, and, less frequently, stitching or seams artefacts can be found. Colour reproducibility, illumination problems, or compression effects are other described problems.

Using Digital Images in Anatomic Pathology

Human Interpretation of Digital Images

Viewers

Due to the special characteristics of large digital slides images, a specific slide viewer is required in most cases to show special file formats and display them efficiently on the screen. Viewing should support fast panning and zooming.

To improve user' experience some viewers use pre-fetching technology to load neighbour areas of the image in the computer memory. Adequate viewing tools, including annotation and image processing are also essential.

Hardware must also be considered. The ideal virtual microscopy workstation should be fast in graphical performance, since users are demanding being able to read large amount of data on the monitor without having the pixelating or mounting effect of the current systems. Special high performance graphics card and mainboard buses may be needed to solve these problems.

Most pathologists have the impression that digital slides are slower than glass slides to review. Optical microscopes cannot be surpassed on image viewing speed because one cannot form an image faster then the speed of light, but some other movements and actions taken when reviewing a slide can be better using digital slides. For instance,

in well focused digital slides, focus change is not necessary, and changing objective is faster and without illumination variations (Zeineh, 2005).

Monitor quality and colour calibration should also be taken into account. Many scanning systems are distributed with a 24" high-resolution LCD (1920 x 1200 pixels). In our experience 3 Mpixels 20.8" (52.8 cm) monitors with a pitch of 0.207 mm and a screen size of 2048 x 1536 pixels and brightness of 500(Dicom)/800 cd/m2 are excellent for routine diagnosis. These medium sized monitors are more efficient than large 30" monitors, which generally have lower brightness and, due to large size (2560 x 1600 pixels), need more time to show images.

Existing viewing software are generally developed to work efficiently only with the corresponding proprietary format. Some companies are developing web-base solutions in open platforms (J2EE) that can be the basis of the future ubiquitous medical imaging for pathology images (figure 3).

Some authors claim that the ideal digital pathology workstation would have three monitors: a small monitor to display clinical data and image metadata; a large, high-resolution monitor with the same aspect ratio as the slide, mounted horizontally for navigation and to provide an uninterrupted, low to middle resolution image of the entire slide; and a high quality, 17–21 inch monitor for high-resolution evaluation of specific areas. In most studies, the mouse and keyboard are felt to be suboptimal for controlling the system (Gilbertson, 2006).

Most digital slide viewers are able to store annotations in an Extensible Markup Language (XML)-based format, describing all parameters such as coordinates, contours, associated label, and magnification, amongst others. However there is no standard in digital slide annotations XML format and annotations are not interchangeable between different manufacturers.

Figure 3. Small bowel biopsy stained with haematoxylin-eosin, showing parasitic infestation by Schistosoma haematobium. Aurora mScope® viewer is able to read multiple virtual slide formats.

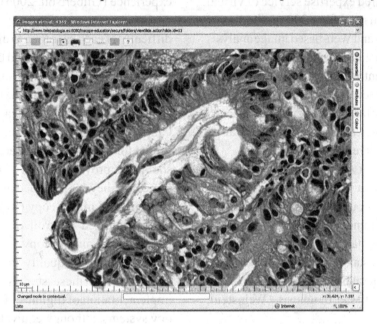

Viewing Digital Images through Internet

Mobile technology in the pathology scenario can be used to securely access medical information without delays from a remote location (Sato, 2007).

Digital slides can be viewed with an Internet connection. After reviewing three different digital viewing systems for web browsers we found that Aperio® viewer (Flash™ player) was very efficient in overview images, but Aurora mScope® viewer (Java applet) was especially efficient in lower magnifications (10x). For larger magnifications (20x and 40x) no significant differences were found between different vendors. Olympus® (Flash™ player) was found to be the most user-friendly interface (Rojo, 2008). Generally, these web-based viewers are less efficient than client-server applications. Two main complains from pathologists are that reading slides at low or medium magnification is too painful and slow, and it is difficult to find areas of interests using overview or low resolution images, which forces to review too many mid or high power fields (Gilbertson, 2006).

A broadband optic fibre network with a capacity of 100 Mbps may be needed in some telepathology applications, when high throughput is needed (Tsuchihashi, 2008).

Different Contexts of Use

Virtual microscopy manufacturers should take into account the main application that different users will make of theses systems. User needs are different if the scanner is being utilized for rapid frozen section intraoperative studies or for education purposes.

In Japan, the primary use of digital imaging and telepathology is frozen section intraoperative studies (63%) whereas in Europe, most telepathology services are used for second opinion consultation and conferences. It is expected that the use in cytodiagnosis will increase in a significant proportion during the next years (Tofukuji, 2007a).

New business models of healthcare services will arise around digital pathology. The current US LABS® (LabCorp, Irvine, California) model focuses on the application of digitized whole slide imaging for the interpretation of immunohistochemical stains and image analysis. This 24-hour operation shared expertise service of virtual immunohistochemistry offers 300 antibodies or combination stains and Web-based image analysis programs for breast cancer and prostate cancer evaluation. This centralized solution proposes access to more subspecialty practitioners by having consultative and collaborative review of cases to prevent misdiagnosis, and can lead to an elevation of the standard of care (O'Malley, 2008).

The University of Arizona College of Medicine and the Arizona Cancer Center in Tucson designed a rapid throughput breast clinic using telepathology for immediate readout of cases by telepathologists as stained slides come off the automated immunostainers. The main benefit is reducing the time it takes a woman with a breast lesion to obtain a tissue diagnosis (Weinstein, 2005).

Diagnostic Accuracy with Digital Slides

With current technology, are digital slides good enough for anatomic pathology diagnosis?

Most existing studies are based in a limited amount of cases and do not reproduce the same conditions in daily anatomic pathology practice with conventional microscopes (e.g. difficulty of cases, pathologist's experience, and special techniques available). In 2002, a critical analysis of 32 published trials of telepathology, some of them about virtual microscopy, including some large prospective studies, concluded that there was strong published evidence for a diagnostic accuracy comparable with glass slide diagnosis, that there was a clear-cut economic argument in favour of telepathology, and that the technique should be integrated into mainstream diagnostic histopathology (Cross, 2002). In routine diagnosis, images produced by existing virtual microscopy devices have enough image quality to allow pathologists to produce accurate, complex, and detailed diagnostic reports, even for difficult and complex cases. Furthermore, pathologists seem

to get better at digital slide interpretation with experience (Gilbertson, 2006).

Concordance rate is more related to the inherent difficulty of each case than to differences between conventional microscope and digital slides, and it may range from 96% in low difficulty cases (superficial spreading melanoma) to 63% in medium difficult cases (palisaded encapsulated neuroma). Clinical correlation and special stains can be essential for the diagnosis of certain cases, and they should be provided for distant diagnosis in the same way they are provided in daily practice with conventional microscopy (RCPA, 2008).

Randomized controlled studies of internet-based virtual microscopy have also been performed in external quality assessment programs. The results of these studies encourage for the implementation of digital slide-based telepathology systems, although equivalence of diagnostic accuracy has not been proved, and financial, legal, professional and ethical factors should also be considered (Furness, 2007).

Similar diagnostic accuracy results have been described with images obtained from array microscope (DMetrix®) scanning systems and lineal (Aperio®) scanners (Weinstein, 2005).

The Royal College of Pathologists of Australasia carried out a pilot survey to determine if virtual microscope images were suitable for use as survey material for the external quality assurance program in anatomic pathology in 2005. The main complaints were related to the poor resolution of fine detail on high power, the difficulty in making a diagnosis from a computer screen compared with a microscope, and some difficulties to launch viewer. The percentage of participants that achieved the target diagnosis with the digital virtual microscope image was similar to that obtained using conventional glass slides, except in some difficult cases, such as biopsies of lung Wegener's granulomatosis (RCPA, 2006).

For teaching activities, virtual microscopy has shown to be at least as effective as traditional microscopy in teaching undergraduate students (Scoville, 2007).

Automated Image Analysis and Computer-Aided Decisions

Anatomic pathology diagnosis is a very complex process that cannot be easily automated or simulated; however, in this process there are some steps that can be addressed in an automated way, to facilitate the decision-making process.

Some of the applications that digitalization of microscopic images allow are the selection of areas of interest, quantification of biomarkers, and measuring structures. Different algorithms can be applied to conventional slides, TMA slides, chromogenic in situ hybridization (CISH), fluorescent in situ hybridization (FISH), polarized light and mutispectral images.

For example, measuring and counting is crucial in the evaluation of certain tumours, like melanoma, and this task can be easier with the use of measuring tools available in digital slide viewers.

Other modes of microscopy, like inverted microscopy of living cells and reflected light microscopy can also benefit from virtual microscopy (Soenksen, 2005).

The main advantages of using digital slides in automated image analysis are:

- Providing a mechanism to share results of experiments with other researchers.
- Unattended automated quantitative analysis
- Removing observer bias
- Providing standards for quality control
- High-throughput analysis
- Software tools for automated analysis (e.g. TMA localization)
- Can be applied to frozen sections, haematoxylin-eosin, special strains, immunohistochemistry (IHQ), FISH, RNA in situ hybridization

Current pharmacology research in fields like oncology is mainly based in the validation for translation of tissue biomarkers from the research lab to the clinical lab. This effort will probably rely heavily on the combination of tissue microarray technology with automated quantitative analysis, but well-designed, thorough validation studies are still needed.

Currently, scanning and image analysis solutions are mainly dedicated to research and training purposes. Some automated image analysis algorithms are USA FDA 510(k)-cleared applications for assessing the level or certain immunohistochemical markers, being the most frequent ones oestrogen receptors, progesterone receptors, and Her-2 membrane staining. In Europe, scanning devices are requested to be compliant with Directive 98/79/EC on in vitro diagnostic medical devices, but this directive is focused on safety requirements, electromagnetic compatibility, software life cycle, information supplied by the manufacturer, performance evaluation, and other related aspects.

Integrating Anatomic Pathology Digital Images into PACS

Digital medical images consist in massive amounts of information that Hospital Information Technology departments should be capable of managing in central repositories. The financial hurdle of this high demand for storage can be optimized by having a single enterprise medical image repository consisting in a well dimensioned picture archiving and communication system (PACS) based on standards.

In radiology, the diagnostic process is patient-driven, an examination (study) usually involves a single image acquisition modality and all images of the study are related to one and only one patient.

Digital imaging in anatomic pathology differs from that in radiology resulting in specific aspects in acquiring, archiving and distributing digital images in anatomic pathology. These specific aspects are key elements to take into account.

In radiology, digital imaging is the main procedure requested by the ordering clinician who is expecting both images and a report. In anatomic pathology, the ordering clinician is mainly expecting a report. It is the initiative of the pathologists to perform digital macroscopic or microscopic images and to make them available to the clinician. Indeed, digital imaging in anatomic pathology is a procedure step ordered by pathologists within the anatomic pathology department. This is an important issue while defining how to integrate acquisition modalities to anatomic pathology information systems.

Moreover, unlike radiology, whenever performed, digital imaging in anatomic pathology usually results in images of different types (gross images, microscopic still images, digital slides, etc) finally gathered in the same imaging study. Many types of imaging acquisition modalities (photo camera, motorized microscope with camera, slide scanners, motorized multispectral microscope, etc) may be involved for a single examination.

While radiologic examination is a patient-centric process, digital imaging in anatomic pathology is a specimen-centric process and images of the same study may be related to different specimen (parts and/or slides) from one or even different patients (e.g. Tissue Micro Array) (Le Bozec, 2007). This point has required main changes in standards in order to integrate properly identified anatomic pathologic images into PACS.

Moreover, unlike in radiology, the "subjects" of digital imaging in anatomic pathology (e.g. slides) are always available to acquire more images, if needed.

Last but not least, the main issue of digital imaging in anatomic pathology is the very large size of virtual slides so that current PACS cannot handle the massive amounts of data being generated by anatomic pathology departments. Besides the storage capacity and network band-width required managing virtual slides, the first barrier is that the current standards cannot handle such images.

Defining Relevant DICOM Objects for Anatomic Pathology

DICOM had several information object definitions (IODs) useful in anatomic pathology including the *visible light photographic image for gross specimens* and the *visible light slide-coordinates microscopic image* for slide-based microscopic imaging. In 1998, minor additions to DICOM Supplement 15 (Visible Light Image) in two existing data types, Pixel Data Type and Curve, were proposed to permit DICOM to be the standard for analytical cytology and its two modalities, digital microscopy and flow cytometry (Leif, 1998).

Some limitations of the DICOM information object definitions (IOD) dedicated to anatomic pathology are currently addressed by the specific DICOM pathology working group (WG26) created in December 2005.

First of all, some types of anatomic pathology digital image (whole-slide images, multispectral images, flow cytometry, etc) do not have applicable DICOM information object definitions.

One of the immediate aims of DICOM WG 26 was creating a mechanism to store, retrieve and view microscope whole slide images within the DICOM framework. Whole-slide images can be larger than 200,000 x 80,000 pixels and are too large in both pixels and byte size to be handled by current DICOM objects. In DICOM there is a limit for maximum values of rows and columns and an image pixel matrix cannot be greater than 64.000 x 64,000. Pixel data attribute is also limited in length. Some workarounds are under development, with the challenge to maintain backwards compatibility of all PACS installed base. One approach could be allowing attributes with a long value representation to be used instead of the existing attributes rows and columns, but only when the value exceeds the existing limits.

Another solution is dividing large images into tiles that can be managed with current DICOM object definition.

An alternative approach is using JPEG2000 and JPEG2000 Interactive Protocol (JPIP) transfer syntaxes that are known to support large images.

Currently, the DICOM standard includes the basic parts of the JPEG2000 standard in Supplements 61 and 105. Supplement 106 (JPEG 2000 Interactive Protocol) describes two JPIP-based Transfer Syntaxes as methods of delivering image pixel data apart from patient data: the non-compressed JPIP Referenced Transfer Syntax and the Deflate-compressed JPIP Referenced Deflate Transfer Syntax.

With the JPIP Transfer Syntaxes, the DICOM-based Picture Archiving and Communication System (PACS) server gives its client a Uniform Resource Locator (URL) string that refers to the virtual slide pixel data provider (i.e., a JPIP server), together with the image name, which can be arbitrary and unrelated to patient data (as shown in figure 4). Upon receiving the pixel data provider reference, the PACS workstation either

uses a built-in JPIP viewer or invokes an external one for retrieving the virtual slide from the specified JPIP server (Tuominen, 2009).

In the regional project of telepathology in Castilla-La Mancha, Spain, it was decided to use DICOM Supplement 106 (JPEG2000 Interactive Protocol) to integrate digital slides with PACS (DICOM WG4, 2006). With this solution, we can send a DICOM object to the PACS, containing all DICOM IOD attributes, and a URL that links this object to the JPIP server. A drawback for this approach is the need to implement two storage servers (PACS and JPIP servers). The Institute of Medical Technology also explored the feasibility of using JPIP to link JPEG2000 WSIs with a DICOM-based Picture Archiving and Communications System (PACS) at the Tampere University Hospital in Finland (Tuominen 2009).

Besides these initiatives, most DICOM systems cannot manage TIFF files with a tiled organization, and/or TIFF files with JPEG or JPEG2000 compression, that are used by some slide scanners manufacturers. Moreover, although some digital slide viewers, like Aura mScope® (http://www.auroramsc.com/en_/Solutions/PatientReord.

Figure 4. Using virtual slides within a DICOM-based PACS over JPIP. (Adapted from Tuominen, 2009)

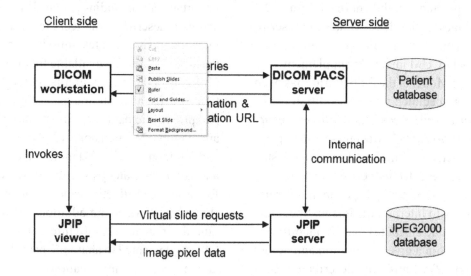

html), Alphelys Inaveo® (http://www.alphelys.com/site/us/pIMG_InaveoVS.htm) or PathFind® (Goode, 2008) are scanner vendor-neutral and are able to show many different formats, including the support of ImageJ image analysis macros, an additional effort should be done by manufacturers and standards bodies to have a universal DICOM viewer able to show digital slides.

Another immediate aim of DICOM WG 26 was updating and extending the data model used to describe anatomic pathologic specimens which are the subject of imaging procedures, The DICOM model did not initially describe specimens in sufficient detail or associate images with specimens with enough precision for the complexity of anatomic pathology practice. In anatomic pathology, a single diagnostic study may involve multiple images of multiple related specimens (parts, blocks, and/or slides) and in some cases, an image can include more than one specimen or even tissue from more than one patient (e.g., tissue microarrays). While the relationship between patient and image is straightforward and accurately captured by DICOM objects, in anatomic pathology there was a need for a new specimen module that formally defines specimen attributes at the image level.

The DICOM WG26 defined the specimen module in a new DICOM supplement (number 122). The specimen module defines formal DICOM attributes for the identification and description of specimens when said specimens are the subject of a DICOM image. In supplement 122, the "DICOM Model of the Real World" has been extended for specimen with the addition of the objects *"specimen," "container," "component"* and *"preparation step."* Attributes of the specimen, container, component, and preparation step objects are represented in the specimen module, which is focused on critical specimen information necessary to interpret the image. Specimen attributes include attributes that (1) identify the specimen (within a given institution and across institutions); (2) identify and describe the container in which the specimen resides as well as each component of the container if required (e.g., a "slide" is a container that is made up of the glass slide, the coverslip, and the "glue" that binds them together); (3) describe specimen collection, sampling, and processing; and (4) describe the specimen or its ancestors when these descriptions help with the interpretation of the image (Daniel, 2009). The specimen module distinguishes the container ID and the specimen ID, making them different data elements to allow maximal flexibility for different situations. Even though the full history of specimen processing is not required in every instance, specimen attributes allow that processing history to be encoded. However, a unique specimen identifier is useful to link a subject specimen to its processing history. Attributes that convey diagnostic opinions or interpretations are not within the scope of the specimen module. The DICOM specimen module does not seek to replace or mirror the pathologist's report.

Although old Specimen Identification Module is retired from all Information Object Definitions (IODs), minimal problems are expected since there were few, if any, actual implementations that used the old specimen identification module (DICOM WG26, 2008).

Besides data related to the specimen, series of important data, including patient data, clinical data and data describing the technical aspects of the image acquisition context must be associated with the digital slides and available for the pathologist (Tofukuji, 2007b). Integrating clinical information and usual anatomic pathology diagnostic and prognostic data with digital slides including annotations, 2-dimensional (2-D) image analysis, and 3-dimensional (3-D) tumour reconstructions and volumetric analysis, can be useful to create, for instance, an effective cancer evaluation system (Petushi, 2008). Some additional efforts are required so that the DICOM Information Definition Objects dedicated to anatomic pathology include all these relevant information.

In practice, current imaging devices in anatomic pathology departments (gross station cameras, digital cameras on conventional microscopes, slide scanners) are not DICOM compliant devices and do not accept DICOM messages or worklists. Also, conventional colour monitors do not include DICOM colour curves or gamma correction.

Specifying Anatomic Pathology PACS

PACS offers reliable long term solution to ensure storage, retrieval, and delivery without error of many types of medical images. The heart of PACS is the image database manager, that must be able to retrieve images for a given patient o specimen when required by hospital or departmental information systems (RIS-radiology information system or PIS-pathology information system) or other systems. These queries are defined by the Digital Imaging and Communications in Medicine (DICOM) standard (Smith, 2006).

The main advantages of using DICOM in pathology are organizational (one central repository of medical images for all medical specialties: PACS), facilitating the integration with EHR, the use of one viewer for all medical images, and the independence of devices manufacturers and proprietary file formats.

Some authors describe the term "pathology PACS" as a storage system to save the results of laboratory tests, including images of patients' laboratory specimens such as digital slides (Weinstein, 2005). The term PACS should only be utilized in those systems having an image archive, a database manager, a workflow/control software (image manager) and an interface with other information system (e.g. radiology information system (RIS), pathology information system(PIS)), and it is able to respond to the queries defined by the Digital Imaging and Communications in Medicine (DICOM) standards. Image manager is an essential part of PACS since it is responsible to ensure that images are stored correctly once received from imaging devices or modalities (Smith, 2006).

With new demands to store images coming from pathology, endoscopy and many other clinical departments, hospitals should establish or redesign their PACS strategic business plan, since these demands will have a significant impact in operational, technical, and financial sections of the PAC strategic plan (Levine, 2006).

In the operational section of the strategic plan, according to Levine (2006) the following components should be considered:

- **Alignment to strategic goals and objectives**: The institution should decide the alignment of including pathology images in the PACS to its strategic goals and objectives. In this sense, some institutions need to move to digital archives because they are running short of room for glass slides, in other cases, the strategic goal may be directed towards educational objectives.

- **PACS readiness assessment**: According to technical infrastructure, departmental culture, and available personnel, a decision should be made if the hospital is ready to implement and manage the change process associated with PACS storage of anatomic pathology images. In most cases, the radiology department of the hospital is already working with PACS, and this model can help to make easier the transitions for pathology.

- **Implementation plan**: The phases of the implementation plan, including primary objectives and benefits of each phase, and plans to reduce expenses (e.g. reduction in sign-out time, or mailing costs reduction).

- **PACS impact analysis**: Improved workflow, productivity, and clinical care at each phase of PACS deployment.

- **Pathology market share analysis**: A description of competitors and the status of their PACS implementation.

- **Meeting future demands needs**: A potent argument for PACS strategic plan is to compare capacity and productivity gains that will make possible future increases in demands for pathology services

There are two technical components of the PACS strategic plan. The first one is the assessment of information technology readiness, including storage technology, clustering design, network infrastructure, installed PC base, and integration interfaces. The second technical component is the discussion of the human resources and contingency plan to successfully support a PACS dimensioned to store large pathology images.

The financial analysis should include a return on investment (ROI) analysis. We must realize that digital slides are not expected to replace conventional glass slides in diagnostic pathology in the medium term, but it may help to reduce turnaround time for pathology reports, optimize archives, decrease errors, reduce transportation costs, decrease teaching costs, and lower quality assurance expenses. The financial analysis should be projected for at least 5 years (Levine, 2006).

Architectural redesign, evolution of technologies underlying PACS, adaptation of existing standards to a broad range of medical imaging and a good PACS strategy (Nagy, 2007) are essential for pathologists to enjoy the benefits of multi-departmental PACS in the near future.

INTEGRATING DIGITAL PATHOLOGY TO THE HEALTHCARE ENTERPRISE

Electronic health records increase the efficiency and quality of medical services, preventing errors and promoting the implementation of clinical guidelines. Anatomic pathology data and images should be an important part of the patient EHR dedicated to patient care. Anatomic pathology also plays a major role in the research activities and anatomic pathology data and images should be also largely integrated to clinical datawarehouses, epidemiological or biomedical research databases and platforms dedicated to translational medicine.

Integrating anatomic pathology to the "healthcare enterprise", as part of e-Health records, can only be achieved with standardization of processes, messages and data following the recommendations of Integrating the Healthcare Enterprise (IHE) Anatomic Pathology Technical Framework. There are several standardization bodies providing complementary efforts to standardize clinical information systems, including DICOM for medical images, Health Level Seven (HL7) for managing data and documents, and SNOMED CT® for terminology (Tofukuji, 2007).

HL7: Health Level Seven

The mission of the HL7 Anatomic Pathology Working Group is to develop and review implementation guides of HL7 standards and to enhance existing HL7 standards to support anatomic pathology use cases.

HL7-Anatomic Pathology Working Group contributed to the DICOM WG26 efforts to define the specimen module in a new DICOM supplement (number 122). The specimen module has been harmonized with the HL7 v2 SPM segment and the HL7 v3 specimen domain information model.

HL7-Anatomic Pathology recent activities have been related to structuring anatomic pathology reports, in order to provide a Clinical Document Architecture (CDA) template for the anatomic pathology report (HL7, 2009).

Another important work item is reporting anatomic pathology to cancer registries and public health repositories, in collaboration with North American Association of Central Cancer Registries (NAACCR) and College of American Pathologists in the United States, and the Association pour le Développement de l'Informatique en Cytologie et Anatomo-Pathologie (ADICAP) in France.

This group is working in the alignment of IHE and NAACCR pathology electronic reporting implementation guides, and a study of terminology, including Logical Observation Identifiers Names and Codes (LOINC®), Systematized Nomenclature of Medicine, Clinical Terms (SNOMED CT®), NAACCR Search Term List, International Classification of Diseases for Oncology 3rd Edition (ICD-0-3), and ADICAP coding system.

IHE: Integrating the Healthcare Enterprise

The Integrating the Healthcare Enterprise (IHE) initiative was started in the United States in 1999, promoted by healthcare professionals and industry, to address the correct use of standards to integrate multivendor electronic medical record systems, initially focused on radiology. IHE is a process based on technical frameworks for the implementation of established messaging standards to achieve specific clinical goals, rigorous testing processes for the implementation of those technical frameworks at a connect-a-thon, and educational sessions and exhibits at major meetings of medical professionals.

IHE promotes the coordinated use of established standards such as DICOM and HL7 (Health Level 7) to address specific clinical needs in support of optimal patient care. Systems developed in accordance with IHE communicate with one another better, are easier to implement, and enable care providers to use information more effectively.

IHE activity in the domain of pathology was started in Japan by the Japanese Association of Healthcare Systems Industry (JAHIS) in January 2004 (Tofukuji, 2007). The first European IHE-Pathology meeting was held at the European Congress of Pathology in Paris, on September 5th, 2005 (Rojo, 2009).

The encouraging integration efforts in pathology from multiple international groups to define a general workflow in pathology information systems materialized in the publication of the IHE Anatomic Pathology Technical Framework,

for trial implementation, at the end of 2008 (http://www.ihe.net/Technical_Framework/index.cfm#pathology).

The Anatomic Pathology Technical Framework aims at the integration of the anatomic pathology laboratory department in the healthcare enterprise. The diagnostic process requires tight consultation and close cooperation between different healthcare providers: pathologists and technicians, surgeons, oncologists, clinicians, radiologists, etc. The ultimate goal is a comprehensive digital pathology record for the patient, of which images are a significant part.

The primary focus will be digital formats for clinical patient management, but digital imaging for research applications may also be addressed as appropriate (dealing with Tissue Micro Arrays (one slide for hundreds of patients) with a link to patient information or dealing with animal experimentation, etc).

The aim is to progressively cover all specialties of anatomic pathology: surgical pathology, clinical autopsy, cytopathology, biopsies and all special techniques (gross examination, frozen section, immunohistochemistry (including TMAs), molecular pathology, flow cytometry, special microscopy techniques (confocal laser scanning, multispectral microscopy), etc.

The IHE Anatomic Pathology Technical Framework comprises two volumes. Volume 1 provides a high-level view of IHE functionality, showing the transactions organized into functional units called integration profiles that highlight their capacity to address specific information technology requirements. Therefore, it is underlined that the diagnostic process in anatomic pathology differs from that in the clinical laboratory since it relies on image interpretation, and it also differs from the process in radiology since pathology is a specimen-driven activity, and a single examination may involve many types of imaging equipments (e.g. gross imaging, microscopic still imaging, whole slide imaging, multispectral imaging) (IHE, 2008a). Volume 2 of the Anatomic Pathology

Technical Framework provides detailed technical descriptions of each IHE transaction or messages used in the existing anatomic pathology profile (IHE, 2008b).

Until now one integration profile (Anatomic Pathology Workflow) have been defined. The Anatomic Pathology Workflow (APW) Integration Profile establishes the continuity and integrity of basic pathology examination data and images exchanged between the systems of the ordering care units, those of the performing anatomic pathology laboratory, and the systems producing, archiving, communicating or presenting images.

In a PACS environment, acquisition modalities (e.g. slide scanners) should be able to receive patient and study-related data from the hospital information system ("Order Placer") and from the anatomic pathology information system ("Order Filler"). DICOM Modality Worklist is the link that transfers this critical information between the acquisition modalities and the HIS or PIS (Gale, 2000). To have the anatomic pathology information system and digital imaging systems interoperate, it is critical that they all be able to reference a particular specimen accordingly to

the same model before associating it with one or more reports or images.

The Anatomic Pathology Workflow (APW) Integration Profile includes 10 transactions (PAT-1 Placer Order Management, PAT-2 Filler Order Management, PAT-3 Order Results Management, PAT-4 Procedure Scheduled and Updated, PAT-5 Query Modality Worklist, RAD-8 Modality Images Stored, RAD-10 Storage Commitment, RAD-14 Query Images, RAD-16 Retrieve Images, and RAD-43 Evidence Document Stored) between nine actors (Acquisition Modality, Department System Scheduler/Order Filler, Evidence Creator, Image Archive, Image Display, Image Manager, Order Placer, Order Filler, and Order Result Tracker) (figure 5). Daniel et al (2009) have described how IHE Anatomic Pathology technical framework can support the basic diagnostic workflow in anatomic pathology departments.

Pathology imaging devices can be adapted to generate DICOMized images that can be sent to the PACS using middleware or integration engines. Non-DICOM compliant imaging devices in pathology departments can be connected to an intermediate information system that transforms

Figure 5. Schematic representation of the anatomic pathology workflow (APW) profile

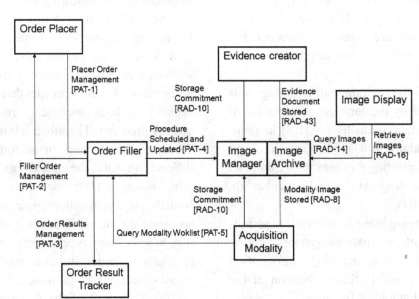

original image formats (TIFF, JPEG, or proprietary digital slide files) in to a DICOM object, performs messaging with PACS and achieves storage commitment.

IHE Anatomic Pathology Technical Framework has been used as a reference to implement standards in some telepathology projects (Rojo, 2009). Even so, we have not been able to implement all transactions defined by IHE since we have to adopt high level rules governing IT infrastructure in our region. For instance, some problems were found to adopt transaction PAT-3 (Order Results Management) in which the PIS should send the pathology report to a report repository using an HL7 ORU^R01 message. However, in the design SESCAM, our public health service, does not agree with sending a copy of the pathology report to a central repository, instead SESCAM prefers sending a message including patient identification, report identification, and report status; and pathology reports are sent directly from the PIS, only when it is requested by the user. This allows having a single instance of the report, always updated.

As multiple actors appear on scene (hospital information system, pathology information system, image repository, and automated immunostainers) a protocol for designing databases is necessary to create a logical model adapted to business requirements. This will avoid inefficiencies like saving the same information in different systems when it is not necessary (Cowan, 2005).

Nowadays, the main efforts of IHE anatomic pathology are focused on how to structure and encode anatomic pathology reports and how to report anatomic pathology results to public health or research repositories.

In conclusion, the use of medical digital image standards (DICOM), compression standards (JPEG2000), messaging and document standards (HL7), are the ground in order to create interoperable solutions. In addition current anatomic pathology information system vendors are only beginning to consider the standard-based integration between the reports generated by the pathologist and its corresponding images, and the role of those standards in virtual microscopy.

Terminology and Data Representation Standards

Terminology standards need to be part of the interoperability of pathology information systems, including digital slides and the rest of the e-Health records.

The Systematized Nomenclature of Medicine-Clinical Terms (SNOMED CT®) is a comprehensive clinical terminology currently adopted as a terminology standard in electronic health information exchange. The January 2009 international release includes more than 310,000 active concepts, 794,000 active English-language descriptions, and over 947,000 relationships.

The U.S. National Library of Medicine Unified Medical Language System (UMLS®) is a complete system to facilitate the development of computer systems for managing biomedicine and health language. The three main components of UMLS are the Methathesaurus, which contains over one million biomedical concepts, their various names, and the relationships among them, from over 100 source vocabularies, including over five million multi-lingual terms or names; the Semantic Network, which defines categories and relationships between them; and the Specialist Lexicon & Lexical Tools, which provide lexical information and programs for language processing (UMLS, 2009).

SNOMED CT® was originally created by the College of American Pathologists (CAP), and as of April 2007, it is owned, maintained, and distributed by the International Health Terminology Standards Development Organisation (IHTSDO) (http://www.ihtsdo.org/). SNOMED CT® (both English and Spanish versions) is included in UMLS Metathesaurus®, where it is linked to many other biomedical terminologies and natural language processing tools (UMLS, 2009). German and Spanish translations are available.

SNOMED CT® is not only the most comprehensive clinical vocabulary available, but also is a well-formed, machine-readable terminology, concept-oriented, with an advanced structure.

SNOMED CT® is more that a controlled vocabulary. It is defined as a controlled clinical terminology with characteristics of interface terminology and reference terminology. As a clinical terminology, it is designed to register clinical data in EHR. As an interface terminology it allows the utilization of users preferred terms, and it has an intuitive and efficient approach in clinical data grouping. Relationships between terms, hierarchies, and mapping to other nomenclatures are valuable tools.

Terminology experts as well as institutional policies do not recommend binding directly clinical statements to reference terminologies, such as SNOMED CT® and support using standard reference terminology concepts - and possibly semantic linkages - for representing commonly used interface terminologies (Rosenbloom, 2006). Rosenbloom et al. investigated how to use SNOMED CT® to represent two interface terminologies (MEDCIN and CHISL) (Rosenbloom, 2009). They encourage terminology developers to create or enrich interface terminologies by using reference terminologies concepts as a starting point but stress out that assembling clinically meaningful compositions, appropriate synonyms and linkage between concepts (related concepts or modifiers) is a labour-intensive approach. Daniel et al propose functional requirements of terminology services for coupling interface terminologies to reference terminologies (Daniel, 2009).

In our experience, user should be offered only a subset of terms that may be useful, and they must be translated into the language of use, without losing meaning. Since different clinical departments have different needs, the creation of a local

interface terminology to SNOMED CT® is recommended also by other groups. With this approach, local classifications and concepts subsets can be mapped to SNOMED CT® (Lopez Osornio, 2007). A significant work is needed to adapt SNOMED CT® in all health areas and specialties, and calls for collaboration and harmonisation are under way in order to achieve multilingual interoperability (Donnelly, 2008).

New diseases are described every year and new techniques are being applied continuously; for that reason, an extensibility mechanism must be considered to include new terms that may not be available in SNOMED CT®. The IHTSDO has set a high priority on the development of a SNOMED CT® concept request submission system, but this system is still under development.

A synoptic reporting system must be part of the pathology information system. This is especially important in the management of cancer. The College of American Pathologists (CAP) Cancer Protocols and Checklists© were created in response to the mandate of the American College of Surgeons Commission on Cancer to use cancer protocols in 2002 (Robert, 2008; Tobias, 2006). Encoding structured pathology protocols or checklists with SNOMED CT® allows enhancing the value of the pathology report, saving user valuable time and reducing coding errors.

In order to facilitate and standardize tissue banks, three main sets of data standards can be used: the College of American Pathologists (CAP) Cancer Checklists©, the protocols recommended by the Association of Directors of Anatomic and Surgical Pathology (ADASP) for pathology data, and the North American Association of Central Cancer Registry (NAACCR) elements for epidemiology, therapy and follow-up data. Combining them it is possible to create a core set of annotations for banked specimens, organized as a set of International Standards Organization (ISO)-compliant Common Data Elements (CDEs) for tissue banking (Mohanty, 2008).

Multidimensional business process modelling can be considered a first step in the interoperability effort.

This normalization effort can also be extended to research efforts, as has been proposed in the tissue microarrays (TMA) data exchange specification (TMA DES).

ORGANIZATION IN DIGITAL PATHOLOGY

In a digital imaging environment, the greatest changes in workflow organization involve three tasks: automation, integration, and simplification (Reiner, 2006). An example of automation in pathology is image analysis software that is able to count with precision the number of oestrogen receptors positive cells in an immunohistochemistry digital slide. Integration between PIS and PACS eliminates the time-consuming steps of transferring gross images from grossing station camera to another computer. Simplification allows converting complex, time-consuming tasks into more straightforward ones. With digital images, pathologists may measure the depth of invasion of a tumour with just a click of a mouse.

Digital pathology includes solutions for pathology primary diagnosis and second opinion, and also includes telepathology solutions.

Most authors agree that pathology images (macroscopic images, digital slides, molecular pathology images) will become an integral component of EHR as part of pathology reports (Weinstein, 2005).

The organization must consider digital pathology as a global integrated effort and provide the adequate infrastructure, including telecommunications. Therefore, it will be necessary not only acquiring all the necessary imaging devices and computer equipment needed in a digital pathology department, or to develop an information system that allows pathology departments to storage and manage the reports and its images, but also they

must consider developing web applications that allows the communication between the different pathology departments, sharing reports and images, facilitating the collaborative work between hospitals.

The development of the digital pathology project must be based on medical standards in accordance with the guidelines described in the IHE Anatomic Pathology Technical Framework.

Since pathology slide images are very large files, a detailed analysis of those cases in which those files must travel through the hospital network should be performed. A different approach to radiology is needed, but the large central storage model delivering images through a very fast network, already used in radiology (Siegel, 2006), can be a good option for pathology.

Access to pathology images for diagnostic and screening purposes requires very fast access to many different areas of the slide. Using the proposed model of central image servers, although current digital slide viewers reduce significantly the size of transmitted data in the network since only the request part of the image to be shown is retrieved from the server, this process may result in a delay in the image to be shown sharp on the monitor. According to local network and server capabilities, each institution should decide if they prefer proprietary solutions versus JPIP standard solutions, or client-server viewers versus web-based viewers to manage digital slide image requests.

Worklists and pre-fetching can also be applied to pathology images. Implementation of DICOM modality worklists management software has been reported to reduce input errors up to 6% in radiology (Siegel, 2006). The advantage of worklists for pathologists are filtering images according to multiple criteria (e.g. accession number, type of image, or date and time), having access to all unread images of all the department, the security improvement eliminating confusion in selecting a wrong slide from a another case, and the ability for multiple pathologists to share responsibility or reading similar types of specimens.

Pre-fetching in radiology is used to store new and historic examinations locally at a workstation to optimize transfers, mainly if they are saved in long term storage (Siegel, 2006). The pathologist may have ready the digital slide files to be read in his/her workstation or in a departmental server before he/she begins reading slides.

A temporal repository of proprietary format files may be needed when essential tools, like image analysis algorithms can only be run using those proprietary files.

Digital slide scanners should be available in small hospitals mainly in those institutions with only one pathologist or without pathologists. Non-specialists technicians and physicians may take the responsibility to put the slide into the scanner. Virtual microscopy avoids the need to select representative images.

In primary diagnosis, the diagnosis responsibility should be on the pathologists. If misdiagnosis occurs as a result of the limits of the telepathology system employed by the client side, some responsibility can be relieved of the client institution. The amount of effort put into overcoming telepathology limitations must be considered in assigning responsibilities. In second opinion, the final diagnostic responsibility lies with the sender, and in return for providing free advice the consultant may be protected from any liability (Ito, 2007).

The use of digital slides in rapid frozen intraoperative studies is expected to increase significantly, not only in hospitals without a pathology department but also in small and medium sized pathology departments due to the special difficulties of these studies that may require an expert opinion. About 5% of surgical procedures require rapid diagnosis (Sawai, 2007b).

Since current scanning systems are not able to expedite the workload of most pathology departments, in our institution, we select those cases that need to be scanned according to the following priority criteria:

1. Before pathology report is available
   a. Frozen section evaluation (consultation to reference hospital)
   b. Cytological smear material adequacy in fine needle aspiration procedures
   c. Second opinion in cytology
   d. Second opinion in histopathology where diagnosis can be made in haematoxylin-eosin stain (e.g. skin biopsies)
   e. Measuring is necessary (e.g. melanomas, distance to borders, or area calculation)
   f. Automated biomarkers counting or image analysis of immunohistochemical stains
   g. Differential diagnosis orientation (counselling for best immunohistochemistry panel to be applied)
   h. Clinicopathological sessions
2. After pathology report sign-out
   a. Identified cases
      i. Patient's request (a copy in DVD)
      ii. Hospital cancer committees
      iii. Second opinion to/from other institutions
      iv. Legal actions
   b. Anonymous cases
      i. Quality assurance program in immunohistochemistry programme (Spanish Society of Pathology)
      ii. Quality assurance programme in diagnosis (Spanish Society of Pathology)
      iii. Collections of interesting cases
      iv. Education
      v. Conferences
      vi. Research

In summary, the technical implementation of a digital pathology project can be divided into two strongly interconnected parts. The first important information system is the Pathology Information

System (PIS) deployed in each hospital, and its main aim is to cover the daily workflow of a pathology department. Included functionalities of this system are:

- Integration with the Hospital Information System (HIS). This allows obtaining the patient demographics data, the scheduled patient appointments and all the order requests associated to the pathological examination performed at the hospital.
- Integration with all image acquiring devices (called modalities) using the DICOM worklist. Each modality will receive a worklist, which contains the information about the specimens that will be digitized.
- Storage all the images generated by the pathology department in the PACS, including digital slides.
- A unique viewer that allows showing, at the same time, gross and microscopic images, including digital slides.
- A reporting system that allows the management of autopsy, biopsy and cytology reports. In addition, it can retrieve from the PACS all the images associated with a report.

The second Information System is a centralized system that consists of a telepathology web portal. Its goal is to offer the following collaborative tools:

- Second opinion: that allows a pathologist to make a consultation about a case with other colleague to obtain a second opinion of the case.
- Consultation forum: the forum is composed of several topics, like skin pathology or soft tissue pathology. The forum allows a pathologist to make a consultation with a group of pathologists belonging to a topic, and then have a discussion about the case.

- Pedagogical public library: A pathology atlas with studies that are of high scientific or teaching interest. All the images and reports showed are anonymous. This tool will be very useful to improve the training of medical students and, in the future, other specialties can be included in the atlas, like dermatology or haematology.

CONCLUSION

The digitalization of anatomic pathology images will allow including them in the electronic health record. This solution will allow other specialists, like dermatologist or haematologist, to have access to this kind of images, as well as improving the training of students and medical residents.

By using teleconsultation and distance diagnosis through digital imaging will offset the shortage of specialists in some countries.

Telepathology services will rapidly grow when all pathology images become available in a digital and standard format. Reviewing pathology reports of patients with certain diseases will allow validation of new physiopathological concepts and therapies.

Digital slides are an important challenge to existing standards. A DICOM standard for whole slide imaging in pathology is needed for interoperability and long term solutions. By using medical informatics standards in the development of a digital pathology project will provide, in the future, an interconnection with others telepathology networks for accessing, exchanging, and upgrading electronic medical records through the Internet.

Nowadays, the use of digital slides is limited by quality factors and the limited 2-D information of the obtained images, which although they are suitable for diagnosis in most situations, in some difficult cases those limitations in current technology can avoid reaching the correct diagnosis. An additional effort should also be made in obtaining 3-D information of the slide, and improving digital slide navigation viewer and hardware, since current software and mouse device are uncomfortable for most pathologists. Internet-based virtual microscopy needs ubiquitous broadband infrastructure.

Digital pathology allows for an unprecedented flexibility in reporting and documenting results, and it is possible to generate different types and formats of reports for different users with different levels of understanding.

Virtual microscopy is an efficient solution for consultation, under- and postgraduate education, clinico-pathological conferences, and it is under study in rapid intraoperative pathology diagnosis and cytological cancer screening.

With the degree of similarity of virtual microscopy with conventional optical microscope most pathologists would be able to transition to digital solutions. Current experts' opinion is that glass slides will remain part of anatomic pathology practice into the predictable future, although pathologists might stop using light microscopes when virtual microscopy becomes a sufficiently advanced technology.

Integrated Digital Pathology solutions will improve the cooperative working relationship between the clinicians and the pathologists in order to increase patient safety, quality of health services and translational medicine

ACKNOWLEDGMENT

This work has been carried out with the support of COST Action IC0604 "EURO-TELEPATH" and the BR-CCM-2006/03 grant from the Foundation for Health Research in Castilla-La Mancha, FISCAM.

REFERENCES

Afework, A., Beynon, M. D., Bustamante, F., Cho, S., Demarzo, A., Ferreira, R., et al. (1998). Digital dynamic telepathology--the Virtual Microscope. In *Proceedings of the AMIA Symposium*, 912-916. Retrieved February 13, 2009, from http://www.pubmedcentral.nih.gov/articlerender.fcgi?artid=2232135

Cowan, D. F. (Ed.). (2005). *Informatics for the Clinical Laboratory. A practical guide for the pathologist*. New York: Springer. doi:10.1007/b99090

Cross, S. S., Dennis, T., & Start, R. D. (2002). Telepathology: current status and future prospects in diagnostic histopathology. *Histopathology*, *41*(2), 91–109. doi:10.1046/j.1365-2559.2002.01423.x

Daniel, C., Buemi, A., Ouagne, D., Mazuel, L., & Charlet, J. (2009, August). *Functional requirements of terminology services for coupling interface terminologies to reference terminologies*. Paper presented at MIE 2009: The XXII International Conference of the European Federation for Medical Informatics, Sarajevo, Bosnia and Herzegovina.

Daniel, C., Garcia-Rojo, M., Bourquard, K., Henin, D., Schrader, T., Della Mea, V., et al. (2009). Standards to Support Information Systems Integration in Anatomic Pathology. *Archives of Pathology & Laboratory Medicine*, 133(11), 1841-1849. Retrieved February 24, 2010 from http://www.archivesofpathology.org/doi/full/10.1043/1543-2165-133.11.1841

Dee, F. R., Donnelly, A., Radio, S., Leaven, T., Zaleski, M. S., & Kreiter, C. (2007). Utility of 2-D and 3-D virtual microscopy in cervical cytology education and testing. *Acta Cytologica*, *51*, 523–529.

DICOM Working Group 26 Pathology (2008). *Digital Imaging and Communications in Medicine (DICOM) Supplement 122: Specimen Module and Revised Pathology SOP Classes*. Rosslyn, Virginia: DICOM Standards Committee. Retrieved February 16, 2009, from ftp://medical.nema.org/medical/dicom/final/sup122_ft2.pdf

DICOM Working Group 4. (2006). *Digital Imaging and Communications in Medicine (DICOM) Supplement 106: JPEG 2000 Interactive Protocol*. Rosslyn, Virginia: DICOM Standards Committee. Retrieved February 17, 2009, from ftp://medical.nema.org/medical/dicom/final/sup106_ft.pdf

Dimech, M., & Beer, T. (2008). *Report of dermatopathology module results SM08-1*. Burwood, Australia: RCPA Quality Assurance Programs Pty Limited. Retrieved February 13, 2009, from http://www.rcpaqapa.netcore.com.au/notices/SM08-1_results.pdf

Dimech, M., & Davies, D. J. (2006). *Report of virtual microscopy pilot survey results 2005*. Burwood, Australia: RCPA Quality Assurance Programs Pty Limited. Retrieved February 13, 2009, from http://www.rcpaqapa.netcore.com.au/notices/VM_pilot_survey_results_VM05-1.pdf

Donnelly, K. (2008). Multilingual documentation and classification. *Studies in Health Technology and Informatics, 134*, 235–243.

Ferreira, R., Moon, B., Humphries, J., Sussman, A., Saltz, J., Miller, R., & Demarzo, A. (1997). The Virtual Microscope. *Proceedings of the AMIA Annual Fall Symposium*, 449-453. Retrieved February 13, 2009, from http://www.pubmedcentral.nih.gov/articlerender.fcgi?tool=pubmed&pubmedid=9357666

Furness, P. (2007). A randomized controlled trial of the diagnostic accuracy of internet-based telepathology compared with conventional microscopy. *Histopathology, 50*(2), 266–273. doi:10.1111/j.1365-2559.2006.02581.x

Gale, M. E., & Gale, D. R. (2000). DICOM modality worklist: an essential component in a PACS environment. *Journal of Digital Imaging, 13*(3), 101–108. doi:10.1007/BF03168381

Gilbertson, J. R., Ho, J., Anthony, L., Jukic, D. M., Yagi, Y., & Parwani, A. V. (2006). Primary histologic diagnosis using automated whole slide imaging: a validation study. *BMC Clinical Pathology, 6*(4). Retrieved February 18, 2009, from http://www.biomedcentral.com/1472-6890/6/4

Goode, A., & Satyanarayanan, M. A. (2008). *Vendor-neutral library and viewer for whole-slide images* (Opendiamond, report). Pittsburgh, PA: Carnegie Mellon University. Retrieved February 13, 2009, from http://diamond.cs.cmu.edu/papers/CMU-CS-08-136.pdf

HL7. (2009). *Work Groups. Anatomic Pathology*. Ann Arbor, MI: Health Level Seven, Inc. Retrieved February 23, 2009, from http://www.hl7.org/Special/committees/anatomicpath/index.cfm

International, I. H. E. (2008). *Anatomic Pathology Technical Framework. Volume 1 (PAT TF-1). Profiles. Revision 1.2 – Trial Implementation*. Retrieved February 17, 2009, from http://www.ihe.net/Technical_Framework/upload/ihe_anatomic-path_TF_rev1-2_TI_vol1_2008-11-24.pdf

International, I. H. E. (2008). *Anatomic Pathology Technical Framework. Volume 2 (PAT TF-2). Transactions. Revision 1.2 – Trial Implementation*. Retrieved February 17, 2009, from http://www.ihe.net/Technical_Framework/upload/ihe_anatomic-path_TF_rev1-2_TI_vol2_2008-11-24.pdf

Ito, M. (2007). Limitations and diagnostic responsibility in telepathology. In T. Sawai (Ed.), Telepathology in Japan. Development and practice (pp. 60-65). Morioka, Iwate, Japan: Celc, Inc.

Kayser, K., Szymas, J., & Weinstein, R. S. (Eds.). (1999). *Telepathology. Telecommunication, electronic education and publication in Pathology*. Berlin: Springer.

Le Bozec, C., Henin, D., Fabiani, B., Schrader, T., Garcia-Rojo, M., & Beckwith, B. (2007). Refining DICOM for pathology-progress from the IHE and DICOM pathology working groups. *Studies in Health Technology and Informatics, 129*(Pt 1), 434–438.

Leif, R. C., & Leif, S. B. (1998). A DICOM Compatible Format for Analytical Cytology Data. In Farkas, D. L., Tromberg, B. J., & Leif, R. C. (Eds.), *Optical Diagnostics of Living Cells II, Advanced Techniques in Analytical Cytology. SPIE Proceedings Series* (*Vol. 3260*, pp. 282–289). A. Katzir Biomedical Optics Series.

Levine, L. A. (2006). Introduction to RIS and PACS. In Dreyer, K. J., Hirschorn, D. S., Thrall, J. H., & Mehta, A. (Eds.), *PACS. A guide to the digital revolution* (2nd ed., pp. 27–44). New York: Springer.

Lopez Osornio, A., Luna, D., Gambarte, M. L., Gomez, A., Reynoso, G., & Gonzalez Bernaldo de Quiros, F. (2007). Creation of a Local Interface Terminology to SNOMED CT. In K.A. Kuhn, J.R. Warren, T.Y. Leong (Eds.), *Medinfo 2007: Proceedings of the 12th World Congress on Health (Medical) Informatics; Building Sustainable Health Systems* (pp. 765-769). Amsterdam: IOS Press.

Mohanty, S. K., Mistry, A. T., Amin, W., Parwani, A. V., Pople, A. K., Schmandt, L., et al. (2008). The development and deployment of Common Data Elements for tissue banks for translational research in cancer - an emerging standard based approach for the Mesothelioma Virtual Tissue Bank. *BMC Cancer*, 8, 91. Retrieved February 16, 2009, from http://www.biomedcentral.com/1471-2407/8/91

Nagy, P. G. (2007). The future of PACS. *Medical Physics, 34*(7), 2676–2682. doi:10.1118/1.2743097

O'Malley, D. P. (2008). Practical Applications of Telepathology Using Morphology-Based Anatomic Pathology. *Archives of Pathology & Laboratory Medicine, 132*(5), 743–744.

Petushi, S., Marker, J., Zhang, J., Zhu, W., Breen, D., & Chen, C. (2008). A visual analytics system for breast tumor evaluation. *Analytical and Quantitative Cytology and Histology, 30*(5), 279–290.

Reiner, B. I., & Siegel, E. L. (2006). Introduction to RIS and PACS. In Dreyer, K. J., Hirschorn, D. S., Thrall, J. H., & Mehta, A. (Eds.), *PACS. A guide to the digital revolution* (2nd ed., pp. 27–44). New York: Springer.

Robert, M.E., Lamps, L., & Lauwers, G.Y., & Association of Directors of Anatomic and Surgical Pathology. (2008). Recommendations for the reporting of gastric carcinoma. *Human Pathology, 39*(1), 9–14. doi:10.1016/j.humpath.2007.05.024

Rojo, M. G. (2009). *Standards in digital pathology and telepathology. IHE-Pathology*. Retrieved February 18, 2009, from http://www.conganat.org/digital/index.htm#ihe

Rojo, M. G., Gallardo, A. J., González, L., Peces, C., Murillo, C., González, J., & Sacristán, J. (2008). Reading virtual slide using web viewers: results of subjective experience with three different solutions. *Diagnostic Pathology, 3*(Suppl 1), S23. doi:10.1186/1746-1596-3-S1-S23

Rojo, M. G., Garcia, G. B., Mateos, C. P., Garcia, J. G., & Vicente, M. C. (2006). Critical comparison of 31 commercially available digital slide systems in pathology. *International Journal of Surgical Pathology, 14*(4), 285–305. doi:10.1177/1066896906292274

Rosenbloom, S. T., Brown, S. H., Froehling, D., Bauer, B. A., Wahner-Roedler, D. L., Gregg, W. M., & Elkin, P. L. (2009). Using SNOMED CT to represent two interface terminologies. *Journal of the American Medical Informatics Association, 16*(1), 81–88. doi:10.1197/jamia.M2694

Rosenbloom, S. T., Miller, R. A., & Johnson, K. B. (2006). Interface terminologies: facilitating direct entry of clinical data into electronic health record systems. *Journal of the American Medical Informatics Association, 13*(3), 277–288. doi:10.1197/jamia.M1957

Sato, K. (2007). Mobile communications in Japan. In T. Sawai (Ed.), Telepathology in Japan. Development and practice (pp. 232-234). Morioka, Iwate, Japan: Celc, Inc.

Sawai, T. (2007a). The state of telepathology in Japan. In T. Sawai (Ed.), Telepathology in Japan. Development and practice (pp. 3-9). Morioka, Iwate, Japan: Celc, Inc.

Sawai, T. (2007b). A survey of telepathology in the public hospitals of Iwate prefecture. In T. Sawai (Ed.), Telepathology in Japan. Development and practice (pp. 105-109). Morioka, Iwate, Japan: Celc, Inc.

Scoville, S. A., & Buskirk, T. D. (2007). Traditional and virtual microscopy compared experimentally in a classroom setting. *Clinical Anatomy (New York, N.Y.), 20*(5), 565–570. doi:10.1002/ca.20440

Siegel, E. L., Reiner, B. I., & Knight, N. (2006). Introduction to RIS and PACS. In Dreyer, K. J., Hirschorn, D. S., Thrall, J. H., & Mehta, A. (Eds.), *PACS. A guide to the digital revolution* (2nd ed., pp. 27–44). New York: Springer.

Smith, G. (2006). Introduction to RIS and PACS. In Dreyer, K. J., Hirschorn, D. S., Thrall, J. H., & Mehta, A. (Eds.), *PACS. A guide to the digital revolution* (2nd ed., pp. 9–25). New York: Springer.

Soenksen, D. G. (2005). A fully integrated virtual microscopy system for analysis and discovery. In J. Gu, R.W. Ogilvie, R.W. (Eds.), Virtual microscopy and virtual slides in teaching, diagnosis, and research. Series Advances in Pathology, Microscopy & Molecular Morphology. (pp. 35-47). Boca Ratón, FL: Taylor & Francis.

Tobias, J., Chilukuri, R., Komatsoulis, G. A., Mohanty, S., Sioutos, N., & Warzel, D. B. (2006). The CAP cancer protocols-a case study of ca-CORE based data standards implementation to integrate with the Cancer Biomedical Informatics Grid. *BMC Medical Informatics and Decision Making, 6*(25).

Tofukuji, I. (2007a). Current implementations of telepathology. In T. Sawai (Ed.), Telepathology in Japan. Development and practice (pp. 39-42). Morioka, Iwate, Japan: Celc, Inc.

Tofukuji, I. (2007b). Virtual slides and telepathology. In T. Sawai (Ed.), Telepathology in Japan. Development and practice (pp. 223-226). Morioka, Iwate, Japan: Celc, Inc.

Tofukuji, I. (2007b). Virtual slides and telepathology. In T. Sawai (Ed.), Telepathology in Japan. Development and practice (pp. 223-226). Morioka, Iwate, Japan: Celc, Inc.

Tofukuji, I. (2007c). Electronic medical records and the Integrating the Healthcare Enterprise initiative. In T. Sawai (Ed.), Telepathology in Japan. Development and practice (pp. 235-238). Morioka, Iwate, Japan: Celc, Inc.

Tsuchihashi, Y., Takamatsu, T., Hashimoto, Y., Takashima, T., Nakano, K., & Fujita, S. (2008). Use of virtual slide system for quick frozen intra-operative telepathology diagnosis in Kyoto, Japan. *Diagnostic Pathology, 3*(Suppl 1), S6. doi:10.1186/1746-1596-3-S1-S6

Tuominen, V. J., & Isola, J. (2009). Linking whole-slide microscope images with DICOM by using JPEG2000 Interactive Protocol. [Epub ahead of print]. *Journal of Digital Imaging*, (May): 5.

U.S. National Library of Medicine. (2009). Unified Medical Language System, Bethesda, MD: National Institutes of Health. Retrieved February 20, 2009, from http://www.nlm.nih.gov/research/umls/

Weinstein, R. S., Descour, M. R., Liang, C., Richter, L., Russum, W. C., Goodall, J. F., et al. (2005). Reinvention of light microscopy. Array microscopy and ultrarapidly scanned virtual slides for diagnostic pathology and medical education. In J. Gu, R.W. Ogilvie, R.W. (Eds.), Virtual microscopy and virtual slides in teaching, diagnosis, and research. Series Advances in Pathology, Microscopy & Molecular Morphology. (pp. 10-34). Boca Ratón, FL: Taylor & Francis.

Yagi, Y. (2007). *Critical comparison of digital pathology systems*. Retrieved February 16, 2009, from http://www.bioimagene.com/pdfs/Study%20Yagi%20et%20al%20070501.pdf

Zeineh, J. (2005). Reinvention of light microscopy. (2005). The Trestle Digital Backbone. In J. Gu, R.W. Ogilvie, R.W. (Eds.), Virtual microscopy and virtual slides in teaching, diagnosis, and research. Series Advances in Pathology, Microscopy & Molecular Morphology. (pp. 77-96). Boca Ratón, FL: Taylor & Francis.

ENDNOTES

[1] IHTSDO®, SNOMED® and SNOMED CT® are registered trademarks of the International Health Terminology Standards Development Organization.

[2] DICOM® is the registered trademark of the National Electrical Manufacturers Association for its standards publications relating to digital communications of medical information.

[3] HL7® is a registered trademark of Health Level Seven (HL7), Inc.

[4] IHE® is a registered trademark of Integrating the Healthcare Enterprise (IHE) International.

[5] LOINC® is a registered trademark of Regenstrief Institute, Inc.

[6] UMLS® and Metathesaurus® are registered trademarks of the National Library of Medicine.

Chapter 23
Content–Based Image Retrieval for Digital Mammography

Issam El Naqa
Washington University School of Medicine, USA

Liyang Wei
Hologic, Inc, USA

Yongyi Yang
Illinois Institute of Technology, USA

ABSTRACT

Content-based image retrieval (CBIR) is an emerging field for computerized detection and diagnosis of breast cancer lesions. The underlying principle of CBIR in mammography is to query mammogram databases for diagnostic information based on the content or extracted features of the images instead of their textual annotation. Potentially, this would provide the radiologist with archived examples that are similar to his/her current case. This chapter reviews recent advances in CBIR technology, discuss its expanding role in medical imaging and its particular application to mammography, provides working examples based on the authors' experience for developing machine-learning methods for CBIR in mammography, and highlights the potential opportunities in this field for computer vision research and clinical decision-making.

INTRODUCTION

Recent years have witnessed burgeoning interest in developing methods for automated image retrieval. This is driven largely by the rapid increase in the size of image collections in various disciplines ranging from industrial, medical, to military applications, and by the steady development of the Internet. There is an increasing demand to retrieve stored pictorial information from these database systems in an efficient manner. Traditionally, these images are retrieved based on some textual annotation. However, in many disciplines, such annotation is neither adequate for capturing the information embedded in the images nor does it provide interactive image understanding for the user because of the following reasons (Niblack, *et al.*, 1993; Smeulders & Worring, 2000; Tagare, Jaffe, & Duncan, 1997):

DOI: 10.4018/978-1-61520-777-0.ch023

Copyright © 2010, IGI Global. Copying or distributing in print or electronic forms without written permission of IGI Global is prohibited.

- The search is solely dependent on the initially stored keywords, and the semantics of knowledge is imprecise to reflect the content of the image.
- Visual properties such as certain textures or geometric shapes are often difficult to describe by text. In addition, spatial information contained in the image data may not be easily expressible in conventional language.
- There is no universally accepted vocabulary yet to describe image characteristics. In medical imaging, diagnostic inference is a continuously evolving lexicon.

Image retrieval is an evolution of traditional information technology that is designed to include and access visual media requests. The main objective in an image retrieval system is the effective "querying" of archived images that match the user's request, where the key challenge is to develop algorithms for automated image-content recognition. This involves a great deal of image understanding and machine intelligence.

Content-based image retrieval (CBIR) has been developed as a visual-based approach to overcome some of the difficulties and problems associated with human perception subjectivity and annotation impreciseness. However, despite the significant developments over the past decade with respect to similarity measures, objective image interpretations, feature extraction, and semantic descriptors (Bustos, Keim, Saupe, & Schreck, 2007; Müller, Michoux, Bandon, & Geissbuhler, 2004), some fundamental difficulties still remain pertaining to CBIR applications. First, it is understood that similarity measures can vary with the different aspects of perceptual similarity between images; the selection of an appropriate similarity measure thus becomes problem-dependent. Secondly, the relation between the low-level visual features and the high-level human interpretation of similarity is not well defined when comparing two images; it is thus not exactly clear what features or com-

bination of them are relevant for such judgment (Bhanu, Peng, & Qing, 1998; El Naqa, Yang, Galatsanos, Nishikawa, & Wernick, 2004). Finally, while the user may understand more about the query, the database system can only guess (possibly through interactive learning) what the user is looking for during the retrieval process. This is an indispensable challenge in information retrieval, where the correct answer may not always be clearly identified.

In Figure 1, we show a diagram to illustrate a typical scenario of image retrieval from mammography databases, where an archive is organized into mammogram images, which in turn is organized into indices (i.e., a data structure of selected image features) for rapid lookup. The user formulates his/her retrieval problem as an expression in the query language (e.g., by presenting the images of the current case as query). The query is then translated into the language of indices and matched against those in the database, and those images with matching indices are retrieved.

In medical applications, there is a strong need to construct medical image databases as a part of a computer-aided diagnosis (CAD) system to serve as a "second reader". Medical images are now produced in ever-increasing large quantities and used for routine diagnostics and therapy. For instance, the Radiology Department of the University Hospital of Geneva alone produced more than 12,000 images a day in 2002 (Müller, *et al.*, 2004). The main objective of a content-based search engine in this case is to find "medically similar" cases with known pathology to the images being evaluated (i.e., the query image) to aid pathological diagnosis (e.g., normal versus disease or disease grade),patient treatment, and medical training. The past few years have witnessed significant interest in developing different types of medical databases for supporting clinical decision-making. This has been assisted by the adoption of the digital imaging and communications in medicine (DICOM) standard in many institutes and by the availability of efficient picture

Figure 1. Image retrieval framework for mammography

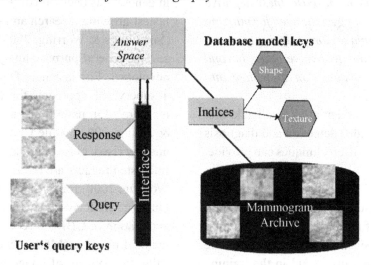

archiving and communication systems (PACS) to store patient's information along with their images (Dreyer, 2006). However, there is still a long way to achieve content-based access to these imaging records. A particularly important class of medical databases that we will focus on in this chapter is the mammographic archive.

Currently mammography is the most effective strategy for early detection of breast cancer. The sensitivity of mammography could be up to approximately 90% for patients without symptoms (Mushlin, Kouides, & Shapiro, 1998). However, this sensitivity varies greatly with the patient's age, the size and conspicuity of the lesion, the hormone status of the tumor, the density of the breast, and the overall image quality and the interpretative skills of the radiologist (Urbain, 2005). Therefore, the overall sensitivity of mammography could degrade from 90% to 70% only (Kolb, Lichy, & Newhouse, 2002). It is difficult to distinguish mammographically benign lesions from malignant ones. It has been estimated that one third of regularly screened women experience at least one false-positive (benign lesions being biopsied) screening mammogram over a period of 10 years (Elmore, *et al.*, 1998). A population-based study that included about 27,394 screening mammograms, interpreted by 1,067 radiologists, showed that the radiologists had substantial variations in the false-positive rates ranging from 1.5 to 24.1% (Tan, Freeman, Goodwin, & Freeman, 2006). Unnecessary histological biopsy is often cited as one of the "risks" of screening mammography. Surgical, needle-core, and fine-needle aspiration biopsies can be expensive, invasive, and traumatic for the patient.

In the last two decades there has been a great deal of research in developing computer aided detection/diagnosis (CAD) tools for detection and diagnosis of breast cancer (Bazzocchi, Mazzarella, Del Frate, Girometti, & Zuiani, 2007; Collins, Hoffmeister, & Worrell, 2006; Hadjiiski, et al., 2006; Malich, Fischer, & Bottcher, 2006). This intensive research has resulted in several FDA approved commercial systems since 1998, which aim to highlight suspicious areas for further review by the radiologist in association with their own reading. Improvement in cancer detection and diagnosis has been reported in retrospective and prospective studies (Dean & Ilvento, 2006; Georgian-Smith, *et al.*, 2007; Yang, *et al.*, 2007). However, this issue was not without controversies (Fenton, *et al.*, 2007). A multi-institutional study of 43 facilities showed that the use of current CAD systems was associated with reduced accuracy of interpretation for screening mammograms

(Fenton, *et al.*, 2007). *In any case, these negative results may strongly suggest the need for utilizing more improved techniques for analyzing mammogram images, which may involve going beyond the limited capacity of detection algorithms into CBIR methodology.*

CBIR has strong potential as a valuable tool for both computer-aided detection and diagnosis in mammography. CBIR techniques can provide, in addition to an estimate of the malignancy likelihood, a list of similar, known cases from the past, which could aid the radiologists in their decision-making of current cases. Besides their potential clinical benefit, CBIR techniques are also expected to be a useful aid in the training of students and residents, allowing them to view images of lesions that appear similar but have possibly differing pathology.

The remainder of this chapter is organized as follows. We provide a background overview of the current role of CBIR in medical imaging in general, and then CBIR for digital mammography in particular. We describe two main types of lesions typically encountered in breast cancer development, followed by characterization of the different image features for each lesion type. Next, we discuss methods for learning perceptual similarity for mammogram retrieval in both offline and online learning modes. This is accompanied by examples from our work using machine-learning techniques based on radiologists' perception of microcalcification (MC) lesions. Afterwards, we discuss some existing issues and problems related to CBIR and recommend possible solutions. In the end, we draw our conclusions and provide suggestions for future work.

BACKGROUND

CBIR in Computer-Aided Diagnosis

Situated at the intersection of database, information retrieval and computer vision, image retrieval in general has been one of the most exciting and fastest growing research areas in the last decade (Smeulders & Worring, 2000). There have been several general-purpose image retrieval systems developed. For instance, Guo *et al.* developed a supervised approach for learning similarity measures for natural images (Guo, Jain, Ma, & Zhang, 2002) while Chen *et al.* investigated unsupervised clustering-based image retrieval. Interested readers are referrred to (Smeulders & Worring, 2000) for further examples on general-purpose CBIR systems. However, an evolving application of CBIR in recent years has been in medical imaging (Müller, *et al.*, 2004). Historically, the concept of image retrieval in medical images was first investigated by Swett *et al.* who developed a rudimentary, rule-based expert system to display radiographs from a library of images as illustrative examples for helping radiologists' diagnosis.

As mentioned earlier, CBIR for medical images is a challenging task due to the complexity in their content in relation to the disease conditions. As a consequence, many of the useful image features in traditional CBIR are no longer adequate. For example, global image features (such as gray-scale histogram) would not be salient for describing the characteristics of pathological regions or lesions which are typically localized in the images (Müller, *et al.*, 2004). In such a case, it is important to derive quantitative features that correlate well with the anatomical or functional information perceived as important for diagnostic purposes by the physicians. Therefore, present medical CBIR systems mostly focus on a specific topic, thus offering support only for a restricted variety of image types and feature sets, such as high-resolution computed tomography (HRCT) scans of the lung (Shyu, *et al.*, 1999). This system was referred to as the ASSERT system, where a rich set of texture features was derived from the disease bearing regions. In (Dy, Brodley, Kak, Broderick, & Aisen, 2003), a new hierarchical approach to CBIR called "customized-queries" approach is applied to lung images. In (Antani, Long, & Thoma, 2004) a system called CBIR2 was developed for retrieval of spine X-ray images. 3D MR image retrieval was studied in (Guimond & Subsol, 1997) based on anatomical structure matching. An online pathological neuroimage retrieval system was investigated in (Liu, Lazar, & Rothfus, 2002) under the framework of classification-driven feature selection. Cai *et al.* (Cai, Feng, & Fulton, 2000) presented a prototype design for content-based functional image retrieval system for dynamic PET images. Tobin *et al.* developed a CBIR system for retrieving diabetic retinopathy cases using a *k*-nearest neighbors based approach (Tobin, et al., 2008). Application to different medical databases such as dermatological images (Dorileo, Frade, Roselino, Rangayyan, & Azevedo-Marques, 2008), cervicographic images (Xue, Antani, Long, Jeronimo, & Thoma, 2007), and microscopic pathology databases (Zheng, Wetzel, Gilbertson, & Becich, 2003) were explored in the literature. More recentlty, there has also been growing interest in retrieving reference images from PACS, and CBIR has now become an important research direction in radiological sciences (Müller, *et al.*, 2004; H. Muller, Rosset, Garcia, Vallee, & Geissbuhler, 2005; Vannier & Summers, 2003).

Despite the extensive research efforts in CBIR, current imaging standards such as DICOM v3.0 still rely on text attributes of images (e.g., study, patient, and other parameters), which are still to date the only information used to select relevant images within PACS (Lehmann, Güld, & Thies, 2003). However, in recent years several research-oriented image retrieval projects and prototypes have been developed for management of medical images for research and teaching purposes. Examples of such systems include: the ASSERT mentioned above; CasImage (Muller, Rosset, Vallee, & Geissbuhler, 2004), which retrieves a variety of images ranging from CT, MR, and radiographs to color photos based on color and textural features; IRMA (image retrieval in

medical applications) (Lehmann, *et al.*, 2004), a development platform of components intended for CBIR in medical applications; NHANES II (the second national health and nutrition examination survey) (Sameer Antani, Lee, Long, & Thoma, 2004) for retrieval of cervical and lumbar spine X-ray images based on the shape of the vertebra. In the rest of this chapter, we will focus on CBIR application to mammography due to its important role in breast cancer management.

Mammography

Breast cancer is the most frequently diagnosed non-skin cancer in women and the second leading cause of cancer death after lung cancer. Early signs of breast cancer include the presence of small bright spots in mammogram images. These small spots represent tiny calcium deposits known as microcalcifications (MCs) and their clustering can be an important indicator of breast cancer. They appear in 30-50% diagnosed cases of mammogram screening (Kopans, 2007). Another important sign is the presence of masses. Masses are typically round shape objects (2-20 mm in diameter), but some masses might have spiculated shapes (having finger-like extensions pointing outwards). As an example, Figure 2 shows a mammogram image with suspected areas highlighted.

Mammograms are low-energy X-ray images of the breast. Typically, they are in the order of 0.7 mSv. A mammogram can detect a cancerous or precancerous tumor in the breast even before the tumor is large enough to be palpable. The results are interpreted according to an American College of Radiology score known as the Breast Imaging Reporting and Data System (BI-RADS) with values ranging from 0 (incomplete) to 6 (known biopsy – proven malignancy) (American College of Radiology, 2003). To date mammography remains the modality of choice for early screening of breast cancer. As mentioned earlier, there has been intensive development of CAD systems for computerized lesion detection; however, this was

Figure 2. A mammogram image with suspected areas highlighted, and a magnified view of a region with clustered microcalcifications.

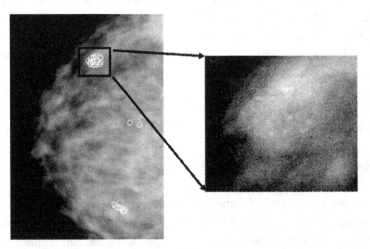

not without controversies about the value of such systems compared to human readers (Fenton, *et al.*, 2007). It is expected that human decision-making is much more complex than what a detection algorithm can provide. *We share the belief that the potential value for application of CAD systems to mammography could be facilitated through the development of information systems based on CBIR.*

CONTENT-BASED IMAGE RETRIEVAL IN MAMMOGRAPHY

Review of Existing Work

Since the pioneering work by Swett and coworkers, there have extensive efforts to apply CBIR to medical imaging in general and mammography in particular (Swett, *et al.*, 1998). Sklansky *et al.* developed a technique that produces a two-dimensional (2D) map based on the decision space of a neural network classifier (Sklansky, *et al.*, 2000), in which images that are close to each other are selected for purposes of visualization; the neural network was trained for separating "biopsy recommended" and "biopsy not recom-

mended" classes. Qi *et al.* (Qi & Snyder, 1999) demonstrated the potential use of CBIR in PACS using a digital mammogram database based on the shape and size information of mass lesions. At about the same time, we started developing our perceptual similarity approach for retrieval of MC lesions in mammograms (El Naqa, 2002; El Naqa, Wernick, Yang, & Galatsanos, 2000, 2002). Giger *et al.* (Giger, *et al.*, 2002) developed an intelligent workstation interface that displays known malignant and benign cases similar to lesions in question (based on one or more selected features or computer estimated likelihood of malignancy), and demonstrated that radiologists' performance, especially specificity, increases with the use of such aid tool. Tourassi *et al.* (Tourassi, Harrawood, Singh, Lo, & Floyd, 2007; Tourassi, Ike, Singh, & Harrawood, 2008; Tourassi, Vargas-Voracek, Catarious, & Floyd, 2003) developed an approach for retrieval and detection of masses in mammograms based on the use of information-theoretic measures (such as mutual information), where a decision index is calculated based on the query's best matches. Zheng *et al.* (Zheng, et al., 2006) applied a multi-feature *k*-nearest neighbor (KNN) algorithm and further used observer-rated spiculation levels to improve the similarity of breast masses, and subsequently investigated the use of mutual information (Zheng, Mello-Thoms, Wang, & Gur, 2007) to improve the similarity measure. An unsupervised learning approach based on Kohonen self-organizing map (SOM) was proposed in (Kinoshita, de Azevedo-Marques, Pereira, Rodrigues, & Rangayyan, 2007). The SOM was trained using a set of 88 features for each mammogram, which included common shape factors, texture and moment features as well as angular projections and morphological features derived from segmented fibroglandular tissues.

Selecting Salient Image Features for Mammogram Lesions

In a typical CBIR system the query and archived images in the database (target images) are represented by a collection of features (see Figure 1). For retrieval, the system compares the similarity between the features of the query and that of target images in the database. How to select the best image features becomes an important problem, particularly when machine-learning algorithms are involved, of which the objective is to reduce the algorithm complexity, decrease the computational burden, and improve efficiency.

As in a typical pattern recognition problem, there is a large number N of features that could be extracted from the mammograms. Therefore, it becomes necessary to select a finite set of features that would cope well with the similarity notion (e.g., diagnostic value) and yield improved retrieval precision. Conceptually, an optimal subset could be determined by using exhaustive search, which would yield as many as $2^N - 1$ possibilities. Instead, there are other (more efficient) alternatives (Kennedy, Lee, Van Roy, Reed, & Lippman, 1998). A conventional approach is to make an educated guess based on experience and domain knowledge, then apply feature transformation (e.g., principle component analysis (PCA) or multidimensional scaling (MDS)), or sensitivity analysis by using

systematic search such as sequential forward selection (SFS), or sequential backward selection (SBS) or combination of both. Other reported methods in the literature include machine learning sensitivity analyses (Guyon & Elissee, 2003; Rakotomamonjy, 2003), genetics algorithms (Vafaie & Imam, 1994), and branch and bound algorithms (Somol, Pudil, & Kittler, 2004).

Typical image features used in CBIR would include geometrical shape, size, and texture descriptors. However, one needs to be cautious when adapting these features toward the endpoint of diagnostic interest. Lesion features in mammography typically intend to represent the descriptions given in the BI-RADS lexicon mentioned earlier. Many features could be used to describe the two main types of mammogram lesions (i.e., microcalcifications and masses). For instance, we have used a set of 12 features for clustered MCs, which were selected from a pool of 33 features by using a sequential feature selection procedure (El Naqa, Yang, Galatsanos, & Wernick, 2004; Wei, Yang, Nishikawa, & Jiang, 2005). The 12 features were: (1) compactness of the cluster, (2) eccentricity of the cluster, (3) the number of microcalcifications per unit area, (4) the average and (5) standard deviation of the inter-distance among cluster points, (6) solidity of the cluster region (regional convexity), (7) the moment signature of the cluster region, (8) the number of MCs in the cluster, (9) the mean effective volume (area times effective thickness) of individual MCs, (10) the relative standard deviation of the effective thickness, (11) the relative standard deviation of the effective volume, and (12) the second highest microcalcification-shape-irregularity measure. The details of these features can be found in (Wei, Yang, Nishikawa, & Jiang, 2005). Other features reported in the literature include morphological features (Nakayama, *et al.*, 1999; Taylor, Fox, & Pokropek, 1999; Zhao, 1993), texture features derived from the gray-level co-occurrence matrix or radial-basis expansions (Chan, et al., 1998; Meersman, Scheunders, & Van Dyck, 1998;

Rogova, Stomper, & Ke, 1999), wavelet decomposition features (Strickland & Hee Il, 1996; Yu & Guan, 2000), as well as patient demographic information (Kallergi, 2004). A combination of morphological and texture was used in (Chan, Sahiner, Kam, Petrick, & Helvie, 1998). Radon domain and granulometric measures were used in (Kinoshita, *et al.*, 2007). The Radon transform yields large values at ray angles and positions that correspond to strong linear features in an image, while granulometric features can characterize the distribution of object sizes in an image (Kinoshita, *et al.*, 2007).

In the case of masses, there is also a large body of features, of which some are used to distinguish spiculated tumors from less probably malignant round masses. Similar to the case of MCs, these features would include texture features (D. Wei, et al., 1995), intensity, iso-density, location, contrast, gradients (te Brake, Karssemeijer, & Hendriks, 2000), and even histological features (Tot, 2005). For a review of these features and others, the interested reader is referred to (Sampat, Markey, & Bovik, 2005). As an example of mass CBIR, the following set of features were chosen in (Zheng, et al., 2006): pixel value (average, standard deviation) in the breast ROI and the background, region conspicuity (contrast), radial length (mean, standard deviation, skew), and gradient metrics. A different approach was proposed in (Tourassi, *et al.*, 2007), where information-theoretic measures such as entropy and divergence measures were used.

LEARNING PERCEPTUAL SIMILARITY FOR MAMMOGRAM RETRIEVAL

Learning is defined in this context as estimating similarity dependencies from data. There are two common types of learning: supervised and unsupervised. Supervised learning is used to estimate an unknown (input, output) mapping from known (input, output) samples (e.g., classification or regression). In unsupervised learning, only input samples are given to the learning system (e.g., clustering or dimensionality reduction) as discussed below.

Supervised Learning Approach

In order for a retrieval system to be useful as a diagnostic aid, the retrieved images must be truly relevant to the query image as perceived by the radiologists, who otherwise may simply dismiss its use as a visual aid. Since 2000 (El Naqa, *et al.*, 2000), we have proposed and investigated a supervised learning approach for modeling the notion of similarity used by radiologists when they interpret mammograms (El Naqa, 2002; El Naqa, *et al.*, 2002; El Naqa, Yang, Galatsanos, Nishikawa, *et al.*, 2004; El Naqa, Yang, Galatsanos, & Wernick, 2004; Wei, Yang, Nishikawa, & Jiang, 2005; Wei, Yang, Nishikawa, Wernick, & Edwards, 2005; Wei, Yang, Wernick, & Nishikawa, 2009). The rationale behind this approach is that the similarity metric must conform closely to the perception of the radiologists. Therefore, simple mathematical distance metrics developed in the context of general-purpose image retrieval (e.g., Euclidean distance (Niblack, *et al.*, 1993), Mahalanobis distance (Hafner, Sawhney, Equitz, Flickner, & Niblack, 1995), the earth mover's distance (Rubner, Tomasi, & Guibas, 1998), etc.) may not adequately characterize clinical notions of image relevance, which are complex assessments made by expert observers. Similarly, standard approaches used in the general CBIR field (e.g., using features based on intensity histograms) may also be inappropriate for specialized clinical applications such as mammographic interpretation.

In our approach, the similarity between two lesion images is modeled as a nonlinear regression function of the features characterizing the lesions, which is determined by using machine learning from examples collected either in human observer studies or from online user feedback (acquired during use of the system). This approach has proven in our preliminary studies to be more effective than alternative similarity measures derived from unsupervised learning such as Euclidean distance, discriminant adaptive nearest neighbor (DANN) (Niblack, *et al.*, 1993), and normalized cut (Ncut) (Chen, Wang, & Krovetz, 2005), as discussed below.

In our approach, the notion of similarity is modeled as a nonlinear function of the image features in a pair of mammogram images containing for instance, microcalcification clusters (MCCs). If we let vectors $\mathbf{u}$ and $\mathbf{v}$ denote the features of two MCCs at issue, the following regression model could be used to determine their similarity coefficient (*SC*):

$$SC(\mathbf{u}, \mathbf{v}) = f(\mathbf{u}, \mathbf{v}) + \zeta \qquad (1)$$

where $f(\mathbf{u}, \mathbf{v})$ is a function determined using a machine learning approach, which we choose to be support vector machine (SVM) learning (Vapnik, 1998), and ζ is the modelling error. The similarity function $f(\mathbf{u}, \mathbf{v})$ in Eq.(1) is trained using data samples collected in an observer study. For convenience, we denote $f(\mathbf{u}, \mathbf{v})$ by $f(\mathbf{x})$ with $\mathbf{x} = [\mathbf{u}^T, \mathbf{v}^T]^T$.

Assume that we have a set of N training samples, denoted by $Z = \{(\mathbf{x}_i, y_i)\}_{i=1}^N$, where y_i denotes the user similarity score for the MCC pair denoted by $\mathbf{x}_i$, $i = 1, 2, ..., N$. The regression function $f(\mathbf{x})$ is written in the following form:

$$f(\mathbf{x}) = \mathbf{w}^T \Phi(\mathbf{x}) + b \qquad (2)$$

where $\Phi(\mathbf{x})$ is a mapping implicitly defined by a so-called kernel funciton which we introduce below. The parameters $\mathbf{w}$ and b in Eq.(2) are determined through minimization of the following structured risk:

$$R(\mathbf{w}, b) = \frac{1}{2}\mathbf{w}^T\mathbf{w} + C\sum_{i=1}^N L_\varepsilon(\mathbf{x}_i) \qquad (3)$$

where $L_\varepsilon(\bullet)$ is the so-called ε-insensitive loss function, which has the property that it does not penalize errors below the parameter ε. The constant C in Eq.(3) determines the trade-off between the model complexity and the training error. In this study the Gaussian radial basis function is used for the SVM kernel function $K(\cdot, \cdot)$, where $K(\cdot, \cdot) = \Phi^T(\mathbf{x})\Phi(\mathbf{x})$. The regression function $f(\mathbf{x})$ in Eq.(2) is characterized by a set of so-called support vectors:

$$f(\mathbf{x}) = \sum_{j=1}^{Ns} \gamma_j K(\mathbf{x}_j, \mathbf{x}) + b \qquad (4)$$

where $\mathbf{x}_j$ are the support vectors, and N_s is the number of the support vectors.

To model the similarity between two feature vectors, we want to learn a symmetric function satisfying $f(\mathbf{u}, \mathbf{v}) = f(\mathbf{v}, \mathbf{u})$, i.e., the notion of similarity is commutative. This can be achieved by duplicating the training image pairs, i.e., first with $(\mathbf{u}, \mathbf{v})$ and then with $(\mathbf{v}, \mathbf{u})$. We can explicitly enforce this property in the SVM cost function as:

$$R(\mathbf{w}, b) = \frac{1}{2}\mathbf{w}^T\mathbf{w} + C\sum_{i=1}^N L_\varepsilon(\mathbf{x}_i) + C\sum_{i=1}^N L_\varepsilon(\mathbf{x}_i^s)$$

$$(5)$$

Here $y(\mathbf{x}_i) = y(\mathbf{x}_i^s)$, $\mathbf{x}_i = (\mathbf{u}_i^T, \mathbf{v}_i^T)^T$, $\mathbf{x}_i^s = (\mathbf{v}_i^T, \mathbf{u}_i^T)^T$.

With this formulation the SVM training algorithm yields the global optimum of a symmetric Lagrangian. The resulting regression function can be written as:

$$f(\mathbf{x}) = \sum_{j=1}^{Ns} \gamma_j [K(\mathbf{x}_j, \mathbf{x}) + K(\mathbf{x}_j^s, \mathbf{x})] + b \qquad (6)$$

That is, if a training sample $\mathbf{x}_j$ is a support vector, i.e, $|y_j - f(\mathbf{x}_j)| \geq \varepsilon$, then its symmetric sample $\mathbf{x}_j^s$ is also a support vector and $\gamma_j = \gamma_j^s$. This will ensure that the solution is symmetric: $f(\mathbf{x}) = f(\mathbf{x}^s)$. A detailed proof of this is given in (Wei, *et al.*, 2009).

Unsupervised Learning Approach

For compraison purposes, we here consider two alternative distance measures based on unsupervised learning: (1) discriminant adaptive nearest neighbor (DANN), and (2) normalized cut (Ncut).

DANN (Hastie & Tibshirani, 1996) is an improved version of the k nearest neighbor (KNN) measure based on the Euclidean distance (Duda & Hart, 1973; Niblack, *et al.*, 1993) for computing the similarity between two images. In DANN, a locally adaptive form of the nearest neighbor measure is used to ameliorate the curse of dimensionality. The distance between a point $\mathbf{x}'$ and a query $\mathbf{x}$ is defined as:

$$D = (\mathbf{x}' - \mathbf{x})^T \Sigma (\mathbf{x}' - \mathbf{x}) \qquad (8)$$

In KNN, the matrix Σ is the identity matrix I. In DANN, with a local discriminant model, the local within- and between-class covariance matrices are used to define the optimal shape of the neighborhood (Σ). In Eq. (8) the matrix Σ is computed as:

$$\Sigma = W^{-1/2}[W^{-1/2}BW^{1/2} + \varepsilon I]W^{-1/2} \qquad (9)$$

where B and W are the between- and within-class covariance matrices, respectively, which are computed from a number k_m of local neighbors around $\mathbf{x}$, and ε is an offset.

Normalized cut (Shi & Malik, 2000) originally is a method for image clustering. When applied for retrieval (Chen, *et al.*, 2005), it retrieves a cluster of images rather than a set of ordered images. Here we adapt this clustering method to mammogram retrieval. In this method, a graph representation of the neighboring target images is defined as $G = (V, E)$, where the nodes $V = 1, 2, ..., n$ represent the images, and the edges $E = (i, j), i, j = 1, 2, ..., n$ are formed between every pair of nodes. Then non-negative weights w_{ij} are defined for the edges according to the similarity (e.g., $w_{ij} = exp(-d(i, j)^2)$) between the nodes. With this method, the images are organized into small groups so that the within-group similarity is high, and the between-group similarity is low. The images in the group where the query image resides are retrieved. Here we can use a two-stage hierarchical fashion as in (Chen, *et al.*, 2005) to speed up the process for mammogram retrieval. In the first stage, the top k nearest neighboring images for a query image are treated as the target images; in the second stage, the Ncut clustering method is applied to the query image and its k nearest neighboring target images to obtain the final retrieval results.

Performance Evaluation

Retrieval systems are typically evaluated using the so-called precision-recall curves (Del Bimbo, 1999). The retrieval precision is defined as the proportion of the images among all the retrieved that are truly relevant to a given query; the term recall is measured by the proportion of the images that are actually retrieved among all the relevant images to a query. Mathematically, they are given by:

$$Precision = \frac{\text{The number of relevant images that are retrieved}}{\text{The total number of retrieved images}}$$
$$Recall = \frac{\text{The number of relevant images that are retrieved}}{\text{The total number of relevant images}}$$

$$(10)$$

The precision-recall curve is a plot of the retrieval precision versus the recall over a continuum of the operating threshold. An example is shown in Figure 3, in which two different machine-learning algorithms (SVM: support vector machine, GRNN: general regression neural networks) are used to learn similarity between MC clusters (El Naqa, 2002). Other metrics to quantify the accuracy of learning a similarity score could be used such as the mean-squared error (MSE) of the model compared to the observer scores. In addition, to evaluate the merit of the learning-based similarity measure for cancer diagnosis, criteria such as cumulative neighbor matching rate could be used (L. Wei, *et al.*, 2009). In the cumulative neighbor matching rate case, for each query image, the ratio of top k images that actually match the disease condition of the query is computed and averaged over all the queries as discussed later.

For statistical validation of the retrieval performance, resampling techniques such as cross-validation and bootstrap are typically used. In cross-validation, the data samples are divided into a number of subsets which are permuted for training and testing in a round-robin fashion, whereas in bootstrap, the data samples are randomly selected for training and testing for many times. Bootstrap could be regarded as a smoothed version of cross-validation. It is thought to be more realistic in modeling real life scenarios (Efron & Tibshirani, 1993).

Finally, we add that besides these rather generic measures used in general information retrieval, it is also necessary to evaluate the retrieval efficiency based on clinical tasks (as further discussed later).

CASE STUDY: SIMILARITY MEASURE FROM EXPERT OBSERVERS

Reader Study

We used a database of mammogram images provided by the Department of Radiology at the University of Chicago. The database consists of a total of 200 different mammogram images of dimension 1024×1024 (a few are 512×512) from 104 patients with known pathology (46

Figure 3. Precision recall curve of MC retrieval using different machine learning methods. Error bars are estimated using the bootstrap method

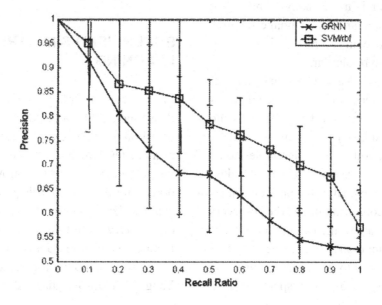

malignant, 58 benign), digitized with a spatial resolution of 0.1 mm/pixel and 10-bit grayscale. All these images contain MC clusters (MCCs). The MCCs in each image have been identified by expert radiologists.

With 200 images we can form as many as 19,900 different image pairs. However, it would be too time-consuming (and also unnecessary) to score all of them in an observer study. Instead, we selected a subset consisting of a total of 600 representative image pairs for the observer study. These image pairs were selected using the following procedure so that they represent the spectrum of the image pairs in terms of similarity. First, the 200 images in the database were partitioned into 10 different groups by the *k*-means method based on the features of their MCCs. The features used were the eight image features in (Wei, Yang, Nishikawa, & Jiang, 2005), which were demonstrated to have high discriminating power for cancer diagnosis. Next, a total of 300 intra-group pairs were randomly selected, of which each pair was formed by images from a common group. Finally, a total of 300 inter-group pairs were randomly selected, of which each pair was formed by images from two different groups. In both cases, the probability that an image was selected was proportional to the size of the group that it was in. Conceivably, an intra-group pair is more likely (though not definitive) to be similar as their image features are closer in distance; in contrast, an inter-group pair is less likely to be similar.

The observer study was carried out by a panel of six expert observers, who scored the 600 pairs based on their perceptual similarity using a scale from 0 (most dissimilar) to 10 (most similar). It consisted of the following different sessions: 1) a "pre-calibration" session, and 2) individual scoring sessions. The goal of the pre-calibration was to establish a consensus among the observers on a uniform measure of the perceptual similarity. In the pre-calibration session, five "anchor" image pairs were used to define the rating scale (their scores were $1, 3, 5, 7, 9$, respectively). In the individual scoring sessions, each observer scored the 600 image pairs separately. In addition, for the purpose of evaluating intra-observer consistency, each observer also scored 30 additional image pairs; these image pairs were presented in a random order, and each pair was scored twice by the same observer.

Statistical analyses were conducted to analyze both intra- and inter-observer consistencies to insure the integrity of the observer data. For intra-observer consistency, Spearman's rank correlation method was used to analyze the two sets of similarity scores from each observer on the 30 image pairs. The values of ρ were 0.5667, 0.6840, 0.7338, 0.3852, 0.5812, 0.7212, respectively for the six observers. It was found that there was statistically significant consistency within each observer with their p-values all below 0.05. For inter-observer consistency, Kendall's coefficient of concordance W was computed, and the result was 0.5317 and there was statistically significant agreement among the observers ($p < 0.0001$). Based on these analyses, we selected the four observers with the highest intra-observer consistency $(2, 3, 5, 6)$, and averaged their similarity scores for each of the 600 image pairs. The resulting scores were used to form training samples for the SVM.

SUPERVISED SIMILARITY LEARNING

In our previous work (El Naqa, Yang, Galatsanos, & Wernick, 2004) a set of 10 features were used based on the geometric distribution of the MCs in a cluster. However, as we mentioned earlier, image features of individual MCs are very important for diagnosis of clustered MCs. To better characterize the similarity data by the experts, in (L. Wei, *et al.*, 2009) we introduced eight additional features which were demonstrated to have high discriminating power for cancer diagnosis (Wei, Yang, Nishikawa, & Jiang, 2005). Consequently, there were a total of 18 features used for describing the MCCs. For the purpose of selecting the most relevant features for similarity learning, as mentioned earlier, we used a sequential feature selection procedure to obtain 12 features for characterizing an MC cluster. In our experiments, all the feature components were normalized to have the same dynamic range $(0,1)$.

The SVM similarity model was trained using the observer data. Besides the human scores for the 600 image pairs, we also added the following pairs for training:

1. $SC(\mathbf{u}, \mathbf{u}) = 10$, and
2. $SC(\mathbf{u}, \mathbf{v}) = 10$ if $\mathbf{u}$ and $\mathbf{v}$ are different views from the same case.

With a leave-one-out procedure, the SVM model achieved a MSE of 0.0334 per image pair compared to the observer scores.

Next, the trained SVM similarity model was tested with the 200 images in the database, where each of the 200 images in the dataset was used in turn as a query image. The average cumulative neighbor matching rate was calculated in the end. Similarly, we also applied the DANN and Ncut measures for retrieval. The test results are summarized in Figure 4 for the different methods, where the average matching rate is plotted against k, which is the number of top retrieved images for each query. In particular, for SVM, the top most similar image can match the disease of the query 72.5% of the time. This is significantly different from the result by random pairing (of which the expected matching rate is 50.75%). As can be seen, the best performance was achieved by the SVM model. The parameter settings for the different methods were chosen by the leave-one-out retrieval procedure and shown as follows: SVM (Gaussian kernel, $\sigma = 1$, $C = 100$, $\varepsilon = 1$),

Figure 4. Cumulative neighbor disease matching rates achieved by different retrieval measures

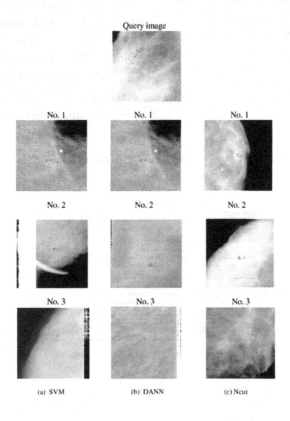

DANN ($k_m = 40$, $\varepsilon = 1$, $k = 5$), and Ncut ($k = 20$).

In Figure 5, we show one retrieval example for a given query image by different similarity measure models. The individual MCs in each mammogram are marked out for better visualization. As can be seen, the learning based similarity measure can indeed achieve meaningful retrieval results and perform better than other similarity measure models.

Relevance Feedback in CBIR Databases

Relevance feedback (RFB) is a post-query process to refine the search by using positive and negative indications from the user regarding the relevance of retrieved images. RFB is a powerful utility that has been applied in text-retrieval systems to improve the results. In text retrieval, the focus is on query expansion, where new terms are added to the original query either manually or automatically. Mathematically, this could be represented according to the so-called *Rocchio* approach in information retrieval as (Grossman & Frieder, 1998):

$$\overline{Q} = aQ + b\sum R - c\sum N, \qquad (10)$$

where Q is the original query features, R is a set of relevant features, N is a set of non-relevant features, and a, b, c are the *Rocchio* weights. This idea was applied in FourEyes system (Rui & Huang). A similar concept was used in our previous work to adjust the learned similarity measure *SC* (El Naqa, Yang, Galatsanos, Nishikawa, *et al.*, 2004):

$$\widetilde{SC}(Q, \mathbf{d}) = (1 - w) \cdot SC(Q, \mathbf{d}) + w \cdot SC(R, \mathbf{d}), \qquad (11)$$

where w is a weighting parameter used to adjust the relative impact of the feedback image R and the targeted database $\mathbf{d}$. The images with the highest weighted *SC*s were then retrieved.

There also exist other approaches using different RFB techniques in the literature. One approach is to use a probabilistic framework to learn the local relevance of features under a given similarity metric. It was shown that using Euclidean distance with RFB could reshape the region around the query (e.g., map a circular region in the feature space into an elliptical one) (Peng, Bhanu, & Qing, 1999). Bayesian approaches were used in PicHunter (Cox, Miller, Minka, Papathomas, & Yianilos, 2000) and in (Su, Zhang, Li, & Ma, 2003) by updating each image probability based

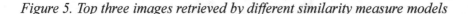

Figure 5. Top three images retrieved by different similarity measure models

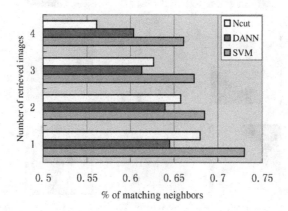

on the user feedback. Jing *et al.* used region-based representation with earth mover's distance to achieve effective online learning capability (Jing, Li, Zhang, & Zhang, 2004).

We also investigated how to incorporate RFB into our supervised learning framework based on the concept of incremental learning (El Naqa, Yang, Galatsanos, & Wernick, 2003). With a new sample, denoted by $(\mathbf{x}_c, y_c)$, which is introduced from online user feedback, the objective is how to modify the existing SVM in Eq. (5) by this newly added information. Conceptually, this could be accomplished by retraining the SVM using the new sample and the old samples $Z = \{(\mathbf{x}_i, y_i)\}_{i=1}^{N}$ altogether. However, this can be excessively expensive in an online application. Therefore, we adopted the incremental learning approach initially developed for online SVM classification (Cauwenberghs & Poggio, 2000), where the SVM solution with the new $(N+1)$-sample training set is developed in terms of the new sample and that of the previous N-sample training set. The key to this procedure is to retain the Karush-Kuhn-Tucker (KKT) conditions of the previous SVM solution, while "adiabatically" (i.e., perturbation without loss or gain) adding the new sample point.

Effect of this method on the CBIR performance is illustrated using the precision-recall curves in Figure 6.

Issues and Recommendations

Despite the increasing number of research systems developed in recent years, the application of CBIR for medical applications is very much still at its infancy. There are some significant, open research issues yet to be addressed. Below we discuss a few of them, which are by no means meant to be complete.

As described earlier, learning similarity from images is a challenging task in its own merit and requires utilization of complex modeling schemes. This may also result in conflict with efficient performance for real-time applications. This is particularly true in the case of medical repositories, which may contain hundreds of thousands of radiologic images and will continue to grow on a rapid pace. This ever-growing volume of images may increase the demand in the precision of a retrieval system and would surely affect its efficiency for real-time processing. To overcome these hurdles, the similarity-learning

Figure 6. Precision-recall curves using relevance feedback for different approaches.

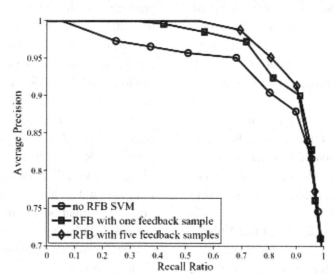

algorithm design (supervised or unsupervised) may need to compromise between effectiveness and efficiency during the retrieval process. Our proposed approach of using perceptual similarity could be used to improve precision in image retrieval. This concept has been studied by other researchers (Li, *et al.*, 2003; Muramatsu, *et al.*, 2006; Muramatsu, *et al.*, 2005). For instance, the results in (Muramatsu, *et al.*, 2006) demonstrate good concordance consistency even among three different types of readers (13 breast radiologists, 10 general radiologists, and 10 non-radiologists), which indicates the reliability of the similarity ratings obtained from observer studies.

On the other hand, problems such as efficient search in a high-dimensional feature space and search in the presence of user-dependent similarity measures are largely unsolved (Smeulders & Worring, 2000). Possible solutions may involve the need to develop faster methods for extracting relevant features from the given query image and to pre-store the image features using efficient data structures (e.g., linked-list tree structures) for rapid retrieval. In addition, one can pre-cluster the cases in the database based on their feature vectors by applying a clustering algorithm, so that non-similar images are distributed in different clusters based on which indexing algorithms for faster retrieval can be developed. To further speed up the retrieval process for an online environment, one can also employ a two-stage approach in which a computationally efficient linear-classifier is used to quickly discard any non-similar entries from further consideration (El Naqa, Yang, Galatsanos, Nishikawa, *et al.*, 2004).

The problem of how to evaluate the retrieval quality is an important topic as well. Retrieval systems need to be compared in order to sort out the different techniques (Müller, *et al.*, 2004). Due to the complexity of medical images, how to construct a common test bed for medical CBIR is an interesting research issue (Wei, Li, & Wilson, 2006). To construct a test bed for medical CBIR, a number of factors such as imaging modalities,

regions, and orientations of images should be taken into account.

To fully evaluate the benefit of a retrieval system, it is desirable to establish a benchmark database which is large enough so that it would maximize the yield of truly relevant images. In practice, this can be an expensive process. In the case study we presented earlier, we used a database collected by the University of Chicago. It is noted that there exist several public domain mammogram databases such as DDSM (Digital Database for Screening Mammography) maintained by the University of South Florida and MIAS (Mammographic Image Analysis Society maintained by the University of Manchester. These databases are mainly used for comparing different CAD systems. It would be beneficial to augment these databases with additional image similarity information so that they could be used as a benchmark for comparing different CBIR systems.

Another issue that may arise in CBIR applications is how to effectively present retrieval results to assist interpretation by radiologists. To serve as a diagnostic aid, the retrieval systems need to demonstrate their performance (i.e., separating benign cases from malignant ones) before it can be accepted by the clinicians. This implies an integration of the systems into daily clinical practice, which is not an easy task (Müller, *et al.*, 2004). To facilitate interpretation of retrieval results, one possible approach would be to use data reduction methods such as multi-diemnsional scaling (MDS). MDS (Borg & Groenen, 1997) is a powerful technique for representation and analysis of a set of objects based on their mutual similarity (or dissimilarity) measurements. In particular, Rubner (Rubner, *et al.*, 1998) applied MDS as a visualization technique for retrieved images based on their texture and color distributions. In evaluation of our retrieval framework, we used MDS to embed the images in a 2D space so that distances in the embedding are reflective of the perceputal simiarlity between the images.

In the MDS plot, both the query and retrieved mammograms are displayed (as thumbnails) in a 2D window according to their similarities, where images similar to each other are closely placed and *vice versa*. Besides being more intuitive, such an MDS approach will be much more informative compared to a conventional approach that lists the retrieved images in their order of similarity to the query. The MDS plot will not only show how similar the retrieved images are to the query, but more importantly, it will also reveal how the retrieved images are similar to each other.

Finally, integration into PACS or even existing Healthcare Enterprise (e.g., post-processing workflow) is an essential step for the clinical use of retrieval systems (Müller, *et al.*, 2004). PACS systems are now widely used in the hospitals to manage the storage and distribution of images. Thus, CBIR is expected to have a great impact on PACS and health database management (Aggarwal, Sardana, & Jindal, 2009). A further important issue in medical practice is to keep patient's private information from any unauthorized access in accordance with the Health Insurance Portability and Accountability Act (HIPAA). Security requirements need to be embedded into to the design of the database system, so that users would have access to data that they only have previldge over. This may add additional burdens to achieve high efficiency for CBIR within the necessary security constraints. Experiences from textual relational database management systems (RDBMS) could be helpful in this regard.

FUTURE RESEARCH DIRECTIONS

For content-based mammogram retrieval, there remain several technical issues that would require further investigation, which may include the following different aspects: 1) how to incrementally improve the retrieval performance through accumulating experts' query log; 2) including semantics-based similarity features such as patient history/age/view/ information besides the low-level image features used to improve retrieval accuracy; 3) investigate advanced relevance feedback techniques to refine the retrieval process, 4) system integration into PACS or other medical image databases; 5) human-computer interaction and usability; 6) performance evaluation framework and standard; 7) validation of many of the proposed methods for clinical use on large databases. These areas could benefit from existing expertise in the computer vision community. If successful, CBIR approaches could realize its potential to improve current clinical decision-making processes for patients with breast cancer.

CONCLUSION

CBIR for mammography is an emerging field for improving automated detection and diagnosis of breast cancer lesions. In this chapter, we provided an overview of recent advances in CBIR technology and its application to mammographic databases. In addition, we presented examples from our expereince in building CBIR systems for mammography. In our approach, we advocated for the use of a supervised learning methodology in content-based mammogram retrieval based on perceptual similarity from expert observers. The proposed similarity model was demonstrated using a set of clinical mammograms. This approach was demonstrated to achieve significant improvement in retrieval performance over competing unsupervised learning methods. Moreover, we also demonstrated that the application of relevance feedback could further improve the CBIR performance during the retrieval phase. We also discussed some of the current problems in the field and highlighted the potential opportunities for future computer vision research and clinical decision-making.

ACKNOWLEDGMENT

This work was partially supported by NIH grants EB009905 and CA128809.

REFERENCES

Aggarwal, P., Sardana, H. K., & Jindal, G. (2009). Content Based Medical Image Retrieval: Theory, Gaps and Future Directions. *ICGST-GVIP Journal*, *9*(2), 27–37.

(2008). *American Cancer Society.* Atlanta: Cancer Facts and Figures.

American College of Radiology. (2003). American College of Radiology (ACR) Breast Imaging Reporting and Data System Atlas (BI-RADS® Atlas). Reston, VA.

Antani, S., Lee, D. J., Long, L. R., & Thoma, G. R. (2004). Evaluation of shape similarity measurement methods for spine X-ray images. *Journal of Visual Communication and Image Representation*, *15*(3), 285–302. doi:10.1016/j. jvcir.2004.04.005

Antani, S., Long, L. R., & Thoma, G. R. (2004). Content-based image retrieval for large biomedical image archives. *Studies in Health Technology and Informatics*, *107*(Pt 2), 829–833.

Bazzocchi, M., Mazzarella, F., Del Frate, C., Girometti, F., & Zuiani, C. (2007). CAD systems for mammography: a real opportunity? A review of the literature. *La Radiologia Medica*, *112*(3), 329–353. doi:10.1007/s11547-007-0145-5

Bhanu, B., Peng, J., & Qing, S. (1998). Learning feature relevance and similarity metrics in image database. *IEEE Workshop Proceedings on Content-Based Access of Image and Video Libraries*, 14-18.

Borg, I., & Groenen, P. J. F. (1997). *Modern multidimensional scaling: theory and applications*. New York: Springer.

Bustos, B., Keim, D., Saupe, D., & Schreck, T. (2007). Content-based 3D object retrieval. *IEEE Computer Graphics and Applications*, *27*(4), 22–27. doi:10.1109/MCG.2007.80

Cai, W., Feng, D. D., & Fulton, R. (2000). Content-based retrieval of dynamic PET functional images. *IEEE Transactions on Information Technology in Biomedicine*, *4*(2), 152–158. doi:10.1109/4233.845208

Cauwenberghs, G., & Poggio, T. (2000). *Incremental and Decremental Support Vector Machine Learning*. Paper presented at the NIPS.

Chan, H.-P., Lam, K., Petrick, N., Helvie, M., Goodsitt, M., & Adler, D. (1998). Computerized analysis of mammographic microcalcifications in morphological and texture feature space. *Medical Physics*, *25*, 2007–2019. doi:10.1118/1.598389

Chan, H. P., Sahiner, B., Kam, K. L., Petrick, N., Helvie, M. A., Goodsitt, M. M., & Adler, D. D. (1998). Computerized analysis of mammographic microcalcifications in morphological and texture feature spaces. *Medical Physics*, *25*, 2007–2019. doi:10.1118/1.598389

Chen, Y., Wang, J. Z., & Krovetz, R. (2005). CLUE: cluster-based retrieval of images by unsupervised learning. *IEEE Transactions on Image Processing*, *14*(8), 1187–1201. doi:10.1109/TIP.2005.849770

Collins, M. J., Hoffmeister, J., & Worrell, S. W. (2006). Computer-aided detection and diagnosis of breast cancer. *Seminars in Ultrasound, CT, and MR*, *27*(4), 351–355. doi:10.1053/j. sult.2006.05.009

Cox, I. J., Miller, M. L., Minka, T. P., Papathomas, T. V., & Yianilos, P. N. (2000). The Bayesian image retrieval system, PicHunter: theory, implementation, and psychophysical experiments. *IEEE Transactions on Image Processing, 9*(1), 20–37. doi:10.1109/83.817596

Dean, J. C., & Ilvento, C. C. (2006). Improved cancer detection using computer-aided detection with diagnostic and screening mammography: prospective study of 104 cancers. *AJR. American Journal of Roentgenology, 187*(1), 20–28. doi:10.2214/AJR.05.0111

Del Bimbo, A. (1999). *Visual information retrieval*. San Francisco, CA: Morgan Kaufmann Publishers.

Dorileo, E. A. G., Frade, M. A. C., Roselino, A. M. F., Rangayyan, R. M., & Azevedo-Marques, P. M. (2008). *Color image processing and content-based image retrieval techniques for the analysis of dermatological lesions*. Paper presented at the Engineering in Medicine and Biology Society, 2008. EMBS 2008. 30th Annual International Conference of the IEEE.

Dreyer, K. J. (2006). *PACS: a guide to the digital revolution* (2nd ed.). New York: Springer.

Duda, R. O., & Hart, P. E. (1973). *Pattern classification and scene analysis*. New York: Wiley.

Dy, J. G., Brodley, C. E., Kak, A., Broderick, L. S., & Aisen, A. M. (2003). Unsupervised Feature Selection Applied to Content-based Retrieval of Lung Images. *IEEE Transactions on Pattern Analysis and Machine Intelligence, 25*(3), 373–378. doi:10.1109/TPAMI.2003.1182100

Efron, B., & Tibshirani, R. (1993). *An introduction to the bootstrap*. New York: Chapman & Hall.

El Naqa, I. (2002). Content-based image retrieval by similarity learning for digital mammography illinois Institute of Technology, Chicago, IL.

El Naqa, I., Wernick, M., Yang, Y., & Galatsanos, N. (2000). *Image retrieval based on similarity learning*. Paper presented at the IEEE Inter. Conf. on Image Processing, Vancouver, CA.

El Naqa, I., Wernick, M., Yang, Y., & Galatsanos, N. (2002). *Content-based image retrieval for digital mammography*. Paper presented at the IEEE Inter. Conf. on Image Processing, Rochester, NY.

El Naqa, I., Yang, Y., Galatsanos, N. P., Nishikawa, R. M., & Wernick, M. N. (2004). A similarity learning approach to content-based image retrieval: application to digital mammography. *IEEE Transactions on Medical Imaging, 23*(10), 1233–1244. doi:10.1109/TMI.2004.834601

El Naqa, I., Yang, Y., Galatsanos, N. P., & Wernick, M. N. (2003). *Relevance feedback based on incremental learning for mammogram retrieval*. Paper presented at the 2003 International Conference on Image Processing, 2003. ICIP 2003.

El Naqa, I., Yang, Y., Galatsanos, N. P., & Wernick, M. N. (2004). *Mammogram retrieval based on incremental learning*. Paper presented at the IEEE International Symposium on Biomedical Imaging: Nano to Macro, 2004.

Elmore, J. G., Barton, M. B., Moceri, V. M., Polk, S., Arena, P. J., & Fletcher, S. W. (1998). Ten-Year Risk of False Positive Screening Mammograms and Clinical Breast Examinations. *The New England Journal of Medicine, 338*(16), 1089–1096. doi:10.1056/NEJM199804163381601

Fenton, J. J., Taplin, S. H., Carney, P. A., Abraham, L., Sickles, E. A., & D'Orsi, C. (2007). Influence of computer-aided detection on performance of screening mammography. *The New England Journal of Medicine, 356*(14), 1399–1409. doi:10.1056/NEJMoa066099

Georgian-Smith, D., Moore, R. H., Halpern, E., Yeh, E. D., Rafferty, E. A., & D'Alessandro, H. A. (2007). Blinded comparison of computer-aided detection with human second reading in screening mammography. *AJR. American Journal of Roentgenology, 189*(5), 1135–1141. doi:10.2214/AJR.07.2393

Giger, M., Huo, Z., Vyborny, C., Lan, L., Bonta, I., & Horsch, K. (2002). *Intelligent CAD workstation for breast imaging using similarity to known lesions and multiple visual prompt aids.* Paper presented at the SPIE.

Grossman, D. A., & Frieder, O. (1998). *Information retrieval: algorithms and heuristics.* Boston: Kluwer.

Guimond, A., & Subsol, G. (1997). Automatic MRI Database Exploration and Applications. *Pattern Recognition and Artificial Intelligence, 11*(8), 1345–1365. doi:10.1142/S0218001497000627

Guo, G. D., Jain, A. K., Ma, W. Y., & Zhang, H. J. (2002). Learning similarity measure for natural image retrieval with relevance feedback. *IEEE Transactions on Neural Networks, 13*(4), 811–820. doi:10.1109/TNN.2002.1021882

Guyon, I., & Elissee, A. (2003). An Introduction to Variable and Feature Selection. *Journal of Machine Learning Research, 3*, 1157–1182. doi:10.1162/153244303322753616

Hadjiiski, L., Sahiner, B., Helvie, M. A., Chan, H. P., Roubidoux, M. A., & Paramagul, C. (2006). Breast masses: computer-aided diagnosis with serial mammograms. *Radiology, 240*(2), 343–356. doi:10.1148/radiol.2401042099

Hafner, J., Sawhney, H. S., Equitz, W., Flickner, M., & Niblack, W. (1995). Efficient color histogram indexing for quadratic form distance functions. *IEEE Transactions on Pattern Analysis and Machine Intelligence, 17*(7), 729–736. doi:10.1109/34.391417

Hastie, T., & Tibshirani, R. (1996). Discriminant Adaptive Nearest Neighbor Classification. *IEEE Transactions on Pattern Analysis and Machine Intelligence, 18*(6), 10. doi:10.1109/34.506411

Jing, F., Li, M., Zhang, H. J., & Zhang, B. (2004). An efficient and effective region-based image retrieval framework. *IEEE Transactions on Image Processing, 13*(5), 699–709. doi:10.1109/TIP.2004.826125

Kallergi, M. (2004). Computer-aided diagnosis of mammographic microcalcification clusters. *Medical Physics, 31*, 314–326. doi:10.1118/1.1637972

Kennedy, R., Lee, Y., Van Roy, B., Reed, C. D., & Lippman, R. P. (1998). *Solving data mining problems through pattern recognition.* Prentice Hall.

Kinoshita, S. K., de Azevedo-Marques, P. M., Pereira, R. R. Jr, Rodrigues, J. A., & Rangayyan, R. M. (2007). Content-based retrieval of mammograms using visual features related to breast density patterns. *Journal of Digital Imaging, 20*(2), 172–190. doi:10.1007/s10278-007-9004-0

Kolb, T. M., Lichy, J., & Newhouse, J. H. (2002). Comparison of the Performance of Screening Mammography, Physical Examination, and Breast US and Evaluation of Factors that Influence Them: An Analysis of 27,825 Patient Evaluations. *Radiology, 225*(1), 165–175. doi:10.1148/radiol.2251011667

Kopans, D. B. (2007). *Breast imaging* (3rd ed.). Baltimore, MD: Lippincott Williams & Wilkins.

Lehmann, T., Güld, M., & Thies, C. (2003). *Content-based image retrieval in medical applications for picture archiving and communication systems.* Paper presented at the Medical Imaging.

Lehmann, T., Guld, M., Thies, C., Plodowski, B., Keysers, D., & Ott, B. (2004). *IRMA - Content-based image retrieval in medical applications.* Paper presented at the 14th World Congress on Medical Informatics.

Li, Q., Li, F., Shiraishi, J., Katsuragawa, S., Sone, S., & Doi, K. (2003). Investigation of new psychophysical measures for evaluation of similar images on thoracic CT for distinction between benign and malignant nodules. *Medical Physics, 30*, 2584–2593. doi:10.1118/1.1605351

Liu, Y., Lazar, N., & Rothfus, W. (2002). *Semantic-based Biomedical Image Indexing and Retrieval.* Paper presented at the *Int'l Conf. on Diagnositc Imaging and Analysis.*

Malich, A., Fischer, D. R., & Bottcher, J. (2006). CAD for mammography: the technique, results, current role and further developments. *European Radiology, 16*(7), 1449–1460. doi:10.1007/s00330-005-0089-x

Meersman, D., Scheunders, P., & Van Dyck, D. (1998). *Classification of microcalcifications using texture-based features.* Paper presented at the 4th International Workshop on Digital Mammography.

Müller, H., Michoux, N., Bandon, D., & Geissbuhler, A. (2004). A review of content-based image retrieval systems in medical applications-clinical benefits and future directions. *International Journal of Medical Informatics, 73*(1), 1–23. doi:10.1016/j.ijmedinf.2003.11.024

Muller, H., Rosset, A., Garcia, A., Vallee, J. P., & Geissbuhler, A. (2005). Informatics in radiology (infoRAD): benefits of content-based visual data access in radiology. *Radiographics, 25*(3), 849–858. doi:10.1148/rg.253045071

Muller, H., Rosset, A., Vallee, J., & Geissbuhler, A. (2004). *Comparing features sets for content-based image retrieval in a medical-case database.* Paper presented at the *PACS and Imaging Informatics*

Muramatsu, C., Li, Q., Schmidt, R., Suzuki, K., Shiraishi, J., & Newstead, G. (2006). Experimental determination of subjective similarity for pairs of clustered microcalcifications on mammograms: observer study results. *Medical Physics, 33*(9), 3460–3468. doi:10.1118/1.2266280

Muramatsu, C., Li, Q., Suzuki, K., Schmidt, R. A., Shiraishi, J., & Newstead, G. M. (2005). Investigation of psychophysical measure for evaluation of similar images for mammographic masses: preliminary results. *Medical Physics, 32*(7), 2295–2304. doi:10.1118/1.1944913

Mushlin, A. I., Kouides, R. W., & Shapiro, D. E. (1998). Estimating the accuracy of screening mammography: a meta-analysis. *American Journal of Preventive Medicine, 14*(2), 143–153. doi:10.1016/S0749-3797(97)00019-6

Nakayama, R., Uchiyama, Y., Hatsukade, I., Yamamoto, K., Watanabe, R., & Namba, K. (1999). Discrimination of malignant and benign microcalcification clusters on mammograms. *J Comp Aid Diag Med Imag, 3*, 1–7.

Niblack, W., Barber, R., Equitz, W., Flickner, M., Glasman, E., & Petkovic, D. (1993). The QBIC project: Querying images by content using color, texture, and shape. *SPIE Proc. on Storage and Retrieval for Image and Video Databases, 1908*, 137–146.

Peng, J., Bhanu, B., & Qing, S. (1999). Probabilistic feature relevance learining for content-based image retrieval. *Computer Vision and Image Understanding, 75*(1-2), 150–164. doi:10.1006/cviu.1999.0770

Qi, H., & Snyder, W. E. (1999). Content-based image retrieval in picture archiving and communications systems. *Journal of Digital Imaging, 12*(2Suppl 1), 81–83. doi:10.1007/BF03168763

Rakotomamonjy, A. (2003). Variable Selection Using SVM-based Criteria. *Journal of Machine Learning Research, 3*(7/8).

Rogova, G., Stomper, P., & Ke, C.-C. (1999). *Microcalcification texture analysis in a hybrid system for computer-aided mammography.* Paper presented at the Medical Imaging: Image Processing.

Rubner, Y., Tomasi, C., & Guibas, L. J. (1998). *A metric for distributions with applications to image databases.* Paper presented at the Sixth International Conference on Computer Vision, 1998.

Rui, Y., & Huang, T. S. (1998). Relevance feedback: A power tool for interactive content-based image retrieval. *IEEE Transactions on Circuits and Systems for Video Technology, 8*(5).

Sampat, M. P., Markey, M. K., & Bovik, A. C. (2005). Computer-aided detection and diagnosis in mammography. In Bovik, A. C. (Ed.), *Handbook of Image and Video Processing* (2nd ed., pp. 1195–1217). Elsevier. doi:10.1016/B978-012119792-6/50130-3

Shi, J., & Malik, J. (2000). REGULAR PAPERS - Perceptual Grouping - Normalized Cuts and Image Segmentation. *IEEE Transactions on Pattern Analysis and Machine Intelligence, 22*(8), 18.

Shyu, C. R., Brodley, C. E., Kak, A. C., Kosaka, A., Aisen, A., & Broderick, L. S. (1999). ASSERT: A Physician-in-the-loop Content-based Retrieval System for HRCT Image Database. *Computer Vision and Image Understanding, 75*(1-2), 111–132. doi:10.1006/cviu.1999.0768

Sklansky, J., Tao, E. Y., Bazargan, M., Ornes, C. J., Murchison, R. C., & Teklehaimanot, S. (2000). Computer-aided, case-based diagnosis of mammographic regions of interest containing microcalcifications. *Academic Radiology, 7*(6), 395–405. doi:10.1016/S1076-6332(00)80379-7

Smeulders, A. W. M., & Worring, M. (2000). Content-Based Image Retrieval at the End of the Early Years. *IEEE Transactions on Pattern Analysis and Machine Intelligence, 22*(12). doi:10.1109/34.895972

Somol, P., Pudil, P., & Kittler, J. (2004). Fast Branch & Bound Algorithms for Optimal Feature Selection. *IEEE Transactions on Pattern Analysis and Machine Intelligence, 26*(7). doi:10.1109/TPAMI.2004.28

Strickland, R. N., & Hee Il, H. (1996). Wavelet transforms for detecting microcalcifications in mammograms. *Medical Imaging. IEEE Transactions on, 15*(2), 218–229.

Su, Z., Zhang, H., Li, S., & Ma, S. (2003). Relevance feedback in content-based image retrieval: Bayesian framework, feature subspaces, and progressive learning. *IEEE Transactions on Image Processing, 12*(8), 924–937. doi:10.1109/TIP.2003.815254

Swett, H. A., Fisher, P. R., Cohn, A. I., Miller, P. I., & Mutalik, P. G. (1989). Expert system controlled image display. *Radiology, 172*, 487–493.

Swett, H. A., & Miller, P. I. (1987). ICON: a computer-based approach to differential diagnosis in radiology. *Radiology, 163*, 555–558.

Swett, H. A., Mutalik, P. G., Neklesa, V. P., Horvath, L., Lee, C., & Richter, J. (1998). Voice-activated retrieval of mammography reference images. *Journal of Digital Imaging, 11*(2), 65–73. doi:10.1007/BF03168728

Tagare, H. D., Jaffe, C. C., & Duncan, J. (1997). Medical image databases: a content-based retrieval approach. *Journal of the American Medical Informatics Association, 4*(3), 184–198.

Tan, A., Freeman, D. H. Jr, Goodwin, J. S., & Freeman, J. L. (2006). Variation in false-positive rates of mammography reading among 1067 radiologists: a population-based assessment. *Breast Cancer Research and Treatment, 100*(3), 309–318. doi:10.1007/s10549-006-9252-6

Taylor, P., Fox, J., & Pokropek, A. (1999). The development and evaluation of CADMIUM: a prototype system to assist in the interpretation of mammograms. *Medical Image Analysis, 3,* 321–337. doi:10.1016/S1361-8415(99)80027-9

te Brake, G. M., Karssemeijer, N., & Hendriks, J. H. (2000). An automatic method to discriminate malignant masses from normal tissue in digital mammograms. *Physics in Medicine and Biology, 45*(10), 2843–2857. doi:10.1088/0031-9155/45/10/308

Tobin, K. W., Abramoff, M. D., Chaum, E., Giancardo, L., Govindasamy, V. P., Karnowski, T. P., et al. (2008). *Using a patient image archive to diagnose retinopathy.* Paper presented at the Engineering in Medicine and Biology Society, 2008. EMBS 2008. 30th Annual International Conference of the IEEE.

Tot, T. (2005). Correlating the ground truth of mammographic histology with the success or failure of imaging. *Technology in Cancer Research & Treatment, 4*(1), 23–28.

Tourassi, G. D., Harrawood, B., Singh, S., Lo, J. Y., & Floyd, C. E. (2007). Evaluation of information-theoretic similarity measures for content-based retrieval and detection of masses in mammograms. *Medical Physics, 34*(1), 140–150. doi:10.1118/1.2401667

Tourassi, G. D., Ike, R. III, Singh, S., & Harrawood, B. (2008). Evaluating the effect of image preprocessing on an information-theoretic CAD system in mammography. *Academic Radiology, 15*(5), 626–634. doi:10.1016/j.acra.2007.12.013

Tourassi, G. D., Vargas-Voracek, R., Catarious, D. M. Jr, & Floyd, C. E. Jr. (2003). Computer-assisted detection of mammographic masses: a template matching scheme based on mutual information. *Medical Physics, 30*(8), 2123–2130. doi:10.1118/1.1589494

Urbain, J. L. (2005). Breast cancer screening, diagnostic accuracy and health care policies. *Canadian Medical Association Journal, 172*(2), 210–211. doi:10.1503/cmaj.1041498

Vafaie, H., & Imam, I. (1994). *Feature selection methods: Genetic algorithms vs. greedy-like search.* Paper presented at the International Conference on Fuzzy and Intelligent Control Systems.

Vannier, M. W., & Summers, R. M. (2003). Sharing images. *Radiology, 228*(1), 23–25. doi:10.1148/radiol.2281021654

Vapnik, V. (1998). *Statistical Learning Theory.* New York: Wiley.

Wei, C., Li, C., & Wilson, R. (2006). *A Content-based approach to medical image database retrieval Database Modeling for Industrial Data Management: Emerging Technologies and Applications* (pp. 258–291). Hershey, PA: Idea Group Publishing.

Wei, D., Chan, H. P., Helvie, M. A., Sahiner, B., Petrick, N., & Adler, D. D. (1995). Classification of mass and normal breast tissue on digital mammograms: multiresolution texture analysis. *Medical Physics, 22*(9), 1501–1513. doi:10.1118/1.597418

Wei, L., Yang, Y., Nishikawa, R. M., & Jiang, Y. (2005). A study on several machine-learning methods for classification of malignant and benign clustered microcalcifications. *IEEE Transactions on Medical Imaging, 24*(3), 371–380. doi:10.1109/TMI.2004.842457

Wei, L., Yang, Y., Nishikawa, R. M., Wernick, M. N., & Edwards, A. (2005). Relevance vector machine for automatic detection of clustered microcalcifications. *IEEE Transactions on Medical Imaging, 24*(10), 1278–1285. doi:10.1109/TMI.2005.855435

Wei, L., Yang, Y., Wernick, M. N., & Nishikawa, R. M. (2009). Learning of Perceptual Similarity From Expert Readers for Mammogram Retrieval. *Selected Topics in Signal Processing. IEEE Journal of, 3*(1), 53–61.

Xue, Z., Antani, S., Long, L. R., Jeronimo, J., & Thoma, G. R. (2007). Investigating CBIR techniques for cervicographic images. *AMIA... Annual Symposium Proceedings / AMIA Symposium. AMIA Symposium*, 826–830.

Yang, S. K., Moon, W. K., Cho, N., Park, J. S., Cha, J. H., & Kim, S. M. (2007). Screening mammography-detected cancers: sensitivity of a computer-aided detection system applied to full-field digital mammograms. *Radiology, 244*(1), 104–111. doi:10.1148/radiol.2441060756

Yu, S., & Guan, L. (2000). A CAD system for the automatic detection of clustered microcalcifications in digitized mammogram films. *IEEE Transactions on Medical Imaging, 19*(2), 115–126. doi:10.1109/42.836371

Zhao, D. (1993). *Rule-based morphological feature extraction of microcalcifications in mammograms.* Paper presented at the Medical Imaging: Image Processing.

Zheng, B., Lu, A., Hardesty, L. A., Sumkin, J. H., Hakim, C. M., & Ganott, M. A. (2006). A method to improve visual similarity of breast masses for an interactive computer-aided diagnosis environment. *Medical Physics, 33*(1), 111–117. doi:10.1118/1.2143139

Zheng, B., Mello-Thoms, C., Wang, X., & Gur, D. (2007). *Improvement of visual similarity of similar breast masses selected by computer-aided diagnosis schemes.* Paper presented at the 4th IEEE International Symposium on Biomedical Imaging: From Nano to Macro.

Zheng, L., Wetzel, A. W., Gilbertson, J., & Becich, M. J. (2003). Design and analysis of a content-based pathology image retrieval system. *IEEE Transactions on Information Technology in Biomedicine, 7*(4), 249–255. doi:10.1109/TITB.2003.822952

Chapter 24
Feature Evaluation and Classification for Content-Based Medical Image Retrieval System

Ivica Dimitrovski
Ss. Cyril and Methodius University in Skopje, Macedonia

Suzana Loskovska
Ss. Cyril and Methodius University in Skopje, Macedonia

ABSTRACT

Image retrieval in general and content-based image retrieval (CBIR) in particular are well-known research fields in information management. A large number of methods have been proposed and investigated in both areas but satisfactory general solution has not still been developed. The aim of this research is to develop highly flexible web-based system for storage, organization and retrieval of medical images. The system besides text and metadata retrieval also supports querying by image to find visually similar images to presented query. Several algorithms and techniques were implemented in the system to support content-based retrieval. For efficient and reliable search machine learning techniques were included in the system.

INTRODUCTION

The number of digital images is rapidly increasing, prompting the necessity for efficient image storage and retrieval systems. The management and the indexing of these large image and information repositories are becoming increasingly complex. Therefore, tools for efficient archiving, browsing and searching images are required.

A straightforward way of using the existing information retrieval tools for visual material, is to annotate records by keywords and then to use the text-based query for database retrieval. Several approaches were proposed to use keyword annotations for image indexing and retrieval (Datta, 2008). These approaches are not adequate, since annotating images by textual keywords is neither desirable nor possible in many cases. Therefore, new approaches of indexing, browsing and retrieval of images are required.

DOI: 10.4018/978-1-61520-777-0.ch024

Copyright © 2010, IGI Global. Copying or distributing in print or electronic forms without written permission of IGI Global is prohibited.

For very large image databases, manual description and annotation of every image is time-consuming and impractical. Rather than relaying on manual indexing and text description for every image, images can be represented by numerical features extracted directly from the image pixels. These features are stored in the database, as a signature together with the images and are used to measure similarity between the images in the retrieval process. This approach is known as Content-based Image Retrieval (CBIR).

The aim of CBIR systems is searching and finding similar multimedia items based on their content. Every CBIR system considers offline indexing phase and online content-based retrieval phase. The visual contents of the database images are extracted and described by multidimensional feature vectors in offline phase. The feature vectors of the database images form the feature database. In the second or online retrieval phase, the query-by-example (QbE) paradigm is commonly used. The user presents a sample image, and the system computes the features vector for the sample, compares it to those vectors for images stored in the database, and returns all images with similar features vectors. The query provided by the user can be a region, a sketch or group of images.

The quality of response depends on the image features and the distance or similarity measure used to compare features of different images. Regarding the features, different approaches are used but the most common for image content representation are color, shape and texture features.

Content-based image retrieval can be applied in various areas (Datta, 2008). The medicine is one of the most prospective application areas, because the growing number of digital image acquisition equipment in hospitals such as: X-ray, computed tomography (CT), magnetic resonance imaging (MR), positron emission tomography (PET), ultrasound, endoscopy and laparoscopy raises demands for new approaches of storing and accessing images. Therefore, the tasks of efficiently storing, processing and retrieving

medical image data have become important research topic.

The medical community proposes inclusion of content-based image retrieval into picture archiving and communication systems (PACS) (Muller, 2003). The PACS integrates imaging modalities and interfaces with hospital and departmental information systems to manage storage and distribution of images to medical personal, researchers, clinics, and imaging centers. The important requirement of PACS is an efficient search function to access required images. A well known standard for medical images is Digital Imaging and Communications in Medicine (DICOM). File header for every image stored in DICOM format, contains information regarding image modality, acquisition device, and patient identification. At present, image search in medicine is carried out according to the alphanumerical order of these textual attributes. But users commonly have the visual content of medical images as starting information. The content of the images is a powerful query which can be used to search for images with similar content. Therefore, content-based approaches are expected to have a great impact on PACS, Radiology Information Systems (RIS), Pathology Information Systems and Hospital Information Systems (HIS). Even medical image databases that are not part of any PACS can benefit from CBIR technology, because CBIR technology supports any work that requires finding images or collections of images with similar contents. For example, medical researchers can use CBIR system to find images with similar pathological areas and investigate their association. Medical student will be provided by a system that enables efficient search for images with given pathological attributes. Additionally, CBIR can be used to collect images for medical books, reports, papers, and CD-ROMs where typical specimens are organized according to the similarity of their features.

This chapter describes the highly flexible web-based system for storing, organizing and retrieving medical images. The chapter is organized as follows. In the first section we present an extensive overview of image features proposed for CBIR and implemented in the system, including features that were proposed in the early days of CBIR and features that were proposed only recently. In the second section we give a quantitative analysis of their performances and direction for improvements using the features for content-based image retrieval in combination with different clustering methods. In the third section we examine the image classification techniques for image organization and retrieval. We present the hierarchical multi label classification and the hierarchical classification scheme for image modality classification.

BACKGROUND

Although content-based image retrieval has frequently been proposed for use in medical image management, only a few content-based retrieval systems have been developed specially for medical images. These systems are mostly research-oriented systems implemented in research institutes.

Automatic Search and Selection Engine with Retrieval Tools (ASSERT) is developed by Purdue University, Indiana University, and University of Wisconsin Hospital, USA (Shyu, 1999). The system uses lung images produced by High-Resolution Computed Tomography (HRCT). The ASSERT system uses a physician-in-the-loop approach to retrieve relevant images. The users mark the outline of the pathology regions and identify anatomical landmarks for each image. Then the system extracts 255 features of texture, shape, edges, and gray-scale properties in pathology regions. The optimization of the retrieval process is done by constructing a multi-dimensional hash table to index the HRCT images.

CasImage is another medical CBIR system (Rosset, 2002). The system is implemented in University Hospital of Geneva, Switzerland. The image database contains variety of images like CT,

MRI, radiographs, and even color images. The CasImage system has been integrated into a PACS environment. It contains a teaching and reference database, and the medGIFT content-based image retrieval system. The medGIFT system is adapted from the open-source GIFT system (Squire, 2000). The medGIFT retrieval system extracts global and regional color and texture features, including 166 colors in the HSV (hue, saturation, value) color space, and Gabor filter responses in four directions each at three different scales. The medical image retrieval is a combination of text based and visual features based retrieval.

Image Retrieval in Medical Applications (IRMA) system developed by Aachen University of Technology, Germany uses various imaging modalities (Lehmann, 2000). The IRMA system is implemented as a platform for content-based image retrieval in medical applications. This system splits the image retrieval process into seven consecutive steps, including categorization, registration, feature extraction, feature selection, indexing, identification, and retrieval.

Moustakas (Moustakas, 2005) presents platform for medical image retrieval based on two-level architecture inspired from human cognitive mechanisms. The first tier of the architecture is concerned with a general description of the images. In the second tier a serial analysis of specific regions of interest is performed. The author uses brain MRI images to prove the usability of this concept as a part of a tool for medical decision support.

The authors in (Moller, 2007) propose system architecture for an automatic large-scale medical image understanding which aims at a formal fusion of feature extraction techniques operating on the bit-level representation of images with formal background knowledge represented in ontology. CBIR methods are often implemented for specific domain or specific type of medical images (Wei, 2005; Zhao, 2004; Dy, 2003). More detailed overview of content-based retrieval in medical application can be found in (Muller, 2003).

FEATURES FOR CBIR

Features can be grouped into the following types: color features, texture features, local features, and shape features. Most of the medical images collections contain various images from gray scale images (X-rays, CT scans, MRI ...) to color images (retionographic, endoscopic, microscopic ...). To differentiate the image types we selected features that capture and describe different aspects of the image content. The color and shape features are used to capture the image content regarding the modality and the anatomic region. Within the modalities the images could be discriminated by structure and texture. We therefore choose several texture features and local features invariant to translation and rotation.

Appearance-Based Image Feature

The most straightforward approach in content based retrieval is direct use of the image pixel values as features. The images are scaled to a common size and compared by Euclidean distance. We used a 32×32 down-sampled representation of the images and this has been compared using the Euclidean distance. It has been shown that for classification and retrieval of medical radiographs, this method serves as a reasonable baseline (Keysers, 2007).

Color Features

Color is an important feature for image representation which is widely used in CBIR systems (Sudhamani, 2007). The performance of the color descriptors highly depends of the color space used in the process of descriptor generation. Although most of the images are represented in the RGB (red, green and blue) color space, this space is rarely used for indexing and querying in CBIR systems because it does not correspond well to the human color perception. Other spaces such as HSV or the International Commission on Il-

lumination (CIE) Lab and Luv spaces suit better to human perception and are more frequently used. We used three color descriptors: color moment, color histogram, and color coherence vector (CCV) in our research.

Color Moments

Color moments are compact representation of the color (Faloutsos, 1994). This descriptor is very suitable for images that contain only one object. It has been shown that most of the color distribution information is captured by three low-order moments. The first-order moment (μ) captures the mean color, the second-order moment (σ) captures the standard deviation, and the third-order moment captures the color skewness (θ). These three low-order moments (μ_i, σ_i, θ_i) are extracted for each of the three color planes, using the following mathematical formulation:

$$\mu_i = \frac{1}{N} \sum_{j=1}^{N} f_{ij}$$

$$\sigma_i = \left[\frac{1}{N} \sum_{j=1}^{N} (f_{ij} - \mu_i)^2 \right]^{\frac{1}{2}}$$

$$\theta_i = \left[\frac{1}{N} \sum_{j=1}^{N} (f_{ij} - \mu_i)^3 \right]^{\frac{1}{3}}$$

where f_{ij} is value of the i-th color component of the j-th pixel of the image, N is the total number of pixels in the image. As a result, we need to extract only nine parameters (three moments for each of the three color planes) to describe the color image. The best results are obtained in combination with HSV color space. The color moments can be used to separate gray scale versus color medical images (Lacoste, 2007). In our case color moments are most suitable for representing gross photography of organ because these images contain only one object.

Color Histogram

The color histogram represents the color content of an image. It is robust to translation and rotation. A histogram is the distribution of the number of pixels in an image. Histograms are made up of bins that represent a certain intensity value range. The histogram is computed by examining all pixels in the image and assigning each pixel to a bin depending on its intensity. The final value of a bin is the number of pixels assigned to it. The number of bins is usually in the order of the square root of the number of pixels. Color histogram is a global property of an image and it does not consider the spatial information of pixels. Therefore, different images may have similar color distributions. Large image database increases the probability two images to have same histogram. To avoid this joint histogram (Pass, 1999) and color coherence vector feature (Pass, 1997) are proposed. The color histogram has limited applicability in medical images but is good to distinguish color images from X-rays and other gray scale images. For example the color histogram can be applied in medical image collections that often contain images with power point presentations of diagnosis or images from medical personal or surgeries.

Color Coherence Vector

In Color Coherence Vector (CCV), each histogram bin is partitioned into two types, coherent and incoherent. If the pixel value belongs to a large uniformly-colored region, it is referred to coherent otherwise it is classified as incoherent pixel (Pass, 1997). In other words, coherent pixels are parts of a contiguous region in an image, while incoherent pixels are not. Each color in the image is represented by coherent and incoherent bins. The color coherence vector gives the best results if it is applied in combination with HSV color space.

Texture Features

Texture has emerged as an important visual primitive for searching and browsing large collection of similar looking patterns. An image can be considered as a mosaic of homogeneous textures so the texture features associated to the image regions can be used to index and retrieve image data (Manjunath, 2001). In medical image retrieval, an effective representation of texture is required to distinguish the images with same modality and layout. We used four texture descriptors: Tamura features, global texture descriptor, wavelets transform coefficients and Gabor features in our research.

Tamura Features

Tamura (Tamura, 1978) proposes six texture features: coarseness, contrast, directionality, line-likeness, regularity, and roughness. Experiments show that the first three features are very important in the context of human perception (Tamura, 1978). So, we use coarseness, contrast, and directionality to create a texture histogram. The histogram consists of 512 coefficients. In the QBIC system (Faloutsos, 1994) histograms of these features are used as well. Tamura features are already used for medical image retrieval in (Gild, 2006).

Global Texture Descriptor

In the system we implemented the global texture feature described in (Terhorst, 2003). The global texture descriptor is 43 dimensional vector. It consists of a value for the fractal dimension, a value for the coarseness, a value for the entropy, 32 values for the difference statistics, and eight values for the circular Moran autocorrelation function. Fractal dimension measures the roughness of a surface and it is calculated using the reticular cell counting method (Rao, 1990). Coarseness characterizes the grain size of an image. It is calculated using the variance of the image. Entropy of pixel values is used as a measure of the disorder in the image. The spatial gray-level difference statistics describe the brightness relationship of pixels within neighborhoods also known as co-occurrence matrix analysis. The circular Moran autocorrelation function measures the roughness of the texture (Gu, 1989). This descriptor has been successfully used for medical images in (Lehmann, 2005).

Wavelets Transform Coefficients

Multi-resolution wavelet analysis provides representations of image data in which both spatial and frequency information are present (Idris, 1997). In multi-resolution wavelet analysis we have four bands for each level of resolution resulting from the application of two filters, a low-pass filter (L) and a high-pass filter (H). The filters are applied in pairs in the four combinations, LL, LH, HL and HH, and followed by a decimation phase that halves the resulting image size. The final image, of the same size as the original, contains a smoothed version of the original image (LL band) and three bands of details. Each band corresponds to a coefficient matrix that can be used to reconstruct the original image. These bands contain information about the content of the image in terms of general image layout (the LL band) and in terms of details (edges, textures, etc...). In our procedure the features are extracted from the luminance image using a three-step Daubechies multi-resolution wavelet decomposition that uses 16 coefficients and producing ten sub-bands (Scheunders, 1998). Two energy features, the mean and standard deviation of the coefficients, are then computed for each of the obtained ten sub-bands, resulting in a 20-valued descriptor. This descriptor is often used in medical CBIR systems (Lamard, 2007) mostly for images from diabetic retinopathy and mammography databases.

Gabor Features

Gabor features have been widely used for texture analysis (Palm, 2000). We extract Gabor features at different scales and directions from the images and calculate the mean and standard deviation of the filter responses. In our system we use five different orientations and five different scales leading to a 50 dimensional vector. Gabor features are mainly used for retrieving medical images from CT scan and MRI. Authors in (Datteri, 2008) and (Jiang, 2008) report good retrieval accuracy of the Gabor features applied for Lung and Hepatic CT images. The authors in (Glatard, 2004) report good retrieval results for cardiac MRIs based on Gabor filter features extraction technique.

Local Features

Many different techniques for detecting and describing local image regions have been developed (Mikolajczyk, 2005). The Scale Invariant Feature Transform (SIFT) was proposed as a method of extracting and describing keypoints which are reasonably invariant to changes in illumination, image noise, rotation, scaling, and small changes in viewpoint (Lowe, 2004). The SIFT algorithm has four major stages.

1) **Scale-space extremes detection**: The first stage searches over scale space using a Difference of Gaussian function to identify potential points of interest.
2) **Keypoint localization**: The location and scale of each candidate point is determined and keypoints are selected according on stability measures.
3) **Orientation assignment**: One or more orientations are assigned to each keypoint based on local image gradients.
4) **Keypoint descriptor**: A descriptor is generated for each keypoint from local image gradients at the scale found in stage 2.

An important aspect of the algorithm is that it generates a large number of features over a broad range of scales and locations. The number of generated features is dependent on image size and content, as well as algorithm parameters. A typical image of 500x500 pixels will generate approximately 2000 keypoints. The dimension of this feature is extremely high because the size of the keypoint descriptor is 128 dimensional vector.

For content based image retrieval good response times are required and this is hard to achieve using the huge amount of data obtained by local features. To reduce the dimensionality we use histograms of local features (Deselaers, 2003). With this approach the amount of data is reduced by estimating the distribution of local features for every image. First a clustering algorithm is applied to a reasonably large set of local features. In the experiments we used the 30 strongest keypoints obtained in the second stage of the algorithm. To create a local feature histogram, the local features are extracted and for every local feature the best representing cluster is selected. Then a histogram of these cluster memberships is created. This process allows simple adjustments of the data amount because the histogram has the same number of bins as the number of clusters. The K-means algorithm was applied in the clustering process, and experimentally we have shown that the optimal number of clusters is 400 (Dimitrovski, 2008). Within the modalities the images are discriminated by structure and texture. Therefore the local features invariant to translation and rotation are crucial for narrowing down the search.

MPEG-7 Features

The Moving Picture Experts Group (MPEG) has defined several visual descriptors in their MPEG-7 standard. An extensive overview of these descriptors can be found in (Manjunath, 2002). The MPEG-7 standard defines features that are computationally inexpensive to obtain and compare and strongly optimizes the features with respect to the required storage memory. In our research we used several MPEG-7 features.

MPEG-7: Color Layout Descriptor

The medical image collections usually contain a large number of gray scale images, such as X-rays and CT scans, with very specific layout. The patients are positioned very precisely to show the area under investigation at the centre of the image. The image layout can be used to indicate both the modality and anatomic region. For this reason visual color layout descriptor was used to detect images with similar layouts. This descriptor represents very compact form of the color spatial distribution in the image (Manjunath, 2002). This characteristic supports high retrieval efficiency with very small computational costs. The descriptor is suitable for queries by sketch because it captures the layout information of color features. This is a clear advantage over other color descriptors. The Color Layout Descriptor (CLD) is calculated by generating an 8x8 grid followed by a discrete cosine transform (DCT) and encoding resulting coefficients. The feature extraction process consists of two parts; grid based selection of representative color and DCT transform with quantization. An input picture is divided into 64 (8x8) blocks and their average colors are derived. The derived average colors are transformed into a series of coefficients using 8x8 DCT. A few low frequency coefficients are selected and quantized to form the descriptor. The color space adopted for CLD is YCrCb.

MPEG-7: Color Structure Descriptor

The Color Structure Descriptor captures both color content and information about the colors spatial arrangement. It is a histogram that counts how many times a color is present in an 8x8 windowed neighborhood, as this window progresses over the image rows and columns (Manjunath,

2002). This enables to distinguish, for example, between images in which pixels of each color are distributed uniformly and an image in which the same colors occur in the same proportions, but are located in distinct blocks. It is extracted in hue, min, max, difference (HMMD) color space with a non-uniform quantization using 256, 128, 64 or 32 bins. Because this feature provides discrimination between images with same global color distribution but different local color structures it is suited for color medical images which tend to have similar overall color but different structure depending on the details of the image. In our research the color structure descriptor was applied for retrieving microscopic images.

MPEG-7: Edge Histogram Descriptor

The distribution of edges is a good texture signature that is useful for image matching even when the underlying texture is not homogeneous. The edge histogram descriptor represents the spatial distribution of five types of edges (four directional edges and one non directional). It consists of local histograms of the edge directions, which may optionally be aggregated into global or semi-global histograms (Manjunath, 2002). The image is divided in 4x4 non-overlapping sub-images where the relative frequencies of five different edge types (vertical, horizontal, 45°, 135°, non-directional) are calculated by 2x2-sized edge detectors for the pixels luminance. The descriptor is obtained with a nonlinear mapping of the relative frequencies to discrete values. The edge histogram descriptor contains 80 bins (five bins for each sub-image). In our research the edge histogram descriptor was used for automatic annotation and retrieval of X-ray images (Dimitrovski & Kocev, 2008).

MPEG-7: Homogenous Texture Descriptor

The homogeneous texture descriptor provides a precise quantitative description of a texture (Manjunath, 2002). The descriptor contains 62 coefficients extracted using a bank of orientation and scale tuned filters modeled by Gabor functions. The first and the second energy moments in the frequency domain in the corresponding sub-bands are used as the components of the texture descriptor. The number of filters is 5x6 = 30 where five is the number of scales and six is the number of directions in the multi-resolution decomposition using Gabor functions. The descriptor is computed by filtering using scale and orientation selective kernels.

MPEG-7: Region Shape Descriptor

An object may consist of a single region, a set of regions or it can contain holes. The region shape descriptor uses all pixels constituting the shape within a frame thus it can describe a complex shape that consists of holes or several disjoint regions. The region shape descriptor is robust to minor deformation along the boundary of the object. The descriptor is characterized by its small size, fast extraction time and matching. The region based shape descriptor belongs to the broad class of shape analysis techniques based on moments (Manjunath, 2002). It uses a complex 2D Angular Radial Transformation and from each shape, as set of ART coefficients are extracted. The region based shape descriptor has 35 coefficients.

CBIR SYSTEM

The architecture of the implemented content-based medical image retrieval system is presented in Figure 1. The system includes two main subsystems: the server and the client sub-system. The server sub-system handles the process of feature extraction, feature matching and system learning or offline phase. The client sub-system handles the process of querying or online phase.

The application was developed by Microsoft Visual Studio 2008™. Images are stored in Microsoft SQL Server 2005™ database. The libraries

Figure 1. Overview of System Architecture

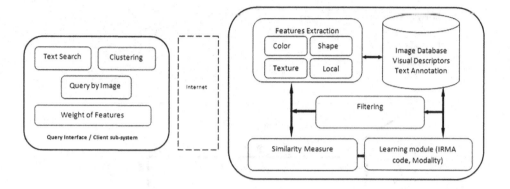

for descriptor generation were implemented in C++ using several image processing libraries as ImageMagick®, OpenCV™, ... The algorithms for machine learning (Support Vectors Machine - SVM, k-means, X-means) were implemented in C++, and the algorithm for the hierarchical multi-label classification was implemented in Java (Dimitrovski & Kocev, 2008).

The image database besides the medical images contains metadata information: format, date of creation and text description for every image. The metadata information enables text retrieval in the system. To add images to the database, the system calculates the color, texture, shape and local features and saves them in the database. The X-ray image classification module enables to store IRMA code for X-ray images in the database, too. The IRMA code allows text based retrieval because in the IRMA coding scheme each code have corresponding text annotation (Muller, 2008). The module for image modality detection classifies images according to modality and eliminates the irrelevant images for the presented query image or text description. This process enables to speedup the retrieval process because in this process the system considers only the images with the same modality as the query image.

The user can retrieve images by providing sample image or text description. The text retrieval is supported by the Microsoft SQL Server 2005 capabilities for text indexing and retrieval. The

user interface supports combination of the text retrieval and content-based retrieval, too. After the user loads a query image, selects the features and sets the weight for these features as presented in Figure 2, the query server receives the query messages.

It passes the image and selected features to the feature extraction, similarity and filtering mechanisms. The feature extraction mechanism will send the feature information of query image to the similarity measure and filtering mechanisms. According to the feature information, the filter mechanism (module for image modality classification) will predict the image modality class and get the feature records of relevant images from the image database. The similarity measure mechanism calculates the similarity of feature information between the query image and database images and returns the results to the interface at the client side.

The system supports integration of new visual descriptors, retrieval metrics or image classification modules for automatic text annotation or modules for decision and diagnosis support because it's modular architecture. The client sub-system (web interface) is independent from the server side application.

Grouping of Visually Similar Images

Image databases with image text annotations (descriptions) are still quite common. A major

Figure 2. Query example based on color feature

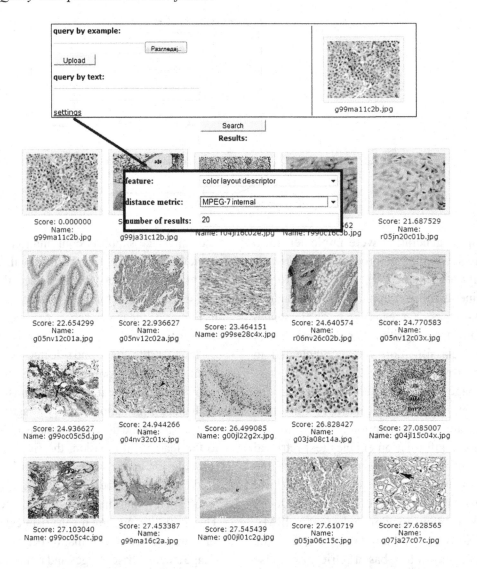

drawback of this method is that annotations are often ambiguous. Even for words with less ambiguity nearly always two groups of images are returned: one group of images that fulfill requirements and the other group without suitable images. To improve the text retrieval we propose to apply methods of computer vision in combination with clustering methods to group results from the text retrieval into groups with visually similar images. The developed application provides access to nearly all features introduced in previous sections and enables selection of Expectation Maximiza-tion (EM) (Carson, 2002), K-means (Kanugo, 2002) and X-means (Pelleg, 2000) clustering algorithms. After the clustering process is finished the images are shown in groups.

BENCHMARK DATABASES FOR CBIR

We used two image bases for feature evaluation. The IRMA-2007 database consists of 12,000 fully annotated radiographs taken randomly from medical routine at the RWTH Aachen University

Figure 3. Example images from IRMA-2007 database

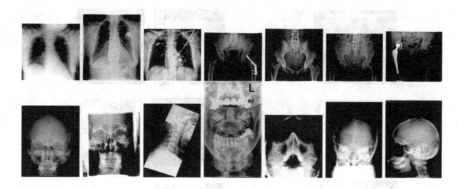

Hospital (Muller, 2008). The images are split into 11000 training and 1000 test images. The images are subdivided into 116 classes based on the hierarchical IRMA code (Lehmann, 2003). This code distinguishes images along the modality, body orientation, body region and biological system axis. For CBIR, the relevance's are defined by the classes. Given a query image from a certain class, all database images from the same class are considered relevant. Figure 3 presents example images.

The image clustering was evaluated by the medical image database available for the Image-Clef 2008 medical retrieval task (Muller, 2008). This database contains 67114 medical images. The images are at different resolution, quality and obtained with various techniques. Example images from this database are presented in Figure 4. Each image has associated XML document that contains the metadata information and text annotation.

PERFORMANCE EVALUATION OF FEATURES

Retrieval Metric

Let the database contains images denoted by $\{x_1,...,x_i,...,x_N\}$ and each image (x_i) is represented by a feature vector $\{x_{i0},...,x_{ij},...,x_{im}\}$. To retrieve similar images to a presented query image q, the system computes the distance function $d(q, x_i)$ for each database image x_i with the query image. The distance function is defined by the distance between the feature vector of the query image and the feature vectors of images in the database. Then, the database images are sorted to fulfill the following distance relation $d(q, x_i) \le d(q, x_{i+1})$ for each pair of images x_i and x_{i+1} in the sequence $(x_1,..., x_i,..., x_N)$.

The distance functions were selected according to previous research and experiments concerning their influence in the retrieval process (Puzicha, 1999). The distances are normalized to be in the same value range and a linear combination of the distances is used to create the ranking.

Several performance measures based on the precision P and the recall R have been proposed for CBIR systems evaluation (Muller, 2001). The precision and the recall are defined by the following equations:

$$P = \frac{\textit{Number of relevant images retrieved}}{\textit{Total number of images retrieved}}$$

$$R = \frac{\textit{Number of relevant images retrieved}}{\textit{Total number of relevant images}}$$

Precision and recall values are usually represented by a precision-recall-graph R -> P(R)

Figure 4. Example images from ImageClef 2008 medical retrieval task

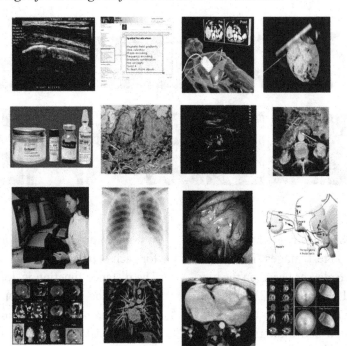

summarizing (R, P(R)) pairs for varying numbers of retrieved images. The most common approach to summarize this graph into one value is the mean average precision (*MAP*). The average precision *AP* for a single query q is the mean over the precision scores after each retrieved relevant item:

$$AP(q) = \frac{1}{N_R} \sum_{n=1}^{N_R} P_q(R_n)$$

where R_n is the recall after the n-th relevant image was retrieved. N_R is the total number of relevant documents for the query. The mean average precision MAP is the mean of the average precision scores over all queries:

$$MAP = \frac{1}{|Q|} \sum_{q \in Q} AP(q)$$

where Q is the set of queries q. An advantage of the mean average precision is that it contains both precision and recall oriented aspects and is sensitive to the entire ranking.

We also calculate the classification error rate *ER* for all experiments. In this performance evaluation we consider only the most similar image from the correct class according to the applied distance function. We consider a query image to be classified correctly, if the most similar retrieved image is from the correct class. Otherwise the query is misclassified. The ER is defined as follows:

$$ER = \frac{1}{|Q|} \sum_{q \in Q} \begin{cases} 0 \ \textit{if the most similar image is (relevant) from the correct class} \\ 1 \ \textit{otherwise} \end{cases}$$

This approach is suitable if the database consists of images labeled with classes like the IRMA database. For databases where images are not classified the corresponding relevant images for selected query image are subjectively chosen by the user. The ER is equal to $1 - P(1)$, where $P(1)$ is the precision after one image retrieved. It was experimentally shown that the error rate and the precision after 50 image ($P(50)$), are correlated

Table 1. Experimental results

Descriptor	ER (%)	MAP (%)
32×32	36.4	53.7
Gray-scale histogram	57.3	37.2
MPEG-7 color layout	59.0	36.7
MPEG-7 edge histogram	31.2	62.6
MPEG-7 homogeneous texture	68.1	34.4
MPEG-7 region-based shape	58.3	34.1
Tamura features	48.5	43.2
Global texture descriptor	72.7	23.0
Gabor vector	51.1	40.7
SIFT histogram	28.5	55.2

Table 2. Results for image clustering

Text query	Image modality	Number of retrieved images	Number of clusters
pulmonary embolism	X-ray, Gross images, CT scan	452	9
giant cell	Microscopic	145	4
tuberous sclerosis	Gross image, MRI, Microscopic	538	11
Merkel cell carcinoma	CT scan	24	1
Budd-Chiari malformation	X-ray	86	3
bone cysts	X-ray	74	3
muscle cells	Microscopic	131	6
MRI or CT of colonoscopy	MRI, CT scan	282	7
CT liver abscess	CT scan	68	3
Fractures	X-ray	533	9

with a coefficient of 0.96 and thus they essentially describe the same property (Deselaers, 2004). The precision oriented evaluation is necessary, because most searching engines, both for images and text, return between 10 and 50 results for a given query.

Experimental Results and Discussion

For all experiments, we report the mean average precision and the classification error rate. Both measures have advantages. The error rate is very strict measure and thus it is the best if relevant images are retrieved early. On the contrary, the mean average precision accounts for the average performance over the complete PR graph.

The results from the feature experiments on the IRMA-2007 database are given in Table 1. It shows that different features perform differently on the selected database. The SIFT histogram is most suitable for the selected database (with error rate equals to 28.5%, and mean average precision approximately equals to 55.2%). The edge histogram that is a part of the MPEG-7 standard also gave good results (error rate equals to 31.2%, and mean average precision approximately equals

to 62.6%). The simple appearance-based feature of 32×32 thumbnails of the images is the second best feature. Among the texture features (Tamura texture histogram, Gabor features, global texture descriptor, MPEG-7 edge histogram and MPEG-7 homogenous texture), the MPEG-7 edge histogram outperforms the others. The global texture descriptor and the MPEG-7 homogenous texture descriptor performed worse and are not suitable for the selected database.

To evaluate the image clustering method we used the query topics from the ImageClef 2008 medical retrieval task (Muller, 2009). The experimental results for the image clustering are presented in Table 2. The table summarizes the text queries used for text based image retrieval, the total number of retrieved images and number of clusters obtained after applying the image clustering.

Several experiments were made to obtain the best combination of feature descriptors and clustering algorithms. The best results were achieved using EM and feature vector formed with concatenation of color structure descriptor and Tamura features. The presented results in Table 2 were obtained using these parameters. Figure 5 shows the first 54 images that are retrieved using the phrase "pulmonary embolism".

Figure 6 shows the result of clustering images queried with "pulmonary embolism". The visually similar images belong to one cluster.

Image Classification

Image classification is advantageous when the image database is well specified, and labeled training samples are available. Domain-specific collections such as medical image databases are examples where categorization can be beneficial. Classification is typically applied for either automatic annotation, or for organizing images into broad categories for the purpose of retrieval.

Hierarchical Annotation of Medical Images

We developed and evaluated method for automatic annotation of medical images. Our goal was to find out how well image modality, body orientation, body region and biological system can be identified by the visual content of the images. With the automatic annotation an image is classified into set of classes. The classes have predefined text annotation and by classification we assign these text annotations to the corresponding images. The results of the classification can be used for multilingual image annotations as well as for DICOM header corrections.

Problem Definition

To evaluate the proposed method for hierarchical image classification we adopted the medical image annotation task of ImageCLEF 2008 (Deselaers, 2009). The objective of this task is to provide the IRMA code for each image of a given set of medical (radiological) images (Lehmann, 2003). 12,076 classified training images are provided for classifier training. According to the IRMA code, a total of 197 classes are defined. The IRMA coding system consists of four axes:

Figure 5. Retrieved images using "pulmonary embolism"

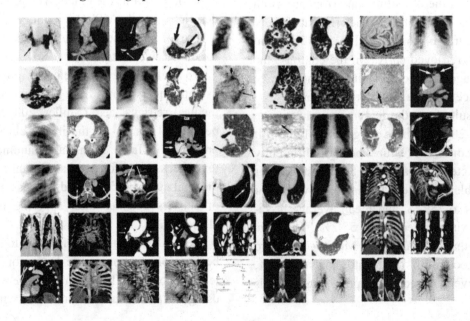

Figure 6. Retrieved images after clustering

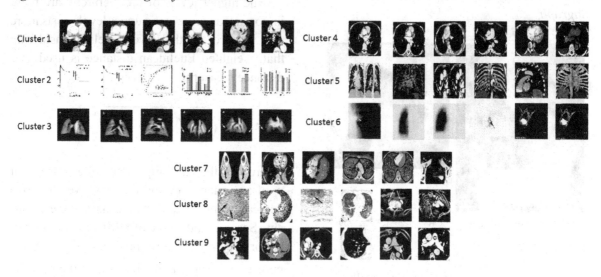

- **T (Technical):** image modality
- **D (Directional):** body orientation
- **A (Anatomical):** body region examined
- **B (Biological):** biological system examined

Every axis is represented by three to four characters that belong to the set {0, …, 9, a, …, z}. This allows a short and unambiguous notation (IRMA: TTTT-DDD-AAA-BBB), where T, D, A, and B denotes a coding or sub-coding digit of the respective axis. Figure 7 presents two examples of unambiguous image classification using the IRMA code.

The image on the left is coded by **1123** (x-ray, projection radiography, analog, high energy) – **211** (sagittal, left lateral descubitus, inspiration) – **520** (chest, lung) – **3a0** (respiratory system, lung). The image of the right is coded by **1220** (x-ray, fluoroscopy, analog) – **127** (coronad, ap, supine) – **722** (abdomen, upper abdomen, middle) – **430** (gastrointestinal system, stomach).

The code is strictly hierarchical – each sub-code element is connected to only one code element. The element to the right is a sub element of the element to the left. For example:

- 2 cardiovascular system
- 21 cardiovascular system; heart
- 216 cardiovascular system; heart; aortic valve

The aortic valve is an element of the heart, which in turn is an element of the cardiovascular system.

To encourage the use of the class hierarchy, the images in the test set belong mainly to classes with only few examples in the training data and thus it is significantly harder to consider this task as a flat classification task. Instead, it is expected that exploiting the hierarchy will lead to large improvements.

Because the classes are organized in a hierarchy we implemented a hierarchical multi-label classification (HMLC) for medical image annotation. We applied Predictive Clustering Trees (PCTs) for HMLC and ensembles of PCTs to accurately classify the images in the IRMA code hierarchy.

Ensembles for PCTs for Hierarchical Multi-Label Classification

In the PCT framework (Blockeel, 1998), a tree is viewed as a hierarchy of clusters: the top-node

Figure 7. IRMA-coded chest and abdomen radiograph

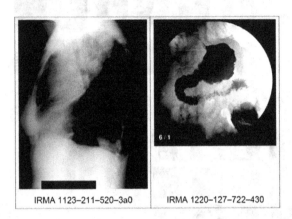

| IRMA 1123–211–520–3a0 | IRMA 1220–127–722–430 |

corresponds to one cluster containing all data, which is recursively partitioned into smaller clusters while moving down the tree. PCTs can be constructed with a standard "top-down induction of decision trees" (TDIDT) algorithm. The heuristic for selecting the tests is the reduction in variance caused by partitioning the instances. Maximizing the variance reduction maximizes cluster homogeneity and improves predictive performance. With instantiation of the variance and prototype function the PCTs can handle different types of data, e.g. multiple targets (Kocev, 2007) or time series (Dzeroski, 2007). A detailed description of the PCT framework can be found in (Blockeel, 1998).

To apply PCTs to the task of HMLC first the example labels are represented as vectors with Boolean components. The i'th component of the vector is 1 if the example belongs to class c_i and 0 otherwise. Then the variance of a set of examples (S) is defined as the average squared distance between each example's label v_i and the mean label $\bar{v}$ of the set, i.e.,

$$Var(S) = \frac{\sum_i d(v_i, \bar{v})^2}{|S|}$$

The higher levels of the hierarchy are more important: an error in the upper levels costs more than an error on the lower levels. Considering that, weighted Euclidean distance is used as a distance measure.

$$d(v_1, v_2) = \sqrt{\sum_i w(c_i)(v_{1,i} - v_{2,i})^2}$$

where $v_{k,i}$ is the i'th component of the class vector v_k of an instance x_k, and the class weights $w(c)$ decrease with the depth of the class in the hierarchy. Second, in the case of HMLC, the notion of majority class does not apply in a straightforward manner. Each leaf in the tree stores the mean $\bar{v}$ of the vectors of the examples that are sorted in that leaf. Each component of $\bar{v}$ is the proportion of examples v_i in the leaf that belong to class c_i. An example arriving in the leaf can be predicted to belong to class c_i if $\bar{v}_i$ is above some threshold t_i. The threshold can be chosen by a domain expert. A detailed description of the PCTs for HMLC can be found in (Vens, 2008).

An ensemble is a set of classifiers constructed with a given algorithm. Each new example is classified by combining the predictions of every classifier from the ensemble. These predictions can be combined by taking the average (for regression tasks) or the majority vote (for classification tasks) (Breiman, 1996; Breiman 2001), or by taking more complex combinations. We consider two ensemble learning techniques that have primarily been used in the context of decision trees: bagging and random forests.

Bagging (Breiman, 1996) constructs the different classifiers by making bootstrap replicates of the training set and using each of these replicates to construct one classifier. Each bootstrap sample is obtained by randomly sampling training instances, with replacement, from the original training set, until an equal number of instances is obtained.

A random forest (Breiman, 2001) is an ensemble of trees, where diversity among the

Figure 8. Precision-recall curves for the T,D,A and B axis, respectively

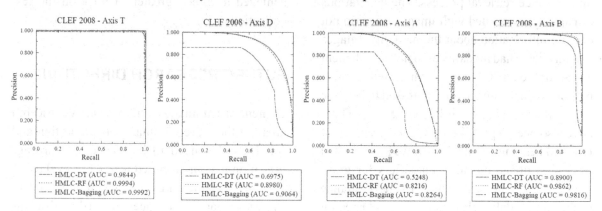

predictors is obtained by using bagging, and by changing the feature set during learning. More precisely, at each node in the decision trees, a random subset of the input attributes is taken, and the best feature is selected from this subset. The number of attributes that are retained is given by a function f of the total number of input attributes x (e.g., $f(x) = 1$, $f(x) = \sqrt{x}$, $f(x) = \lfloor \log_2 x \rfloor + 1$,...). By setting $f(x) = x$, we obtain the bagging procedure. The PCTs for HMLC are used as base classifiers. Average is applied to combine the different predictions because the leaf's prototype is the). To compare the performance of a single tree and an ensemble we use Precision-Recall (PR) curves. The curves presented in Figure 8 are obtained with varying the threshold value: a given threshold corresponds to a single point from the PR-curve. For more information, see (Vens, 2008). To select an optimal threshold value (t), 10-fold cross validation on the training set is performed. From the PR curves, few thresholds can be selected and the predictions of the models for every threshold can be evaluated.

The results from the experiments are shown in Figure 8. For every axis we present a PR curves for the three methods. From the curves we can note the increase of the predictive performance for ensembles over the single tree. The lift in performance that ensembles give to their base classifier was previously noted in the cases of classification and regression (Breiman, 1996; Breiman 2001)

and multiple targets prediction (Kocev, 2007). The excellent performance for the prediction task for axes T and B (AUPRC of 0.9994 and 0.9862) is due to the simplicity of the problem. The hierarchies along these axes contain only few nodes (9 and 27, respectively). This means that in each node in the hierarchy there are nice portion of the examples, thus learning a good classifier is not a difficult task. The classifiers for the other two axes have high predictive performance (AUPRC of 0.9064 and 0.8264), but the predictive task is somewhat more difficult (especially for axis A). The sizes of the hierarchies for axes A and D are 110 and 36 nodes, respectively.

A successful image annotation system highly depends of the performance of its two main components: the feature extractor and the classifier. The feature extraction process should provide a vector of features that best reflects the different aspects for distinguishing one class from the others. When such features are given to a classifier that is able to capture the nature of the task, then the predictive performance of such a classifier will be very high.

AUTOMATIC IMAGE MODALITY BASED CLASSIFICATION

Image modality is an important visual characteristic that can be used to improve and speed up the image retrieval process. The annotations or captions associated with images often do not capture information about the modality. Images that may have had modality associated with them as part of the DICOM header can lose that information when the image is compressed to become a part of a teaching or on-line collection. There have also been reported errors in the accuracy of DICOM headings (Guld, 2002). We have created automatic image modality classifiers for gray-scale and color medical images. The performance of the two modality classifiers was evaluated on the ImageClefMed 2008 database. Both classifiers were created using Support Vector Machines (SVM) for learning. We employed a supervised machine learning approach to problem of medical image modality classification using the hierarchical classification scheme presented in (Kalpathy-Cramer, 2007).

Gray-scale medical images are classified in the following classes: angiography, computerized tomography scans (CT), X-ray, Magnetic resonance (MRI), ultrasound, and scintigraphy. A similar scheme was used to create the modality classifier for color medical images. The color images are categorized into six categories as microscopic, gross photography of organ, EEG/ECG or other charts, power-point slides, endoscopic images and other.

The classification system was created using SVM. Low level color and texture based feature vectors were extracted to train the classifiers. For the gray-scaled images we used combination of texture and intensity histogram features. The classifier for color images was trained using texture and color histogram features extracted in Luv color space. The texture feature was generated using wavelet transformation.

The classifiers were trained on 1500 randomly selected images for every class from the entire database. The 1500 images in the database were randomly split into a training set of 1200 images and a test set of 300 images. Both classifiers

achieved accuracy greater of 96% on the test collections.

FUTURE RESEARCH DIRECTIONS

Content-based image retrieval is active research area but there are still many open question and problems that need to be solved. Feature aggregation in content-based image retrieval using multiple visual features is a challenging problem as various features distances are not directly comparable with each other. In our work we consider only a linear combination of the selected features. Further work in this direction would include implementation of different feature aggregation schemes and adaptation of the feature aggregation schemes to the user queries.

One major obstacle to the development of the CBIR technology is the semantic gap between the extracted low level visual features and users conceptual interpretation of the images. The challenge in bridging this semantic gap is one of the most actively studied areas in CBIR research. Users of CBIR systems are often only interested in specific regions of the image. These regions may capture certain semantic attributes such as objects or events. Unfortunately, these attributes are not well represented using low level visual features. More information is usually required to translate low level features to semantic concept and more abstract representation that correspond to user's perception of the images. In the previous work we consider only automatic image annotation for mapping the low level image characteristics into semantic concepts represented by text description. In the future we must consider integration of relevance feedback technique. The idea is to calculate the discriminate ability of each image feature by using training samples gathered through the relevance feedback cycles. After the feature selection cycle, selected features are used to analyze the rest of the image database and statistical discriminate analysis can be used to adjust the weight of each of the selected features.

Although most of the content-based medical image applications consider large image archives with images from various medical domains, a specialization of the retrieval systems for domains such as dermatology or pathology will be necessary to include as much domain knowledge as possible into the retrieval. This will be necessary for decision support systems such as systems for case based reasoning. Such a specialization can be easily done because of the modularity of our retrieval system. The retrieval process can be considerably improved by image segmentation algorithms and by defining region of interest in the image. This will help to find new relationships among images and certain diseases and multimedia data mining will also be made possible.

CONCLUSION

This chapter describes a content-based medical image retrieval system. For it, we have implemented and tested various feature extraction algorithms. The CBIR system supports metadata and text retrieval and query by image retrieval. The query interface supports inclusion of more than one descriptor in the retrieval process. Through the web interface the user can provide weights for the selected descriptors. Our experiments showed that it is possible to achieve good retrieval performance on a medical image collection using a CBIR approach. The results also show that CBIR can be used as a useful first step in medical image retrieval.

To improve the retrieval performance we include supervised learning mechanism in the retrieval process. Hierarchical multi label classification procedure was proposed for automatic annotation of medical images. The experiment described in the section Image classification shows that clinically relevant information can be extracted out of the images without any user

supervision and parameter tuning for a specific purpose. It demonstrates that some semantic interpretation of the image can be accomplished through low-level feature extraction and classification, although high level query tools will need to add domain-specific knowledge to perform queries responding to specific clinical requests.

REFERENCES

Blockeel, H., De Raedt, L., & Ramon, J. (1998). Top-down induction of clustering trees. In *15th International Conference on Machine Learning* (pp. 55–63)

Breiman, L. (1996). Bagging predictors. *Machine Learning Journal, 24*(2), 123–140. doi:10.1007/BF00058655

Breiman, L. (2001). Random Forests. *Machine Learning Journal, 45*(1), 5–32. doi:10.1023/A:1010933404324

Carson, C., Belongie, S., Greenspan, H., & Malik, J. (2002). Blobworld: Image Segmentation Using Expectation-Maximization and its Application to Image Querying. *IEEE Transactions on Pattern Analysis and Machine Intelligence, 24*(8), 1026–1038. doi:10.1109/TPAMI.2002.1023800

Datta, R., Joshi, D., Li, J., & Wang, J.Z. (2008). Image Retrieval: Ideas, Influences, and Trends of the New Age. *ACM Transactions on Computing Surveys, 40*(5).

Datteri, R., Raicu, D., & Furst, J. (2008). Local versus global texture analysis for lung nodule image retrieval. Medical Imaging 2008: PACS and Imaging Informatics, Vol. 6919 (pp. 691908-691908-9).

Deselaers, T. (2003). *Features for Image Retrieval. Master's theses*. Germany: RWTH Aachen University.

Deselaers, T., & Deserno, T. M. (2009). Medical Image Annotation. ImageCLEF 2008, CLEF Workshop 2008 / Evaluating Systems for Multilingual and Multimodal Information Access (CLEF2008), Aarhus, Denmark.

Deselaers, T., Keysers, D., & Ney, H. (2004). Classification Error Rate for Quantitative Evaluation of Content-based Image Retrieval Systems. In *International Conference on Pattern Recognition: Vol. 2* (pp. 505–508). Cambridge, UK.

Dimitrovski, I. (2008). *System for content-based medical image retrieval. Master's theses, University Ss.* Macedonia: Cyril and Methodius.

Dimitrovski, I., Kocev, D., Loskovska, S., & Dzeroski, S. (2008). Hierarchical annotation of medical images. In 11th International Multiconference, Information Society – IS 2008, Data Mining and Data Warehouses (pp. 170–174). Ljubljana, Slovenia.

Dy, J., Brodley, C., Kak, A. C., Broderick, L., & Aisen, A. (2003). Unsupervised Feature Selection Applied to Content-Based Retrieval of Lung Images. *IEEE Transactions on Pattern Analysis and Machine Intelligence, 25*(3), 373–378. doi:10.1109/TPAMI.2003.1182100

Dzeroski, S., Gjorgjioski, V., Slavkov, I., & Struyf, J. (2007). *Analysis of Time Series Data with Predictive Clustering Trees. Lecture Notes in Computer* (pp. 63–80). Berlin, Heidelberg: Springer.

Faloutsos, C., Barber, R., Flickner, M., Hafner, J., Niblack, W., Petkovic, D., & Equitz, W. (1994). Efficient and Effective Querying by Image Content. *Journal of Intelligent Information Systems, 3*(3/4), 231–262. doi:10.1007/BF00962238

Gild, M. O., Thies, C., Fischer, B., & Lehmann, T. M. (2006). *Content-Based Retrieval of Medical Images by Combining Global Features* (pp. 702–711). LNCS.

Glatard, T., Montagnat, J., & Magnin, I. E. (2004). Texture based medical image indexing and retrieval: application to cardiac imaging. In *Proceedings of ACM Multimedia 2004, Workshop on Multimedia Information Retrieval* (pp. 135–142). New York, USA.

Gu, Z. Q., Duncan, C. N., Renshaw, E., Mugglestone, M. A., Cowan, C. F. N., & Grant, P. M. (1989). Comparison of Techniques for Measuring Cloud Texture in Remotely Sensed Satellite Meteorological Image Data. *Radar and Signal Processing, 136*(5), 236–248.

Guld, M. O., Kohnen, M., Keysers, D., Schubert, H., Wein, B. B., Bredno, J., & Lehmann, T. M. (2002). Quality of DICOM header information for image categorization. *Proceedings of the Society for Photo-Instrumentation Engineers, 4685*, 280–287.

Idris, F., & Panchanathan, S. (1997). Storage and retrieval of compressed images using wavelet vector quantization. *Journal of Visual Languages and Computing, 8*, 289–301. doi:10.1006/jvlc.1997.0041

Jiang, L., Luo, Y., Zhao, J., & Zhuang, T. (2008). Hepatic CT image retrieval based on the combination of Gabor filters and support vector machine. *Chinese Optics Letters, 6*, 495–498. doi:10.3788/COL20080607.0495

Kalpathy-Cramer, J., & Hersh, W. (2007). Automatic Image Modality Based Classification and Annotation to Improve Medical Image Retrieval. In *12th World Congress on Health (Medical) Informatics, Building Sustainable Health Systems* (pp. 1334–1338).

Kanungo, T., Mount, D. M., Netanyahu, N., Piatko, C., Silverman, R., & Wu, A. Y. (2002). An efficient k-means clustering algorithm: Analysis and implementation. *IEEE Transactions on Pattern Analysis and Machine Intelligence, 24*, 881–892. doi:10.1109/TPAMI.2002.1017616

Keysers, D., Deselaers, T., Gollan, C., & Ney, H. (2007). Deformation Models for Image Recognition. *IEEE Transactions on Pattern Analysis and Machine Intelligence, 29*(8), 1422–1435. doi:10.1109/TPAMI.2007.1153

Kocev, D., Vens, C., Struyf, J., & Dzeroski, S. (2007). Ensembles of Multi-Objective Decision Trees. In 18th European conference on Machine Learning (LNAI 4701, pp. 624–631). Warsaw, Poland.

Lacoste, C., Chevallet, J.-P., Lim, J. H., Le Thi Hoang, D., Wei, X., Racoceanu, D., et al. (2007). Inter-Media Concept-Based Medical Image Indexing and Retrieval with UMLS at IPAL. In Evaluation of Multilingual and Multi-Modal information retrieval (LNCS 4730, pp. 694-701).

Lamard, M., Cazuguel, G., Quellec, G., Bekri, L., Roux, C., & Cochener, B. (2007). *Content Based Image Retrieval based on Wavelet Transform coefficients distribution* (pp. 4532–4535). Engineering in Medicine and Biology Society.

Lehmann, T. M., Guld, M.-O., Deselaers, T., Keysers, D., Schubert, H., & Spitzer, K. (2005). Automatic Categorization of Medical Images for Content-based Retrieval and Data Mining. *Computerized Medical Imaging and Graphics, 29*(2), 143–155. doi:10.1016/j.compmedimag.2004.09.010

Lehmann, T. M., Schubert, H., Keysers, D., Kohnen, M., & Wein, B. B. (2003). The IRMA code for unique classification of medical images. *In SPIE Medical Imaging 2003. PACS and Integrated Medical Information Systems: Design and Evaluation, 5033*, 440–451.

Lehmann, T. M., Wein, B., Danmen, J., Bredno, J., Vogelsang, F., & Kohnen, M. (2000). Content-based image retrieval in medical applications: A novel multi-step approach. In Storage and retrieval for media databases Vol. 3972 (pp. 312–320). San Jose CA, USA.

Lowe, D. G. (2004). Distinctive Image Features from Scale-Invariant Keypoints. *International Journal of Computer Vision, 60*(2), 91–110. doi:10.1023/B:VISI.0000029664.99615.94

Manjunath, B. S., Salembier, P., & Sikora, T. (Eds.). (2002). *Introduction to MPEG 7: Multimedia Content Description Language.* Chichester, UK: John Wiley, Sons, Inc.

Mikolajczyk, K., Leibe, B., & Schiele, B. (2005). Local features for object class recognition. In *tenth IEEE International Conference on Computer Vision, Vol. 2* (pp. 1792–1799). Beijing, China.

Moller, M., & Sintek, M. (2007). A Generic Framework for Semantic Medical Image Retrieval. In 2nd international conference on Semantics And digital Media Technologies (SAMT), Knowledge Acquisition from Multimedia Content (KAMC) Workshop. Genova, Italy.

Moustakas, J., Marias, K., Dimitriadis, S., & Orphanoudakis, S. C. (2005). *A Two-Level CBIR Platform with Application to Brain MRI Retrieval* (pp. 1278–1281). Amsterdam, Netherlands: ICME, Multimedia and Expo.

Muller, H., Deselaers, T., Kim, E., Kalpathy–Cramer, J., Deserno, T. M., & Hersh, W. (2008). Overview of the ImageCLEF 2007 Medical Retrieval and Annotation Tasks. Advances in Multilingual and Multimodal Information Retrieval 8th Workshop of the Cross-Language Evaluation Forum, Vol. 5152. Budapest, Hungary.

Muller, H., Kalpathy-Cramer, J., Kahn, C. E., Jr., Hatt, W., Bedrick, S., & Hersh, W. (2009). Overview of the ImageCLEFmed 2008 medical image retrieval task. CLEF Workshop 2008 / Evaluating Systems for Multilingual and Multimodal Information Access (CLEF2008), Aarhus, Denmark.

Muller, H., Michoux, N., Bandon, D., & Geiss-buhler, A. (2003). A Review of Content-Based Image Retrieval Systems in Medical Applications - Clinical Benefits and Future Directions. *International Journal of Medical Informatics, 73*(1), 1–23. doi:10.1016/j.ijmedinf.2003.11.024

Muller, H., Muller, W., Squire, D. McG., March-and-Maillet, S., & Pun, T. (2001). Performance Evaluation in Content-Based Image Retrieval: Overview and Proposals. [Special Issue on Image and Video Indexing]. *Pattern Recognition Letters, 22*(5), 593–601. doi:10.1016/S0167-8655(00)00118-5

Palm, C., Keysers, D., Lehmann, T., & Spitzer, K. (2000). Gabor Filtering of Complex Hue/Saturation Images for Color Texture Classification. In *International Conference on Computer Vision, Pattern Recognition, and Image Processing, Vol. 2* (pp. 45–49). Atlantic City, NJ.

Pass, G., & Zabih, R. (1999). Comparing Images Using Joint Histograms. *Multimedia Systems-Special issue on video content based retrieval, 7*(3), 234–240.

Pass, G., Zabih, R., & Miller, J. (1997). Comparing images using color coherence vectors. In Fourth ACM international conference on Multimedia Proceedings (pp. 65–73).

Pelleg, D., & Moore, A. W. (2000). X-means: Extending K-means with Efficient Estimation of the Number of Clusters. In *Proceedings of the Seventeenth International Conference on Machine Learning* (pp. 727–734).

Puzicha, J., Rubner, Y., Tomasi, C., & Buhmann, J. (1999). Empirical Evaluation of Dissimilarity Measures for Color and Texture. In *International Conference on Computer Vision, Vol. 2* (pp. 1165–1173). Corfu, Greece.

Rao, R. (1990). *A Taxonomy for Texture Description and Identification*. New York: Springer-Verlag.

Rosset, A., Ratib, O., Geissbuhler, A., & Vallee, J. P. (2002). Integration of a Multimedia Teaching and Reference Database in a PACS Environment. *Radiographics, 22*, 1567–1577. doi:10.1148/rg.226025058

Scheunders, P., Livens, S., Van de Wouwer, G., Vautrot, P., & Van Dyck, D. (1998). Wavelet-based texture analysis. *Journal Computer Science and Information management, 1*(2) 22-34.

Shyu, C. R., Brodley, C. E., Kak, A. C., Kosaka, A., Aisen, A. M., & Broderick, L. S. (1999). AS-SERT: A Physician-in-the-Loop Content-Based Retrieval System for HRCT Image Databases. *Computer Vision and Image Understanding, 75*(1–2), 111–132. doi:10.1006/cviu.1999.0768

Squire, D. McG., Muller, W., Muller, H., & Pun, T. (2000). Content based query of image databases: inspirations from text retrieval. *Pattern Recognition Letters (Selected Papers from The 11th Scandinavian Conference on Image Analysis SCIA '99), 21*(13–14), 1193–1198.

Sudhamani, M. V., & Venugopal, C. R. (2007). Grouping and Indexing Color Features for Efficient Image Retrieval. *International Journal of Applied Mathematics and Computer Sciences, 4*(3), 150–155.

Tamura, H., Mori, S., & Yamawaki, T. (1978). Textural Features Corresponding to Visual Perception. *IEEE Transactions on Systems, Man, and Cybernetics, 8*(6), 460–472. doi:10.1109/TSMC.1978.4309999

Terhorst, B. (2003). *Texturanalyse zur globalen Bildinhaltsbeschreibung radiologischer Aufnahmen (Research project)*. Aachen, Germany: RWTH Aachen, Institut fur Medizinische Informatik.

Vens, C., Struyf, J., Schietgat, L., Dzeroski, S., & Blockeel, H. (2008). Decision trees for hierarchical multi-label classification. *Machine Learning Journal, 73*(2), 185–214. doi:10.1007/s10994-008-5077-3

Wei, C. H., Li, C. T., & Wilson, R. (2005). A general framework for content-based medical image retrieval with its application to mammograms. In SPIE, Medical Imaging 2005: PACS and Imaging Informatics Vol. 5748 (pp. 134–143). San Diego, CA, USA.

Zhao, C. G., Cheng, H. Y., Huo, Y. L., & Zhuang, T. G. (2004). Liver CT-image retrieval based on Gabor texture. In *26th Annual International Conference, Engineering in Medicine and Biology Society.*

Chapter 25
Virtual Reality as an Experiential Tool:
The Role of Virtual Worlds in Psychological Interventions

Alessandra Gorini
Istituto Auxologico Italiano, Italy

Andrea Gaggioli
Istituto Auxologico Italiano, Italy

Giuseppe Riva
Istituto Auxologico Italiano, Italy

ABSTRACT

The present chapter illustrates the past and the future of different virtual reality applications for the treatment of psychological disorders. After a brief technical description of the virtual reality systems, the rationale of using virtual reality to treat different psychological disorders, as well as the advantages that the online virtual worlds offer to the promising field of the virtual therapy will be discussed. However, challenges related to the potential risks of the use of virtual worlds and questions regarding privacy and personal safety will also be discussed. Finally, the chapter introduces the concept of "Interreality", a personalized immersive form of e-therapy whose main novelty is a hybrid, closed-loop empowering experience bridging physical and virtual worlds. The main feature of interreality is a twofold link between the virtual and the real world: (a) behavior in the physical world influences the experience in the virtual one; (b) behavior in the virtual world influences the experience in the real one. This is achieved through: (1) 3D shared virtual worlds; (2) bio and activity sensors (that connect the real to the virtual world); (3) mobile internet appliances (that connect the virtual to the real world).

INTRODUCTION

Virtual Reality (VR) is more than a fancy technology: it is an advanced form of human–computer interface that allows users to interact with and become immersed in a computer-generated environment in a naturalistic way. Using visual, aural or haptic devices, the human operator can move and interact with the virtual world, experiencing

DOI: 10.4018/978-1-61520-777-0.ch025

Copyright © 2010, IGI Global. Copying or distributing in print or electronic forms without written permission of IGI Global is prohibited.

the environment as if it were a part of the real world. From a technological point of view, VR is made possible by the capability of computers to synthesize a 3D graphical environment from numerical data. Different input devices sense the subjects' reactions and motions, while the computer modifies the environment accordingly, giving subjects the illusion of interacting with, and being immersed in it.

From a psychological point of view, VR can be considered an advanced imaginative system: an experiential form of imagery that is as effective as reality in inducing a wide range of cognitive and emotional responses. As discussed later in this chapter, this feature makes VR an innovative instrument to assess and treat a wide range of mental disorders.

After an introductory description of the technological components of a VR system, the chapter will be organized in two main sections: the first one will explain the rationale of using VR as an advance form of exposure therapy for the treatment of anxiety disorders, while the second part will discuss the potential of the on-line virtual worlds for the creation of shared therapeutic environments accessible by different users who are physically distant one from the others. Pros and cons of the "virtual approach" will be also discussed.

VIRTUAL REALITY: THE TECHNOLOGY

A typical VR system is made of the following components:

Hardware

- **The computational device:** a desktop or a laptop pc equipped with an advanced image graphic card;
- **Different peripheral devices** (visual, aural or haptic devices);

- **A non immersive or immersive image display system:** a screen or a head mounted display (HMD);
- **A motion sensor** (or tracking device), usually integrated in the HMD, that tells the computer where the user is looking at on the basis on his/her head movement;

Software

- *the VR application*, According to the hardware and software included in a VR system it is possible to distinguish between different kinds of virtual settings:
- *desktop VR*, based on subjective immersion: in these systems the feeling of immersion can be improved through stereoscopic vision tools. Users interact with the virtual world using a mouse, a joystick or other VR peripherals such as datagloves;
- *fully immersive VR*: users appear to be fully immersed in the computer generated environment. This illusion is produced by providing them immersive output devices (HMD, force feedback robotic arms, etc.) and a system of head/body tracking to guarantee the exact correspondence and coordination of users' movements with the feedback of the environment;
- *CAVE*: a CAVE is a small room where a computer-generated world is projected on the walls. The projection is made on both front and sidewalls. This solution is particularly suitable for collective VR experiences because it allows different people to share the same experience at the same time;
- *telepresence systems*: users can influence and operate in a world that is real even if they are in a different location. They can observe the current situation with remote cameras and achieve actions via robotic and electronic arms;

- *augmented reality*: it is based on the combination of real and virtual stimuli. This system blurs the line between what is real and what is computer-generated by enhancing what users see, hear, feel and smell adding graphics, haptics and smell to the natural world as it exists.

Today computers are as powerful as supercomputers of the early 1990s and cost incredibly less. This huge advance in technology combined with the reduction in costs have made the VR hardware available to anyone. Unfortunately, this is not true for the VR softwares, that are still very expensive, not easily customizable by the users, and usually based on not user-friendly interfaces that require continual maintenance and technical support. When used for clinical and therapeutic purposes, their limitations also include the limited possibility of tailoring the virtual environments to the specific requirements of the clinical or the experimental setting, as well as the low availability of standardized protocols that can be shared by the community of researchers and clinicians.

A first significant step to address these challenges has been performed by Riva and coll. (Riva, 2005) who have designed and developed NeuroVR (http://www.neurovr.org), a cost-free VR platform based on an open-source software, that allows non-expert users to easily modify a virtual environment and visualize it using either an immersive or non-immersive system. The NeuroVR platform is implemented using open-source components that provide advanced features including an interactive rendering system based on OpenGL for high quality images. The NeuroVR Editor is realized by customizing the User Interface of Blender, an integrated suite of 3D creation tools available on all major operating systems, under the GNU General Public License; this means that the program can be distributed with the complete source code. Thanks to these features, clinicians and researchers can run, copy, distribute, study, change and improve the NeuroVR software, to create the environments they need and to share them with the whole VR community.

As we will discuss below, in the very last years, the diffusion of the Web 2.0 has further on facilitated the creation of fully customizable virtual environments that can be used for many different purposes, including therapy. The decreased costs of technology together with the enormous diffusion of the Web 2.0 are the main reasons of increased use of VR in clinical practice.

VIRTUAL REALITY: THE EXPERIENCE

In a VR system, hardware and software concur in generating the so called "sense of presence" (Riva & Davide, 2003; Steuer, 1992), that is the key of any virtual experience. Presence is usually defined as the "sense of being there" (Steuer, 1992) or the "feeling of being in a world that exists outside the self" (Riva, 2004). As shown by different papers, the level of presence is directly connected to the level of emotions and the quality of actions experienced in the virtual environment (Riva et al., 2007).

Experiencing presence, VR users become not simply external observers of images provided by a computer screen, but active participants within a computer-generated 3D virtual world. This process is fundamental to make the subject able to transfer the knowledge acquired in the virtual environment to the real world. After having identified an enriched environment that contains functional real-world demands, the technology is used to enhance the level of presence of the subject in the environment and to induce an *optimal* experience, that is defined as a positive, complex and rewarding state of consciousness (Csikszentmihalyi, 1975, 1990). Once the subject reaches this optimal experience, he/she will be able to transfer this new knowledge in his/her behavior, by linking the experience acquired in the virtual world to his/her actual experience in the real one. This is the key factor that makes VR a successful therapeutic instrument.

VIRTUAL REALITY IN CLINICAL PRACTICE

Although it is difficult to trace the origins of VR's application to mental health disorders, most people agree that Myrron Krueger was one of the first to apply it. In one of his books (Krueger, 1991) Krueger discussed the idea that patients may use an artificial experience in combination with a traditional psychotherapy to overcome the inhibition usually present in real life. In particular, he suggested that, at least in some cases, patients are more comfortable relating to and interacting with computers, a finding that has been supported in a number of subsequent studies (Joinson, 1999, 2001; Richman, Kiesler, Weisband, & Drasgow, 1999) and particularly evident after the introduction of the on-line virtual worlds. Kruger can be also considered a pioneer in the use of VR for exposure therapy since he was the first to suggest that a virtual environment can be used to *gradually* introduce elements of change during a traditional therapeutic intervention.

On the basis of his observations, in the early to mid-1990s different clinicians started to use VR to treat patients; in particular, virtual exposure therapy was immediately demonstrated to be effective in the treatment of specific phobias, such as acrophobia (Lamson, 1997), social phobia and agoraphobia (Camara, 1993). These studies pointed out that even though the VR environments were at that time primitive, the user could become immersed in the virtual world having a meaningful experience (Bard, 1991). They also suggested that, in a virtual world, the therapist can accompany the patient to assist him/her in the desensitization process and to better understand how he/she processes and responds to information coming from specific threatening environments and situations.

And most important, using virtual environments the therapist can control the speed and intensity of the therapeutic process, tailoring the virtual experience to each patient's specific needs.

Advantages of Using VR in the Treatment of Anxiety Disorders

Virtual exposure therapy consists in exposing patients to virtual environments created ad hoc for specific disorders (for example, specific phobias) under the direct supervision of the therapist. The patient undergoes the therapeutic sessions in the therapist office where the virtual sessions substitute both *in vivo* and *imaginative* exposure. Psychological therapies based on VR have been demonstrated to be effective in the treatment of anxiety disorders as confirmed by two different meta-analyses (Parsons & Rizzo, 2008; Powers & Emmelkamp, 2008) that have shown that VR-based treatments are more effective than no treatment, but also slightly but significantly more effective than in vivo and imaginative exposure therapy. They also suggest that VR treatments have a statistically large effect on all affective domains and that these effects are significant (Cohen, 1992).

Compared to the traditional exposure-based approaches, virtual therapy presents great advantages related to the ratio between costs and benefits. In a clinical setting costs refer not only to the expenditure in money and time, but also in emotional involvement requested to the patient. On the other side, benefits regard to the effectiveness of the treatment, that can be defined as the achievement of the target set in the shortest time possible.

In particular, compared to *in vivo* and *imaginative* exposure, VR presents the following advantages:

- guarantees the vividness of exposure: in the imaginative condition patients are trained to visualize the anxiety-provoking stimuli through mental images, but they often fail in doing that because they have difficulties in visualizing stressful scenes in a vivid way. VR provides a real-like experience that may be more emotionally engaging than imaginative exposure;

- increases the controllability of experience: during in vivo exposure subjects experiences anxious situations and are exposed to phobic stimuli in semi-structured situations. The therapist can not fully control the real-life events and the patient's reactions, with the high risk of provoking too much stress in the patient. On the contrary, VR gives the therapist the opportunity to recreate a structured and controlled hierarchy of real-like situations specific for the disorder that must be treated;

- during the virtual exposure, nothing the patients fear can "really" happen to them. With such assurance, they can freely explore, experiment, feel, live, and experience feelings and/or thoughts related to the anxious stimuli. Thus VR becomes a very useful intermediate step between the therapist's office and the real world;

- using the VR exposure the single fear components can be isolated more efficiently than in vivo exposure. For instance, treating the fear of flying, if landing is the most fearful part of the experience, it can be repeated as often as necessary without having to wait for the airplane to take-off several times.

Putting together, these observations highlight how the VR exposure therapy is effective in reducing costs and increasing benefits for both the therapist and the patient. In particular, the flexibility of the virtual environments allows the patient to overpractice in situations that are often much worse and more exaggerated than those that are likely to be encountered in real life. This allows

patients to develop a sense of mastery and the confidence to carry out the task successfully.

ONLINE VIRTUAL WORLDS: THE NEW FRONTIER FOR VIRTUAL THERAPY

As mentioned above, the most expensive and less easily customizable component of a VR system is the software. This problem has been partially solved by the introduction of Web 2.0 in 2004 (Graham, 2005), that has produced a huge increase in the potential of web applications, allowing users to create, modify and share contents from multiple computers in various locations. In particular, Web 2.0 represents the trend in the use of World Wide Web (WWW) technology aimed to enhance information sharing and collaboration between users, so that they can do more than just retrieve static information. These innovative features have led to the development of web-based communities, social-networking sites, wikis, blogs, and three dimensional (3-D) online virtual worlds that represent one of the most successful applications of the Web 2.0.

On-line 3-D virtual worlds are computer-based simulated environments mainly modelled by their users that can create and manipulate elements and thus experiences telepresence to a certain degree (F. Biocca, 1995). Such modelled worlds may appear similar to the real world or instead depict fantasy worlds, and can be used for many different aims: game and pleasure, social interaction, education, research, commercial and business, e-commerce, and so on. Differently from the previously described VR applications, on-line virtual worlds admit multiple user interactions based on 3-D objects, text, graphical icons, visual gestures, sound and voice. Second Life, There, IMVU and Active World are some of the 3-D virtual worlds where every day millions of users interact each others through their avatars, that is to say, three dimensional graphical representations of themselves. Today Second Life is the 3-D virtual world with the greater number of registered users, counting approximately 18 million of subscribers with a daily concurrency between 70 and 80 thousand users worldwide. Everyone can download a free client software called *Second Life Viewer* that enables its users, called Residents, to interact with each others through motional avatars, providing an advanced level of a social network service. Residents can explore the different worlds, meet other Residents, socialize, join individual and group activities, play, create and mutually trade items and services. Within Second Life, avatars can communicate using text-based chat or voice. There are two main ways of text-based communication: local chat, and global instant messaging (IM). Chatting is used for public localized conversations between two or more avatars and can be heard (seen messages) within 20 meters, while IM is used for private conversations, either between two avatars, or among the members of a group. Second Life and other online virtual worlds are sometimes referred to as games, but this description does not fit the standard definition, because they really allow a lot of various activities other than games.

Recent experimental studies performed on avatar-based interactions in on-line virtual worlds have shown that these kinds of virtual relations are able to convey such as feelings of social presence, that users undergo the experience of inhabiting a shared space with one or more, while their awareness of mediation by technology recedes into the background (F. Biocca, Harms, & Burgoon, 2003). As suggested by Casanueva and Blake (Casanueva & Blake, 2001), users develop a sense of social presence consisting in the belief that the other subjects in the virtual environment are real and really present, and that they and the others are part of a group and process. Moreover, compared to other kinds of communicative methods, such as phone calls or chat, avatar-based interactions significantly increase level of social presence (G.

Bente, Rüggenberg, & Krämer, 2004; G. Bente, Rüggenberg, & Krämer, 2005), elicit strong emotional responses and increase the sense of community (Fabri, Moore, & Hobbs, 1999), even in those avatars with rather primitive expressive abilities.

According to these studies avatar platforms offer new potentials to overcome many of the restrictions related to audio and video communication modes. In particular, they suggest that virtual worlds and avatars play a critical role in contextualizing social interaction and fostering the salience of nonverbal information by providing active filtering and contingency management systems as opposed to being just the virtual equivalents of call or video conferencing systems. These features are fundamental in facilitating and making functional social interaction between users that are physically distant one from the other. Through their avatars (that usually remain stable over time) users can meet friends, colleagues, students or teachers, clients, and so on, share with them a common virtual space and discuss about their interests in real time, without the necessity to reach a specific place somewhere in the physical world. Today, many companies, universities, organizations and private individuals use Second Life and other parallel universes to make their business and activities. Computer-generated realities are also becoming a fertile terrain for researchers and psychologists, who can analyze what people do when freed physical and social constraints from real-world (G. Miller, 2007). As in the off-line VR environments, also in the on-line virtual worlds all users' behaviors can be tracked and recorded by external observers (psychologists, therapists, etc.) and everything happens in "ecological" environments that reflect the real ones. Moreover, the possibility for users to create a fully personalized avatar allows psychologists to study the way in which people self-conceptualize and how they use information from online virtual worlds to understand themselves in the real worlds.

Considering the discussed advantages offered by the online virtual worlds, including the possibility for multiple users to share a common virtual environment at the same time, even when they are physically distant, to have digital characters that represent themselves, to communicate in real time using chat or voice in public or private way, and to experience a greater sense of presence than the one experienced using phone or chat, as well as the fact that the avatars' virtual behaviors often affect the subsequent real-world behaviors (Yee & Bailenson, 2007) there is no doubt that on-line virtual worlds also show a great potential for therapeutic purposes (Gorini, Gaggioli, & Riva, 2007). In particular, Second Life currently features a number of medical and health education projects. By way of example, the Nutrition Game proposed by the Ohio University simulates choices a user can make in various restaurants and informs the player about the health impacts of those choices. The Heart Murmur Sim (Kemp, 2006) provides an educational virtual world for cardiac auscultation training that enables clinical students to tour a virtual clinic and test their skills at identifying the sounds of different types of heart murmurs. The Second Life Virtual Hallucinations Lab (Yellowlees & Cook, 2006) aims to educate people about schizophrenic hallucinations. The Gene Pool is an interactive genetic lab and learning area featuring simulated lab experiments, tutorials, and simple videos to enhance the learning experience. The Virtual Neurological Education Centre (VNEC) demonstrates a virtual simulated online experience where people are able to actively expose themselves to the most common symptoms that a person suffering from a neurological disability may encounter, and the HealthInfo Island is funded by the US National Library of Medicine (NLM) to provide consumers health information services. All these virtual initiatives are mainly centred on the promotion of an innovative form of public health consisting of the diffusion of medical information and the education of therapists and patients (Boulos,

Hetherington, & Wheeler, 2007). But virtual worlds can be also used to treat patients with psychological disturbances in a very innovative and quite unexplored way consisting in creating on-line, protected virtual spaces in which patients, using their avatars, can meet other patients or their therapist without being in the same physical place. Different psychologists and counsellors are already using online virtual worlds to work with patients in their virtual offices. Some of them do not personally know their patients, having met them for the first time in the virtual world, while some others use the virtual therapy with patients who started a face-to-face therapy and then moved to an online therapy.

For those who choose to offer a psychological support without physically meet the patient, the lack of physical presence is a great advantage because it allows the patient to be less inhibited, so it is a much faster way of working. At the same time, the lack of visual feedback from a client's real world means that the therapist needs to be explicit in asking how his clients are. On the contrary, those who consider the online virtual therapy as an adjunct to the traditional one affirm that the virtual therapy can never be a complete substitute for face-to-face therapy and refuse to start a therapy without knowing the patient in the real life. A face-to-face relationship – they say – is absolutely relevant to create a good therapeutic relationship between the patients and their therapist.

What is clear from the discussed applications of the on-line 3-D virtual worlds is that they represent a good opportunity to create innovative online health services based on the following features:

- an extended sense of presence (Lee, 2004; Riva, 2007; Riva, Anguera, Wiederhold, & Mantovani, 2006): 3-D virtual worlds transform health guidelines and provisions into experience. In the virtual environments users do not receive abstract information but live meaningful experiences;

- an extended sense of community (social presence): on-line worlds use hybrid social interaction and dynamics of group sessions to provide each user with targeted—but also anonymous, if required—social support in both the physical and virtual world.

From a clinical perspective, the advantages offered by the 3-D avatar-based interactions serve to facilitate the communication process between therapists and patients, to positively influence group cohesiveness in group-based therapies and to create greater levels of interpersonal trust, which is a fundamental requirement to establish a successful therapeutic alliance.

3-D On-Line Worlds for Virtual Reality Exposure Therapy

Compared to the traditional virtual worlds, the on-line worlds appear to have much to offer to the virtual exposure therapy. Since they allow multiplayers' interactions, the therapist and the patient can share the same online virtual space. This means that the therapist can accompany the patient through a particular threatening experience just by logging onto a specific website and adopting a preferred avatar. The way of interaction as well as the surrounding environment can be easily modified on the basis of the patient's therapeutic needs. In the case of social phobia, for example, after practicing with the therapist within a closed environment (ie, the therapist's virtual office), the patient can be taken to a virtual world populated by other avatars and asked to initiate a conversation and obtain feedback from them in real-time audio. Similarly, patients with agoraphobia can be exposed to a variety of unfamiliar worlds different from those the clinician can provide in an office setting, while patients suffering from addiction disorders (eg, drug abuse, pathological gambling, food craving) can be exposed to specific kinds of dangerous stimuli without running the risk of "succumbing to temp-

tation" (Wiederhold & Wiederhold, 2004). These are just few examples describing the promising potential of on-line virtual worlds in the field of psychological therapy.

3-D On-Line Worlds for Creating Virtual Communities of Patients

On-line virtual worlds may also have the potential to bring several innovative features to virtual communities of patients by providing mediated environments with appropriate social, nonverbal, and contextual information that previous web applications (Web 1.0) were unable to convey.

Winkelman and Choo (Winkelman & Choo, 2003) surmised that patients with chronic diseases possess a particular tacit knowledge gleaned from their personal experience of illness and experientially acquired by having to cope with the daily challenges and needs posed by a chronic disease. These needs include information on diseases, treatment side effects, treatment plans, professional contacts, as well as supportive information for family and friends. According to the authors, if this tacit knowledge can be shared or socialized through a program, tool, or medium, the patient's sense of self-efficacy can improve, and positively affects health outcomes as well as social functioning. This approach argues for a shift in the role of chronic disease patients from external consumers of health care services to a community of practice of internal customers. Introduced by Wenger (1998), communities of practice are social constructs that bring learning into lived experience of participation in the world. They are defined as self-organizing, informal groups whose members work together toward common goals, face common needs, share best practices, and have a common identity. Drawing on these concepts, Winkelman and Choo (Winkelman & Choo, 2003) suggest that, gaining access from the expertise of peers, patients integrate others' experiences of living with chronic disease into their self-management. In particular, they claim that virtual patients communities can become effective tools of communication if (1) members have common interests, needs, goals, as well as an aspiration for mutual communication, and (2) they are able to supplement already existing face-to-face communication opportunities. The possibility to share specific virtual environments from different parts of the world and to interact via customizable avatars can presumably facilitate the development and the diffusion of online communities of practice allowing an efficient exchange of medical and experiential information between patients and experts.

Second Life and Psychotherapy: An Exploratory Case Study

One of the greatest advantage of using on-line virtual worlds in clinical practice is represented by the possibility offered to the users to share a common virtual space, even when they are far away one from the other. This means that people with physical disabilities, or those who cannot easily reach their therapists, or people who live in underserved geographical areas, can virtually meet a therapist or other patients without moving themselves in a certain physical place.

Following the original suggestion of Kahan (Kahan, 2000) we proposed to use on-line virtual worlds not only for cognitive-behavioural oriented therapies, such as exposure therapies, but also for dynamic psychotherapy drawing on psychoanalytic principles. This idea was previously introduced by Harris in 1994 (Harris, 1994) who theoretically discussed the potential of virtual reality experiences on our conscious being. "Those experiences - he says - can become part of a perceptual and an emotional background that changes the way we see things. At its best, virtual reality can allow us to transcend our limitations and to expand our emotional lives".

Starting from these considerations, we asked an analytic oriented psychiatrist to conduct the following exploratory study using Second Life as virtual setting. As this way to conduct psychological interventions is to be considered very innovative, our main aim was to investigate its feasibility from the side of both the patient and the therapist, analyzing their reactions to this kind of approach. For this reason we will describe the characteristics of both of them, analyzing the different aspects regarding the therapeutic dyad during their interactions in the virtual world.

The Patient

C.B. (these are the initials of her avatar's name) is a 47-year-old woman with a scientific academic degree. She has been married since 1995 and has one 8-year-old son. In 2002 she received a diagnosis of dependent personality disorder (DSM-IV) also characterized by obsessive-compulsive traits and severe physical somatizations that needed a pharmacological treatment. C.B. is defined by her therapist as a clever and affective woman, highly motivated to deeply elaborate her insecure adult attachment style and her difficulties in forming secure adult relationships. From 2002 to 2006 she underwent a psychoanalytic treatment based on two sessions per week that produced a significant symptomatic remission and an increasing in self and work efficiency. Though from the end of the psychoanalytic treatment up to now C.B. has undergone only sporadic consultation sessions, in the last few months she has expressed her therapist the desire to start a second phase of analytic-oriented treatment. At the beginning her request seemed incompatible with her work engagement which often demanded her to move from Milan (Italy) – her usual home place – to far-away destinations, in Italy and abroad. C.B. has a basic knowledge of the main Windows applications, is not used to play videogames and has never experienced virtual reality systems before.

The Therapist

The therapist involved in the study, both psychiatrist and psychoanalyst, is a 51-year-old man, who has matured a full experience as a trainer and a deep personal interest in studying the relationship between human mind-body and technological devices. He joined this experimental study in accordance to the Freudian concept of *Junktim,* the unbreakable link between clinical and research aspects. Similarly to C.B., the therapist has a good knowledge of the main Windows applications, is not use to play videogames and has never had experiences with virtual reality systems before. He has recently changed his home place and life-style, living for half a week in Milan (Italy) and the rest of the time in another Italian city, located about 300 Km far from Milan. The difficulty in combining their working commitments and the physical distance (at least for half week) have been some of the reasons pushing C.B. and her therapist to try this innovative therapeutic approach.

In order to guarantee that no one else other than the patient and the therapist participated to the sessions, all the chat transcriptions were countersigned by both of them.

Assessment

In order to evaluate their imaginative abilities, their confidence with technology and virtual reality, and the sense of presence elicited by the use of Second Life, both the patient and the therapist were asked to fill out the following questionnaires:

- Betts questionnaire (adapted from: (Betts, 1909), revised by (Sheehan, 1967), and previously used in Italy by (Cornoldi et al., 1991)) (administered before the beginning of the protocol);
- Computer knowledge and experience questionnaire (administered before the beginning of the protocol);
- Barfield Presence questionnaire (Barfield & Weghorst, 1993; Hendrix & Barfield, 1996) (administered every 15 days from the beginning of the protocol)

The Second Life Virtual Office

The psychiatrist's virtual office is located inside the Eureka Island (152,184,44), a private Second Life land owned by Istituto Auxologico Italiano. The island includes a place called "experience

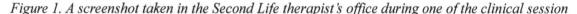

Figure 1. A screenshot taken in the Second Life therapist's office during one of the clinical session

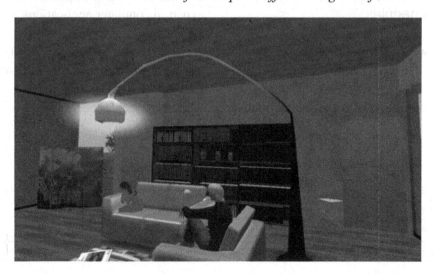

area" in which patients can do different virtual therapeutic experiences. This area is composed of a bar, a restaurant and a house (that are interactive environments useful to treat patients suffering from alcohol or food addiction) and also includes the psychiatrist's office. This is a small house, composed of two rooms. The first one, immediately after the entrance, is the place where the patient and the therapist met each other. This area was created by a graphical expert following the suggestions of the therapist in order to obtain an appropriate therapeutic setting (see fig.1).

Differently from the other island areas, this place can be accessed only by invited avatars, and people not authorized are rejected. These settings can be modified only by the administrator of the island and are defined in order to guarantee the privacy of the therapeutic sessions.

The patient and the therapist interact through their avatars and communicate using the IM (instant message) channel so that their conversation is audible only from selected avatars. All chats are recorded and automatically saved on a.txt file together with date and time.

Before the beginning of the protocol, the patient and the therapist are guided by an expert through the creation of their personal avatars, and instructed about the use of Second Life in general, and about the privacy issues in particular.

Treatment Schedules

The treatment was based on two virtual sessions (45 minutes each) per week plus one face-to-face session per month. The patient and the therapist agreed on date and time of the virtual appoint-

ments with the same modalities they used for real ones.

Technical Requirements

Both the therapist and the patient used a laptop with Windows as operating system and a DSL internet connection.

Quantitative Data

The Betts questionnaire reveals that the therapist has slightly higher imaginative abilities (43/70) than the patient (39/70). Imaginative abilities are usually correlated with high sense of presence.

The Computer knowledge and experience questionnaire, administered before the beginning of the protocol, shows that the level of experience in computer managing is "sufficient" (2/5) for C.B. and "good" (3/5) for the psychiatrist, and that both of them have had at least one previous experience with stereoscopic images. They have never played with videogames before and none of them have ever used a virtual reality system and know how it works. Their scores regarding the sense of presence are reported in table 1.

Qualitative Observations

Since neither the therapist nor the patient were expert in computer applications, the first virtual appointment was characterized by a certain degree of slowness that was easier ridden out in the following sessions. Analyzing the text-chats obtained from the different sessions, the psychiatrist noticed that their formal aspects and the relation style of

Table 1. The barfield presence questionnaire

Questions	C.B.	Psychiatrist
If your level in the real world is 100, and your level of presence is 1 if you have no presence, rate your level of presence in this virtual world.	50	60
How strong was you sense of presence, "being there", in the virtual environment (1-5 scale)?	3	3

the virtual interactions were comparable to those observed during the face-to-face sessions. Starting from the first session, the patient conveyed her emotional contents and reactions, made free associations, reported her recent dreams and expects the therapist's interpretation exactly with the same expressive modalities she uses when she is sitting in front of him. Apparently, there were no signs of inhibition caused by the presence of a technological medium between the therapist and the patient. The "fundamental rule" of psychoanalysis that urges that patients say "whatever comes into their heads, even if they think it is unimportant or irrelevant or nonsensical...or embarrassing or distressing" (Freud's Psycho-Analytic Procedure" (1904a [1903] p. 251) is respected.

Forcing the physical distance between the therapist and the patient, the virtual setting also represents a good opportunity to practice, at least from a physical point of view, another important analytic rule: the "rule of abstinence". This rule designates a number of technical recommendations that Freud stated regarding the general framework of the psychoanalytic treatment, including, for example, the prescription to have no physical or gaze contacts with the patient. In our study the therapist referred that the application of the rule of abstinence in the virtual setting did not interfere with the therapeutic relationship, since they had already practiced it during the traditional sessions. On the contrary, it could contribute to maintain a favorable tension potential, which is assumed to keep the therapeutic process in motion.

Another important point regards the constancy of setting: virtual reality offers the therapist the possibility to create a therapeutic environment more stable than any other real physical setting, other than to maintain the avatar's aspect unchanged over time. Starting from the very first sessions, the therapist and the patient met each other always in the same place, recognizing their respective avatars as the "virtual incarnation" of their real interlocutor.

The only critical point emerged during the virtual sessions regards the patient's concern about privacy. A certain number of times she asked the therapist the following question: "Doctor, are you sure we are alone?". This doubt did not really invalidate the session, because immediately after the therapist's answer it was regularly performed.

Conclusions

Even if these results come from few virtual sessions, we can start to draw some preliminary positive conclusions about this innovative experience. Both the therapist and the patient experienced a quite high sense of presence and did not find particular problems or limitations in the use of Second Life as therapeutic setting. On the contrary, analyzing what the patient said, and listening to the psychiatrist's comments, it seems that the physical barriers imposed by the virtual setting contributed to knock down the psychological resistances that tend to emerge during face-to-face interactions. As discussed above, this is not just an experimental protocol, but also a way to allow the patient to have frequent meeting with her therapist, that should not be possible if they were forced to meet twice a week somewhere in a physical place. If we will be able to demonstrate the effectiveness of this approach, its potentialities could be enormous, especially for all patients who have difficulties to physically reach their therapists, such as those with specific mental, physical or social disabilities.

Issues, Controversies, Problems

Although the therapeutic potential of on-line virtual worlds is quite promising, there are important challenges that need to be addressed. First, if it is true that people can explore threatening aspects of reality in a virtual safe environment, it is also true that if the use of on-line worlds becomes excessive, there is a risk that it will prevent people from forming meaningful real-world contacts and relationships. In fact, as observed by Allison et al. (Allison, Wahlde, Shockley, & Gabbard, 2006), an increased substitution of cyberspace-based relationships at the expense of face-to-face interaction may create a developmental double-edged sword. In the case of socially anxious patients, for example, the Internet is useful to modify peer group interactions, while it does little to foster the development of genuine intimacy. Exposing patients to virtual environments, therapists should always consider the risk of web addiction and encourage patients to participate in real-life social interaction as much as possible.

Another critical point regards anonymity: the chance to remain anonymous offers a less intimidating opportunity for social interaction and psychological reflection and would allow more people to discreetly seek help on their own. On the other side, anonymity represents a significant risk for patients and therapists. The computer-based interface does not guarantee that the person on the other side of the screen is really who we expect, and anybody can enter the virtual environment and interact with patients, producing negative effects on their experience and introducing uncontrollable and disturbing variables in the environment. These aspects can be overcome, for example, by creating private servers specific for controlled environments designed and dedicated to therapy and using protection codes personally given by the therapist to the patients.

Regarding the therapists, they need to first conduct self-assessment and then enhance their knowledge and skills in using these alternative forms of therapy (Glueckauf, Pickett, Ketterson, Loomis, & Rozensky, 2003) because the provision of on-line therapeutic services is not simply a click of the mouse (Koocher & Morray, 2000).

Besides the previous clinical considerations, there are also some very challenging issues that need to be resolved to ensure the safe and ethical use of web-based therapy in general. These include complex and interrelated questions of security, confidentiality, and privacy; licensure requirements; competency; standards of care; and reimbursement that must be considered by practitioners, researchers, consumers, health care organizations, managed care companies, and federal and state legislatures (Jerome et al., 2000). The American Psychological Association (APA) has published a statement entitled "Services by Telephone, Teleconferencing, and Internet" (American Psychological Association, 1997). This statement stipulates that in the absence of specific e-health standards, psychologists must take reasonable steps to ensure competence in providing services and to protect patients, clients, and research participants from harm. The APA is also developing recommendations for the board regarding ethical, legal, and clinical concerns related to the practice of e-health, with the aim of providing practitioners with information about electronic activities. While conducting interventions via on-line applications, patients may believe that the Internet sessions are secure and completely private and confidential. To safeguard against a breach in confidentiality, therapists and clinicians should fully inform patients of the limits of confidentiality associated with e-health and other forms of telecommunications.

FUTURE RESEARCH DIRECTIONS

The future of health technology will probably include two main features: portability and inter-reality. Portability refers to the use of portable devices (PDAs and smartphones) to provide VR everywhere. Having the possibility to run a VR system on a pocket device will allow patients to practice the skills learned in therapist's office by themselves and without limitations.

More complex, is the concept of *interreality* (Gorini, Gaggioli, Riva, 2007; Riva, 2009) a personalized immersive e-therapy whose main novelty is the creation of a hybrid, closed-loop, empowering experience bridging both the physical and virtual worlds. The main feature of interreality is a twofold link between the virtual and the real world:

- *Behavior in the physical world influences the experience in the virtual world.* For example:
  - *If my emotional regulation during the day was poor, some new experiences in the virtual world will be unlocked to address this issue.*
  - *If my emotional regulation was okay, the virtual experience will focus on a different issue.*
- *Behavior in the virtual world influences the experience in the real world.* For example:
  - *If I participate in the virtual support group I can SMS during the day with the other participants.*
  - *If my coping skills in the virtual world were poor, the decision support system will increase the chance of possible warnings in real life and will provide additional homework assignments.*

The bridge between the real and the virtual world can be achieved using the following technologies (see Figure 2):

- **3-D Individual and/or Shared Virtual Worlds**: immersive (in the health care center) or non-immersive (at home) role-playing experiences in which one or more users interact each other within a 3-D world. A 3-D world enables its users to interact one with the others through motional avatars, providing an advanced level of a social network service combined with general aspects of fully immersive 3D virtual spaces. Residents can explore, meet other users, socialize, and participate in individual and group activities.
- **Personal Biomonitoring System (from the real world to the virtual world):**

typically 3-D virtual worlds are closed worlds and do not reflect in any way the real activity and status of the users. In interreality, instead, bio and activity sensors (Personal Biomonitoring System – PBS) are used to track the emotional/health status of the user and to influence his/her experience in the virtual world (aspect, activity and access). The link between the real and virtual worlds will be both in real-time - allowing the development of advanced dynamic biofeedback settings - or not, to ensure health tracking also in situations where an internet connection is not immediately available.

- **Mobile Internet Appliances (from the virtual to the real one):** In interreality, the social and individual user activity in the virtual world has a direct link with the users' life through a mobile phone/digital assistant.
  - *Follow-up (warnings and/or feedbacks)*: it is possible to assess/improve the outcome of the virtual experience through the PDA/phone, eventually using the info coming from the bio and activity sensors.
  - *Training/Homework*: thanks to the advanced graphic/communication capabilities now available on PDAs/ Smarthphone, they can be used as training/simulation devices to facilitate the real-world transfer of the knowledge acquired in the virtual world.
  - *Community*: the social links created in the virtual world can be continued in the real world even without revealing the real identity of the user.

Even if the concept of interreality is quite new, Google Inc. is developing different free tools that can transform it in reality very soon (Figure 2):

Figure 2. The interreality approach using Google tools

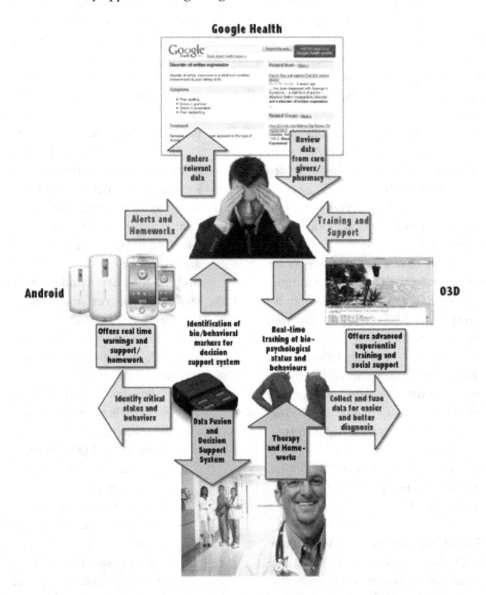

- ***O3D Application Programming Interface (API)***: O3D is an open-source web API for creating rich, interactive 3D applications in the browser using JavaScript. The O3D API is intended for web developers who are familiar with JavaScript and have some background in 3D graphics. Because the O3D application runs as a browser plug-in, users do not have to overcome the hurdles of downloading and running standalone application code on their systems. The O3D API maximizes performance by programming to the GPU's shader language directly, an advantage over pure software rendering. In essence, it tries to provide the flexibility and speed of a low-level graphics API like OpenGL or Direct3D, while addressing the constraints of running inside the browser.

- ***Android***: Android delivers a complete set of software for mobile devices: an operating system, middleware and key mobile applications. The Android Software Development Kit (SDK) provides the tools and APIs necessary to begin developing applications that run on Android-powered devices. Android breaks down the barriers to building new and innovative applications. For example, a developer can combine information from the web with data on an individual's mobile phone - such as the user's contacts, calendar, or geographic location - to provide a more relevant user experience. With Android, a developer can build an application that enables patients to view the location of their caregivers and be alerted when they are in the vicinity giving them a chance to connect.

- *Google Health*: Google Health is a personal health record (PHR) that offers a single web-based location to consolidate and store medical records and personal health information. Specifically, it is a patient-directed information tool that allows the patient to enter and gather information from a variety of healthcare information systems such as hospitals, physicians, health insurance plans, and retail pharmacies. PHRs allow people to access and coordinate their health information and share it with those who need it. Through Google Health it is also possible to access a host of online services and tools, from a variety of third-party companies.

CONCLUSION

This chapter addresses a broad and emerging idea in the field of e-health: the use of 3-D virtual worlds for online mental health applications. As we have recently discussed elsewhere (Gorini et al., 2007), 3-D online worlds have become not only a fertile ground for psychologists exploring human behavior (G. Miller, 2007), but they are also starting to play an emergent role in health services. Why should this be so? Compared with traditional communicating systems (videoconferencing, email, telephone, Web 1.0 applications, etc) and other available technologies (eg, CD or DVD), 3-D virtual worlds provide users with a more immersive and socially interactive experience, as well as a feeling of embodiment that has the potential to facilitate the clinical communication process and to positively influence group interaction and cohesiveness in group-based therapies. Moreover, unlike the available VR software, 3-D virtual worlds, being Internet-based applications, can be used by different people from different places without physical limitations.

Although this new medium has the potential to improve the existing e-health applications, there are several challenges that need to be addressed. First, more basic psychological research is needed in order to gain a clearer understanding of psychological, communicative, and interpersonal aspects of avatar-based interactions and of the differences between this and other interaction modes. Second, to date, there are some encouraging qualitative observations (Alcaniz et al., 2003; Fildes, 2007; Goldfield & Boachie, 2003; T. W. Miller, Kraus, Kaak, Sprang, & Burton, 2002; Nelson, Barnard, & Cain, 2003; SecondLife_Live2give), but no experimental or controlled data about the therapeutic effectiveness of on-line virtual worlds in patients with mental health disorders. Third, 3-D on-line virtual worlds were not built with clinical purposes in mind. This means that clinicians and researchers have to create specific and protected environments to meet their clinical needs as well as the needs of patients. Further, as for any kind of e-health system, it is important to define international guidelines for the development of 3-D virtual world–based clinical applications in order to reduce the risk of abuse and to guarantee appropriate levels of privacy.

In conclusion, despite a number of controversial issues, we suggest that 3-D virtual worlds, used as an adjunct to face-to-face settings, may represent a valid opportunity for the future developments of e-health tools. More, the emerging concept of interreality, bridging virtual and real world, may open a new breed of e-health applications. In fact, by creating a bridge between virtual and real worlds, interreality allows a full-time closed-loop approach actually missing in current e-health approaches:

- *the assessment is conducted continuously throughout the virtual and real experiences:* it enables tracking of the individual's psychophysiological status over time in the context of a realistic task challenge;
- *the information is constantly used to improve both the appraisal and the coping skills of the patient*: it creates a conditioned association between effective performance state and task execution behaviours.

In particular, the free tools developed by Google Inc. - O3D, Android and Google Health – are a clear path towards this vision.

Our hope is that the present chapter will stimulate a discussion within the research community about potential, limitations, and risks of virtual reality in the treatment of psychological disorders.

ACKNOWLEDGMENT

The present work was supported by The European Union IST Programme (Project "INTREPID – A Virtual Reality Intelligent Multi-sensor Wearable System for Phobias' Treatment" – IST-2002-507464; Project "INTERSTRESS" - Interreality in the management and treatment of stress related disorders - FP7-ICT-247685). A special thanks to Glenn Rotaru (John Alonzo in the real life), who daily helps us to discover the incredible world of Second Life (even if we have never met him personally!)

REFERENCES

Alcaniz, M., Botella, C., Banos, R., Perpina, C., Rey, B., & Lozano, J. A. (2003). Internet-based telehealth system for the treatment of agoraphobia. *Cyberpsychology & Behavior*, *6*(4), 355–358. doi:10.1089/109493103322278727

Allison, S. E., Wahlde, L., Shockley, T., & Gabbard, G. O. (2006). The Development of the Self in the Era of the Internet and Role-Playing Fantasy Games. *The American Journal of Psychiatry*, *163*, 381–385. doi:10.1176/appi.ajp.163.3.381

American Psychological Association. E. C. (1997). Services by telephone, teleconferencing, and Internet [Electronic Version], from http://www.apa.org/ethics/stmnt.01html

Bard, S. R. (1991). Virtual reality: an extension of perception. Noetic Sciences Review(Autumn), 7-16.

Barfield, W., & Weghorst, S. (1993). The sense of presence within virtual environments: A conceptual framework. In Salvendy, G., & Smith, M. (Eds.), *Human-computer interaction: Applications and case studies* (pp. 699–704). Amsterdam: Elsevier.

Bente, G., Rüggenberg, S., & Krämer, N. C. (2004). *Social presence and interpersonal trust in avatar-based, collaborative net-communications.* Paper presented at the 7th Annual International Workshop Presence 2004, Valencia.

Bente, G., Rüggenberg, S., & Krämer, N. C. (2005). *Virtual encounters. Creating social presence in net-based collaborations.* Paper presented at the 8th International Workshop on Presence.

Betts, G. H. (1909). *The distribution and function of mental imagery.* New York: Teachers College.

Biocca, F. (1995). *Communication in the Age of Virtual Reality.* Lawrence Erlbaum Associates.

Biocca, F., Harms, C., & Burgoon, J. (2003). Toward a More Robust Theory and Measure of Social Presence: Review and Suggested Criteria. *Presence (Cambridge, Mass.), 12*(5), 456–480. doi:10.1162/105474603322761270

Boulos, M. N. K., Hetherington, L., & Wheeler, S. (2007). Second Life: an overview of the potential of 3-D virtual worlds in medical and health education. *Health Information and Libraries Journal, 24*, 233–245. doi:10.1111/j.1471-1842.2007.00733.x

Camara, E. (1993). Virtual reality: applications in medicine and psychiatry. *Hawaii Medical Journal, 52*(12), 332–333.

Casanueva, J. S., & Blake, E. H. (2001). *The Effects of Avatars on Co-presence in a Collaborative Virtual Environment*. South Africa: Department of Computer Science, University of Cape Towno.

Cohen, J. (1992). A power primer. *Psychological Bulletin, 112*, 155–159. doi:10.1037/0033-2909.112.1.155

Cornoldi, C., De Beni, R., Giusberti, F., Marucci, F., Massironi, M., & G., M. (1991). The study of vividness of images. In R. H. Logie & M. Denis (Eds.), *Mental images in human cognition*. Amsterdam: North Holland.

Csikszentmihalyi, M. (1975). *Beyond Boredom and Anxiety*. San Francisco: Jossey-Bass.

Csikszentmihalyi, M. (1990). *Flow: The psychology of optimal experience*. New York: Harper Collins.

Fabri, M., Moore, D. J., & Hobbs, D. J. (1999). The Emotional Avatar: Nonverbal Communication between Inhabitants of Collaborative Virtual Environments. In Braffort (Ed.), *Gesture-Based Communication in Human-Computer Interaction* (LNCS 1739, pp. 245-248).

Fildes, J. (2007). Virtual treatment for US troops. Retrieved from http://news.bbc.co.uk/2/hi/science/nature/6375097.stm

Glueckauf, R. L., Pickett, T. C., Ketterson, T. U., Loomis, J. S., & Rozensky, R. H. (2003). Preparation for the Delivery of Telehealth Services: a Self-Study Framework for Expansion of Practice. *Professional Psychology, Research and Practice, 34*(2), 159–163. doi:10.1037/0735-7028.34.2.159

Goldfield, G. S., & Boachie, A. (2003). Delivery of family therapy in the treatment of anorexia nervosa using telehealth. *Telemedicine Journal and e-Health, 9*(1), 111–114. doi:10.1089/153056203763317729

Gorini, A., Gaggioli, A., & Riva, G. (2007). Virtual worlds, real healing. *Science, 318*(5856), 1549. doi:10.1126/science.318.5856.1549b

Graham, P. (2005). Web 2.0. Retrieved from http://www.paulgraham.com/web20.html

Harris, L. D. (1994). Psychodynamic effects of virtual reality. *The Arachnet Electronic Journal on Virtual Culture, 2*(1).

Hendrix, C., & Barfield, W. (1996). Presence within virtual environments as a function of visual display parameters. *Presence (Cambridge, Mass.), 5*, 274–289.

Jerome, L. W., DeLeon, P. H., James, L. C., Folen, R., Earles, J., & Gedney, J. J. (2000). The coming of age of telecommunications in psychological research and practice. *The American Psychologist, 55*(4), 407–421. doi:10.1037/0003-066X.55.4.407

Joinson, A. (1999). Social desirability, anonymity, and Internet-based questionnaires. *Behavior Research Methods, Instruments, & Computers, 31*(3), 433–438.

Joinson, A. (2001). Self-disclosure in computer-mediated communication: the role of self awareness and visual anonimity. *European Journal of Social Psychology*, *31*(2), 177–192. doi:10.1002/ejsp.36

Kahan, M. (2000). Integration of Psychodynamic and Cognitive–Behavioral Therapy in a Virtual Environment. *Cyberpsychology & Behavior*, *3*(2), 179–183. doi:10.1089/109493100316021

Kemp, J. (2006). Second Life Heart Murmur Sim video demonstration. Retrieved from http://it.youtube.com/watch?v=xJY2Iwbzop4

Koocher, G. P., & Morray, E. (2000). Regulation of Telepsychology: A survey of state attorneys general. *Professional Psychology, Research and Practice*, *31*, 503–508. doi:10.1037/0735-7028.31.5.503

Krueger, M. W. (1991). *Artificial reality II*. New York: Addison-Wesley.

Lamson, R. J. (1997). *Virtual therapy*. Montreal, Canada: Polytechnic International Press.

Lee, K. M. (2004). Why Presence Occurs: Evolutionary Psychology, Media Equation, and Presence. *Presence (Cambridge, Mass.)*, *13*(4), 494–505. doi:10.1162/1054746041944830

Miller, G. (2007). The promise of parallel universes. *Science*, *317*(5843), 1341–1343. doi:10.1126/science.317.5843.1341

Miller, T. W., Kraus, R. F., Kaak, O., Sprang, R., & Burton, D. (2002). Telemedicine: a child psychiatry case report. *Telemedicine Journal and e-Health*, *8*(1), 139–141. doi:10.1089/15305620252933482

Nelson, E. L., Barnard, M., & Cain, S. (2003). Treating childhood depression over videoconferencing. *Telemedicine Journal and e-Health*, *9*(1), 49–55. doi:10.1089/153056203763317648

Parsons, T. D., & Rizzo, A. A. (2008). Affective outcomes of virtual reality exposure therapy for anxiety and specific phobias: a meta-analysis. *Journal of Behavior Therapy and Experimental Psychiatry*, *39*(3), 250–261. doi:10.1016/j.jbtep.2007.07.007

Powers, M. B., & Emmelkamp, P. M. (2008). Virtual reality exposure therapy for anxiety disorders: A meta-analysis. *Journal of Anxiety Disorders*, *22*(3), 561–569. doi:10.1016/j.janxdis.2007.04.006

Richman, W. L., Kiesler, S., Weisband, S., & Drasgow, F. (1999). A meta-analytic study of social desirability distortion in computer-administered questionnaires, and interviews. *The Journal of Applied Psychology*, *84*, 754–775. doi:10.1037/0021-9010.84.5.754

Riva, G. (2004). Immersive Virtual Telepresence: virtual reality meets eHealth. *Studies in Health Technology and Informatics*, *99*, 255–262.

Riva, G. (2005). Virtual reality in psychotherapy [review]. *Cyberpsychology & Behavior*, *8*(3), 220–230, discussion 231–240. doi:10.1089/cpb.2005.8.220

Riva, G. (2007). Virtual reality and telepresence. *Science*, *318*(5854), 1240–1242. doi:10.1126/science.318.5854.1240d

Riva, G. (2009). Interreality: A new paradigm for E-health. *Studies in Health Technology and Informatics*, 144.

Riva, G., Anguera, M. T., Wiederhold, B. K., & Mantovani, F. (Eds.). (2006). *From Communication to Presence: Cognition, Emotions and Culture towards the Ultimate Communicative Experience*. Amsterdam: IOS Press.

Riva, G., & Davide, F. (Eds.). (2003). *Being there: concepts, effects and measurements of user presence in synthetic environments*. Amsterdam, The Netherlands: IOS Press.

Riva, G., Mantovani, F., Capideville, C. S., Preziosa, A., Morganti, F., & Villani, D. (2007). Affective interactions using virtual reality: the link between presence and emotions. *Cyberpsychology & Behavior, 10*(1), 45–56. doi:10.1089/cpb.2006.9993

Sheehan, P. W. (1967). A shortened form of Bett's questionnaire upon mental imagery. *Journal of Clinical Psychology, 23*, 386–389. doi:10.1002/1097-4679(196707)23:3<386::AID-JCLP2270230328>3.0.CO;2-S

Steuer, J. S. (1992). Defining virtual reality: dimensions determining telepresence. *The Journal of Communication, 42*(4), 73–93. doi:10.1111/j.1460-2466.1992.tb00812.x

Wiederhold, B. K., & Wiederhold, M. D. (2004). *Virtual Reality Therapy for Anxiety Disorders*. American Psychological Association Press.

Winkelman, W. J., & Choo, C. W. (2003). Provider-Sponsored Virtual Communities for Chronic Patients: Improving Health Outcomes through Organizational Patient-Centred Knowledge Management. *Health Expectations, 6*(4), 352–259. doi:10.1046/j.1369-7625.2003.00237.x

Yee, N., & Bailenson, J. N. (2007). The Proteus effect: Self transformations in virtual reality.

Yellowlees, P. M., & Cook, J. N. (2006). Education about hallucinations using an internet virtual reality system: a qualitative survey. *Academic Psychiatry, 30*(6), 534–539. doi:10.1176/appi.ap.30.6.534

Chapter 26
Use of Clinical Simulations to Evaluate the Impact of Health Information Systems and Ubiquitous Computing Devices Upon Health Professional Work

Elizabeth M. Borycki
University of Victoria, Canada

Andre W. Kushniruk
University of Victoria, Canada

ABSTRACT

Health information systems, and in particular ubiquitous computing devices (UCD), promise to revolutionize healthcare. However, before this can be widely achieved UCD need to be adapted to fit the information, workflow and cognitive needs of users of such devices. Indeed systems and devices that are not developed appropriately may inadvertently introduce error in healthcare ("technology-induced error"). This chapter describes an approach to applying clinical simulations to evaluate the impact of health information systems and ubiquitous computing devices on health professional work. The approach allows for an assessment of "cognitive-socio-technical fit" and the ability to modify and improve systems and devices before they are released into widespread use. The application of realistic clinical simulations is detailed, including the stages of development of such simulations (from the creation of representative clinical environments to subject selection and data collection approaches). In order to ensure the success and widespread adoption of UCD, it is argued that greater emphasis will need to be placed on ensuring such systems and devices have a high degree of fit with user's cognitive and work processes.

DOI: 10.4018/978-1-61520-777-0.ch026

Copyright © 2010, IGI Global. Copying or distributing in print or electronic forms without written permission of IGI Global is prohibited.

INTRODUCTION

Health information systems (HIS) and in particular ubiquitous computing devices (UCD) have promised to revolutionize healthcare. Early research in this area demonstrated the value of integrating varying HIS and UCD into clinical settings in terms of improving the quality of patient care and reducing medical error rates (e.g. Bates et al., 1999; Chaudry et al., 2006). More recent research has called into question some of these findings. Some researchers have identified that poor cognitive, social and technical fit may influence some implementations of HIS and UCD and be the cause of health professional adoption and appropriation failures (Borycki et al., 2009a). In healthcare the hospital and clinic costs associated with implementing and re-implementing a HIS and UCD can be significant. There is a need to develop new evaluation methodologies that allow for testing of differing constellations or groupings of HIS and UCD prior to their implementation in clinical settings to reduce the likelihood of costs being associated with health professional adoption and appropriation failure. The authors of this book chapter will introduce a novel methodology that can be used to evaluate the cognitive-socio-technical fit of HISs and UCD prior to their implementation in real world clinical settings. This may prevent poor adoption and appropriation of these technologies. The authors will begin this chapter by first introducing the reader to the literature involving HIS and UCD successes and failures. This will be followed by a brief introduction to the theory of cognitive–socio-technical fit as applied to HIS and UCD in clinical settings. Following this, the authors of the book chapter will describe the new and emerging area of HIS evaluation involving the use of clinical simulations. This section of the book chapter will not only describe the background and rationale for using clinical simulations to

evaluate HIS and UCD, but will also describe the steps in the evaluation method and provide examples from the authors' work. The authors will use examples from their previous research to illustrate the use of clinical simulations as an evaluation methodology for HIS and UCD.

The application of clinical simulations to the evaluation of HIS and UCD was pioneered by the authors and builds upon their previous work in the areas of clinical simulation and usability engineering (e.g. Borycki et al., 2009b; Kushniruk et al., 1992). Clinical simulations as applied to HIS and UCD evaluation in health informatics have their origins in the medical education and usability engineering literatures. Clinical simulations, when applied to the evaluation of a technology(ies), borrow from medical education, where clinical simulations are used to train physicians and evaluate their competency as health care practitioners (Issenberg et al., 1999). The author's work also extends the usability literature to clinical simulation by using many of the methods and analysis approaches employed by usability engineers to collect, record and analyze data involving HIS and UCD. Unlike the clinical simulation and usability literatures, clinical simulation when applied to the evaluation of HIS and UCD involves a more holistic evaluation of technology's impact upon the cognitive-socio-technical fit of health professionals' work. Lastly, this work also adds to the scientific knowledge in health informatics by identifying a new methodological approach that can be used by health informaticians to evaluate cognitive-socio-technical fit prior to HIS and UCD release and implementation. This approach has not been described elsewhere in the mainstream health informatics evaluation literature (e.g. Anderson & Aydin, 2005; Friedman & Wyatt, 2006; Shortliffe & Cimino, 2006) and is emergent in nature.

UNDERSTANDING THE NEED FOR APPLYING CLINICAL SIMULATIONS TO THE EVALUATON OF HEALTH INFORMATION SYSTEMS AND UBIQUITOUS COMPUTING DEVICES

The published research literature demonstrating the ability of HIS and UCD to improve patient and health care system processes and outcomes has been mixed. For example, Chaudry et al. (2006) in his systematic review of the health informatics literature found that HIS in conjunction with varying devices: (a) improved physician use of guidelines, (b) monitoring and surveillance of patient disease, and (c) decreased medication error rates (but only in healthcare organizations where home grown systems were being used). There were no proven improvements in the quality of patient care associated with the use of commercial HIS. As well, Chaudry and colleagues found that research on the cost-effectiveness of HIS/UCDs was limited and the findings that had been published in the literature were inconclusive. Eslami and colleagues in their 2007 and 2008 systematic reviews of the literature had similar findings. Eslami et al. (2007; 2008) found that implementing a computerized physician order system (i.e. the ordering of medications via computer) increased physician adherence to guidelines in outpatient settings, but that there was a lack of evidence to support the system's ability to improve patient safety and reduce the costs of providing patient care in outpatient care settings. Lastly, Ammenwerth et al. in her 2008 systematic review found that HIS/UCD may reduce the risk of medical errors when used by physicians, but at the same time acknowledged there is a need for more research in this area as the quality of the studies published to date are variable.

Other researchers found that some types of HIS and UCD may facilitate medical errors (e.g. Koppel et al. 2005). Koppel et al. (2005) found HIS system features and methods of implementing could facilitate medical errors in real-world settings if not designed and implemented properly. Kushniruk et al. (2005) suggested the interaction between HIS and UCD (i.e. handheld devices) could potentially lead to technology-induced errors (e.g. where interface design features may induce users to unknowingly prescribe medications incorrectly and UCD features may influence decision making). Lastly, Schulman et. al. (2005) found that while some types of errors were reduced by HIS, new types of errors were also introduced or emerged with the introduction of the technology. This has lead some researchers (e.g. Borycki & Kushniruk, 2008; Koppel & Kreda, 2009) and healthcare organizations (e.g. The Joint Commission for Health Care Quality, 2008) to suggest there is a need to exercise caution and apply rigorous evaluation when implementing HIS and UCD in healthcare organizations. In response to these suggestions researchers have begun to call for the evaluation of differing constellations of HIS and UCD cognitive-socio-technical fit to prevent medical errors involving patients and health professionals from occurring (Borycki & Kushniruk, 2005; Borycki et al., 2009a). As Berg (1999), Kushniruk et al. (1992) and Koppel et al. (2005) suggest improving this fit may reduce the likelihood of unintended consequences.

When a healthcare organization (e.g. hospital or clinic) identifies that a HIS and UCD affects the quality of patient care, the organization's leadership typically tries to address these HIS and UCD issues (Koppel et al., 2005). However, there are high costs associated with modifying a HIS and/or replacing a UCD after a hospital or clinic has implemented it. Yet, in healthcare, HISs and/or UCDs often require modification and/or reimplementation in order to address the above mentioned issues and improve the cognitive-socio-technical fit of the system with health professional work (i.e. physician, nurse and other allied health professional work) (Ash et al., 2004; Borycki et al., 2009b). In some cases, where systems have not achieved full cognitive-socio-technical fit with health professional work, physicians and nurses have chosen to boycott the HIS and/ or UCD (LaPoint & Rivard, 2005; LaPoint & Rivard, 2006). In other cases health professionals have chosen to not use many of the HIS and UCD features and functions that would have lead to significant reductions in medical errors or improvements in patient outcomes (Granlien et al., 2008; Kushniruk et. al., 2006). As a result, some organizations have "turned off" HISs and/ or removed some types of UCD from the clinical setting, instead attempting to redesign HIS or select new UCD and then re-implement them at a later date and time (thereby improving fit and health professional adoption and appropriation) (Ash et. al., 2004).

Some health informaticians have suggested there is a 65% failure rate associated with implementing HIS and their associated devices (Rabinowitz et al., 1999). Others have suggested this failure rate may be higher when one considers the number of HIS and/or UCD that are not used to their fullest extent (i.e. in terms of their features and functions) (Granlien et al., 2008). Therefore, there is a need for new approaches that can be used to evaluate the cognitive-socio-technical fit of HIS and UCD. As well, poor software and hardware designs (including UCD), and poor implementations can lead to significant healthcare organizational costs (e.g. hospital or clinic) (LaPoint & Rivard, 2005; LaPoint & Rivard, 2006). Costs arise from HIS/UCD device removal, redesign and/or reimplementation (including costs associated with retraining health professional staff) when such failures occur. In a time where there is a scarcity of healthcare resources (i.e. financial and human) to provide patient care such expenditures can have a significant impact upon regional health authority and federal healthcare budgets. This has led some policy makers and researchers to also conclude that there is a need for new evaluation methods that can be used to inform systems/UCD design and implementation prior to deployment in order to reduce the need for costly redesign and

reimplementation (Ash et al., 2004; Borycki et al., 2009a; Borycki & Kushniruk, 2006).

THE THEORY OF COGNITIVE-SOCIO-TECHNICAL FIT, HEALTH INFORMATION SYSTEMS AND UBIQUITOUS COMPUTING DEVICES

Assessing cognitive-socio-technical fit involves examining the degree of integration between cognitive, social and technical aspects of work. The effects of poor cognitive-socio-technical fit are often significant. The process of evaluating cognitive-socio-technical fit involves taking an integrated, holistic approach towards understanding how differing constellations of HIS and UCD interact in healthcare settings and identifying those HIS and UCD constellations that best match work processes. Cognitive-socio-technical fit addresses the cognitive aspects of fit involving health professionals' cognition, the social aspects of fit including social interactions that take place between health professional, patient and technology and the use of the technology to provide patient care. Research suggests poor cognitive-socio-technical fit often leads to unintended consequences that were not expected by either the technology's designer or the organization that procured and implemented the HIS and/or UCD (Borycki et al., 2009a). Poor cognitive-socio-technical fit may result in health professional process and outcomes changes. Process changes include those changes that alter how work is done when a new technology(ies) is implemented. As outcome changes arise from process changes (McLaughlin & Kaluzny, 2006), outcome changes include those changes that affect a patient's health and wellness and are as a direct result of interactions between the health professional, the HIS/UCD that supports work and the social systems of the organization (e.g. hospital or clinic) (Borycki et al., 2009a).

Research has found cognitive-socio-technical fit affects processes and has led to health professionals bypassing some HIS and UCD functions (Kuwata et. al., 2006; Patterson et al., 2002) or experiencing increased cognitive load (Borycki et. al. 2009b; Shachuk et al., 2009), and/or experiencing cumbersome workflows (Kuwata et al., 2006; Patterson et al., 2002). For example, research has shown that that introducing a computer workstation into a physician's office affects the nature of physician-patient communication and physician workflow (Ludwick & Doucette, 2009; Shachuk et al., 2009). Ludwick and Doucette (2009) found that the positioning of a computer workstation in typical physician office led some physicians to modify their workflow and in some cases affected their ability to conduct sensitive communications about health issues with their patients. In such cases, the physicians chose to not document in the electronic patient record on the workstation in the examination room, instead choosing to document on a paper patient record. In another study Shachuk et al., (2009, p.345) found that 92% of physicians found that having an electronic medical record in the exam room "disturbed" their communication with patients in some way. In order to overcome some of these issues physicians developed new skills (i.e. used blind typing) or used templates to improve the workflow that emerged from interactions between the workstation, electronic medical record and the patient. Shachuk et al. (2009) also noted the positioning of a computer workstation in a clinic setting (i.e. social context) influenced workflow and increased cognitive work.

These findings are not unique to the physician office setting. Poor workflows emerging from interactions between UCD-HIS and organizational context (i.e. environment) are also present in the hospital setting. For example, wireless carts that provide ubiquitous access for health professionals to electronic patient records may provide timely patient information, but when used to provide certain types of patient care (i.e. medication administration), they may lead health professionals to develop unplanned workarounds. Publications by Granlien et al. (2008), Kushniruk et al. (2006),

Kuwata et al., (2005) and Patterson et al., (2004) reveal wireless carts in conjunction with medication administration systems (i.e. systems that support nurse administration and documentation of medications administered to patients), bar code scanners, patients, and the hospital environment may lead clinicians to undertake significant workarounds and bypassing of some system functions in order to provide timely patient care. Each of these studies has identified that there is a need to better understand the cognitive-socio-technical fit between the worker and system/UCD in order to optimize fit and improve adoption and appropriation of these technologies (Borycki et al., 2009a; Granlien et al., 2008).

Cognitive-Socio-Technical Fit and Healthcare Processes and Outcomes

The theory of cognitive-socio-technical fit involving HIS and UCD influences healthcare processes and subsequent outcomes. According to the healthcare quality improvement literature, process improvements may lead to significant improvements in outcomes (McLaughlin & Kaluzny, 2006). Along these lines, process changes may also lead to workarounds or bypassing of system functions (if not effectively changed), thereby leading to poor or unintended outcomes such as no reductions in health professional error rates or improvements in patient health status) (Koppel et al., 2005; Kushniruk et al., 2005). Healthcare process changes arising from poor cognitive-socio-technical fit include the development of new unintended interactions (not expected by the technology's designer nor the adopting organization) between a HIS, the UCD and the health professional that in turn influences patient outcomes. For example, in some cases HIS have failed to reduce medication error rates projected by procuring organizations (Koppel et al., 2005). In other cases researchers have reported that the attributes of UCD (e.g. small screen size) have served as a barrier to clinicians use of the UCD (e.g. a handheld device, cellular phone) in the clinical practice setting (Chen al., 2004). Lastly, still other researchers have found that interactions between HIS and UCD can introduce a new class of "unintended" consequences (Ash et al., 2004) such as technology-induced errors (Kushniruk et al., 2005). These unintended consequences have their origins in the interactions between the HIS and the UCD within a given healthcare organizational context. In these cases HIS and UCD have introduced new types of errors to the organization. Such instances of poor cognitive-socio-technical fit need to be identified and addressed to prevent harm from occurring to patients prior to HIS and UCD implementation in real-world settings (Borycki & Kushniruk, 2008). In summary poor-cognitive-socio-technical fit involving HIS, UCD, the healthcare organization and the patient can have significant impact upon healthcare processes and patient outcomes. The substantive costs associated with addressing "unintended" process and outcome changes arising from poor cognitive-socio-technical fit following the introduction of HIS and UCDs in healthcare requires that researchers develop new methods of identifying potential process and outcome changes before a HIS/UCD is implemented to prevent unintended consequences from occurring.

According to Boehm's seminal research (1976), the relative costs of repairing software errors increase exponentially the further the software product moves through the design, coding, testing and implementation phases of the software development lifecycle (SDLC). Although this work focuses on software products, the quality improvement literature in healthcare identifies introducing new processes using HIS and UCD can also lead to significant costs - costs associated with modifying the HIS to meet UCD specifications or the need to identify a new UCD that has high cognitive-socio-technical fit with health professional work (McLaughlin & Kaluzny, 2006). Lastly, the adverse events literature in healthcare identifies the human cost of death and disability arising from software

and UCD failure during medical treatment (Levenson, 1995). In summary it is important to detect unintended consequences associated with using HIS and UCD early in the SDLC, rather than during the operations and maintenance phase (i.e. when HIS and UCD are implemented in a hospital or clinic) and they may lead to medical errors. In the next section of the book chapter the authors will discuss the use of clinical simulations, a methodology for evaluating the impact of HIS and UCD upon health professional work.

CLINICAL SIMULATIONS: A METHODOLOGY FOR EVALUATING THE IMPACT OF HEALTH INFORMATION SYSTEMS AND UBIQUITOUS COMPUTING DEVICES UPON HEALTH PROFESSIONAL WORK

One emerging methodology that may be an effective approach to evaluating the impact of a HIS and UCD upon health professional work processes and patient outcomes is clinical simulation as applied to the evaluation of HIS and UCD in healthcare. Clinical simulations involve the use of real-world examples of complex clinical work activities involving health professionals (e.g. doctors or nurses) being observed as they carry out a work task involving a HIS and UCDs in a hospital or clinic. In the next section of this book chapter, the authors will describe the development and history of clinical simulations in healthcare, their subsequent application and use in health informatics in the evaluation of HIS and UCD, and their use in detecting "unintended" consequences associated with poor cognitive-socio-technical fit.

History of the Use of Clinical Simulations is Healthcare

Clinical simulations have been used in the healthcare industry for many years. Several researchers have successfully developed and utilized clinical simulations as a way of preparing medical and nursing students for real-world practice. Initially, instituted as a method for providing clinicians with opportunities to practice clinical skills and procedures in preparation for work involving live patients, clinical simulation has become an accepted methodology for training physicians and nurses prior to their real-world encounters with patients (Issenberg et al. 2005; Kneebone et al., 2005). Research examining the effectiveness of clinical simulation as a training methodology has shown that student participation in clinical simulations can improve the quality of their clinical decision-making and practice. Clinical simulation can also provide opportunities for students to develop expertise in a given clinical area as well as learn about how to manage a patient's states of health and illness in a safe environment where there are no live patients and instructors can provide constructive feedback (Issenberg et al., 1999; Issenberg et al., 2005; Kneebone et al., 2005).

Clinical simulations may take many forms. For example, a clinical simulation may involve live actors who are "playing" the part of an ill patient – acting out the signs and symptoms of a disease such as pain or melancholy. In such clinical simulations health professional students such as medical students have the opportunity to practice skills such as patient interviewing while an instructor observes and later provides feedback. Instructors review the medical students' performance and provide feedback aimed at improving the health professionals' diagnostic and procedural skills. Simulations may also take the form of interactions with a mannequin (that represents a patient) in a laboratory setting. The health professional has the opportunity to perform procedures on the mannequin that would typically be done on a patient in the clinical setting. Procedures are practiced until the health professional achieves competence in performing the activity, skill or

procedure (Issenberg et al., 2005; Kneebone et al., 2005).

Clinical Simulations and Health Professional Education

In the laboratory setting instructors can observe students applying theory to practice using such clinical simulations. For example, an instructor can observe a student performing an activity or a procedure that was discussed in the classroom. Once the student has completed the activity or procedure, the instructor can provide the student with constructive feedback and thereby help the student to achieve a higher level of knowledge and improve the student's ability to perform the activity or procedure. More recently, the tools used in training health professionals (e.g. physicians and nurses) have improved significantly. Instead of using unresponsive mannequins', health professional training programs are using computerized mannequins and actors to help build clinician skills. Mannequins have been developed that can simulate real patient signs and symptoms of disease over time. Furthermore, these computerized mannequins can be used to train health professionals to respond to life critical events (such as heart attacks) and to perform complex procedures within the context of simulated, life threatening events. This gives the health professional student an opportunity to experience events that are more representative of the real-world and an opportunity to learn about how to respond to these events over time as the patient's condition deteriorates or improves in response to student interventions. Once competencies are achieved, health professionals can move to assessing actors playing the role of a patient. Following this students can learn to manage real patients and perform procedures on real patients in real-world clinical settings under the supervision of a health professional (having practiced these activities on a mannequin and with actors) (Cioffi, 1997; Issenberg et al., 2005).

APPLICATION OF CLINICAL SIMULATIONS TO THE EVALUATION OF HEALTH INFORMATION SYSTEMS AND UBIQUITOUS COMPUTING DEVICES

Researchers have begun to apply key learning's gained from clinical simulation research involving medical and nursing students to the testing and evaluation of HIS and UCDs prior to their implementation in real-world clinical settings. Initial research in this area has employed clinical simulations as a methodology for evaluating the impact of systems and UCDs upon physician cognition and work. Early research in this area took place in the 1990's. Cognitive researchers attempted to determine what effect a HIS deployed on a desktop computer would have upon physician-patient interviews and a physician's cognition. The researchers simulated a typical physician office and asked physician subjects to conduct an interview with an actor, while using the HIS. The researchers found the introduction of a HIS had significant cognitive implications for physicians, as the HIS altered the nature of the patient-physician interview, caused some physicians to become "screen driven" (Kushniruk et al., 1992) and in some cases altered diagnostic reasoning processes (Patel et al., 2000).

More recent research has extended this work to evaluate the impact of HIS deployed on differing UCDs (i.e. hand held UCDs). In one line of research, researchers asked physician subjects to perform a number of prescribing tasks in a simulated clinical environment using a prescription writing system on a personal digital assistant (PDA). The researchers studied the effects of the HIS/UCD upon physician prescribing error rates. In the clinical simulation the researchers were able to observe interactions between a HIS and a hand held computing UCD upon physician prescribing and subsequent medical error rates. The researchers observed that HIS and UCD usability problems led to technology-induced errors.

They were able to identify a number of hand held UCD and HIS interface features that could lead to errors. In addition to this, the researchers noted that the size of the UCD and its responsiveness influenced subject error rates, demonstrating an interaction effect between the HIS and UCD. This research was successful in predicting differing types of technology-induced errors prior to HIS/UCD deployment and implementation (Kushniruk et al., 2005).

In a subsequent study the researchers extended their work to additional health professionals (i.e. nurses and physicians) to evaluate the use of a mobile wireless medication cart with a laptop and a barcode scanner. Subjects were asked to administer medications (i.e. oral medications, injectible medications and intravenous medications) to a mannequin who was wearing a bar-coded bracelet for identification. In this study the researchers again conducted a clinical simulation where health professionals were asked to administer the medications and document their administration on a HIS using a laptop on a mobile cart. The researchers noted the interactions between the health professional, HIS, UCDs (i.e. laptop and bar code scanner) and the mannequin (who took the place of the patient). The researchers observed that the medication administration task involving the UCD and system in the clinical environment led to the development of cumbersome workflows involving the UCD, system and patient. In addition to this, the researchers found the interactions between the subject, UCD, system and patient could lead to increased cognitive load. In some cases subjects engaged in cumbersome and confusing workarounds in order to be able to successfully complete the task of medication administration (including documentation) (Borycki et al., 2009a; Kushniruk et. al. 2006). The researchers were able to provide the healthcare organization that was implementing the HIS/UCDs with feedback about how the system/UCDs could be modified, how to simplify some of the emergent workflows arising from using systems/UCDs and how to improve health professional training so that health professionals spent less time learning about how to use the integrated system (Kushniruk et al., 2006). In summary the use of clinical simulations in the evaluation of interactions between health professionals, HIS, UCDs and patients has demonstrated the value of using clinical simulations to improve health professional work processes while at the same time identifying key ways outcomes can be improved when using HISs/UCDs (i.e. reducing the likelihood of technology-induced errors or unintended consequences). In the next section of this chapter the authors will provide an overview of the clinical simulation methodology.

The Clinical Simulation Methodology

In order for clinical simulations to be effectively used in evaluating the process and outcome impacts of implementing a HIS and its associated UCDs, researchers need to ensure that clinical simulations have a high level of ecological validity. Ecological validity refers to the ability to create clinical simulations that are representative of the real-world settings so that the results of the clinical simulations are generalizable (Vogt, 1999). Therefore, ecological validity ensures the quality and value of the clinical simulation results when they are used to: (1) redesign a system/UCD, (2) procure a system, (3) understand the effects of system customization in conjunction with UCD selection and (4) as an aid to providing technology trainers with information about how to train individuals to use such systems/devices to increase the speed of learning how to use the HIS/UCD in a given clinical setting. In the next section of the chapter we will discuss a sequence of steps that can be used to create clinical simulations that can test aspects of cognitive-socio-technical fit in more detail. This involves creating representative clinical environments (that would typically be found in healthcare organizations where the HIS/UCD would be designed for or deployed). This involves: (1) using representative equipment

from that organization, (2) selecting a range of representative tasks health professionals would typically engage in, (3) developing a range of representative scenarios, and (4) inviting a range of representative health professional subjects to participate in the clinical simulations as part of the evaluation.

Creating Representative Clinical Environments

The complexity of representative clinical environments required for clinical simulations in health informatics where a HIS/UCD is being evaluated varies from low to high fidelity. A low fidelity clinical environment somewhat approximates the real world. In a high fidelity clinical simulation every attempt is made to imitate the real world. In creating high or low fidelity environments there is a need to attend to ecological validity (as outline earlier). As part of creating an ecologically valid environment, the essential features of a real-world environment would need to be re-created so that the subject that is participating in the clinical simulation responds as they would in the real-world when confronted with a similar situation. Therefore, creating a representative organizational or clinical environment is critical to ensuring the ecological validity of the clinical simulation and the validity and value of the results. High ecological validity will lead to representative results in terms of observed impacts of systems and UCDs upon health professional processes and outcomes where as low ecological validity will not.

Tangible and Intangible Aspects of Creating Representative Clinical Environments

Clinical environments (e.g. hospital rooms, nursing stations) have both tangible and intangible components. Tangible aspects of organizations include those visible structures that can be easily replicated such as the physical layout of a hospital room, desks, chairs, hospital beds, intravenous equipment, oxygen equipment etc. Intangible aspects of an organization include those that are not readily visible such as underlying organizational policies, procedures, social norms and culture. Intangible aspects of the clinical environment are difficult to identify and replicate, yet they have a significant impact upon how work is done within an organizational context (Shortell & Kaluzny, 2006).

Tangible aspects of a clinical environment should be evaluated and judged by experts to be representative of typical clinical settings to ensure the setting's ecological validity (Haimson & Elfenbein, 1985; Shortell & Kaluzny, 2006). Experts with clinical, management and health information technology backgrounds should be used to evaluate the ecological validity of a clinical environment in conjunction with health informaticians (Shamian, 1988). Clinical and management experts can be used to judge the representativeness of the simulated clinical environment in terms of layout, furniture and equipment. Information technology and health informatics experts can be used to judge the representativeness of the systems/UCDs that will be used or are currently being used in a "typical" clinical environment. These experts will also be expected to select the "ideal" or planned UCDs for use in the clinical simulation and integrating the system/UCDs for the simulation. For example, if the intent of a clinical simulation is to re-create a representative hospital environment that is "typical"(where the system/UCD would be implemented) of a hospital room with healthcare equipment, this can be done in a laboratory setting. The results of this clinical simulation would be generalizable to most typical hospital environments, but may not be typical of the organization where the HIS/UCDs would actually be implemented (Borycki et al., 2009b; Haimson & Elfenbein, 1985).

Alternatively, if the intent of the clinical simulation is to create a representative hospital environment that is ecologically valid and to ensure the

results of the clinical simulation are representative of the local healthcare organization (e.g. hospital) every effort should be taken to conduct the clinical simulation in the local organization (Haimson & Elfenbein, 1985; Kushniruk & Borycki, 2005; Shortell & Kaluzny, 2006). For example, if a hospital is implementing a specific HIS/UCD that has been customized for the hospital, an empty hospital room can be used with the HIS/UCD to be tested (Kushniruk & Borycki, 2005). As a result, both the tangible and intangible aspects of the organizational environment are replicated in using an empty hospital room within the local organization. In conducting the clinical simulation in the organizational environment where the HIS/UCD will be deployed there will be full replication of the tangible aspects of the organization in the clinical simulation (e.g. room layout, hospital equipment etc.). As well, the intangible aspects of the organizational environment will also be present in the clinical simulation (e.g. organizational culture, social norms in behaviour etc.). The health professionals who participate in the simulation within the context of their own local organization may engage in those organizational and practice norms that underlie all health professional practice and are unique to that organizational context. It must be noted that if a health professional participates in the clinical simulation and they are not familiar with the intangible aspects of the organization they may not practice according to local organizational practices and thereby influence the quality of the clinical simulation results for the local organization. Alternatively, if the health professional participates in a clinical simulation outside their organization (i.e. in a laboratory setting) they may not use the same organizational cultural and behavioural norms. This will also influence the quality of the clinical simulation results (Haimson & Elfenbein, 1985; Shortell & Kaluzny, 2006). Therefore, ecological validity is necessary in order to ensure the process and outcomes changes that are observed during the clinical simulation are representative of those involving the HIS/UCD. Furthermore, there is a need to attend to the tangible and intangible aspects of an organization. Tangible and intangible aspects of organizations may influence health professional activities, practices and behaviours during a clinical simulation and therefore, the quality of the simulation outcomes are affected.

Use of Representative Equipment

The complexity of the equipment used in clinical simulations varies depending on whether the clinical simulation is low or high fidelity. As a low fidelity clinical simulation roughly approximates the real-world, the equipment is often not complex and may be limited to only the HIS/UCDs that are to be evaluated. Alternatively, as we increase the fidelity of the clinical simulation the equipment that is added to the clinical simulation is more representative of the clinical environment. For example, a clinical simulation in an empty hospital room would also include the use of equipment that would typically be used by health professionals in managing a patient's care such as a hospital bed, bedside table, IV poles, oxygen equipment etc. As well, the HIS/UCD that is planned for use would also be used in the clinical simulation environment. This might include the use of a computer workstation placed beside the patient's bed with a copy of the patient's electronic patient record available for viewing during the clinical simulation (Kushniruk et al., 2006; Kuwata et al., 2005).

Use of Representative Patients and Other Health Professionals

The use of representative patients and other health professionals will also range from low to high fidelity. In a low fidelity clinical simulation a mannequin may be used to represent the patient. As the fidelity of the clinical simulation increases a computerized mannequin (that simulates the signs and symptoms of disease) may be used to represent the patient. The fidelity may further

increase with instructors controlling the signs and symptoms of disease that the mannequin is experiencing and providing the mannequin with a "voice" via a speaker or instructor from the control room. Lastly, a high fidelity situation may be constructed where the health professional interacts with an actor playing the part of a patient, other health professionals as well as the systems/UCDs that will be evaluated.

The authors of the book chapter have found that one can create clinical simulations that can be used to evaluate the HIS/UCD. Low and high fidelity simulations have been created by the authors. Low and high fidelity simulations involving a health professional, HIS and UCD can be easily created for as little as $2000 (to evaluate cognitive-socio-technical fit). These simulations involve using real-world equipment and health professionals that can be found in any healthcare facility globally (see Kushniruk & Borycki, 2006). Simulations involving computerized mannequins can also be constructed in facilities that employ such technology to train medical and nursing students as they are now an important part of the training these health professionals globally. Here, such simulations can be conducted in a medical school, nursing school or government organization that uses such technology to train health professionals or a teaching hospital where such equipment resides (Issenberg et al. 2005; Kneebone et al., 2005).

Use of Scenarios

Scenarios are an important component of clinical simulations. Careful attention should be paid to the attributes or qualitative dimensions of each scenario used in the clinical simulation. Scenarios are used to select or create the environment where the clinical simulations will take place (e.g. a hospital room, an operating room, a hallway). Scenarios are also used to set out the context for the clinical simulation. Scenarios should include varying levels of complexity and urgency. For example, if the researcher wishes to examine the ability of a system to address subject information needs in time limited, demanding environments, he or she may observe the subject attempting to acquire information from the system given varying time constraints and urgency (e.g. 5 minutes use of the system to address an information need about a patient's condition versus 20 minutes of possible system use to make a decision about a patient's condition after a clinic visit). Scenarios should take into account routine and atypical cases. For example, in conducting evaluations involving medication order entry systems, the evaluator may include routine cases (e.g. the prescribing of medication in a physician's office to a patient with a chronic illness) (as illustrated in Kushniruk et al, 2005) to atypical cases (e.g. a physician giving medications immediately (i.e. stat) during a critical, life threatening event such as a patient experiencing a myocardial infarction (see Kushniruk et al., 2006 for more details).

Scenarios should be representative of a range of situations that would be encountered by subjects. They should also outline possible sequences of activities that will take place. This will serve as a comparison point between existing processes and outcomes and those that are expected as a result of introducing the technology and those that emerge during a scenario as unintended consequences once the HIS/UCD are introduced (Borycki et al., 2009b; Orlinkowski, 1992). For example, when studying the adequacy of a HIS in addressing information needs, the researcher must first select scenarios that stimulate subjects' need for information such as the need to assess a patient's condition (e.g. Borycki & Lemieux-Charles, 2009). Then the researchers might compare what is routinely done by health professionals in a paper environment to that done to complete the same work in a HIS/UCD environment.

Scenarios can involve low fidelity, simple written medical case descriptions that are given to subjects to read and respond to. Higher fidelity clinical simulation scenarios can involve more

complex scenarios involving computer controlled mannequins that display preset programmed signs and symptoms of disease over time for health professionals to respond to. Even higher fidelity simulations may involve actors with specifically developed scripts that engage the health professional and involve the HIS/UCD to be evaluated. For example, a simple clinical simulation may involve presenting physicians with a short written case description of a patient and asking them to enter the information about the patient into a patient record system. A high fidelity simulation would reproduce more closely the real world situation being studied. This might involve actors playing the roles of patients and staff in a clinic exam room in a study of how doctors' use of an electronic patient record system on a hand held UCD. Such a study may involve multiple recordings of UCDs to precisely document all subject interactions (e.g. audio and video recording of all verbalizations, computer activities and the hospital room or clinic environment as a whole to document actions). For example, in studying the impact of hybrid electronic-paper environments upon novice nurse information seeking, Borycki et al., (2009b) recreated a typical nursing unit environment that would be found in a hospital (i.e. desk, telephone, chairs, workstation, software and paper and electronic sources of nursing and medical information about a typical patient). In order to capture the effects of the hybrid environment upon novice, nurse information seeking the researcher recorded each nurses' verbalizations while reviewing their patient's information by using an audio recorder. The nurses' actions and interactions with their environment were recorded by using a video camcorder. Lastly, the nurses' interactions with the software and hardware (i.e. the workstation) were recorded using Hypercam®, a screen recording program.

Selecting Representative Tasks

This stage involves the selection of representative tasks users are expected to undertake when using the system and UCD under study. A range of tasks should be selected (Kushniruk & Patel, 2004). Ideally, tasks should be in keeping with the environment where the task will be performed and the scenario that has been constructed (Borycki et al., 2005). For example, a nurse may be asked to administer routine medications to a patient in a hospital room. Tasks that are part of this scenario include: logging on to the electronic medication administration system (eMAR), searching for a patient that will be receiving the medication in the electronic medication administration system (eMAR), electronically identifying the patient, identifying the medications that need to be administered at that time, scanning the patients' identifying bar-coded bracelet with a bar code scanner, scanning the medication package, pouring the medication, verifying the patient's identity verbally, giving the medication to the patient and then documenting the administration of the medication in the eMAR that is provided on a laptop mounted on a portable medication administration cart (Altman, 2004; Patterson et al., 2002). This process ensures the medication that is being given by the nurse is given to the correct patient, is the correct medication, is in the correct dose, and is provided by the correct route (e.g. by mouth). This process also ensures the administration of the medication is documented in the eMAR (Altman, 2004).

Inviting Representative Participants

This step involves the identification and selection of representative subjects for the simulation. Subjects should be representative of end users of the system under study in terms of level of disciplinary, domain and technology expertise. Research suggests health professional background can have a significant impact upon processes that involve patient care, systems and UCDs and patient and health professional outcomes (e.g. medical error rates). For example, health professionals of differing disciplinary backgrounds may respond differently to the same scenario (Johnson & Turley, 2006). Research has also demonstrated that a domain of expertise will influence health professional behaviours and outcomes (Lammond et al., 1996). For example, a medical nurse will attend to differing types of information as compared to a surgical nurse when presented with the same task - searching an electronic patient record. Organizational experience has also been shown to have an effect upon worker behaviours (Jablin & Putnam, 2001). Lastly, more recent research by Patel and colleagues (2000) reveals computer expertise can have a significant impact upon health professional use of systems. In addition to this, research suggests experience with differing UCDs may have an impact upon health professional behaviours and outcomes. Evaluators must take into account disciplinary, domain, organizational and technology expertise when selecting representative participants. Ideally a range of participants should be selected to understand differing users' responses to the system/UCD. If the intent is to study user ability to learn about the new HIS/UCD constellation or group of software and devices, then novice users are best to be invited to participate in the clinical simulations (Borycki et al., 2009b).

Data Collection

The authors of this book chapter recommend that audio and video data be collected. Individuals may be asked to "think aloud" as they work with the HIS/UCD individually. Groups of health professionals working with the system/UCD should have their conversations recorded. Audio data of individual's thinking aloud or the conversations of groups of users working with the system/UCD is essential. Audio data provides insights as to what information in the system representative participants are attending to as well as data about potential usability issues arising from system and UCD attributes while the individual or group is working with the HIS and UCD constellation (Kushniruk & Patel, 2004). Other forms of data may include video recordings of subjects interacting with systems, UCDs, other health professionals and simulated patients. Video data allows the researcher to observe emergent workflows arising from interactions between system, UCD and technology (Borycki & Kushniruk, 2005). Computer screen recordings of participants interacting with the system allow the researchers to identify sources of poor or cumbersome workflows. Screen recordings also illuminate human computer interaction issues and issues arising from poor system usability (Kushniruk et al., 2006).

Video data and computer screen recordings can be triangulated with the audio data. Increasingly, the role of computer screen recordings and video data has been found to inform and contextualize information (Borycki et al., 2009). These two types of data have provided researchers with additional insights and understanding of the underlying cognitive processes of subjects and the effects of systems and UCDs upon them. For example, in a recent study by the author that examined the relationship between medical error and system usability, video and computer screen data was used to inform audio transcripts of subjects' "thinking aloud" while interacting with a system on a hand held device. During analysis, audio data indicated subjects were under the impression they had entered the correct prescription data when using an electronic prescribing program on a hand held device. Corresponding video data and computer screen recordings revealed subjects had not entered the correct information and they experienced usability issues. As a result, subjects unknowingly entered the wrong prescription (Borycki & Kushniruk, 2006; Kushniruk et al., 2005).

As described above, clinical simulations as a methodological approach can be used to study the effect of systems and UCDs upon health profes-

sional work processes and outcomes. Clinical simulation unlike other evaluation approaches in health informatics (e.g. randomized clinical control trials) allow one to observe clinicians (e.g. physicians or nurses) interacting with HIS/UCDs under simulated conditions. Clinical simulations allow one to study the effects of the system, UCD, health professional and patient interactions upon clinical processes and outcomes. Clinical simulations can be conducted early in the software development lifecycle to inform design, development, customization, procurement, implementation, operation and maintenance of software and hardware. It must be noted that clinical simulations conducted in a laboratory setting offer significant insights into interactions between UCD, systems and health professionals within an organizational environment (e.g. a hospital). In conducting clinical simulations (as outlined above) all aspects of the interaction are recorded. Researchers can make observations about cognitive-socio-technical fit and changes can be made to the UCD/system to improve fit (Borycki & Kushniruk, 2006). Recordings allow multiple researchers to review the collected data. Inter-rater reliability can be calculated as a result. Researcher reviews of video and audio recordings can prevent researcher and subject recall bias and researcher recording bias. Subject's may experience recall bias – being unable to remember all the interactions between the system, UCD and organizational environment, if other forms of data collection are used such as semi-structured interviews or focus groups. In such cases subjects may not be able to recall all the events that occurred in their interactions with the UCD and system within in a given organizational environment (Jackson & Verberg, 2006). Researcher bias involves a researcher not being able to physically record all of the information when taking notes or being selective about the information that is recorded during observations of subjects interacting between the UCD and technology.

Some researchers have attempted to conduct

these types of studies in naturalistic settings involving real-world interactions between patients, health professionals, systems, UCDs and organizational contexts. Many of these studies (e.g. Ash et al., 2004) have involved semi-structured one-on-one interviews and focus groups with key informants (i.e. health professionals who have been affected by these UCD/HIS implementations). As well, researchers have conducted observational analyses of subjects working in these environments. Researchers observed subjects while they were performing tasks and took notes.

Data Analysis

Data analysis, where clinical simulations are concerned, is both qualitative and quantitative in nature. Data can be qualitatively coded using empirically accepted coding schemes to identify subject patterns of interactions with a system, workflow issues, usability problems and recurring system issues. Audio, video and computer screen data can be qualitatively coded. Data can be coded using inductive, deductive and mixed method approaches. Deductive approaches involving the coding of qualitative data involve the use of existing empirically accepted coding schemes, model(s) or theory (ies) (Ericsson & Simon, 1993). Alternatively, when inductive approaches are used, data drives coding scheme development (e.g. grounded theory approaches) (Kuziemsky et al., 2007). Mixed method approaches towards the analysis of qualitative data combine both inductive and deductive methods. Here inductive and deductive approaches are combined. Empirically validated coding schemes from the research are used while at the same time new codes can emerge from the data as prior empirical work may not be sufficient to fully inform the coding of the data. In combining the approaches, transcripts of audio, video and computer screen recordings are initially coded using existing empirically validated coding schemes, models or theories. Then, inductively extensions are made to the empirically validated

coding schemes, models or theories (Borycki et al., 2009b; Ericsson & Simon, 1993; Kushniruk & Patel, 2004; Patel et al., 2000).

Qualitative data are not limited to coded audio, video or computer screen data. Video data and computer screen recordings can be reviewed. Workflow and data flow diagrams can be constructed to observe for differences in before and after HIS/UCD use. Such diagrams allow the evaluator to identify cumbersome workflows as well as interactions between HIS/UCDs that increase the complexity of work and cognitive load (Borycki et. al., 2009a). Qualitative data (i.e. coded verbal transcripts, actions on the computer screens and observed behaviours) can be quantified (Borycki & Lemieux-Charles, 2008). Coded verbal data may be reduced to individual items "intended to mean on thing" (Sandelowski, 1999, p. 253). Frequencies can be tabulated for each code in the transcribed data. Then, inferential statistics can be done (Borycki & Lemieux-Charles, 2008; Ericsson & Simon, 1993).

In summary clinical simulations in health informatics involve imitating real-world situations in a laboratory setting or a organizational environment (e.g. a clinic, hospital room or operating room). Clinical situations are used to assess the impact of new software, UCDs and interactions between the two upon health professional work. In health informatics clinical simulations allow health informaticians to observe health professionals with differing backgrounds (e.g. nurses or physicians) while they perform tasks typical of their profession as they would perform them in real-world settings while engaging with other health professionals and patients. In addition to aiding in the assessment of these UCDs, clinical simulations allow one to assess differing constellations of HIS and UCDs in laboratory or real-world environments to be tested and evaluated prior to their real-world or organization wide implementation - in the process reducing the risk to the healthcare organization by minimizing the likelihood of an institution wide redesign and reimplementation arising from poor cognitive-socio-technical fit. In undertaking clinical simulations in health informatics, HIS and UCD designers as well as the organization's where these systems and UCDs are implemented are able to assess the impact of the system and UCD upon health professional processes and outcomes without patient involvement and without placing the health professional in a situation where the new system and UCD may impact upon their ability to work with other health professionals or with a patient. In this case, the health professional encounters difficulties while working with the HIS and UCD when using the system/device in the context of a "safe" laboratory environment and clinical situation (i.e. not involving patients).

FUTURE RESEARCH DIRECTION

Future research involving the use of clinical simulations will involve applying the methodology to new and emerging types of UCD and HIS. For example, many healthcare organizations are attempting to determine the UCDs that would best meet the needs of clinicians in the hospital and clinical setting. In addition to this as UCDs have become more prevalent in healthcare, HIS that have historically been made available to clinicians via desktop workstations will need to be evaluated in terms of their ability to support the cognitive and social aspects of health professional work using varying types of UCD/HIS in combination. This will help to identify the best constellations of HISs and UCDs that lead to improvements in health care processes and the quality of patient care while at the same time reducing the likelihood of a medical error occurring. The authors are currently working on developing advanced simulations to assess potential issues in the integration of electronic health records with a range of physical devices (e.g. monitoring devices, bar coded patient bracelets etc). Lastly, there will be a need to identify the range of routine to urgent

and typical to atypical situations that can be used to test HIS and UCD.

CONCLUSION

Clinical simulations in health informatics have allowed software and hardware vendors as well as healthcare organizations to better customize HIS to the local organizational environments prior to implementation. Clinical simulation also allows organizations to assess the impact of HIS and UCD constellations upon health professionals cognitive-socio-technical fit. Such knowledge is significant as it influences the design and development of software and UCDs at the vendor level. Such knowledge also influences the customization of software by organizations and their procurement of software and UCDs for use in the clinical setting. Lastly, such information offers organizations the opportunity to develop training strategies for health professionals that take into account the cognitive-socio-technical learning needs of health professionals as they learn to use the new HIS and the UCDs that will be used in conjunction with the HIS in a real-world setting.

The outcomes of using clinical simulations to evaluate HIS and UCDs are significant. Clinical simulations have been effectively used to evaluate the impact of a technology (i.e. HIS and UCDs) upon health professional processes such as patient interviews (involving actors who are playing the role of patient) (Kushniruk et al., 1996), information seeking (Borycki et al., 2009b), decision-making (Patel et al., 2000), knowledge organization, reasoning (Patel et al., 2001), workflow (Borycki et. al., 2009a), and patient safety (Kushniruk et al., 2005). They have also been used to evaluate the impact of interactions between UCDs, HIS and health professionals where patient care processes and outcomes are concerned (Kushniruk et. al., 2005; Patel et. al., 2000). Clinical simulations when applied to the evaluation of cognitive-socio-technical fit involving HIS and UCDs can provide significant benefit to technology designers and organizations who are procuring these systems and UCDs. They allow technology designers to evaluate the impact of systems/UCDs upon health professional work prior to systems implementation (thereby preventing possible system/UCD implementation failures or failures to fully use HIS/UCD functionality). From an organizational perspective, clinical simulations allow organizations to evaluate the interactions between HIS, UCD, organizational environment and health professional. The use of clinical simulations ensures that organizations achieve a strong cognitive-socio-technical fit for health professionals. This lessens the likelihood of implementation failure and poor health professional adoption and appropriation of technology(ies). Such use of clinical simulation is needed to evaluate HIS/UCD cognitive-socio-technical fit with health professional work. Such evaluation is important to prevent the need for the modification of HIS/UCDs after implementation when the cost of implementation is significantly higher. The use of clinical simulations in the evaluation of HIS/UCDs is a significant advancement over an evaluation of HIS/UCD after implementation using semi-structured interviews or observation of clinicians in the healthcare work environment (as both these methodologies are prone to recall and researcher recording bias) and may not allow for full documentation of the interactions. This is a new and emerging methodology that extends work in the area of usability engineering by borrowing methods of recording data and applying those recording methods to the evaluation of cognitive-socio-technical fit involving HIS and UCDs. This work also borrows methods from the training of health professionals and extends them for use in evaluating the effects of HIS/UCDs upon cognitive-socio-technical fit involving organizational processes and outcomes.

REFERENCES

Altman, G. (2004). *Delmar's fundamental and advanced nursing skills* (2nd ed.). Toronto: Thompson Delmar Learning.

Ammenwerth, E., Schnell-Inderst, P., Machan, C., & Siebert, U. (2008). The effect of electronic prescribing on medication errors and adverse drug events: A systematic review. *Journal of the American Medical Informatics Association, 15*(5), 585–600. doi:10.1197/jamia.M2667

Anderson, J. G., & Aydin, C. E. (2005). *Evaluating the organizational impact of healthcare information systems*. New York: Springer Verlag. doi:10.1007/0-387-30329-4

Ash, J. S., Berg, M., & Coiera, E. (2004). Some unintended consequences of information technology in health care: The nature of patient care information system related errors. *Journal of the American Medical Informatics Association, 11*(2), 121–124.

Bates, D. W., Teich, J. M., Lee, J., Seger, D., & Kuperman, G. J., Ma'Luf, N., Boyle, D., Leape, L. (1999). The impact of computerized physician order entry on medication error prevention. *Journal of the American Medical Informatics Association, 6*(4), 313–321.

Berg, M. (1999). Patient care information systems and health care work: A sociotechnical approach. *International Journal of Medical Informatics, 55*(2), 87–101. doi:10.1016/S1386-5056(99)00011-8

Boehm, B. W. (1976). Software engineering. *IEEE Transactions on Computers, ▪▪▪*, C-25.

Borycki, E. M., & Kushniruk, A. W. (2006). Identifying and preventing technology-induced error using simulations: Application of usability engineering techniques. *Healthcare Quarterly (Toronto, Ont.), 8*, 99–105.

Borycki, E. M., & Kushniruk, A. W. (2008). Where do technology induced errors come from? Towards a model for conceptualizing and diagnosing errors caused by technology. In Kushniruk, A. W., & Borycki, E. M. (Eds.), *Human and Social Aspects of Health Information Systems* (pp. 148–166). Hershey, PA: IGI Global.

Borycki, E. M., Kushniruk, A. W., Kuwata, S., & Kannry, J. (2006). Use of simulation in the study of clinician workflow. *AMIA Annual Symposium Proceedings* (pp. 61-5).

Borycki, E. M., Kushniruk, A. W., Kuwata, S., & Watanabe, H. (2008). Using low-cost simulation approaches for assessing the impact of a medication administration system on workflow. *Studies in Health Technology and Informatics, 136*, 567–572.

Borycki, E. M., Kushniruk, A. W., Kuwata, S., & Watanabe, H. (2009a). Simulations to assess medication administration systems. In Staudinger, B., Hob, V., & Ostermann, H. (Eds.), *Nursing and Clinical Informatics* (pp. 144–159). Hershey, PA: IGI Global.

Borycki, E. M., & Lemieux-Charles, L. (2008). Does a hybrid electronic-paper environment impact on health professional information seeking. *Studies in Health Technology and Informatics, 136*, 505–510.

Borycki, E. M., Lemieux-Charles, L., Nagle, L., & Eysenbach, G. (2009b). Evaluating the impact of hybrid electronic-paper environments upon novice nurse information seeking. *Methods of Information in Medicine, 2*, 1–7.

Chaudhry, B., Wang, J., Wu, Sh., Maglione, M., Mojica, W., & Roth, E. (2006). Systematic review: Impact of health information technology on quality, efficiency and costs of medical care. *Annals of Internal Medicine, 144*, E-12–E22.

Chen, E. S., Mendonca, E. A., McKnight, L. K., Stetson, P. S., Lei, J., & Cimino, J. J. (2004). PalmCIS: A wireless handheld application for satisfying clinician information needs. *Journal of the American Medical Informatics Association, 11*(1), 19–28. doi:10.1197/jamia.M1387

Cioffi, J., & Markham, R. (1997). Clinical decision making by midwives: Managing case complexity. *Journal of Advanced Nursing, 23*, 265–272. doi:10.1046/j.1365-2648.1997.1997025265.x

Elmes, D. G., Kantowicz, B. H., & Roediger, H. L. (1981). *Research methods in psychology* (2nd ed.). St. Paul: West Publishing Company.

Ericsson, KA, Simon, HA. *Protocol analysis: Verbal reports as data* (2nd ed.). Cambridge, Massachusetts: MIT Press.

Eslami, S., Abu-Hanna, A., & deKeizer, N. F. (2007). Evaluation of outpatient computerized physician medication order entry systems: A systematic review. *Journal of the American Medical Informatics Association, 14*(4), 400–406. doi:10.1197/jamia.M2238

Eslami, S., deKeizer, N. F., & Abu-Hanna, A. (2008). The impact of computerized physician medication order entry in hospitalized patients: A systematic review. *International Journal of Medical Informatics, 77*, 365–376. doi:10.1016/j.ijmedinf.2007.10.001

Friedman, C. P., & Wyatt, J. C. (2006). *Evaluation methods in biomedical informatics*. New York: Springer.

Granlien, M. F., Herzum, M., & Gudmundsen, J. (2008). The gap between actual and mandated use of an electronic medication record three years after deployment. *Studies in Health Technology and Informatics, 136*, 419–424.

Haimson, B. R., & Elfenbein, M. H. (1985). *Experimental methods in psychology*. Toronto: McGraw-Hill.

Issenberg, S. B., McGaghie, W. C., Hart, I. R., Mayer, J. W., Felner, J. M., & Petrusa, E. R. (1999). Simulation technology for health care professionals skills training and assessment. *Journal of the American Medical Association, 282*(9), 861–866. doi:10.1001/jama.282.9.861

Issenberg, S. B., McGaghie, W. C., Petrusa, E. R., Gordon, D. L., & Scalese, R. J. (2005). Features and uses of high-fidelity medical simulations that lead to effective learning: A BEME systematic review. *Medical Teacher, 27*(1), 10–28. doi:10.1080/01421590500046924

Jablin, F. M., & Putnam, L. L. (2001). *The new handbook of organizational communication: Advances in theory, research and methods*. New York: Sage.

Jackson, W., & Verberg, N. (2006). *Methods: Doing social research* (4th ed.). Toronto: Pearson Prentice Hall.

Johnson, C. M., & Turley, J. P. (2006). The significance of cognitive modeling in building healthcare interfaces. *International Journal of Medical Informatics, 75*, 163–172. doi:10.1016/j.ijmedinf.2005.06.003

Joint Commission for Health Care Quality. (2008). Safely implementing health information and converging technologies. Retrieved April 14, 2009 from http://www.jointcommission.org/SentinelEventAlert/sea_42.htm

Kneebone, R. (2005). Evaluating clinical simulation for learning procedural skills: A theory-based approach. *Academic Medicine, 80*(6), 549–553. doi:10.1097/00001888-200506000-00006

Koppel, R., & Kreda, D. (2009). Health care information technology vendors' "hold harmless" clause: Implications for clinicians. *Journal of the American Medical Association, 301*(12), 1276–1278. doi:10.1001/jama.2009.398

Koppel, R., Metlay, J. P., Cohen, A., Abaluck, B., Localio, R., Kimmel, S. E., & Strom, B. L. (2005). Role of computerized physician order entry systems in facilitating medication errors. *Journal of the American Medical Association, 293*(10), 1197–1203. doi:10.1001/jama.293.10.1197

Kushniruk, A. W., Borycki, E., Kuwata, S., & Kannry, J. (2006). Predicting changes in workflow resulting from healthcare information systems: Ensuring the safety of healthcare. *Healthcare Quarterly (Toronto, Ont.), 9*, 114–118.

Kushniruk, A. W., & Borycki, E. M. (2006). Low-cost rapid usability engineering: Designing and customizing usable healthcare information systems. *Healthcare Quarterly (Toronto, Ont.), 9*(4), 98–100, 102.

Kushniruk, A. W., Kaufman, D. R., Patel, V. L., Levesque, Y., & Lottin, P. (1992). Assessment of a computerized patient record system: A cognitive approach to evaluating an emerging medical technology. *M.D. Computing, 13*(5), 406–415.

Kushniruk, A. W., & Patel, V. L. (2004). Cognitive and usability engineering methods for the evaluation of clinical information systems. *Journal of Biomedical Informatics, 37*, 56–76. doi:10.1016/j.jbi.2004.01.003

Kushniruk, A. W., Triola, M. M., Borycki, E. M., Stein, B., & Kannry, J. L. (2005). Technology induced error and usability: The relationship between usability problems and prescription errors when using a handheld application. *International Journal of Medical Informatics, 74*, 519–526. doi:10.1016/j.ijmedinf.2005.01.003

Kuwata, S., Kushniruk, A., Borycki, E., & Watanabe, H. (2006). Using simulation methods to analyze and predict changes in workflow and potential problems in the use of bar-coding medication order entry systems. *AMIA Annual Symposium Proceedings*, 994.

Kuziemsky, C. E., Borycki, E. M., Black, F., Boyle, M., Cloutier-Fisher, D., Fox, L., et al. (2007). A framework for interdisciplinary team communication and its implications for information systems design. wcmeb. *Eighth World Congress on the Management of eBusiness* (pp. 14).

Lammond, D., Crow, R., Chase, J., Doggen, K., & Sinkels, M. (1996). Information sources used in decision making: Considerations for simulation development. *International Journal of Nursing Studies, 33*(1), 47–57. doi:10.1016/0020-7489(95)00064-X

Lapointe, L., & Rivard, S. (2005). Clinical information systems: Understanding and preventing their premature demise. *Healthcare Quarterly (Toronto, Ont.), 3*(4), 92–99.

Lapointe, L., & Rivard, S. (2006). Getting physicians to accept new information technology: Insights from case studies. *Canadian Medical Association Journal, 174*(11), 1573–1578. doi:10.1503/cmaj.050281

Levenson, N. (1995). *Safeware: System safety and computers*. Reading, Massachusetts: Addison-Wesley.

Ludwick, D. A., & Doucette, J. (2009). The implementation of operational processes for Alberta Electronic Health Record: Lessons for Electronic Medical Record Adoption in primary care. *Healthcare Quarterly (Toronto, Ont.), 7*(4), 103–107.

McLaughlin, C. P., & Kaluzny, A. D. (2006). *Continuous quality improvement in healthcare: Theory, implementations and applications* (3rd ed.). Toronto: Jones and Bartlett.

Orlikowski, W. J. (1992). The duality of technology: Rethinking the concept of technology in organizations. *Organization Science, 3*(3), 398–427. doi:10.1287/orsc.3.3.398

Patel, V. L., & Groen, G. J. The general and specific nature of medical expertise: A critical look. In Ericsson, K. A., & Smith, J. (Eds.), *Toward a general theory of expertise prospects and limits. New York* (pp. 93–125). Cambridge.

Patel, V. L., Kushniruk, A. W., Yang, S., & Yale, J.-F. (2000). Impact of a computer-based patient record system on data collection, knowledge organization, and reasoning. *Journal of the American Medical Informatics Association, 7*(6), 569–585.

Patterson, E. S., Cook, R. I., & Render, M. L. (2002). Improving patient safety by identifying side effects from introducing bar coding in medication administration. *Journal of the American Medical Informatics Association, 9*(5), 540–553. doi:10.1197/jamia.M1061

Rabinowitz, E. (1999). Is there a doctor in the house? *Managed Care (Langhorne, Pa.), 8*(9), 42–44.

Sandelowski, M. (1991). Combining qualitative and quantitative sampling, data collection and analysis techniques in mixed-method studies. *Research in Nursing & Health, 23*, 2046–2255.

Shachak, A., Hadas-dayagi, M., Ziv, A., & Reis, S. (2009). Primary care physicians' use of an electronic medical record system: A cognitive task analysis. *Journal of General Internal Medicine, 24*(3), 341–348. doi:10.1007/s11606-008-0892-6

Shamian, J. (1988). The effect of the teaching of decision analysis on student nurses' clinical intervention decision making. Unpublished doctorial dissertation. Case Western Reserve University, Clevland, Ohio.

Shortell, S. M., & Kaluzny, A. D. (2006). *Health care management: Organization design and behaviour* (5th ed.). Canada: Thompson Delmar Learning.

Shortliffe, E. H., & Cimino, J. J. (2008). *Biomedical Informatics: Computer Applications in Healthcare and Biomedicine*. New York: Springer.

Shulman, R., Singer, M., Goldstone, J., & Bellingan, G. (2005). Medication errors: A prospective cohort study of hand-written and computerized physician order entry in the intensive care unit. *Critical Care (London, England)*, *9*(8), 516–521. doi:10.1186/cc3793

Vogt, W. P. (1999). *Dictionary of statistics and methodology* (2nd ed.). Thousand Oaks: Sage.

ADDITIONAL READING

Ammenwerth, E., Schnell-Inderst, P., Machan, C., & Siebert, U. (2008). The effect of electronic prescribing on medication errors and adverse drug events: A systematic review. *Journal of the American Medical Informatics Association*, *15*(5), 585–600. doi:10.1197/jamia.M2667

Ash, J. S., Berg, M., & Coiera, E. (2004). Some unintended consequences of information technology in health care: The nature of patient care information system related errors. *Journal of the American Medical Informatics Association*, *11*(2), 121–124.

Borycki, E. M., & Kushniruk, A. W. (2008). Where do technology induced errors come from? Towards a model for conceptualizing and diagnosing errors caused by technology. In Kushniruk, A. W., & Borycki, E. M. (Eds.), *Human and Social Aspects of Health Information Systems* (pp. 148–166). Hershey, PA: IGI Global.

Borycki, E. M., Kushniruk, A. W., Kuwata, S., & Watanabe, H. (2009a). Simulations to assess medication administration systems. In Staudinger, B., Hob, V., & Ostermann, H. (Eds.), *Nursing and Clinical Informatics* (pp. 144–159). Hershey, PA: IGI Global.

Borycki, E. M., Lemieux-Charles, L., Nagle, L., & Eysenbach, G. (2009b). Evaluating the impact of hybrid electronic-paper environments upon novice nurse information seeking. *Methods of Information in Medicine*, *2*, 1–7.

Chaudhry, B., Wang, J., Wu, Sh., Maglione, M., Mojica, W., & Roth, E. (2006). Systematic review: Impact of health information technology on quality, efficiency and costs of medical care. *Annals of Internal Medicine*, *144*, E-12–E22.

Eslami, S., Abu-Hanna, A., & deKeizer, N. F. (2007). Evaluation of outpatient computerized physician medication order entry systems: A systematic review. *Journal of the American Medical Informatics Association*, *14*(4), 400–406. doi:10.1197/jamia.M2238

Eslami, S., deKeizer, N. F., & Abu-Hanna, A. (2008). The impact of computerized physician medication order entry in hospitalized patients: A systematic review. *International Journal of Medical Informatics*, *77*, 365–376. doi:10.1016/j.ijmedinf.2007.10.001

Koppel, R., Metlay, J. P., Cohen, A., Abaluck, B., Localio, R., Kimmel, S. E., & Strom, B. L. (2005). Role of computerized physician order entry systems in facilitating medication errors. *Journal of the American Medical Association*, *293*(10), 1197–1203. doi:10.1001/jama.293.10.1197

Kushniruk, A. W., & Borycki, E. M. (2006). Low-cost rapid usability engineering: Designing and customizing usable healthcare information systems. *Healthcare Quarterly (Toronto, Ont.)*, *9*(4), 98–100, 102.

Kushniruk, A. W., Triola, M. M., Borycki, E. M., Stein, B., & Kannry, J. L. (2005). Technology induced error and usability: The relationship between usability problems and prescription errors when using a handheld application. *International Journal of Medical Informatics*, *74*, 519–526. doi:10.1016/j.ijmedinf.2005.01.003

KEY TERMS AND DEFINITIONS

Clinical Simulation: A re-creation or imitation of the key characteristics of a real-world healthcare environment or setting (e.g. hospital room, emergency room, physician office) for the purpose of evaluating a group of HIS/UCD.

Cognitive-Socio-Technical Fit: Cognitive-socio-technical fit refers to the cognitive aspects of fit involving health professionals' cognition, the social aspects of fit including social interactions that take place between the health professional(s), patient and technology and the use of the technology to provide patient care.

Computerized Physician Order Entry (CPOE): Computerized physician order entry is a health information system that allows for the electronic entry of physician orders for patients under a physician's care. These orders are sent over a computer network to other health professionals so that they may be fulfilled.

Ecological Validity: Ecological validity refers to the ability to create clinical simulations that are representative of real-world healthcare settings (e.g. hospitals and clinics) so that the results of a clinical simulation are generalizable to the real-world.

Electronic Medication Administration Record (eMAR): An electronic medication administration record is an electronic health information system that uses bar code reader technology, an electronic medication record system and a wireless medication cart to aid in the process of medication administration.

Intended Consequences: Those real-world processes and outcomes that HIS and UCD are expected to change by the technology's designers or the organization that implemented the HIS/UCD after the HIS/UCD has been implemented.

Technology-Induced Error: A new type of medical error that arises from the introduction of a technology or from the interactions that take place between a technology, a health professional and a real-world healthcare environment.

Unintended Consequences: Those real-world processes and outcomes of HIS and UCD that were not predicted and that did not change as was originally expected by the technology's designers or the organization that implemented the HIS/UCD.

Chapter 27
Technology and Human Resources Management in Health Care

Stefane M. Kabene
University of Western Ontario, Canada

Lisa King
University of Western Ontario, Canada

Candace J. Gibson
University of Western Ontario, Canada

ABSTRACT

Health care has lagged behind most industries and businesses in its adoption of information and communication technologies (ICT). Many of the current information technologies and those to be deployed and developed over the next few years (e.g. electronic health records, telehealth applications, elearning technologies, social networking via Web 2.0) could be of benefit in health care delivery and improvement of the quality, efficiency and effectiveness of health care services. The uses of technology in human resources management (HRM) can help improve the medical care that health professionals provide to their patients. For instance, technology can be used to maximize communication, collaboration and support between health professionals separated by distance, as well as provide immediate and up-to-date patient care information. ICT can also be used for distance training and education for those facing geographic isolation and provide a medium through which continued education can be maintained for both rural and urban health professionals. However, due to the differences in barriers to ICT use found for each group, such as computer illiteracy, geographic isolation or poor infrastructure, different steps need to be taken in order to ensure the successful implementation and use of information technologies in both urban and rural communities in developed and developing regions across the world.

DOI: 10.4018/978-1-61520-777-0.ch027

Copyright © 2010, IGI Global. Copying or distributing in print or electronic forms without written permission of IGI Global is prohibited.

INTRODUCTION

Human resources management (HRM) includes the selection and recruitment of personnel, their retention (which is affected by compensation, benefits, quality of work life, and support), their training and development, career progression and promotion. Human resources planning and effective human resources management are essential within a single institution or institutions, a local region or even at the national level to meet organizational objectives, requirements and needs. Within the health care field HRM is focused on making sure that the right mix of health care providers is in place to meet the health care needs of citizens, on adequate recruitment and retention (i.e. encouraging more people to enter the health care field and improving working conditions to retain them), and increasingly on new paradigms that adjust the way in which health professionals are educated and practice in interprofessional health care teams (Kabene et al, 2006).

New information and communication technology(ies) (ICT), and the growing use of computers and the Internet, can address many of the information, communication, and training issues faced by health professionals and human resources managers. HRM itself relies on information systems and information needs. All of the activities in health HR management rely on the existence of information systems that can provide high-quality data that are timely, accurate, comparable, accessible and relevant. Priority information areas for HRM are information on the demographics of the workforce, their education/training, geographical distribution, migration or non migration-related attrition, and employment or practice characteristics (Dussault & Franceschini, 2006; Henderson & Tulloch, 2008; Hongoro & McPake, 2004; Wibulpolprasert & Pengpaibon, 2003). The focus of this discussion though relates to the use of ICT to assist in the training, recruitment and retention of health professionals.

Additionally an unbalanced distribution of health professionals both within countries (urban versus rural) and between countries (developed versus developing) has been recognized as a widespread global problem. In this discussion 'urban developed' refers to city centers in Westernized regions; 'rural developed' regions are those found in Westernized remote locations; 'urban developing' refers to city centers in non-industrialized or low resource/income countries; and rural areas of the developing world would be considered to have an increased level of poverty, poor transportation and fewer specialized services and organizations to provide health care (Goldsmith et al, 1995). These disparities have been attributed to individual, organizational, and economic issues – the lack of coordinated national health human resources policies being one (Dussault & Franceschini, 2006). Although not a panacea, ICT presents a tool to both manage and improve aspects of human resources including satisfaction and retention of personnel, recruitment, training, improved working conditions and access to needed information. Telemedicine or telehealth, the utilization of telecommunication technology for delivery of health services at a distance (that is, for diagnosis, treatment, and patient care, as well as training and continuing education), can "provide expert-based health care to understaffed remote sites and to provide advanced emergency care through modern telecommunication and information technologies" (Lin, 1999, p. 28).

Information technologies encompass any technology which processes and communicates data. It includes: computers, voice, data and image sensing and communications devices, graphics devices, multi-media storage, et cetera. ICT hardware devices include those used for sensing (e.g. bar code scanners, keyboards, mice), communication (fax, cellular phones, local or wide area networks (LANs and WANs)), analysis (computers - micros, minis, mainframes), and display (monitors, printers, voice output, television) and the software applications (operating systems, end-user applications) needed to provide theses services.

In analyzing the HRM literature we have concentrated on looking at those areas where information technology can reinforce and improve some of the resource management issues, e.g. increased retention of health professionals through improved working conditions by providing health information where and when it is needed, providing clinical guidance and support, improved training and educational opportunities (both initial training and in continuing professional education), and improved geographic distribution by providing support for rural physicians and professionals in low income countries in the developing world. This review of the effects of these telecommunication services and current status and use among health care professionals highlights and emphasizes HRM's use of technology in health care and suggests where improvements can be made.

THE INTERSECTION OF ICT AND HRM IN HEALTH CARE

ICT and HRM Issues in Urban-Developed Regions

The practice of medicine is an information-based, knowledge intensive business. Experienced physicians use about two million bits of information to manage their patients (Smith, 1996). It is estimated in the US that about a third of a doctor's time is spent recording and synthesizing information and about a third of hospital costs are spent on personal and professional communications (Smith, 1996). With an increasing number of medical journals and articles (for example over 14 million citations and abstracts to articles in over 5,000 life sciences journals appear in PubMed/Medline with about 10,000 to 20,000 added weekly) (MEDLINE – Fact Sheet, 2007); over 5,000 systematic reviews in the Cochrane Collaboration library database

(Cochrane Collaboration – http://www.cochrane.org), and over 20,000 prescription drugs (e.g. Health Canada – Drug Product Database - http://www.hc-sc.gc.ca/dhp-mps/prodpharma/databasdon/index-eng.php) it is impossible for the average physician to keep that information "in their heads" to effectively diagnose, prescribe and treat patients.

The term "information needs" refers to the knowledge required for health care professionals "to carry out patient care and professional duties" (Dorsch, 2000, p. 347). According to Westberg and Miller (1998), information needs in clinical practice fall on two axes: formal to informal and general to specific. An example of formal information is peer reviewed literature from controlled scientific studies. Examples of informal information would be unwritten, common practices followed at a clinic. Knowledge that is widely available and applies to several categories of patients is general knowledge; while findings in a patient's chart, for example, would be local or specific knowledge.

In terms of access to information resources all health professionals can be divided into the following three groups (Dorsch, 2000): the served, underserved, and the unserved. Common among all groups is that information is underused, all face barriers to optimal information use, and all prefer referring to colleagues or personal library collections over bibliographical sources for acquiring information. Moreover, "information literacy is the ability to recognize the need for information; to find, organize, evaluate and use such information for effective decision making or problem solving; and to apply these skills to independent, life-long learning" (Sheppard and Mackintosh, 1998, p. 192).

For both urban and rural health care professionals, the primary reasons for seeking information are related to patient health care. In the ordinary course of patient care family doctors ask a number of questions dealing with diagnosis, treatment and management of diseases. The most frequently asked questions relate to the causes of symptoms, what tests may be indicated, doses of drugs, and how a disease should be managed or treated (Dorsch, 2000; Ely et al, 1999). Answers to most of these questions (64%), with the exception of drug prescribing, are not immediately pursued and for those that are, doctors spent an average of less than 2 minutes pursuing an answer. Their preference for resource material to answer these questions was readily available print or text sources and human resources (a nearby colleague) (Dorsch, 2000; Ely et al, 1999). Few questions generated either a computer-based search on the Internet or with a CD-ROM resource. Previous studies have shown that most computer applications were too slow or cumbersome to use at the bedside or point of care.

During the next decade, we will undoubtedly see the development and deployment of comprehensive electronic health information systems incorporating all aspects of in-hospital and out-of-hospital care. These systems will allow health providers at all levels and across geographic distances to access information quickly and share information, improving both patient care outcomes and operational efficiency. Health information technologies that are being implemented and newly emerging technologies that will have an impact on health care, health services delivery and HRM include:

1. electronic lifetime health records (EHR) to store data from many sources (e.g., text and voice notes, medical images, laboratory values, patient demographics), with available access from any locale;

2. mobile computing technologies such as hand-held computing devices (or personal digital assistants, PDAs), mobile clinical assistants designed for both provision and entry of relevant health information at the point of care (Adatia & Bedard, 2002; 2003);

3. picture archiving and communication systems (PACS) that capture, store and provide access to diagnostic images (X-ray films, magnetic resonance images, computed tomography scans) from any location;

4. radio frequency identification (RFID) systems will use radio waves to wirelessly track hospital patients, and microchips to carry information on medications, laboratory tests, imaging studies and medical devices;

5. automated inventory systems to track and manage pharmaceuticals and other medical and general hospital supplies;

6. computerized provider order entry systems for laboratory tests, diagnostic images, drug prescribing;

7. decision support systems that will give health care providers real-time advice on diagnosis and treatment options based on continuously updated information and best evidence (Anvari, 2007; Westberg & Miller, 1999).

Use of new electronic record systems will improve the quality of patient care by streamlining processes, reducing duplication of orders and tests, and minimizing the risk of medical errors, such as administration of the wrong drug or dosage, or even the performance of a wrong surgery.

What makes the HR responsibilities of these evolving technologies more difficult is that there are as yet no hard-and-fast answers to formulate best-practice guidelines. For example, identification cards with radio frequency identification devices for employees allow employers to better maintain a secure workplace, but privacy advocates say that employers can (and do) abuse RFIDs by tracking employee movements at any or all times, which may modify potential deviant employee behaviour (Vilamovska et al, 2009). This technology also has the potential to help with health-care applications when used to carry an employee's medical records.

Case studies suggest that security and public safety trump personal privacy; such that securing the workplace, investigating instances of theft or misconduct, and accounting for employees after emergencies, plus providing effective responses to medical problems are the priorities favoured in designing and operating the systems that use RFIDs (Vilamovska et al, 2009). Key human resource issues regarding technology and health care are the dual responsibilities of supervised access to personnel (and personal) data from a standpoint of both database security and medical ethics (i.e. monitored access for quality assurance purposes, outcome assessments and disease surveillance) (Anvari, 2007).

Similarly the benefits of a fully electronic record in improved quality of care – increased adherence to care guidelines, enhanced monitoring and surveillance, decreased medication errors and decreased utilization of care may outweigh the risks of breaches of privacy and confidentiality particularly when safeguards using the technology itself can be built in (e.g. audit trails, levels of authorization and access, consent documentation) (Chaudry et al, 2006; McGraw et al, 2009). The benchmark studies on benefits of ICT exist primarily in academic institutions in urban centres that have often implemented internally developed information systems; whether or not, and when, other institutions with commercially available software solutions can achieve similar benefits, and at what cost are not clear.

As technology becomes more pervasive in urban, developed centres, new found mobility will allow a greater dispersion of medical knowledge and human capital. HRM will need to adopt technology as a strategy to acquire and retain knowledgeable, well trained staff.

Technology can also be used in simple yet innovative ways to solve human resources problems. One real-life example is the following story found at St. Peter's Health Care Services, a hospital in Albany, NY. St. Peter's typically filled its nursing requirement shortages by hiring agency-based temporary nurses, each costing the hospital approximately $54 per hour. These nurses were seldom familiar with procedures specific to

St Peter's, creating inefficiencies financially and procedurally (Robinson, 2003). To address this problem, human resources management, using an idea borrowed from Priceline.com and eBay, put together a team of people from information technology and patient care services to develop the "shift-bidding" system. Two months later, the hospital launched "St. Peter's Jobs Online." When shifts were open, a nurse manager added the shifts to the website. Qualified staff hospital nurses or other pre-approved independent nurses bid on their preferential shifts for the best qualifying rate per hour; perhaps even earning more than sharing fees with an agency. The results showed that for the St. Peter's case, everybody benefited. In 2003 the bidding system filled 43,400 of St. Peter's available shift-hours at an average of $37 per hour, saving the hospital nearly $750,000 over the course of a year (Robinson, 2003). Shift bidding and scheduling systems are now widely used to ease staffing shortages and result in decreased agency use and cost savings, improved employee recruitment and retention, reduced administrative time spent scheduling and improved staffing practices that optimize the use of the existing workforce (Kulma & Springer, 2006).

ICT and HRM Issues in Rural Developed Regions

Those health professionals characterized as part of the underserved group are primarily the rural health professionals in developed regions. This group faces significant barriers to acquiring information, especially when compared to their urban counterparts (Dorsch, 2000). In this survey of information needs, rural health professionals ranked what they perceived to be major barriers to acquiring information. They included: lack of time, geographic isolation, lack of a library, technology illiteracy, lack of equipment (computers), and cost.

As was found with most health professionals, rural health professionals preferred their colleagues or personal libraries over bibliographical sources as information sources; for example 63.1% would discuss a decision with a colleague before adopting clinical methods, while only 17% would search the literature for more information. Moreover, when judging the scientific soundness of medical information, 90% compared the findings to their personal experiences, rather than appraising "the findings based on study methodology and statistical significance" (Dorsch, 2000, p. 347). The average age of health professionals in rural areas in this study was 46 years old, with 17 years of work experience (compared to the average age of urban health professionals of 38 years old with 9 years of work experience). Of those who had been in practice for less than ten years, 80.6% owned computers equipped with CD-ROM drives, however, among those who had been practicing for more than 30 years, the percentage of computer ownership was only 32.4% (Dorsch, 2000). Throughout the 1990s, use of electronic information resources among rural health professionals remained constant. For instance, 40% used MEDLINE, 25.6% used CD-ROMs for literature searching and 44.9% for accessing medical texts. More than half (52%) also used the CD-ROM for entertainment (Dorsch, 2000).

In the field of health care, continuing education is essential and necessary for all health professionals in order to ensure that quality health care is being provided and that access to the most up-to-date and best medical evidence for practice and care is available. Since health professionals prefer their colleagues as an information source above all else, a better means of facilitating communication among all health care professionals is needed.

Due to the barriers specifically cited by rural health professionals, some technologies may be more useful than others. Those most useful are audioconferencing (even simple teleconferencing), videoconferencing, and CD-ROMs (compact disc-read only memory) (Curran, 2006; Sheppard & Mackintosh, 1998). The Internet provides

networks with access to medical databases and online communities of practice, as well as electronic mail (e-mail) (Coma del Coral et al, 2005; Curran, 2006). Studies have also shown that, although awareness of telemedicine's applications and capabilities among health professionals in rural areas is minimal, the attitudes towards its adoption are favourable (Lin, 1999). The delivery of tele-education programs via ICTs enables the timely dissemination of new developments, provides training opportunities for hospital staff and employees, and can enhance educational experiences for primary care practitioners via consultations with specialists and/or attendance at virtual grand rounds (Curran, 2006). The use of these technologies can alleviate some of the isolation felt by rural health professionals and reduce the costs, travel time and staff absences associated with attendance at distant continuing education programs.

ICT and HRM Issues in Urban Developing Regions

Effective human resource practice is crucial for improving the efficiency of the health care system in developing countries. Because developing nations have the heaviest burden of disease, it is even more important to use human resources management to increase the overall quality of health care and to balance health workforce deployment with where it is most needed (i.e. usually in rural communities). It is often more difficult for people in developing countries and low income nations to provide effective and efficient health care than those in industrialized countries due to the failure or inability to provide appropriate social infrastructure for health care due to limited financial resources and budgets, as well as adequate funding for training or education of health care workers. For example, of the approximate 8.8 million new tuberculosis (TB) infections in 2005, 7.4 million (84%) were concentrated in Asia and sub-Saharan Africa. Nigeria has the highest TB burden in Africa, fifth highest in the world, while Kyrgyzstan has the second highest tuberculosis burden in Central Asia, after Kazakhstan (Awofeso et al, 2008). The main human resource issues affecting effective TB control are insufficient quality, quantity and distribution of health workers (Awofeso et al, 2008).

From 2004 to 2007, "government annual budgets for tuberculosis control in Nigeria and Kyrgyzstan averaged US\$ 14 million and US\$ 1 million respectively, barely enough for staff salaries, let alone training" (Awofeso et al, 2008, p. 2). Training/retraining programs for tuberculosis workers may be used as an incentive to influence distribution patterns; either by preferentially funding applicants from high TB prevalence regions or by developing and funding distance learning and on-site training programs for workers in these regions. These can include high tech solutions through Internet or web-based programs as well as low tech solutions such as correspondence courses and the use of radio or TV narrow casts (Zarocostas, 2008).

According to Henderson and Tulloch (2008), the main causes of health care labour shortages in low income countries include a lack of effective planning, limited health budgets, limited employment opportunities, low salaries, poor working conditions, weak support and supervision, and limited opportunities for professional development.

The lack of effective human resource practices also result in recruitment and retention problems, or even brain drain, which make the shortages of local health care workers even worse. The high demand for doctors and nurses in Western countries attract health care professionals from developing countries to migrate with the promise of better working conditions, higher remuneration, and additional work opportunities for family members. From 1985 to 1997, in Ghana, it was estimated that the cumulative average annual emigration rate was about 14%, which meant that half of medical graduates emigrated within

4.5 years, mainly to the United Kingdom and the United States. During the same period, 25% of Thai doctors immigrated to the United States, and most of them never returned (Wibulpolprasert & Pengpaibon, 2003).

Although technology innovation may not bring as significant change to low income countries as to developed countries, the health care system in developing countries does benefit from this, especially in urban areas because of the comparably better social infrastructure. One important aspect that technology can do to enhance the effectiveness of HRM is to provide a broader scope of training. Virtual universities, networks of institutions and professional associations, international standards of certification and distance learning give people in developing countries more channels to access higher education and training. An example of such a distance learning approach for tuberculosis control and training of doctors and nurses was developed jointly by the International Council of Nurses, the International Hospital Federation, and the World Medical Association in 2006 (Awofeso et al, 2008). This provides efficient and high quality tuberculosis training for health care workers internationally at a reduced cost.

E-health innovations such as electronic health records, telehealth, health knowledge management, health information systems, and clinical databases have brought significant change to HRM in health care in developing countries. First, the globalization of communication and the advances in information technology offer unprecedented opportunities to improve public health worldwide. Videoconferences, telecommunication, and professional institution networks give health care professionals in developing countries the opportunity to discuss problems with those in industrialized nations, and can also create a medical network within their own countries. In Thailand, for example, "the launch of the country's first communications satellite allowed for the implementation of a nationwide telemedicine network by the Ministry of Public Health, currently linking 19 hospitals with health facilities all over the country" (Dussault & Franceschini, 2006, p. 10).

Information and communication technology can also help to address the shortage of health care professionals through international volunteering programs. These programs, which are supported by large corporations, can connect with each other and contact governments in order to send volunteer health care professionals from developed countries to the places where they are most needed. For example, the Pfizer Global Health Fellows program sent 72 Pfizer employees to work with organizations in 19 countries such as Uganda, Kenya, Ghana, South Africa and India from 2003 to 2005, with a goal of promoting better health by "improving the service delivery capacity of local partners in poor countries" (Vian et al, 2007, p. 2). Many of these fellows imparted skills or enhanced operations of non-governmental organizations in HIV/AIDS and other health programs providing training to clinical and research personnel; strengthening laboratory, pharmacy, financial control, and human resources management systems; and helped to expand organization networks. Local staff also reported the program changed their work habits and attitudes (Vian et al, 2007). Although transferring volunteer health care professionals to low income countries cannot completely solve the shortage problem, it does relieve, to some extent in the short term, the human resource burden in developing countries.

ICT and HRM Issues in Rural Developing Regions

As we've seen over and over again, human resources are a crucial part of the health care industry and the assurance of the delivery of quality health care with improved health outcomes; however health professionals remain in critically short supply in developing countries, particularly in rural regions (Hongoro & McPake, 2004). One strategy to address this shortage of human resources is to make

use of the capacity within the developed world by the promotion of distance learning opportunities or provision of training staff through networks or twinning of medical schools with developing countries. These efforts may be hampered however by the lack of interest or funding or cultural sensitivity in the developed world.

General literacy levels within a country may be a major hurdle in recruitment and training of any rural workers. Literacy rates in Pakistan are very low (only 38.6% of the population can read or write) and little of the national budget is spent on education (only 2.9%). Although training facilities to improve literacy have been attempted in rural Pakistan, they have largely failed due to a lack of perception of the populations' need or a clear strategy of what benefits would be gained. Within the rural community agriculture forms the basis of the local economy. An innovative model proposing the introduction of rural kiosk machines (RKM) within rural community centres and schools has been proposed to provide text, audio and video material on agricultural crops and to provide training to rural farmers in their use.. Machines will be connected via wireless connections to a central department for regular updates of the information. The kiosks will serve at least two purposes, one to provide valuable information to enhance the growth and sustainability of crops and two to help raise the literacy levels in rural communities (Sattar, 2007). This kiosk technology could be easily adapted to provide health information to rural communities.

Within rural communities shifting of tasks to health workers with less training may provide needed preventive health services, basic treatment services, and serve as a liaison between the community and more highly skilled workers in short supply. Well designed programmes using such community health workers with proper support and supervision have been successful and may even reduce the number of medical consultations and hospitalizations (Dussault & Franceschini, 2006). However some professional bodies may themselves prove an impediment to this potential solution of task shifting. It was noted that in rural Uganda many rural midwives only supervised one birth per day, yet there was a very high need for those midwives to be cross-trained as nurses to do the regular nursing tasks involved in primary care (Hongoro &McPake, 2004). Although the larger problem of providing training to these rural and often remote areas remained, there was also a level of protectionism against such cross-training from professional nursing organizations in Uganda (Hongoro & McPake, 2004).

The World Health Organization indicated that poor human resources information systems hinder the proper deployment of health workers to where they are needed and reliable numbers of properly trained workers (Awofeso et al, 2006). Incomplete reporting of where TB cases and on the distribution of health care workers in general are hampers the ability to send trained health workers to areas of high prevalence of TB where they are most needed. Also in Nigeria where training for front-line workers was well provided, the financial and travel incentives to be trained removed these rural workers away from their duties for a significant period of time. The adverse impact of training on availability of workers could be minimized by developing and funding distance learning and on-site training programs.

Trouble filling nursing postings as well as a migration away from rural, developing areas has also been a large problem in South Africa particularly in addressing the need for large scale antiretroviral treatment programs among the large number of HIV/AIDS cases (van Rensberg, 2008). Introduction of new positions in an ART program resulted in an increased recruitment of nurses, but often at the expense of other existing facilities or regions – no new nurses were recruited, nurses simply moved from one facility to another or one department to another. Supporting health care employee's with appropriate information systems to track HIV patients and drugs is also critical, yet often lacking in rural, developing areas due

to technological limitations (Fraser et al,2004). A simple, web based medical record system linking remote areas in rural Haiti was used to track clinical outcomes, laboratory tests, and drug supplies. The use of open source software and satellite and wireless technologies linked through a central location kept costs low (Fraser et al, 2004). Health workers were also able to conduct consultations by contacting more experienced colleagues, and share images and efficiently manage patient information and test results.

In Afghanistan, coordination of health human resources was transformed by an outstanding director of Human Resources in the Ministry of Public Health (Schiffbauer et al, 2008). A central database containing information on about 24,500 health workers was established to identify the numbers, types and locations of health workers and determine their level of competency. Training is being provided to refresh the skills of health workers and train new workers including female doctors, nurses and midwives that are needed in rural communities (Schiffbauer et al, 2008). Similarly centralized HR programs in South Africa and southern Sudan have used similar strategies; development of a comprehensive HR policy, establishment of HR units in the ministries of health and training of HR managers, nationwide health HR information systems, expanded recruitment, training, testing and certification of health workers, and revision of pre-service training curricula for doctors and nurses (Schiffbauer et al, 2008).

Once human resources were moved to a national level in Afghanistan it allowed for a consistent training basis and also allowed for a coordination amongst other governmental agencies. Across a number of countries in east and southern Africa the development of HRM systems and HR information systems have improved health care workers satisfaction and retention by being able to better manage resources and personnel and provide incentives to maintain staffing needs (Dambisya, 2007). Such incentives can have a great impact, for instance in Uganda such changes resulted in a considerable reduction in turnover and growth in patient services by 50%.

SUMMARY: SOLUTIONS AND RECOMMENDATIONS

While some of the benefits of information and communication technologies have been realized in the health care field, the full impact across many disciplines will be more fully realized as it is applied in a more systematic form, rather than in the current patchy and uneven implementation. To date, technological advances such as electronic health records are typically instituted by larger institutions in urban centres with significant resources capable of aligning funding with available technological expertise. However over time this technology will facilitate the decentralization of, and access to, expert medical equipment and staff (e.g. telerobotic surgery, telementoring or distance education). Other changes, such as personnel and shift management, as well as core medical practices (i.e. evidence-based practice, health care teams and interprofessional collaboration) are facilitated by technology.

Additionally, as technology advances, the types of medical care provided are likely to change drastically over time, such as minimally invasive surgical interventions, gene therapy and personalized medicine (Anravi, 2006). This will have an impact on the shift of medical health care professionals from one sub-specialty to another and new roles for health professionals on the health care team. Also, this will undoubtedly impact the type of health care coverage HR professionals will offer for their employees, and may even evolve further to define specific benefit coverage for certain high-impact employees.

As the joining of technology and health care moves forward, patient transfers will be replaced by the transfer of medical expertise from one health center to another, e.g. from urban centres to rural communities, and across even greater distances across countries from the developed world to the developing world. Along with this comes the potential accessibility of private patient medical information anywhere in the world. The implications of the information benefit versus privacy duality are huge. Medical records perhaps represent the most personal and private information regarding patients or employees. As such, the responsibility and care of these records require priorities of security from both a technical and ethical perspective.

Differences in information needs and preferences do not differ greatly from rural to urban health professionals, rather, it is more dependent on the type of practice whether solo or group practice or family physician versus specialist (Dorsch, 2000). However, there is a difference in the frequency of information use in that rural health professionals were found to search for answers to clinical questions and use information sources less frequently than their urban counterparts (Dorsch, 2000). Rural health professionals face more significant barriers for meeting their information needs, such as accessibility issues (i.e. the lack of libraries, technological illiteracy, and the lack of equipment). Demographic barriers may also play a part; for instance, rural health professionals tended to be older and had been in practice longer. When compared to urban health professionals, those in rural areas on average had lower computer use and spent less time pursuing clinical questions and were, therefore, less likely to use information. The nature of the health care profession requires that all health professionals remain up to date on current methods and research findings. Therefore, it is crucial that rural health professionals are able to bypass such barriers in order to maintain their quest for continued education. Technology in the form of audioconferencing (both by conventional telephone and voice over IP), videoconferencing, CD-ROMs, and Web-based resources can provide a link to urban resources and colleagues.

Audioconferencing is an ideal tool for rural health professionals because it provides a simple and convenient means of communication between groups or individuals and its interactive nature provides a means to get instant information, support, and feedback (Curran, 2006; Shepherd & Mackintosh, 1998). Videoconferencing provides the opportunity to add a visual link as well as the audio link for simultaneous communication between two or more sites. It can be used to deliver lectures, show practical techniques, or demonstrate clinical procedures; hence making it a great tool for continued education (Curran, 2006). However, rural health professionals need to have access to a videoconferencing site or be able to access via their own computers, either of which may not be available. Installation of computers and broadband transmission of videos can also be a financial burden, especially for the small practices or small community hospitals found in rural areas.

CD-ROMs are disc packages that contain information usually found in medical texts, but can provide far greater interactivity than the usual medical text since it can contain still and animated graphics, as well as video sections. Interactive features can also provide users with question and review sections, as well as immediate feedback regarding their performance. CD-ROM packages are especially useful for rural health professionals because they provide information that can be easily received at great distances (packages can even be delivered by regular mail service). One drawback is the data on CD-ROMs is not regularly updated, which means health professionals must continue to purchase new packages in order to stay up to date. The Internet and the Web browser interface facilitates the creation of virtual networks which enable a group of users who share a common aspect of knowledge (such as health care) to gather and post relevant information or hold discussions on specific topics. They are "universal, free of language or geographical boundaries and [are] open to all interests" (Coma del Corral et al, 2005, p. 2). These networks provide rural health professionals with a means to maintain communication and collaboration with their colleagues by use of chat rooms, text conferencing, e-mail lists, and access to medical databases (e.g. MEDLINE, PubMed, or online publications).

Research shows that the use of such networks has achieved positive changes in medical care in rural areas. Studies have shown a decrease in the total average of hospital stays due to increased access to information on patient care (Coma del Corral et al, 2005). E-mail provides easy and immediate contact with colleagues and can reduce time spent waiting for missed or returned calls. In addition, e-mail allows health professionals to send and receive documents quickly, efficiently, and in a cost effective way. Secure networks and/or encryption can be used to ensure privacy and confidentiality of transmitted health information. E-mail lists are also beneficial to rural health professionals because they allow one to build a larger network of colleagues and professionals for information sources and feedback. Networks, such as UniNet, allow for continued medical education; communication tools, such as video or text conferencing, and reduced costs (such as long distance phone calls or purchasing costs for acquiring books and other materials).

Because developing countries often have limited budgets to invest in education and training of health care professionals, distance education is a feasible option due to its comparably lower cost and equivalent or higher quality. Students and trainees can access advanced knowledge and skills from Western countries without going abroad or even leaving the community. The use of information technology to provide online learning can generate a larger pool of qualified health care workers and assist in alleviating the problem of worker shortages. However, poor infrastructure in low income countries may still limit the application of technology, particularly, as in the West, outside of urban centres.

Although the advances in information and communication technology can greatly increase the efficiency of HRM in health care in developing countries, problems still exist. Brain drain is one of the leading causes of health care professional shortages. While Internet-based distance studies provide higher education and training to people in developing countries, these individuals tend to leave their home country after they become professionals in order to find better working and living conditions. It is difficult for governments in low income countries to retain health care workers by providing financial incentives or increased remuneration due to their limited financial budgets. As a result, solving the problem of health care worker shortages is a long term process. Developing countries need to focus on improving infrastructure that allows for information sharing, training and development through technology in order to retain their human capital.

Distance learning abilities such as wireless technology is an opportunity that should not be overlooked by human resource professionals in order to meet training needs. It allows remote access to human capital and creates opportunities for remote training where there once may have been little recourse but to remove the worker to a centralized location. In rural areas that have limited health workers to start with, removing workers for training for significant amounts of time could mean a significant reduction in services and care for the population they serve. Wireless technology such as wireless local area networks and mobile technologies requires only a modest investment at a central area, and little in the way of remote access.

Ensuring information is focused on the needs of a rural population allows not only the information but the technology to be successfully transferred and sustained. This is critical for a long-term commitment in recruitment and training. Use of the Internet for distance learning or even use of cell phones can facilitate learning yet keep the worker on the front lines as well as minimize costs. In extremely remote locations use of technology is not always feasible. In such cases radio communications or even mail can be used to substitute for those learning opportunities

(Awofeso, 2008). Television is another low cost opportunity of training workers in rural environments. In South Africa the use of televised communications allowed the department of health to facilitate some of its training from a centralized location without having to transport workers to a training facility (van Rensburg, 2008).

A proper human resource information system that collects data on the training quality and support given to workers is another key success factor in rural, developing areas. A human resource information system can be used to predict and manage levels of recruitment, training, delivery and production needs (Dambisya, 2004). Through the use of such tracking and monitoring systems, appropriate training can be given to workers while being able to maintain staffing needs. A strong commitment to rural areas in training is vital as it shows not only workers, but the population that they do not need to migrate away from rural areas to urban centers to get the quality training they need. Monetary incentives remain a popular way of retaining and recruiting health care workers in rural developing areas, however other incentives can be vitally important. This includes housing, transportation, security and promotion prospects. All of these can then be used to retain and recruit workers in rural, developing areas. These non-financial incentives create an incentive for health care workers to not only stay in the country, but to stay in rural areas, as most developing countries are unable to compete on wages alone.

Moving human resources management to a state level and no longer spread between various regions in the country and developing a comprehensive national HRM policy was a first step to a more efficient system in Afghanistan. This set the stage for a database to track training and other government agency initiatives; a centralized agency working with all levels of government has a better chance of fulfilling its HR obligations.

THE FUTURE: TRAINING AND EDUCATION

Information and communication technologies continue to expand and improve. New dimensions of interactivity offered through social networking and increased connectivity will have an influence on human resources and HRM in health care as well. Once again these technologies will first be rolled out in urban centres and offer improved ways of training and education of health professionals and these urban centres will be able to provide these tools to rural and remote regions.

Within medical schools adoption of computer technology has been initially slow. In most cases introduced to assist in administrative functions medical schools are increasingly turning to computer-assisted learning in one form or another (Gordon et al, 1999; Riva, 2000, Ward et al, 2001). The spectrum of computer usage runs from simple use of email as a communication tool between students and teachers to posting links to helpful web sites, posting course notes, posting interactive quizzes, animations that supplement lecture material or provide diagrammatic understanding of more complex mechanisms, to the use of computer-based simulations or virtual reality. Information and communication technology is now seen as an integral part of the medical school enterprise and often expected by its students as part of the mode of content delivery. What differentiates medicine though from other forms of learning is the interaction with patients and the need to acquire practical skills (physical examination, e.g. assessment of heart and lung sounds, palpation; procedures, e.g. injections, inserting IV, suturing, surgical techniques). Can these tasks be supplemented or addressed by computer-based tools?

LEARNING WITH VIRTUAL PATIENTS

The University of Minnesota's Medical School Virtual Clinic with 70 virtual patients is set up as a web-accessible electronic medical record with tabs that include health history, lab results, medications ordered, images (e.g. X-rays), progress notes and links to teaching items. The virtual clinic is used by first year medical students, and is also to be used in the IVIMEDS virtual patient panel (Voelker, 2003). Students 'attend' the weekly clinic by logging into the virtual clinic and see a group of simulated patients representing a variety of conditions and cultural backgrounds and follow them over time. The underlying tools facilitate a variety of educational links for any item of information from simple popup windows for definitions to illustrative images and interactive student exercises. At the same time it provides an introduction to certain informatics practices including basic security and use of an EMR for patient care (Speedie & Niewoehner, 2003).

More advanced virtual patients, e.g. cyberPatient by CyberActive Technology Ltd (Qayumi & Qayumi, 1999), provides not only virtual patient cases but the opportunity for the learner to conduct a physical examination with auscultation and palpation modalities, order laboratory tests (blood tests, EKGs, X-rays, etc), offer a diagnosis, plan treatment and if necessary simulate a surgical procedure. Feedback can be provided immediately by the 'chief surgeon' or physician, or at the end of the case. Patients can be followed up for months or years after their treatment and management; thus students can revisit patients and appreciate the long-term follow-up that occurs with 'real' patients. Student responses can be tracked making this virtual patient simulation suitable for testing purposes.

Computational advances in natural language processing, 3-D modeling and database repositories have led to the development of even more sophisticated virtual patients that can respond with emotions and answer questions with natural language (Hubal et al, 2000). Physical signs are again available in terms of heart and lung sounds, etc. The virtual standardized patient provides feedback, tracking and recording of responses.

MEDICAL SIMULATIONS

One more step of complexity introduces a 'simulated' patient or mannequin linked to a multimedia computer system to more closely approximate the bedside learning experience and to allow students to practice in a stress-free environment in situations where wrong decisions may literally mean life or death. One of the most fully developed simulators is 'Harvey' a cardiology patient simulator developed at the University of Miami Centre for Research in Medical Education (CRME) (Gordon et al, 1999; http://www.crme.med.miami.edu/harvey_findings. html). Harvey is programmed to present with lifelike vital signs including blood pressure, arterial and venous pulses, heart and lung sounds (with accompanying multimedia instruction), access to laboratory data, pathology, and treatment choices. Harvey has been used by medical students, nursing students, primary care physicians, cardiologists, EMTs, firemen and other health professionals.

Successful simulations/simulators now exist for anesthesia, emergency medicine, and surgery. In the latter it may be far more preferable to develop skills in a simulation environment for a new or complex medical procedure rather than in the traditional apprenticeship model on real patients (Gorman et al, 2000). Surgical training has been extended with the marriage of virtual reality or 3-D modeling into the simulation exercise. Manipulations are performed through haptic interfaces that not only convey a rich three-dimensional depiction of the tissue, but can also simulate touch and pressure. Examples include laparoscopic camera and cholecystectomy simulators, a VR-based needle-driving simulator for suturing technique, a Web-based surgical training system for abdominal aneurysm stent graft deployment and a Web-based CardioOp system that allows for the composition of multimedia fragments that can be reused to suit the needs of individual learners in cardiac surgery (Gorman et al, 2000).

"Future physicians will be able to rehearse an operation on a projectable palpable hologram derived from patient-specific data, and deliver the data set of that operation with robotic assistance the next day" Gorman et al, 2000, p. 353

Another example weds all of these elements into the learning environment (i.e. simulation, an immersive virtual reality environment, Internet technology) to "overcome geographic barriers for delivery of tutorial sessions to medical students pursuing rotations at remote sites" (Jacobs et al, 2003; Project TOUCH (Telehealth Outreach for Unified Community Health – http://hsc.unm.edu/touch). This multi-year collaboration between the University of New Mexico and the University of Hawaii uses case scenarios as virtual models to make the learning of critical concepts relevant and more life-like. Students are fully immersed in a representational virtual environment and can see fellow students or team members and interact as if they were physically present even when separated by significant distances. The "Flatland' environment allows real-time exploration and manipulation of 3-D objects and images within the virtual world. The application is displayed using the Access Grid – a broadband Internet2 videoconferencing, multicasting network that allows real-time distribution of the learning environments across academic medical centers and distant training centers.

Second Life (http://secondlife.com) is a popular virtual world platform that is being used for medical and health education. On the "Healthinfo island" (Second Life Medical and Consumer Health Libraries), for instance, librarians have provided extensive consumer health information services that users can wander through in a virtual environment (Boulos et al, 2007).

COMMUNITY OF LEARNERS/ COMMUNITIES OF PRACTICE

The Internet can offer a variety of modes for establishing communities of learners via discussion boards, chat rooms, virtual seminars and I.P. videoconferencing. Peer-to-peer learning is enhanced and encouraged in these settings and faculty can also act as mentors for students at a distance. Virtual advisors were linked to students from North American and international medical schools with experienced emergency medicine faculty mentors in which encounters relied on electronic or voice correspondence depending on their geographical location and preferences. Feedback was positive for both advisors and advisees (Coates et al, 2004).

Canada's first new medical school in over three decades, the Northern Ontario School of Medicine, is a collaborative effort between Laurentian University in Sudbury, ON and Lakehead University in Thunder Bay, ON. It uses a distributed learning network with advanced information technology support to facilitate small group learning for students seeing patients in rural, northern, underserviced and Aboriginal communities (Rourke, 2002). Components of the technology include an e-learning (virtual learning) environment, online collaboration and telehealth (using the existing NORTH network infrastructure), a medical school information portal (on a high-speed Intranet – the ORION network that connects the two universities), e-library (health information resources centre), administrative infrastructure (that include student/faculty/staff access and IT support services) and IT research support. The goal is to provide faculty and students with secure, reliable access to curriculum, cohorts, coaches, and faculty regardless of geographic location.

INTERNATIONAL VIRTUAL MEDICAL SCHOOL (IVIMEDS)

This represents a 'revolutionary' approach to medical education leaving the notion of a physical medical school associated with a teaching hospital far behind (Harden, 2000; Harden & Hart, 2002; http://www.ivimeds.org/). Based in

Dundee, Scotland and formally launched in 2003 IVIMEDS builds on the successful experiments with virtual degrees and virtual universities (Pritchard, 2003). An international group of 30 to 40 medical schools (from the US, UK, Europe, Australasia) is exploring the feasibility of establishing a virtual medical school with a broadly-based consortium of dozens of medical schools that will contribute shared learning resources and expertise to teach medical students at a distance. Their aims are to apply innovative thinking and new learning technologies (e.g. e-learning via the Internet, CD-ROM, virtual reality), new approaches to curriculum planning and instructional design (e.g. curriculum mapping, outcomes-based education, electronic study guides, peer-to-peer learning, a bank of reusable learning objects), and the development of a flexible curriculum that will meet the needs of different students in many different geographic locations to a new medical school open to students from around the world (Harden & Hart, 2002). Two central features of the model are the curriculum map and reusable learning objects. The curriculum map identifies what, where, when and how students can learn and in essence they will be able to follow their own map through the curriculum. On each node of the map learning resource material related to that node is identified. This material is contained in a learning repository which contains small, discrete self-contained learning objects. Benefits of this program are seen to be an increased accessibility of medical education globally and improved medical education that is more responsive to community needs.

The use of digital technologies through the Internet and world wide web interface continue to influence and affect the delivery of health care and health services and with regard to HRM can provide the venue for training and education of health workers, access to the medical literature and knowledge databases providing best evidence for clinical care and clinical care guidelines, continuing education opportunities and invaluable links to colleagues and mentors that will improve the retention of health professionals in remote and rural regions. Considerable progress and use of these technologies has been made, as we have discussed, and in the next generation the so-called Web 2.0 technologies will have an even greater impact on these activities with their emphasis on social connection and collaboration.

Web 2.0 technologies take the original Web based resources beyond the simple provision of text, images and video and add a dimension of interactivity and social networking that enhance professional, patient and consumer interactions (Boulos & Wheeler, 2007). More common applications in health and medical education include the use of wikis, web information sites that are editable by anyone; blogs or web logs or online journals that can offer text or multimedia–based discussions in one-way or two-way environments; and podcasts or audio files that can be downloaded to a user's computer or audio device and listened to anywhere, anytime (Boulos et al, 2006; Boulos & Wheeler, 2007). Media sharing sites such as You Tube contain a number of video presentations of educational material available for widespread use and the social networking sites, MySpace and FaceBook, have become areas where patients can find support from fellow patients, students can share work and learning, and researchers and health professionals can find like-minded individuals to share information and establish connections across the world. Examples of each of these technologies in health education exist, (e.g. Ganfyd a collaborative medical knowledge database that anyone can read and medical professionals can edit – http://ganfyd. org; Clinical Cases and Images blog from the Cleveland Clinic - http://clinicalcases.org/; Johns Hopkins Medical Podcasts for health professionals and the public - http://www.hopkinsmedicine. org/mediaII/Podcasts/index.html; medical school pathology lectures on YouTube – http://www. youtube.com).

It is still early days in the use of these technologies in training and education, and research is still needed into how these technologies best fit into undergraduate, postgraduate and continuing education of health professionals (Boulos et al, 2006; Sandars & Schroter, 2007). A recent survey of 3,000 medical students and 3,000 medical practitioners in the UK found that although there was familiarity with these Web 2.0 technologies for both personal and educational use, there was little actual use of these technologies. Medical students had both greater familiarity and use, especially of instant messaging, media sharing and social bookmarking. There was interest in the use of Web 2.0 technologies for education by all groups but both practitioners and students wanted more training in their use. Other barriers for use in education were different learning preferences, concern about quality of resources, lack of time and difficulties with ICT access (Sandars & Schroter, 2007).

Since these are interactive tools and developed collectively by a community of interested participants the resulting quality can vary greatly. Although some proponents profess a "darwikian" theory of survival of the fittest or best, that is not always the case (for example, good content can be replaced by poor content or by misinformation, sites can be hijacked by groups of users with selective points of view) (Boulos & Wheeler, 2007). In some cases those perils can be lessened by the presence of a moderator or access restricted to only certain individuals, but to a certain extent that defeats the purpose of the original idea of social networking and building free and open collaborative networks.

Many of these web tools require quite high bandwidth and high connectivity speeds, infrastructure that may be readily available in urban centres, but may still not be available to those in remote regions or in low income countries. ICT use and penetration continues to expand across the globe with the greatest increases over the past several years seen in mobile cellular technologies and networks. In the developing world mobile phones had reached an estimated 49.5% penetration rate by the end of 2008 (from almost zero ten years ago) (ITU, 2009, p. 1). Fixed Internet access in developing countries is still limited and where available is often slow and expensive. Although there is still a digital divide the latest indicators of ICT use and prevalence indicate that it is slightly closing between countries with high and low ICT levels (which are in turn correlated to high (Europe and North America) and low income countries (central and southern Asia, sub-Saharan Africa)) (ITU, 2009, p. 1-2). One encouraging sign for the coming decade is the increase in, and adoption of, national eHealth policies that provide a framework for developing and using ICT in the health sector. Although industrialized countries still show the highest rates of adoption of eHealth policies, African regions projected a doubling of adoption of policies and ICT development by the end of 2008 (WHO, 2006, p. 18-20, 31)..Accompanying the introduction of policies and infrastructure is the recognition of the need for building capacity, i.e. the need to train the health workforce in use of the eHealth applications being deployed. ICT training of both health science students and continuing education for health professionals is relatively stable across all geographic regions with roughly two thirds of countries reporting they have introduced some form of university level and continuing education in ICT (WHO, 2006, p. 46-47). The need to build human resources capacity in health informatics and eHealth was reported by responding countries and often cited as a barrier to full eHealth implementation (WHO, 2006, p. 19).

HUMAN RESOURCES: NEW ROLES

The introduction of new technologies and changes in practice will also have an impact on the types of health professionals needed in the workforce in the future. As already mentioned there will be a need for increased training in the use of ICT for all health professionals and an increased need for health informatics specialists to develop, maintain and use these technologies and manage the massive amounts of health data that will be available across shared data repositories.

Multidisciplinary and interprofessional health care teams will be supported by improved technologies. The introduction of robotics and minimally invasive surgical techniques, pharmacogenetics, and bioinformatics will mean the addition of new health professionals to the health care team with expertise in the use of these new technologies and their integration into a fully electronic health information system (Anvari, 2006). Technology, in some instances, will also lead to the disappearance of jobs (e.g. medical transcriptionists, radiology film technicians, health records clerks).

Shifting of care from the hospital and health facilities to the community and home will also mean an increased need for community and home health care workers and expanded roles for family and community-based physicians, nurse practitioners, and even patients in controlling and monitoring their own conditions and health. In many countries there is a lack of national health human resources policies and planning to address these current and future needs.

CONCLUSION

Technology in health care overcomes barriers for health professionals in all regions. It minimizes distance and accessibility issues, providing a medium whereby information is easily and immediately attained. Technology furthermore maintains communication between health professionals and academic sources/centres which allows for continued education and training. In addition, it enhances the ability to recruit and select qualified personnel from all regions for optimal deployment of human resources by the use of HR information systems. Computer and Internet access to health professionals in rural regions have provided a better means of access to critical medical information, distance training and continuing education and have improved medical care services to patients. Although initial set up costs may be substantial, such investments indicate long term HRM benefits. In developing areas, governments – specifically those in urban and rural developing regions – need to improve technological infrastructures in order to provide better telecommunication services. In rural developing areas, centralized management will ensure consistent information is being provided to health professionals, and will provide well developed HRM strategies in all areas of the government pertaining to health care management.

REFERENCES

Adatia, F., & Bedard, P. L. (2003). Palm reading: 2. Handheld software for physicians. *Canadian Medical Association Journal, 168,* 727–734.

Adatia, F. A., & Bedard, P. L. (2002). Palm reading: 1. Handheld hardware and operating systems. *Canadian Medical Association Journal, 167,* 775–780.

Anvari, M. (2007). Impact of Information Technology on Human Resources in Healthcare. *Healthcare Quarterly, 10,* 84-88. Retrieved November 9, 2008 from http://www.longwoods.com/product.php?productid=19320&cat=513&page=1

Awofeso, N., Dalhatu, A., & Schelokova, I. (2008). Training of Front-line Health Workers for Tuberculosis Control: Lessons from Nigeria and Kyrgyzstan. *Human Resources for Health, 6*(20). Retrieved October 28, 2008 from http://www.human-resources-health.com/content/6/1/20

Boulos, M. N., Marimba, I., & Wheeler, S. (2006). Wikis, blogs and podcasts: a new generation of Web-based tools for virtual collaborative clinical practice and education. *BMC Medical Education, 6,* 41–49. doi:10.1186/1472-6920-6-41

Boulos, M. N. K., Hetherington, L., & Wheeler, S. (2007). Second Life: an overview of the potential of 3-D virtual worlds in medical and health education. *Health Information and Libraries Journal, 24,* 233–245. doi:10.1111/j.1471-1842.2007.00733.x

Boulos, M. N. K., & Wheeler, S. (2007). The emerging Web 2.0 social software: an enabling suite of sociable technologies in health and health care education. *Health Information and Libraries Journal, 24,* 2–23. doi:10.1111/j.1471-1842.2007.00701.x

Chaudry, B., Wang, J., Wu, S., Maglione, M., Mojica, W., & Roth, E. (2006). Systematic Review: Impact of health information technology on quality, efficiency, and costs of medical care. *Annals of Internal Medicine, 144,* 742–752.

Clements, A. (2008). It's Good to Get a Second Opinion. *Human Resources, 66.* Retrieved November 9, 2008 from http://proquest.umi.com/pqdweb?did=1582613671&sid=7&Fmt=3&clientId=77774&RQT=309&VName=PQD

Coates, W. C., Ankel, F., Birnbaum, A., Kosiak, D., Broderick, K. B., & Thomas, S. (2004). The virtual advisor program: linking students to mentors via the world wide web. *Academic Emergency Medicine, 11,* 253–255. doi:10.1111/j.1553-2712.2004.tb02205.x

Coma del Corral, M. J., Luquín, P. A., Guevara, J. C., Movilla, A. O., Torres, G. T., & Garcia, J. L. (2005). Utility of a thematic network in primary health care: a controlled interventional study in a rural area. *Human Resource for Health, 3,* 4-11. Retrieved November 9, 2008 from http://www.human-resources-health.com/content/3/1/4

Curran, V. R. (2006). Tele-education. *Journal of Telemedicine and Telecare, 12*, 57–63. doi:10.1258/135763306776084400

Dambisya, Y. A. (2007). Review of Non-financial Incentives for Health Care Worker Retention in East and Southern Africa. *Regional Network for Equity in Health in East and Southern Africa,* 1-72. Retrieved October 30, 2008 from http://www.equinetafrica.org/bibl/docs/DIS44HRdambisya.pdf

Dorsch, J. L. (2000). Information needs of rural health professionals: a review of the literature. *Bull Med Libr Assoc, 88*(4): 346-354. Retrieved November 9, 2008 from http://www.pubmedcentral.nih.gov/articlerender.fcgi?tool=pubmed&pubmedid=11055302

Dussault, G., & Franceschini, M. C. (2006). Not Enough There, Too Many Here: Understanding Geographical Imbalances in the Distribution of the Health Workforce. *Human Resources for Health,* 4, 12-28. Retrieved November 18, 2008 from http://www.human-resources-health.com/content/4/1/12

Ely, J. W., Osheroff, J. A., Ebell, M. H., Bergus, G. R., Levy, B. T., Chambliss, M. L., & Evans, E. R. (1999). Analysis of questions asked by family doctors regarding patient care. *BMJ (Clinical Research Ed.), 319*, 358–361.

Fraser, H. S. F., Jazayeri, D., Nevil, P., Karacaoglu, Y., Farmer, P. E., Lyon, E., et al. (2004) An information system and medical record to support HIV treatment in rural Haiti. *BMJ,* 329, 1142-1146. Retrieved October 30, 2008 from http://www.bmj.com/cgi/content/full/329/7475/1142.

Goldsmith, H., Manderscheid, W., & Merwin, E. (1995). Human Resource Issues in Rural Mental health Services. *Community Mental Health Journal,* 31, 525-537. Retrieved October 28, 2008 from http://www.springerlink.com/content/p68r402563qp0755/fulltext.pdf

Gordon, M. S., Issenberg, S. B., Mayer, J. W., & Felner, J. N. (1999). Developments in the use of simulators and multimedia computer systems in medical education. *Medical Teacher, 21*, 32–36. doi:10.1080/01421599980002

Gorman, P. J., Meier, A. H., Rawn, C., & Krummel, T. M. (2000). The future of medical education is no longer blood and guts, it is bits and bytes. *American Journal of Surgery, 180*, 353–356. doi:10.1016/S0002-9610(00)00514-6

Harden, R. M. (2000). Evolution or revolution and the future of medical education: replacing the oak tree. *Medical Teacher, 22*, 435–442. doi:10.1080/01421590050110669

Harden, R. M., & Hart, I. R. (2002). An international virtual medical school (IVIMEDS): the future for medical education? *Medical Teacher, 24*, 261–267. doi:10.1080/01421590220141008

Heeks, R., Jang, S., Ko, K., & Lee, H. (2008). Analysing South Korea's ICT for Development Aid Programme *The Electronic Journal of Information Systems in Developing Countries,* 35, 1-15. Retrieved October 28, 2008 from http://www.ejisdc.org/ojs2/index.php/ejisdc/article/viewFile/496/252

Henderson, L. N., & Tulloch, J. (2008). Incentives for Retaining and Motivating Health Workers in Pacific and Asian Countries. *Human Resources for Health,* 6, 18-37. Retrieved November 18, 2008 from http://www.human-resources-health.com/content/6/1/18

Hongoro, C., & McPake, B. (2004). How to Bridge the Gap In Human Resources for Health. *Lancet, 364*, 1451–1456. doi:10.1016/S0140-6736(04)17229-2

International Telecommunication Union (ITU). (2009). *Measuring the Information Society: The ICT Development Index, 2009 Edition. Geneva, Switzerland.* Retrieved April 21, 2008 from http://www.itu.int/ITU-D/ict/publications/idi/2009/material/IDI2009_w5.pdf

Jacobs, J., Caudell, T., Wilks, D., Keep, M. F., Mitchell, S., & Buchanan, H. (2003). Integration of advanced technologies to enhance problem-based learning over distance: Project TOUCH. *The Anatomical Record, 270B*, 16–22. doi:10.1002/ar.b.10003

Kabene, S. M., Orchard, C., Howard, J. M., Soriano, M. A., & Leduc, R. (2006). The importance of human resources management in health care: a global context. *Human Resources for Health, 4*, 20–36. doi:10.1186/1478-4491-4-20

Kulma, M., & Springer, B. (2006). Easing the bottom-line impact of staffing shortages: A case study in shift bidding. *Healthcare Financial Management, 60*, 92–97.

Lin, J. C. (1999) Applying telecommunication technology to health-care delivery. *Engineering in Medicine and Biology Magazine, IEEE*, 28-31. Retrieved November 9, 2008 from http://ieeexplore.ieee.org/xpls/abs_all.jsp?arnumber=775486

McGraw, D., Dempsey, J. X., Harris, L., & Goldman, J. (2009). Privacy As An Enabler, Not An Impediment: Building Trust Into Health Information Exchange. *Health Affairs, 28*, 416–427. doi:10.1377/hlthaff.28.2.416

Pritchard, L. (2003). Great Scots! *Medical Education, 37*, 493–494. doi:10.1046/j.1365-2923.2003.01529.x

Qayami, A. K., & Qayami, T. (1999). Computer-assisted learning: cyperPatient™ - A step in the future of surgical education. *Journal of Investigative Surgery, 12*, 307–317. doi:10.1080/089419399272296

Riva, G. (2000). From telehealth to e-health: Internet and distributed virtual reality in health care. *Cyberpsychology & Behavior, 3*, 989–998. doi:10.1089/109493100452255

Robinson, K. S. (2003). Online Bidding Fills Nursing Jobs. HRMagazine. Alexandria, 44.

Rourke, J. T. B. (2002). Building the new Northern Ontario Rural Medical School. *The Australian Journal of Rural Health, 10*, 112–116.

Sandars, J., & Schroter, S. (2007). Web 2.0 technologies for undergraduate and postgraduate medical education: an online survey. *Postgraduate Medical Journal, 83*, 759–762. doi:10.1136/pgmj.2007.063123

Sattar, K. (2007). A Sustainable Model for Use of ICTs in Rural Pakistan. *International Journal of Education and Development using Information and Communication Technology, 3*, 89-97. Retrieved October 30, 2008 from http://proquest.umi.com/pqdweb?did=1409299671&Fmt=4&clientId=11263&RQT=309&VName=PQD

Schiffbauer, J., O'Brien, J. B., Timmons, B. K., & Kiarie, W. N. (2008). The Role of Leadership in HRH Development in Challenging Public Health Settings. *Human Resources for Health, 6*, 23. Retrieved October 30, 2008 from http://www.human-resources-health.com/content/pdf/1478-4491-6-23.pdf

Sheppard, L., & Mackintosh, S. (1998). Technology in education: what is appropriate for rural and remote allied health professionals? *Aust J Rural Health, 6*, 189-193. Retrieved November 9, 2008 from http://www3.interscience.wiley.com/journal/119830096/abstract

Smith, R. (1996). What clinical information do doctors need? *BMJ (Clinical Research Ed.), 313*, 1062–1068.

Van Rensburg, D., Steyn, F., Schneider, H., & Loffstadt, L. (2008). Human Resource Development and Antiretroviral Treatment in Free State Province, South Africa. *Human Resources for Health, 6,* 15. Retrieved October 28, 2008 from http://www.human-resources-health.com /content/6/1/15

Vian, T., Richards, S. C., McCoy, K., Connelly, P., & Feeley, F. (2007). Public-Private Partnerships to Build Human Capacity in Low Income Countries: Findings from the Pfizer Program. *Human Resources for Health, 5,* 8-19. Retrieved November 18, 2008 from http://www.human-resources-health.com/content/5/1/8

Vilamovska, A. M., & Hatziandreu, E. Schindler, H.R., van Oranje-Nassau, C., de Vries, H., & Krapels, J. (2009). Study on the requirements and options for RFID application in healthcare: Identifying areas for Radio Frequency Identification deployment in healthcare delivery: A review of relevant literature. Rand Europe, European Commission. Retrieved May 4, 2009 from http://www.rand.org/pubs/technical_reports/TR608/

Voelker, R. (2003). Virtual patients help medical students link basic science with clinical care. *Journal of the American Medical Association, 290,* 1700–1701. doi:10.1001/jama.290.13.1700

Ward, J. P. T., Gordon, J., Field, M. J., & Lehmann, H. P. (2001). Communication and information technology in medical education. *Lancet, 357,* 792–796. doi:10.1016/S0140-6736(00)04173-8

Westberg, E. E., & Miller, R. A. (1998). The Basis for Using the Internet to Support the Information Needs of Primary Care. *Journal of the American Medical Informatics Association, 6,* 6–25.

Wibulpolprasert, S., & Pengpaibon, P. (2003). Integrated Strategies to Tackle the Inequitable Distribution of doctors in Thailand: Four Decades of Experience. *Human Resources for Health, 1,* 12. Retrieved November 18, 2008 from http://www.human-resources-health.com/content/1/1/12

World Health Organization (WHO). (2006) *Building Foundations for eHealth: Progress of Member States: Report of the Global Observatory for eHealth.* Geneva, Switzerland; WHO. Retrieved November 9, 2008 from http://www.who.int/ehealth/resources/bf_full.pdf

Zarocostas, J. (2008). World Medical Association scales up training for multidrug resistant tuberculosis to fight epidemic. *BMJ (Clinical Research Ed.), 336,* 1155. doi:10.1136/bmj.39584.662130.DB

Section 5
The Future

Chapter 28

Enabling Technologies and Challenges for the Future of Ubiquitous Health:
The Interoperability Framework

Donald W. M. Juzwishin
Juzwishin Consulting Inc., Canada

ABSTRACT

Web 2.0 and Web 3.0 emerge at a time when health care reforms are stymied. Current barriers to an effectively functioning health care system are linked to the historical, political and social institutions and processes that are preventing health system interoperability causing issues with access (to service and information), continuity of care, safety and the assessment of program delivery. An interoperability framework, identifying citizens, providers, policy makers and researchers is developed and related to the improvement of understanding, access, trust, discourse, and practice for the purpose of moving toward a high performing health care system. Web 2.0 and Web 3.0 offer great promise as an eHealth platform to synergistically catalyze significant improvements to health care delivery, however, caution is advised about uncritical adoption. Barriers to progress and opportunities for advancement are identified and questions for future research are posited.

INTRODUCTION

Canada lags other nations in the introduction and use of the electronic medical record (EMR) and the electronic health record (EHR). Progress is slow and Canada ranks last in EMR adoption compared to many other countries (Davis, Doty, Shea, & Stremikis, 2009). Two primary reasons for the lack of progress are a slow rate of adoption

and system interoperability (Archer, 2009). The federal government made a commitment to Canada Health Infoway to advance the adoption of the EMR and EHR with funding of $1.6 billion in 2001 and another $500 million in 2009. In addition to these funds the provincial and territorial governments have leveraged national funds with commitments of their own to advance the eHealth agenda. Some successes have been achieved but as of 2006 only 23% of Canadians have an EMR (Davis, Doty, Shea, & Stremikis, 2009, p. 241). Should we be

DOI: 10.4018/978-1-61520-777-0.ch028

Copyright © 2010, IGI Global. Copying or distributing in print or electronic forms without written permission of IGI Global is prohibited.

concerned with lack of progress in Canada? What are the barriers to interoperability and adoption? What are some of the ingredients for success? How can they be achieved?

This chapter is based on the premise that the constituent elements of the health care system must be effectively interoperative for electronic interoperability to be achieved. Political, social and policy interoperability of the health system's functioning are factors for improving electronic interoperability. The emergence of Web 2.0 and the attendant initiatives Health 2.0 and Medicine 2.0® look promising and are stimulating discussion in the field because they advance the concept of the patient at the center of care and the personal health record (PHR) as a way to accelerate adoption and interoperability. Despite how much money is spent on eHealth in Canada the process of health care delivery must be integrated and coordinated so that the relationships and interactions among physicians, hospitals, home care services and pharmacies, to name a few, are working together on behalf of the patient in order for electronic interoperability to be achieved. The question of whether Web 2.0 offers more promise than peril, value rather than vapor, and hope rather than hype is currently being contested. This chapter will address these questions. It will critically describe and analyze barriers to the advancement of eHealth and health reforms generally as they relate to the creation, use and exchange of electronic data, information and knowledge. Its focus will be to determine whether and how Web 2.0 and its successor Web 3.0 can catalyze and stimulate the changes necessary to achieve interoperability of the health care systems on the one hand and information interoperability on the other. Although Canada may be a laggard in the advancement of the eHealth agenda the emergence of Web 2.0 may be timely to catalyze and stimulate progress in the near future and leapfrog Canada to catch up to its European counterparts (Archer, 2009).

The objectives of this chapter are to:

- Provide a background to health care reform and identify the contemporary challenges of system interoperability;
- Describe and define Web 2.0, Web 3.0, Health 2.0 and Medicine 2.0;
- Develop a framework for thinking about advancing health care reforms through interoperability and identify potential opportunities offered by Web 2.0;
- Describe and critically review the issues arising from Web 2.0 enabling new and emerging technologies and systems in health care;
- Propose areas for future research in Web 2.0, interoperability, health informatics, health technology assessment, and health care policy.

BACKGROUND

The emergence of new technologies and techniques in health care intervention, delivery and systems is a two edged sword; they often make remarkable contributions to the successful treatment of disease but they also raise new social, political and ethical issues. Technologies and their purveyors can unwittingly create the illusion that technology alone can remedy contemporary health care issues. The EHR and EMR are perfect examples and are victims of having over promised and under delivered. The EHR and EMR alone cannot facilitate health care reforms to achieve coordination and integration of health care services however they can be important tools to help governance, management, and policy makers achieve a high performing health care system.

In 2004 Coiera identified that all of the technical improvements in health informatics were not sufficient to successfully achieve the required health care reforms. Information and communication technologies were necessary but they alone were not sufficient to achieve the reforms. Coiera professed:

If health care is to flourish in the coming setting of diminished resources and increased demand, then it will do so because we have explicitly designed and implemented new systems of care that are fundamentally sustainable. Given the likely enormity of that task, it may require nothing less than the reinvention of health care. (Coiera, 2004, p. 1197)

A multitude of commissions, task force reports and reviews of the Canadian health care systems have pointed toward necessary health care reforms, many of which are well underway, however much remains to be done as was pointed out in the Health Council of Canada five year review of progress of health reform in Canada (Health Council of Canada, 2008a). Common criticisms of the health care system are that citizens and patients cannot get access to the services or information they require when they need them. Examples are waits for surgery or patients having to repeat their histories to multiple care providers in different care settings that are in the same community. Patients and health care providers are inundated with a plethora of information and available service alternatives but are uncertain which information is reliable and which services are effective, in other words, how can they best understand what is available and what information can they trust. Citizens and patients today are less likely to be complacent and accepting of the traditional paternalistic approach to health care service delivery, they want to be treated as equal partners in the care process, engaging in discourse, making informed decisions and choices along the way. Policy makers face a barrage of multiple expectations from citizens and health care providers often with conflicting objectives. Researchers who create and disseminate the new knowledge of how to improve health care services or policies are often stymied by not having access to the necessary information. These are just a selection of the many challenges facing contemporary health care systems.

Current analysis of Canadian health care systems confirms that structural reforms do not deliver improved health care functioning. Commenting on the effect of provincial restructuring efforts Elson observes,

From a structural perspective... Ontario has made it extremely challenging for the LHINs to address their system management and integration role. The multitude and diversity of organizations that report individually to the LHINs means that in reality they have neither a coherent nor manageable number of organizations with which to engage in operational or service integration from a systems perspective.... In balance, structural regionalization can be seen as a necessary but insufficient condition to deliver on the promise of system-wide health services integration at the local or regional level. It does not have a direct impact on the frontline delivery of care, but it does establish the conditions that facilitate the more substantive and systemic work of integrating the delivery of health care. (Elson, p. 8)

Alberta, in contrast to Ontario, has collapsed its governance structure into one health board thereby setting the stage for one organization to advance health care reforms. Whether this is the approach that helps remedy the process and informatics interoperability challenges remains to be seen.

Web 2.0 displays promising characteristics that may ameliorate many of the issues and challenges identified above. They look promising because taken in concert with Health 2.0 and Medicine 2.0 they are not simply a technical solution but have deep and penetrating social contexts and consequences that are respectful of today's prized values of collaboration, sharing, peering, openness and global action (Tapscott & Williams, 2006). In 2004 Coiera published four rules for the reinvention of health care:

1. Technical systems have social consequences;
2. Social systems have technical consequences;
3. We don't design technology, we design sociotechnical systems; and
4. To design sociotechnical systems, we must understand how people and technologies interact (Coiera, pp. 1198-1199).

The rules are a helpful reminder that to be successful with health care reform a strictly technical, social or political solution is not enough. An iterative synergy is necessary between them. Taken together Web 2.0 and Web 3.0 approaches embrace Coiera's rules.

PROMISE OR PERIL?

Evidence for the fact that Web 2.0 is being taken seriously is reflected in several recent developments. In April 2009 the third successful Health 2.0 conference, bringing together eHealth enthusiasts was held in San Francisco (Health 2.0). On April 16, 2009 the Economist released a special report highlighting the promising potentials of Health 2.0, digital medicine and the digitization of medical records (Economist, 2009). Kevin Leonard, an advocate for patients having a greater role in eHealth, drew more than 100 participants to a "One Patient, One Record" symposium in April 2009 at which patients, policy makers and researchers explored how to achieve a health system where patients could successfully have a comprehensive and accurate personal health care record (Leonard, 2009). Telus, a Canadian telecommunications giant, purchased MyChart® personal heath record system from its developer, Sunnybrook Hospital, for a cost of approximately $3 million (Shaw, 2009). In May 2009 Telus and Microsoft announced a joint program of advancing HealthVault® in Canada. The 2nd world congress on social networking and Web 2.0 on health and medicine will be held in Toronto in September 2009 (Medicine 2.0, 2009).

The enthusiasm for Web 2.0 and Web 3.0 should not be mistaken for proven effectiveness. As this is being written Web 3.0 or the semantic web are emerging as a more sophisticated successor to Web 2.0. We must be cautious; eHealth is merely one tool in health care reform. It is not the goal itself. The goal is to improve citizens' health outcomes and population health. EHealth is more likely to be a successful strategy if it takes into account citizen and patient preferences and needs (Sarasohn-Kahn, 2008). The current structural and process challenges in the health care system leave room for it to be safer, less expensive and more effective; thus it would be unwise to uncritically computerize a system to simply magnify the weaknesses. Improvements to the health care system must come from reforms to its structure and processes coupled with the promise of Web 2.0 and Web 3.0 not by imposing eHealth on an archaic artifact. Health informatics is necessary for health reform to be successful but it alone is not sufficient, as Coiera reminds us, a cultural revolution is necessary and Web 2.0 can be a catalyst to quicken the revolution (Coiera, pp. 1197-1199).

WEB 2.0, WEB 3.0, HEALTH 2.0, AND MEDICINE 2.0 AND A NEW WAY OF THINKING

To define and understand the relevance of Web 2.0 it is necessary to compare it to Web 1.0. Web 1.0 refers to the Internet before the dot-com crash which took place in 2001 and was characterized by static pages instead of dynamic interactive content and graphics interchange format (GIF). Web 2.0 is an evolutionary development increasing the technical capability and content complexity of web pages toward more sophisticated visual and audio sources married with content that is more interactive. Giustini tells us that Web 2.0 "brings people together in a more dynamic, interactive space. This new generation of internet services and devices-often referred to as social software-can be leveraged to enrich our web experience, as information is continually requested, consumed and reinterpreted" (Giustini, 2006, p. 1283). It represents a social and cultural revolution that captures the emerging character of the Internet and society generally and is designed to maximize creativity, communications, secure information sharing, collaboration and functionality of the web and is continually changing. The O'Reilly Radar states that "Web 2.0 is a set of economic, social and technology trends that collectively form the basis of the next generation of the Internet – a more mature, distinctive medium characterized by user participation, openness, and network effects" (Musser, 2006, p. 4). Web communities have developed with social networking sites, video sharing, podcasts, mashups, wikis, blogs, twittering and folksonomies.

Following on the heels of Web 2.0 is Web 3.0, sometimes called the semantic web. Whereas Web 2.0 provided a platform for interaction between computers and people, Web 3.0 facilitates meaningful interaction between computers. "An important feature of Web 3.0 is that it enables computers to talk to each other so that they can perform the tasks necessary for us to do our work. However, a primary feature of Web 3.0 is that it uses metadata-data about data" (Giustini, 2007, p. 1273). According to Giustini, Web 3.0 provides improved control over information, moves us from the 'wisdom of the crowd' to the 'wisdom of the expert', from searching for information to finding information and from an anarchic and lawless environment to one more controlled with standards, protocols and rules (Giustini, 2007, p. 1273).

Web 2.0 and Web 3.0 are emerging at the same time as health care reforms are advancing the adoption of the EMR, EHR, improvements to the quality and safety of health care delivery, evidence based practice by health care providers, improved access, integration and coordination of

services and information, as well as greater accountability for explicit performance indicators from the policy makers and politicians who are responsible for the health care delivery systems. The very sustainability of the health care system has come into question as a recent report analyzed what sustainability in public health care *really* means (Health Council of Canada, 2008b). Simultaneous with the emergence of Web 2.0 and Web 3.0, citizens and patients began to look to new and more effective ways of interacting with their health care providers. Policy makers began to explore how they could encourage the effective delivery of health care services using the electronic medium. Social and political changes were taking place in society that sparked the emergence of Web 2.0 and Web 3.0 thereby providing a venue for Health 2.0 and Medicine 2.0.

Health 2.0 and Medicine 2.0 are recently coined terms whose definitions are still developing. They represent the possibilities that emerge from synergies that arise between and among health care, eHealth and Web 2.0. Ian Furst suggests, "Health 2.0 is participatory healthcare characterized by the ability to rapidly share, classify and summarize individual health information with the goals of improving health care systems, experiences and outcomes via integration of patients and stakeholders" (Furst, 2009). The key words in the definition are "improving" and "integration of patients and stakeholders". The term Health 2.0 emerged because of its general and limitless potential for participation of citizens to achieve improved health outcomes in what is currently a fragmented and disjointed health care delivery system.

According to Eysenbach:

Medicine 2.0 applications, services and tools are Web-based services for health care consumers, caregivers, patients, health professionals, and biomedical researchers, that use Web 2.0 technologies as well as semantic web and virtual reality tools, to enable and facilitate specifically social networking, participation, apomediation,

Table 1. Comparison of old thinking and new thinking about chronic disease management

Old think	Rethink
Institutions have impenetrable boundaries	Institutions boundaries are permeable facilitating interoperability, networking and collaboration
Doctors, nurses and administrators are in charge	The patient is the care leader supported by care givers
Health care providers are purveyors of knowledge	Citizens and patients pursue knowledge and are partners in knowing
Health care providers are purveyors of care	Citizens and patients participate in self care
Researchers extract knowledge and truth	Researchers engage and interact with the world
Policy makers pronounce policy	Policy makers engage citizens and providers in policy making

collaboration, and openness within and between these user groups. (Eysenbach G., 2008, p. 4)

Medicine 2.0 does for the health care provider community what Health 2.0 does for health care consumers – it brings them closer together within an open and collaborative environment. Because the fields are emerging there is significant fragmentation among the groups advocating their ideas, however, there is an overall commitment to the principles of collaboration, networking and openness. The terms Health 2.0 and Medicine 2.0 will be conflated into the term Web 2.0 in the remainder of the paper unless a distinction is necessary to make a specific point.

Health 2.0 and Medicine 2.0 are a departure from traditional approaches and catalyze a paradigm shift that reflects the contemporary values and expectations of citizens, providers, researchers and policy makers. We can compare and contrast the old way of thinking, "old think", about health care and the emerging way "rethink" which is becoming increasingly more prominent and influential. Examples of the two contrasting views using chronic disease management are noted in Table 1.

Shifting our thinking to a new paradigm and using Web 2.0 and Web 3.0 may be very powerful; however, unbridled enthusiasm for technology to solve social or political problems without a sober second thought often leads to disappointment. We encourage a critical approach to the development and application of Web 2.0 and Web 3.0 so that potentially undesirable consequences can be anticipated and averted.

HEALTH TECHNOLOGY ASSESSMENT: A CRITICAL APPROACH TO ASSESSING EFFECTIVENESS

All forms of health care intervention can be thought of as a technology. We define health technology as "any intervention that may be used to promote health, to prevent, diagnose or treat disease or for rehabilitation or long-term care. This includes the pharmaceuticals, devices, procedures and organizational systems used in health care" (Facey, Topfer, & Chan, p. 26). In order to fully understand and explicate the relationship between health care technology and Web 2.0 we must take a broad societal perspective. We also need to take a critical perspective and posit that health care interventions and the attendant heath information systems must be beneficial and therefore effective (clinically and economically) to individual citizens, patients and the general population. Information technologies are often differentiated from health care technologies; however information technologies today are inextricably an integral part of health technologies and systems.

To protect the public's health and interest as well as facilitate an appropriate diffusion of heath care technologies, a policy instrument or mechanism is needed to identify the issues, assess the risks and benefits, and adjudicate on the appropriateness for the introduction of the technology. The field of health technology assessment emerged to fill this void. The role of health technology assessment is to critically appraise the effectiveness of technologies with a view to ensure that their introduction and diffusion serves the best interests of citizens. Health technology assessment (HTA) is defined as:

...the systematic evaluation of properties, effects, and/or impacts of health care technology. It may address the direct, intended consequences of technologies as well as their indirect, unintended consequences. Its main purpose is to inform technology-related policymaking in health care. HTA is conducted by interdisciplinary groups using explicit analytical frameworks drawing from a variety of methods. (Facey, Topfer, & Chan, p. 27)

HTA is rarely used to assess the effectiveness of computerized health care because it is not an intervention – it is however an inextricable component of care delivery.

The emergence of Web 2.0 and Web 3.0 as a new media of interaction and mediation between and among citizens, providers, researchers, and policy makers to promote health system reforms and improved population health is both simplistic and complex. It is simplistic because on the surface it appears as though the characteristics are synergistic with necessary health reforms. On closer examination we find barriers, issues and problems associated with adapting a new way of mediating between citizens, providers, researchers and policy makers with a system still steeped in traditional structures, processes, incentives, disincentives and relationships.

A NEW PARADIGM FOR THINKING ABOUT HEALTH SYSTEM INTEROPERABILITY

Thinking about a problem differently can give rise to new solutions where none appeared before. We will use the paradigm of the values espoused by Web 2.0 to think about how to effectively accelerate health care reforms to achieve system integration, coordination and interoperability. For the paradigm to be manageable we will break it up into a series of actors, values and actions. We divide the health care system into 4 primary actors;

- citizens, patients or consumers
- health care providers
- researchers, and
- health care policy makers and decision makers

There are other actors such as health care supply manufacturing firms, consultants, software development companies and pharmacy businesses but we will exclude them as they function, alongside but admittedly, outside of the public enterprise and follow a different set of motivations and goals.

The emergence and development of Web 2.0 is synergistic with the following values;

- informed choice
- collaboration
- openness
- provider commitment to excellence of practice (peering)
- researcher autonomy
- fair and egalitarian state direction based on the principle of social solidarity.

Although there are many challenges for Web 2.0 to be to be an effective catalyst, it provides an important stimulus toward the following:

Table 2. Using Web 2.0 to improve understanding, access, trust, discourse, practice and behavior in the health care system

Dimensions for Improvement	Citizens	Providers	Researchers	Policy makers
Understanding	What mechanisms exist or are emerging?			
Access	How can the mechanisms be improved?			
Trust	What are the issues and problems?			
Discourse	What are the opportunities?			
Behavior/practice	What research is necessary?			

- Improving citizen knowledge, access and choice regarding effective health care interventions to benefit their personal health care status;
- Improving provider autonomy and practices to best serve the interests and health outcomes of patients and the health of the population;
- Improving researchers' capability and capacity to bridge between the creation of new knowledge and contributing to its application; and
- Improving the state's direction of the health care system through better data, information and knowledge thereby improving health care policy making.

Web 2.0 can serve as the mediating dimension leading to more informed citizens, providers, policy makers and researchers. These more informed actors undertake improved practices, policies and behaviors leading to improved health of citizens and a higher functioning health care system.

These representations are not a direct reflection of reality but are an approximation of reality that can help us organize and categorize our thinking about how best to harness the positive characteristics of Web 2.0 to advance health care reforms oriented toward improving system interoperability at the functional and informational levels.

Table 2 below is a construct that takes the dimensions of understanding, access, trust, discourse and behavior & practice and sets them against

each of the actors. We will examine each of the dimensions and interrogate how each actor might be impacted by Web 2.0. This table informs the structure of the remainder of the chapter.

IMPROVING UNDERSTANDING

The first theme of our framework examines how Web 2.0 can become a powerful platform to help citizens, providers, researchers and policy makers improve their understanding of the health care system and how they can turn that understanding into behaviors, practices, research endeavors and policies that improve the functioning of the health care system. 'Seek first to understand' is the first tenant of reform and interoperability demands understanding.

Improving Understanding of Citizens

The Internet has become an important source of information to the public on topics of health and diseases. In a survey in January 2009 Ipsos Reid found that almost three-quarters (70%) of online Canadians have visited a health care website in the past year (Ipsos Reid, 2009). In 2001 Eysenbach and Jadad published an article ushering in the era of consumer health informatics. In the article they identify the rise of computers and information technology claiming that it will give the public unprecedented access to information and provide the opportunity to participate and interact with evidence based health care (Eysenbach & Jadad,

2001). McDaniel reinforces the importance of consumer health informatics and underlines its importance as a medium of information exchange (McDaniel, Schutte, & Keller, 2008). Both authors point to the potential opportunities that lie in the power of Web 2.0 to help transform health care delivery to be much more respectful and responsive to the consumer. In spite of the promising opportunities these very same attributes raise concerns about the quality of online health information. Indeed, a 2002 systematic review found that quality, completeness, and accuracy of health information were problems in the majority of studies (Eysenbach, Powell, Kuss, & Sa, 2002). This paradox of having access to a plethora of information and the challenge of differentiating between what is of high quality and what is not, is a serious problem.

In spite of the relative ubiquity of health information there are several barriers that prevent the public from becoming full partners participating in evidence based or informed decision making. Eysenbach and Jadad identify that some providers jealously guard their knowledge acting as "owners" and "filters" of information. Some providers give information to the citizen but do not engage in a discourse that would allow informed decision making. An approach that is gaining prominence is participative and collaborative discourse where the citizen, researcher and provider engage in a dialogue to evaluate the pros and cons of different interventions (health technology assessments for example) and what would be most appropriate for the individual. As a medium, Web 2.0 lends itself to connecting the providers, researchers and patients both in spirit and substance. The challenge is to restructure today's work processes to supplement communication channels and skills, and to find the time, resources and financial incentives so that citizen, researcher and provider linkages can be made more effective.

In the past health professionals were overloaded with information. Today the public are inundated with information through mass media advertising, self support groups, and the Internet. In addition they now have access to data bases previously restricted to medical professionals such as PubMed, a peer reviewed collection of high quality articles ranging from genomics to population health (U.S. National Library of Medicine) and the Cochrane Library which provides high quality systematic reviews assessing the effectiveness of health care interventions (Canadian Cochrane Centre).

The challenge for the public is twofold: understanding the information, and differentiating between information that is of high quality and that which is not. With the explosion of Internet sites offering information on health, diseases and interventions how are the public to separate the 'wheat from the chaff'? Information that has been peer reviewed and is from a reputable source which has a good standing and credibility in society can often be accepted at face value. One approach is to provide independent external credentialing of web sites such as that provided by the Health on the Net Foundation (HON), a non-governmental organization in Switzerland, who developed a code for improving the quality of information for patients and health care providers. The mission of the HON is to improve "the quality of information intended to both patients and medical professionals for facilitating quick access to the most relevant and up-to-date medical discoveries. (Health on the Net Foundation, 2009)

Web 2.0, because of its ubiquitous, collaborative and open nature, provides significant opportunities for advancing the exchange of high quality information between citizens, providers, policy makers and researchers. The challenge will be to provide each of the actors with the ability to access, understand, interpret and evaluate the information to best serve their needs. In the case of citizens this will involve providing access to the Internet, increasing their literacy so that they can understand and evaluate the information, and providing them with the linkages to the knowledgeable health care provider community.

A critical approach to systematically evaluating the validity and generalizability of the information to their context will be an important skill for actors to develop. Health technology assessments, Cochrane reviews and systematic critical reviews are examples of the types of information that can be helpful.

Improving Understanding of Providers

The health care provider communities have begun to reap significant benefits from the application of Web 2.0. Just as citizens can become more knowledgeable about the effectiveness of health care interventions so can providers use the Internet to increase their knowledge and skills. One sound application of the interactive nature of Web 2.0 is for Internet based education. It allows learners to participate at a convenient time and place (podcasts), is universally accessible, can be updated and can be delivered to the provider's site of clinical activity. Learners can customize learning requirements by selecting the content as well as the pace and place of learning. Cost can be minimal and the multimedia format provides a selection of presentation styles and the ability to create interactive clinical cases providing instantaneous feedback.

Internet based education has become a popular approach in health care education however questions have arisen as to whether it is as effective as other forms of teaching. David Cook and colleagues undertook to systematically review, summarize and assess through a meta-analysis the effect of Internet based education for health profession learners compared with no intervention and with non-Internet interventions. Cook and colleagues concluded that "Internet based learning is associated with large positive effects compared with no intervention. In contrast, effects compared with non-intervention instructional methods are heterogeneous and generally small, suggesting effectiveness similar to traditional methods" (Cook,

Levinson, Garside, Dupras, Erwin, & Montori, 2008, p. 1181). The findings support the view that computer assisted instruction is neither inherently better nor worse than traditional methods but further study is required to determine whether a different form of computer assisted instruction may improve effectiveness. The challenge is that users need to have the skill and hardware to access the Internet and navigate it effectively, be aware of the web resources and how they can be helpful. Curricula need to be developed that are valid and captivating to the audience. Research needs to be advanced to determine how to integrate learning into the work place or the work flow of the busy clinician. The provider community will need to adopt existing credentialing or accreditation processes or establish standards, guidelines and codes for ensuring that information is reliable and can be trusted.

Improving Understanding of Researchers

Researchers play an important role advancing the frontier of knowledge and its application to everyday issues and problems. To do this effectively and efficiently researchers need access to data and information that is anonymous but linked to existing data bases as well as to new ones created to provide a comprehensive understanding of the health and diseases within the population, its health care needs, utilization patterns, human resource and health technology distribution as well as the outcomes from the interventions. Researchers need to have mechanisms in place to easily and appropriately gain access to the communities, organizations, networks, families and individuals that may be the subject of their research. To maintain their methodological prowess researchers require access to knowledge and data bases to inform the approaches and methods of their research activities. The interactive capability of Web 2.0 permits instantaneous communication and collaboration between and among those in the research communities over vast distances and in either asynchronous or synchronous mode. Web 2.0 permits researchers to advance their techniques for gathering data through surveys or interaction with focus groups on the web. Mashups that collate information from different data banks and present the results in a new form provide significant promise for increasing our understanding of the relationships among variables that affect health and disease.

Improving Understanding of Policy Makers

To achieve a better understanding of the health of the population as well as the performance of the health care system, policy makers need access to valid and reliable data that can be analyzed and interpreted to structure a health policy framework that will best address health needs of citizens. The setting of the policy agenda is only one stage of the policy cycle. Polling and surveying the population from an interactive Web 2.0 platform can provide insight into health issues that concern the public as well as provide an insight into the effectiveness of health system performance.

Information for the identification and formulation of policy options, assessing policy options through interactive and dynamic modeling or simulation, choosing the option, making transparent the assumptions at play, predicting the possible consequences, developing an implementation strategy and program are all necessary for the policy process. Policy makers will be more successful if they achieve an improved understanding of citizens' health needs and how they can more effectively intervene to reduce health disparities in the population. There are many policy initiatives supported by Web 2.0 that we could examine but we will choose two, (1) population health, and (2) the effectiveness of health care system functioning.

Population health is defined as "the health outcomes of a group of individuals, including the distribution of such outcomes within the group" (Kindig & Stoddart, p. 380). Unlike traditional approaches of medicine and public health focusing on the health of individuals, population health aims to improve the health of an entire population by reducing health inequities among population groups. It does this by addressing the broad range of contributors, called social determinants of health, that impact health on a population level such as environment, social structure, and resource distribution. A population health perspective looks beyond being free from disease to the ability of people to live to their full potential. Policy makers working within the population health paradigm approach health issues by looking to individual, organization and cultural interventions to improve health status. An example of a population health management approach would entail the analysis and understanding of income and education gradients and barriers that contribute to the relative morbidity and mortality rates leading to the introduction of remedial policy actions. The creation and maintenance of data on population health status indicators, historical citizen health care utilization experience, and distribution of health care providers can be collated into mashups to provide powerful tools for health care planning and management. Health goals with measureable health outcomes could be established to monitor and report on progress.

Policy makers can improve their understanding of the effectiveness of the health care system by using Web 2.0 to monitor, report on and evaluate performance. At peak performance the health care system is universally accessible, clinically effective, cost effective, safe, efficient, patient centered, integrated, coordinated and population health oriented. Policy makers are expected to provide leadership for identifying the means for achieving a high performing health care system. They can look to organizations like the Canadian Institute for Health Information (CIHI) whose role it is to provide timely, accurate and comparable information to inform health policies, support the effective delivery of health services and raise awareness among Canadians of the factors that contribute to good health. CIHI data and reports focus on health care services, health spending, health human resources and population health. CIHI also identifies and promotes national health indicators to measure life expectancy, spending per capita and health system performance. In addition to producing reports CIHI contains repositories of data on health services utilization by case mix, which is available for policy makers and researchers to interrogate and answer health policy questions. Web 2.0 provides an interactive platform for policy makers to extend the contribution CIHI could make informing important policy questions by providing unfettered access to anonymous data to researchers.

Several provinces have established institutes to conduct and disseminate research on the effectiveness of health care interventions. The Institute for Clinical Evaluative Sciences (ICES) provides unique scientific insights to help policymakers, managers, planners, practitioners and other researchers shape the future direction of the Ontario health care system. ICES unbiased, evidence-based knowledge and recommendations, profiled in atlases, investigative reports, health technology assessments, and peer-reviewed journals, are used to guide decision-making and inform changes in health care delivery and policy making. ICES is able to produce valuable reports for policy makers because of their ability to anonymously link population-based health information on an individual patient basis, using unique ICES identifiers that ensure the privacy and confidentiality of health information. Linked data allows researchers to obtain a more comprehensive view of specific health care issues than could be achieved with unlinked data. In Alberta the Institute of Health Economics (IHE) produces and disseminates health research findings from health economics, health policy, health technology assessment and comparative effectiveness to improve the delivery and sustainability of health care.

Policy makers that advance the effective application of the population health paradigm to study and influence the health of citizens coupled with models of high performing health care systems will find that Web 2.0 provides significant leverage to effectively achieve improved health for Canadians.

IMPROVING ACCESS

The second theme of our framework looks to how Web 2.0 can be a catalyst for citizens, providers, researchers and policy makers to improve their access to the health care system and the choices that they make.

Improving Access of Citizens

Web 2.0 can empower citizens to make wise choices regarding access within the health care system that is appropriate to their needs at a specific point in time. British Columbia was the first followed by several others that have introduced province wide information sourcing programs that are available to citizens 24/7. The program, HealthLink BC, provides British Columbians with trusted non-emergency health information and services they can access through the Internet or by calling 811 on their telephone. The service permits the citizen to discuss their symptoms with a nurse, consult with a pharmacist, or get healthy eating advice from a dietitian. The service also helps identify the health services or resources needed and how the person would go about accessing them (HealthLinkBC, 2009).

Access to health care services has been an ongoing challenge for the health care delivery system in Canada as was highlighted in the Health Council of Canada review of health care reforms (Health Council of Canada, 2008a). Citizens want access to health care within a time frame that does not have negative consequences on their health or well-being. They desire a system that is fair, responding to the sickest people with the quickest access to care without compromising access for those whose needs may be less urgent but are none the less real. The desire by the public for quick access to health care for elective procedures has come into conflict with the state's ability to deliver. The reasons for this are complex but some of it is based on the inability of the structures and functions of health care delivery to adapt to the new expectations of citizens. One notable example is people queuing in the hospital emergency departments to see a physician for a non emergent matter because there is no other option such as a clinic open when they require the service. Establishment of 24/7 community primary health clinics serve as an alternative to emergency departments but these are only recently emerging.

A big challenge for wait list management and interoperability generally is developing a common language, definitions and terminology for dealing with the different types of wait list for service. A common set of definitions is essential if measurement of success against a set of objectives is to be achieved with accountability and transparency. To address and advance these challenges the Health Council of Canada developed recommendations for a common framework for wait lists (Health Council of Canada, 2005). Policy makers taking the leadership and working collaboratively and cooperating with counterparts across the country would go some distance to make sense of the wait list issue for Canadians.

The province of Saskatchewan has introduced the surgical care network which creates a transparent surgical wait list system for the province (Saskatchewan Surgical Care Network). In Ontario a similar approach has been undertaken (Ministry of Health and Long-Term Care). Citizens can view on the web site wait time for a procedure by hospital. Armed with this information they may chose to request their doctor refer them to a specialist or hospital where they would get treatment more quickly. The Ontario website differentiates between information of interest to citizens versus

that of providers with the information for providers being more detailed. Web 2.0 provides an opportunity to build on these innovative initiatives to provide citizens with the appropriate information to advance their ability to interact with the health care system.

Improving Access of Providers

Providers can help citizens access the health care system more effectively and appropriately. The Ontario website noted above has a section directed to providers to help them explain and interpret the data to interested patients. An approach that shows great promise for advancing the access of citizens to health care is the continuous quality improvement paradigm, a quality improvement project that led to the introduction of a new and innovative scheduling program to the offices of providers. The quality improvement paradigm offers a way to have providers, managers and patients work together on changing the structure and function of care delivery. In Saskatoon, urologist Dr. Visvanathan, introduced a quality improvement project and formed a team to brainstorm how they could improve patient flow in their clinic. The team used an Advanced Access® scheduling system for shortening the wait time for appointments in physician practices. They were able to free up appointment slots by assessing which patients truly need follow-up with the urologist and which could be seen by their own physician. Dr. Visvanathan says that for initiatives like this to be adopted more widely, the health care system needs to enable improvement efforts. "Physicians need support from QI specialists...They are too busy to learn QI from scratch and their clinical time would be wasted on the administrative side of QI. Ultimately, the fee-for-service system is poisoning QI. Alternate funding plans will be necessary to move forward with any momentum." (Saskatchewan Health Quality Council, 2007). The quality improvement project led to the introduction of a clinic scheduling website that patients could visit and make an appointment. Examples such as these where structural and process changes are used to stimulate new approaches to use Web 2.0 should be strongly encouraged.

Improving Access of Researchers

For researchers to be effective they must have access to valid and reliable data. The data must be linked in time, along a continuum of care and provide analysis along several dimensions. Web 2.0 is revolutionizing access to data and information through web modalities such as 'Delicious' for social bookmarking and 'flickr' for tagging photographs. Another opportunity is presented with unprecedented global access to knowledge bases of primary and secondary studies which often become the object of study for systematic critical reviews or meta-analysis. A third dimension of access is the barriers to access to information, knowledge and services. Identifying remedies to the access issues is both relevant and timely.

Several sources of health care data are available nationally at Statistics Canada and the CIHI as well as the provinces of Ontario, Manitoba and British Columbia but the linkages remain weak and their breadth is not as broad as they should or could be. Policy makers will need to consider what policy frameworks provide access to the greatest breadth and depth of data, ensure the privacy and confidentiality of citizens and make them available to researchers. For researchers to undertake timely and relevant studies to inform questions of interest and utility for citizens and policy makers, they require access to citizens, providers and policy makers so that they can collaborate and work on projects that require multiple disciplines and perspectives.

Access and linkage to global reservoirs of data, information and knowledge is necessary to create a research environment that facilitates the opportunity for broad epidemiological analysis, economic analysis, and sociological studies as well as basic and secondary research in health

informatics. Researchers must also give consideration to what will make their contributions more accessible (literally and substantively) to citizens, providers, policy makers and one another.

Improving Access of Policy Makers

The use of Web 2.0 by the policy community is in its infancy. CIHI has recently published comparative data on the hospital standardized mortality rates. Making the data available publicly has caused a stir by those who have taken positions defending their high rates and why they are not correct. Policy makers in Ontario have introduced a new program that allows citizens to find health care close to home on the Internet. The information about local health services is available at the Ontario Ministry of Health and Long-Term Care website. Using this site citizens can find the nearest walk-in and after-hours clinics, urgent care centres, family health teams, general practitioners and emergency rooms by typing in their postal codes. The service is updated regularly and is intended to be expanded to offer information on all front-line health services in Ontario including community care access centres, laboratories and long term care homes. Opportunities to use the Web 2.0 platform to build secure data banks of biomedical information ranging from genomic to population health accessible to researchers is a challenge for the future.

IMPROVING TRUST

Canadians have ranked health care as one of their top three issues of concern. Concern with access to services and the future sustainability of the health care system have compromised the public's trust in whether the services will be there when they require them. The third theme of our framework looks to how Web 2.0 may help citizens, providers, researchers and policy makers improve the respective trust they hold in one another. On the other hand the platform can also be viewed as a significant threat to the security of information and data on the Internet. Ways to build trust and reduce the risk of harm through a breach will be a major endeavor for Web 2.0.

Improving Trust of Citizens

The quality of health information on the Internet is of great concern to citizens, providers, researchers and policy makers. Citizens may be misled to undertake interventions that are not effective and may be dangerous and providers may need to spend time with patients dispelling wrong advice or information. Policy makers may fall into the same trap of being influenced by opinions not supported by the scientific evidence. Eysenbach and colleagues undertook the first systematic and comprehensive review of the quality of health information in the Internet. They conclude that "due to differences in study methods and rigor, quality criteria, study population, and topic chosen, study results and conclusions on health – related Web sites vary greatly" (Eysenbach, Powell, Kuss, & Sa, p. 2691). They call for operational definitions of quality criteria to be developed and applied to websites.

What health information can citizens trust? Previously we mentioned the HON guidelines but more specific assurances are necessary. The Canadian Public Health Association (CPHA) website provides advice to consumers wishing to be critical and differentiate between high quality information and poor information. The following are pointers to evaluate the quality of information on the Internet:

- Does the website say who is responsible for the information and how you can contact them? Look for links that say *about us, about this site,* or *contact us.*
- Is the purpose of the website to give information, or is it to sell something?

- Health information should be unbiased and balanced, based on scientific evidence and not opinion. The most trustworthy health information is based on medical research. Are there references to articles in medical journals or other sources to back up its health information?
- Health information for the public should be easy to understand. Technical or unfamiliar terms should be clearly explained.
- When was the information prepared and updated?
- Consult a health professional about the health information you find on websites that may be conflicting (Canadian Public Health Association, 2008)

Citizens should be concerned about the security, privacy and risk of breach of their confidential information on the Internet. Caution is advised about providing personal information on the Internet. Some websites collect and sell personal information to other organizations. Such concerns can be a significant barrier to the widespread sharing of citizen eHealth records. In response legislation has been enacted to establish the rules on the use, disclosure and collection of personal information. In Canada this is the Personal Information Protection and Electronic Documents Act (PIPEDA) and provinces have enacted their own health sector implementations of the act. The privacy threat posed by network interoperability is a key concern and needs to be treated seriously so that the privacy of individuals can be assured. The interest of citizens in personal health records (PHR) will invariably require the use of the Internet to link with patient records located on private networks – raising the possibility of a breach without appropriate safeguards. As the citizen becomes the owner of the PHR (a trend of Web 2.0 and Web 3.0) maintaining privacy and confidentiality will likely transfer to the owner rather than it being under the control of medical practitioners. Mechanisms for facilitating the patient's access to and control of their health record without risking breach of privacy will need to be resolved and assured.

Improving Trust of Providers

Broad use of information technology and the transformation it can bring to health care will only occur with widespread participation and trust of consumers which will depend upon their confidence that their information will be protected. This assurance can only be established if we have strong and harmonized information policies that guide the development and use of new electronic tools that emerge from Web 2.0 and subsequently Web 3.0.

Health care providers and researchers are working together to establish trusted sites which provide the strongest scientific evidence in respect to the effectiveness of health care interventions. One, mentioned above, is the Cochrane Collaboration, an international not-for-profit and independent organization, dedicated to making up-to-date, accurate information about the effects of healthcare readily available worldwide. It produces and disseminates systematic reviews of healthcare interventions and promotes the search for evidence in the form of clinical trials and other studies of interventions. A second important organization for addressing the effectiveness of less clinical and more social interventions is the Campbell Collaboration (Campbell Collaboration). Its mandate is to help people make well-informed decisions by preparing, maintaining and disseminating systematic reviews in education, crime, justice, and social welfare. It is a sister organization to the Cochrane Collaboration and supports an international research network that produces systematic reviews of aspects of social interventions.

Improving Trust of Researchers

The integrity, credibility and reputation of researchers are based on the high quality of their research and the maintenance of that standard of practice. Once researchers have established their reputation and credibility they begin to gain the trust of citizens, providers and policy makers. In addition to their commitment to a high standard of methodological excellence researchers gain trust if they have a reputation of being unbiased. The removal of bias from research is one of the strongest characteristics researchers aspire toward in building trust relationships with their peers and other actors. The added value arising from the work of researchers is that it rises above the partisan positioning in the community. Citizens, providers and policy makers are looking for an objective assessment and pronouncement as to the efficacy, effectiveness and efficiency of various health care interventions.

The research community will need to develop peer review processes that citizens, providers and policy makers can trust. The health informatics research community should consider the establishment of a Cochrane-like organization to serve as a clearing house and repository of trusted and helpful information to inform the question of the efficacy and effectiveness of health information technologies.

Improving Trust of Policy Makers

Policy makers have the task of balancing between the preservation of individual privacy and confidentiality on one hand and aggregating citizen data to the greatest community benefit on the other. These goals can come into conflict. An approach has been developed by two Australian researchers, Peter and Jasmine Croll, which can help address the dichotomy of concerns. In their paper entitled "Investigating risk exposure in e-health systems", they propose an integrated model aiming at providing a framework to help build trustworthy solutions for the individual and the community. The method proposed focuses on the identification of pertinent issues that determine the risk exposure of a given system. An important result of their work relates to the interdependency of factors influencing the safety of the system. Their approach called QUiPS (Quality, Usability, Privacy and Safety) provides a framework that helps identify causes that could lead to a safety incident and demonstrates their interdependencies. A valuable point of their work is the practical outcomes validated on two large Australian projects (Croll & Croll, 2007).

Croll & Croll point out that policy makers must satisfactorily address the following issues of public concern:

- Abuse of genetic data (disclosure to insurance companies)
- Release of sensitive information (e.g. sexual, mental health)
- Government control of personal data
- Use of data integrity (information accurately recorded or records mismatched)
- Inadequate safeguards (any access by unauthorized people).

The biggest risk faced is in understanding the complex environments that our health services present and ensuring the users appreciate and comply with any policies set. Numerous divergent approaches continue to provide practical, secure and compliant solutions that protect health data privacy. Convergence towards a viable universal solution is not imminent therefore trust in e-health is decidedly more fragile as compared with many other industry sectors. Hence, any policies that data custodians follow need to be flexible and updated on a regular basis to allow for changes. (Croll & Croll, p. 464)

Since policy makers will be setting the stage for the societal approach to ensuring that Web 2.0 is safe and secure for the use of citizens, providers and researchers they will need to be explicit about

how this is to be achieved to gain and maintain the trust of citizens

IMPROVING DISCOURSE

The fourth theme of our framework looks to how Web 2.0 can be a stimulus to help citizens, providers, researchers and policy makers improve the respective discourses within their domains and among them in order to improve population health and the functioning of the health care system. In looking to the characteristics that maximize the value of the discourse it must be open, honest, multi-disciplinary, timely and relevant.

Improving Discourse of Citizens

Web 2.0, and on its heels Web 3.0, provide a powerful platform for citizens to engage in conversations among themselves, with the provider community, researchers and policy makers. Citizens are exploring the use of the Internet for social networking to share information with one another on their experiences with health care. This has the action of making explicit and open what might have been private conversations in the past. The fact that they appear on the Internet presents an opportunity to help inform but also raises issues of propriety surrounding what kind of information is being shared and whether it is being done with discretion. Opportunities for the abuse of individuals and reputations could become an issue and due care and attention must be taken to ensure that societal rules and laws that apply in the public sphere are adhered to on the Internet.

Citizens are using the Internet and Web 2.0 as a social support network. One recent phenomenon was that of Jason Boas who established a blog to share his experience in dealing with cancer. The-boasblog was established to follow his progress in his battle against cancer. After his death the No Surrender Charitable Trust was established to help cancer sufferers all over the world and includes a global social network for cancer patients (No Surrender) Another example of a very popular interactive patient support is PatientsLikeMe where citizens can share their experiences with diseases and health care treatments (PatientsLikeMe).

The Web 2.0 development of mashups show promising opportunities for increasing the understanding and discourse of citizens and health care providers. Mashups are a web application with the ability to provide information automatically by combing data banks on the Internet and extracting the information or functionality of interest and combining that with other forms of information that are illustrated and analyzed. Examples of two Mashups are those created to track the Avian Flu globally and more recently to track the spread of the Swine Flu (H1N1).

Another popular form of interaction of the public on the Internet is the use of blogs. A Blog is a website maintained by an individual who posts regular entries of commentary, descriptions of events with complementary graphics or video. Citizens are invited to comment on the blog or to discuss the pros and cons of the point of view posted by the writer. There are several health care blogs that the public have a great interest in. Seeman recently reviewed the content quality and governance of the most popular health care blogs. Seeman observes "health blogs are positive tools that create meaningful, informed news and exchange for consumers and health professionals" (Seeman, 2008, p. 101). Seeman observes that many blogs are 'niche blogs' meaning that they exist to support a very narrow interests for example diabetes management. Other blogs such as the Wall Street Journal Health Blog, Kevin M.D. Medical Web Blog and The Health Care Blog (THCB) are much broader and deal with a wide variety of issues. These blogs are important examples of where Web 2.0 Health 2.0 and Medicine 2.0 have converged to become a very powerful source of information to stimulate discourse among citizens, providers, policy makers and researchers.

Improving Discourse of Providers

Provider communities have begun to a build a forum of discourse among one another on the Internet. The capability of Web 2.0 permits sophisticated interaction and communications to take place on the Internet to build solutions using open source. One example of this is the voluntary organization of physicians who have organized under the name OSCAR (Open Source Clinical Application Resource) and have dedicated themselves to assisting colleagues interested in the Open Source movement to develop an electronic medical record for their office practices (OSCAR).

A second emerging practice for providers is to use search engines such as Google as a clinical support to assist with diagnosis. Tan and Ng undertook a blind study to determine how often searching with Google would lead doctors to the same diagnose as those published in the New England Journal of Medicine and found that the Google searches revealed the correct diagnosis in 15 of 26 cases (58%, 95% confidence interval 38% to 77%). The authors concluded that the Internet can be an important clinical tool for physicians especially in diagnosing difficult cases (Tan & Ng, 2006).

Web 2.0 may also serve as a platform on which collaborative discourse among multi-disciplinary providers interact on the Internet to integrate and coordinate the care plans for patients in health care settings or in their homes. Health care providers are using the blogosphere and mashups extensively to advance the sharing of information and knowledge among themselves as well as with citizens, policy makers and researchers.

Improving Discourse of Researchers

The research community can realize significant benefits from the emergence of Web 2.0. The ubiquity of data and information from secure protected sources could serve as the focus of collaboration among researchers from different parts of the globe to study, analyze and interpret health data though the electronic medium of exchange. Text is not the only form of communications to be shared; it is possible to share video and audio clips as well. Researchers from one part of the world can engage in discussions around the world.

Although language translation programs may still be in their infancy, researchers are using them to access and extract information and knowledge contained in foreign published articles. Care and attention is required to ensure that interpretation is accurate but it opens up the opportunity for taking into account the usual limitation of conducting literature searches and reviews that are restricted to one language.

Application programming interface (API) is another potential initiative of Web 2.0 that may have significant implications for advancing the discourse and research agendas within the health care system. An API is a set of routines, data structures, object classes and/or protocols provided by libraries and or operating system services in order to support the building of applications (Wikipedia, 2009). Examples of API are Google Maps, Java APIs, and iPhone API. Google maps have already been used effectively to report and monitor the spread of contagious diseases.

Discourse among researchers can be facilitated by Web 2.0 but it can also enable the interaction with citizens, providers and policymakers. Web 2.0, can facilitate interviews with subjects, the recording of audio files for transcription, the recording of video files for purposes of capturing expressions and nuance of conversation that cannot be easily captured in other formats.

Improving Discourse of Policy Makers

Policy makers are becoming attuned to the power of the Internet and its qualities of ubiquity, collaboration, and integration. A forward thinking policy maker, the Deputy Minister of Health in Saskatchewan, is exploring ways in which the

internet can be used to advance the health policy discourse in his province. One of the initiatives introduced in 2008, called the Patient First Review was to interact with Saskatchewan residents about the delivery of health care services in the province and how they might be changed so that the experiences of patients is improved. The review includes a website where citizens can complete a workbook documenting their experiences with the health care system. Policy makers review the data and draw conclusions from their findings (Patients First Review, 2009). One of the first blogs introduced in a large health care provider organization in Canada was that of the CEO of the Alberta Health Services Board who communicates with 90,000 staff, 7,200 physicians and 18,700 volunteers on a regular basis (Duckett, 2009).

IMPROVING BEHAVIOR AND PRACTICE

The fifth theme of our framework looks to how Web 2.0 can become an important stimulus to help citizens, providers, researchers and policy makers improve their behavior and best practice in how to use the health care system effectively, what health care interventions to choose in discussion with a health care provider or to support the citizen with their self care in the home.

Improving Behavior and Practice of Citizens

Armed with the appropriate information, resources and support, patients can glean great benefit from Web 2.0 applications. Studies have demonstrated that interactive applications for chronic health conditions have a positive effect on consumer knowledge, increase perceived social support, and improve clinical outcomes (Murray, Burns, Tai, Lai, & Nazareth, 2005). This is an important finding if one begins to explore ways in which the sustainability of the health care system can be maintained through better self management of health by citizens. Another promising example is the Comprehensive Health Enhancement and Support System (CHESS), first developed in 1989. This system provides information resources and social support through online discussion forums and live chats, and decision support services via multimedia technology on a web-based platform (Gustafson, Hawkins, Boberg, McTavish, Owens, & Wise, 2002).

Smart house technology using embedded sensors and surveillance devices to allow the elderly and disabled to remain independent is another Web 2.0 initiative showing promise. Studies have shown that technology can enable social support networks for patients and caregivers who are isolated due to geographical distance, stigma, or the burden of illness. This work was pioneered by Brennan who developed the ComputerLink® system. Brenan demonstrated that computer-mediated communication among home-bound individuals can increase perceived social support and decrease caregiver strain (Brennan, 1992).

Another initiative touched on above is online support groups for cancer patients. The support groups are common and may enhance coping skills among participants. Web 2.0 technology is creating a sea of change in social networking on the Internet, particularly among young people. The ability to create and post multimedia content (e.g., YouTube), interact with friends (e.g., MySpace, Facebook), and navigate within virtual environments such as Second Life are increasingly common.

Improving Behavior and Practice of Providers

Web 2.0 offers great potential to facilitate and encourage improved behaviors and best practices of providers. Many health care professional organizations have established their own websites for their associations and colleges. Individual providers have established their own websites

providing information and interactive capability to consumers. Provider organizations may be responsible for the representation of their members in society while others are responsible for their admission to practice, maintenance of credentials and discipline of the profession. Web 2.0 offers an approach for health care professionals to be open and transparent with the respective responsibilities of their organizations.

The challenge for a health care provider to stay abreast of the explosion of knowledge in the health sciences is impossible under the traditional approaches of information dissemination. The information about new pharmaceuticals, techniques, procedures and diseases is an unending avalanche of information for health care providers. The challenge is to find ways to have the right information available to the right individuals at the right time. One way forward is to introduce new Web 2.0 "knowledge management technologies" and automated "sensemaking" approaches which can assist health care providers in their decision making at the bedside, in the board room and at the policy table.

Improving Behavior and Practice of Researchers

Web 2.0 affords opportunities for improving the behavior and best practice of researchers. The quality of research is directly related to the standards of the research design and how it is carried out and adheres to the standards of research in the discipline, field or domain. Standards of research are accessible on the Internet and communications and linkage among the members of the research community can be achieved easily and quickly. World experts on topics of their areas of expertise are accessible to those wishing advice on their research design or methodology. Mentoring is possible over vast distances using video and interactive audio capabilities. Researchers are aided by the emergence of eHealth grids for medical research that will provide powerful computing and data management capabilities to manage large amounts of heterogeneous data.

The credibility and reputation of researchers and their work can add significant value to advancing improvements in health care delivery if their approach is critical. In the past health information systems have not been the focus of health technology assessments or critical reviews because the field was emerging and methods of evaluation were in their infancy. However, with the scarcity of resources and the pressure for innovative and effective new approaches to health care delivery upon us, researchers are becoming much more critical and not accepting at face value information technology solutions as being effective by mere fact of their existence or their marketing brochures. Usability analysis for example has emerged as a method for the evaluation of clinical information systems (Kushniruk & Patel, 2004).

Improving Behavior and Practice of Policy Makers

The policy and decision making communities are embracing the contribution that Web 2.0 can make to improve the functioning of the health care system. An important advancement is the ability for policy makers to make accountable and transparent to citizens the monitoring and reporting on the performance of the health care system.

EHealth can make a contribution to continually improving health care delivery in the form of quality, efficiency, effectiveness and access however it requires that citizens, providers and policy makers work together to extract those benefits. Some of the opportunities that lay untapped are the delivery of care that is customized to individual patients where eHealth enables more informed decision making based on patient specific data and the global best evidence. Evidence based practice can be used to reduce errors and undertakings introduced to improve the diagnostic accuracy of tests and appropriate interventions pursued. Citizens and patients can be empowered to partner more

effectively in treatment decision making and for self care. Health care delivery processes can be streamlined, wait times and waste reduced in an effort to improve efficiency.

Health policy makers must become familiar with the global literature in effective strategies and health care policies around the world and undertake comparisons to determine if there are applications that can help advance the agenda in their local settings. Publication of the results of the comparative analysis being posted on the Internet for the world's policy community to review and critique would help advance knowledge of what is found to work and what does not. Blogs are becoming a popular way for the policy community to monitor what is taking place in the broader health care community. Some of the more popular blogs followed by the public and policy makers are the Wall Street Journal Health Blog, Kevin M.D. Medical Weblog and The Health Care Blog.

FUTURE RESEARCH DIRECTIONS

The full potential of the social and political implications of Web 2.0 and Web 3.0 on the health care system are only beginning to be understood and exploited. The nature and qualities of Web 2.0 and 3.0 are changing the way we think about health care services and how they should be delivered. Web 2.0 emerged at a time that health reforms were gridlocked in structural and process improvements. Web 2.0 and now Web 3.0 are catalyzing the opportunity for traditional barriers and hindrances to be addressed. However, as promising as eHealth is there are many issues and challenges to its effective use. In spite of a growing evidence base for effective health care delivery there is a lack of rigorous and generalizable evidence of the effectiveness and cost effectiveness of eHealth applications. Development of a rigorous research base of evaluation and technology assessment of eHealth applications is essential if it is to effectively contribute to the improvement of health system performance and improved population health. The complexity of human beings and their interactions in organizations requires that future research consider the human relations and organization factors of implementing eHealth initiatives that take into account the perspectives and needs of providers, citizens and policy makers. Health 2.0 and Medicine 2.0 encourage multidisciplinary collaborative team approaches to care and research will be required to identify the barriers that exist and enablers that would help address these challenges – particularly from an eHealth perspective. A major challenge for advancing the implementation of eHealth systems into care and management processes are the insufficient levels of systems interoperability. Research in providing a better understanding of the dynamics and iterative nature of health care reforms with eHealth and how they can be advanced through strategic policy making to create a high performing health care system will be essential if we are to achieve a sustainable health care system. The legal and ethical implications of using eHealth in clinical and management settings as decision support systems is not yet clearly understood and resolved. Research to identify what Web 2.0 and Web 3.0 mechanisms should be developed and applied to reduce harm and risk to citizens and patients should be encouraged. Further research will be necessary to fully understand the effects that eHealth, Web 2.0 and Web 3.0 have on patient behavior and the relationship between providers and patients. Studies of how the care process between providers and patients might be enhanced through Web 2.0 and Web 3.0 should be undertaken. Research into the methods and approaches to create new and time saving communications between citizens, patients and providers would be of significant benefit. Not all citizens have access to the Internet, those who are disabled, financially challenged, or not Internet literate are particularly disadvantaged. Research into how those barriers might be mitigated with facilitators will be necessary. Research into better understanding the role of trust and how it can be

nurtured in the health care system, particularly as it relates to Web 2.0 and Web 3.0 would help to advance a high performing system. As our social, political and technical capabilities in effectively harnessing the opportunities afforded by Web 2.0 are captured we should also be aware and vigilant of the opportunities that Web 3.0 may offer in the future and how we can bridge effectively to them.

CONCLUSION

The emergence of Web 2.0, Web 3.0, Health 2.0, and Medicine 2.0 at a time when health care reform appears to be in a gridlock is opportune. Web 2.0 has lead to the emergence and introduction of new forms of social interaction among patients, providers, researchers and policy makers which promise to improve the effectiveness of the care delivery process to individual patients. We have identified how Web 2.0 can be instrumental in advancing health care actors understanding, access, trust, discourse, practice and behaviour of the health care processes, interrelationships and systems. On the other hand the new social phenomena also raise difficult issues which will require careful study and resolution. If resolved satisfactorily the future of ubiquitous health can be assured and built upon with Web 3.0.

Web 2.0, Health 2.0, and Medicine 2.0 require integration, collaboration and coordination if they are to become a significant force for improving the functioning of the health care system. Web 2.0 and 3.0 cannot be helpful or successful without effective health care reform and health care reform cannot be successful without Web 2.0 and Web 3.0. Returning to Coiera's rules we must be mindful of the necessity for an iterative linkage to be encouraged between the social cultural environment we dream of achieving and how the technical information and communications systems can help us get there.

Web 2.0 and 3.0 are an emerging phenomenon in society encouraging the reduction in information asymmetry between citizens, providers, researchers and policy makers and is helping to create an environment where the actors can openly and transparently collaborate to work toward a high performing health care system. By making the current barriers and hindrances explicit all actors can work together to remove them and advance the agenda. There are however pitfalls, and critical thinking and behavior will be required to assure that promises are held to account, benefits are realized, discourse is respectful and trust is not breached. Supporting a platform in which health information technologies and communications encourage social and technical interoperability supporting open and honest discourse that promotes excellence in behavior and the best practice of health care providers should be the goal of all in the service of patients.

REFERENCES

Archer, N. (2009). System Interoperability and Adoption in eHealth: Perspectives for the Canadian Healthcare System. *MCETECH 4th International Conference on eTechnologies*. Ottawa: MECTECH 2009.

Brennan, P. (1992). Computer Networks Promote Caregiving Collaboration: the ComputerLink Project. *Procedings Annual Symposium Computer Application Medical Care* (pp. 156-160). Baltimore: American Medical Informatics Association.

Campbell Collaboration. (n.d.). *What Helps? What Hurts? Based on What Evidence?* Retrieved May 15, 2009, from The Campbell Collaboration (C2): http://www.campbellcollaboration.org

Canadian Cochrane Centre. (n.d.). *The Cochrane Library*. Retrieved April 30, 2009, from Canadian Cochrane Centre: www.ccnc.cochrane.org

Canadian Public Health Association. (2008). *Health Literacy Portal*. Retrieved January 23, 2009, from Canadian Public Health Association: http://www.cpha.ca/en/portals/h-l.aspx

Coiera, E. (2004). Four Rules for the Reinvention of Health Care. *British Medical Journal, 328*, 1197–1199. doi:10.1136/bmj.328.7449.1197

Cook, D., Levinson, A., Garside, S., Dupras, D., Erwin, P., & Montori, V. (2008). Internet-based Learning on the Health Professions: A Meta-analysis. *American Medical Association Journal, 300*(10), 1181–1196. doi:10.1001/jama.300.10.1181

Croll, P. R., & Croll, J. (2007). Investigating Risk Exposure in e-Health Systems. *International Journal of Medical Informatics, 76*, 460–465. doi:10.1016/j.ijmedinf.2006.09.013

Davis, K., Doty, M. M., Shea, K., & Stremikis, K. (2009). Health Information Technology and Physician Perceptions of Quality of Care and Satisfaction. *Health Policy (Amsterdam)*, 239–246. doi:10.1016/j.healthpol.2008.10.002

Duckett, S. (2009). *News and Views from the President/CEO*. Retrieved May 20, 2009, from Alberta Health Services Internal Blog: http://iblogs.albertahealthservices.ca/ceo/

Economist. (2009, April 16). A Special Report on Health Care and Technology. *The Economist*. London, Britain, UK: The Economist.

Elson, S. (2009). Regionalization of Health Care from a Political and Structural Perspective. *Healthcare Management Forum*, 6–11.

Eysenbach, G. (2008). Medicine 2.0: Social Networking, Collaboration, Participation, Apomediation, and Openness. *Journal of Medical Internet Research, 10*(3), 1–14. doi:10.2196/jmir.1030

Eysenbach, G., & Jadad, A. (2001, June). Evidence-based Patient Choice and Consumer Health Informatics in the Internet Age. *Journal of Medical Internet Research,* ▪▪▪, 1–14.

Eysenbach, G., Powell, J., Kuss, O., & Sa, E. (2002). Empirical Studies Assessing the Quality of Health Information for Consumers on the World Wide Web: a Systematic Review. *Journal of the American Medical Association,* 2691–2700. doi:10.1001/jama.287.20.2691

Facey, K., Topfer, L., & Chan, L. (2009). *Glossary.* Retrieved February 14, 2009, from INAHTA Health Technology Assessment Glossary: http://www.inahta.org/GO-DIRECT-TO/Members/

Furst, I. (2009). *Wait Time & Delayed Care.* Retrieved February 14, 2009, from Wait Time & Delayed Care: http://waittimes.blogspot.com

Giustini, D. (2006, December 23-30). How Web 2.0 is Changing Medicine. *British Medical Journal,* –1284. doi:10.1136/bmj.39062.555405.80

Giustini, D. (2007, December 22-29). Web 3.0 and Medicine. *British Medical Journal, 335,* 1273–1274. doi:10.1136/bmj.39428.494236.BE

Gustafson, D., Hawkins, R., Boberg, E., McTavish, F., Owens, B., & Wise, M. (2002). CHESS: 10 years of Research and Development in Consumer Health Informatics for Broad Populations Including the Underserved. *International Journal of Medical Informatics,* 167–177.

Health 2.0. (n.d.). *The Next Conference.* Retrieved April 29, 2009, from Health 2.0: http://health2con.com

Health Council of Canada. (2005). *Ten Steps to a Common Framework for Reporting on Wait Times.* Toronto: Health Council of Canada.

Health Council of Canada. (2008a). *Rekindling Reform: Health Care Renewal in Canada 2003 - 2008.* Toronto: Health Council of Canada.

Health Council of Canada. (2008b). *Sustainability in Public Health Care: What Does it Mean? A Panel Discussion Report.* Toronto: Health Council of Canada.

Health on the Net Foundation. (2009, March 9). *HONcode.* Retrieved May 15, 2009, from Health on the Net Foundation: http://www.hon.ch

HealthLinkBC. (2009). *HealthLink BC.* Retrieved May 15, 2009, from HealthLinkBC: www.healthlinkbc.ca

Ipsos Reid. (2009). *Online Healthcare: Coming of Age.* Calgary: Ipsos Reid.

Kindig, D., & Stoddart, G. (2003). What is Population Health? *American Journal of Public Health,* 380–383. doi:10.2105/AJPH.93.3.380

Kushniruk, A., & Patel, V. (2004). Cognitive and Usability Engineering Methods for the Evaluation of Clinical Information Systems. *Journal of Biomedical Informtics,* 56-76.

Leonard, K. (2009, January 30). *One Patient, One Record (OPOR).* Retrieved April 29, 2009, from Patient Destiny: http://patientdestiny.typepad.com

McDaniel, A., Schutte, D., & Keller, L. (2008). Consumer Health Informatics: from Genomics to Population Health. *Nursing Outlook,* 216–223. doi:10.1016/j.outlook.2008.06.006

Medicine 2.0. (2009). *Medicine 2.0.* Retrieved April 29, 2009, from Medicine 2.0 2009: http://www.medicine20congress.com

Ministry of Health and Long-Term Care. (n.d.). *Ontario Wait Times.* Retrieved April 12, 2009, from Government of Ontario: http://www.health.gov.on.ca/transformation/wait_times/wait_mn.html

Murray, E., Burns, J., Tai, S., Lai, R., & Nazareth, J. (2005). *Interactive Health Communication Applications for People with Chronic Disease.* Oxford: Cochrane Collboration.

Musser, J. (2006, Fall). *Web 2.0 Principles and Best Practices.* Retrieved April 24, 2009, from O'Reilly Radar: http://oreilly.com/catalog/web2report/chapter/web20_report_excerpt.pdf

No Surrender. (n.d.). Retrieved April 12, 2009, from No Surrender Charitable Trust: http://www.no-surrender.org

OSCAR. (n.d.). *Welcome to OSCAR Canada Users Society.* Retrieved May 17, 2009, from OSCAR: http://www.oscarcanada.org/

Patients First Review. (2009, January). Retrieved April 10, 2009, from Government of Saskatchewan: http://www.patientfirstreview.ca/

PatientsLikeMe. (n.d.). *PatientsLikeMe: Patients Helping Patients Live Better Every Day.* Retrieved April 10, 2009, from www.Patientslikeme.com

Sarasohn-Kahn, J. (2008). *The Wisdom of Patients. California Healthcare Foundation.* Oakland: California Healthcare Foundation.

Saskatchewan Health Quality Council. (2007). *Finding the Time to Shorten the Wait Time for Patients.* Retrieved January 23, 2009, from Health Quality Council: https://www.hqc.sk.ca/portal.jsp;jsessionid=uyam4ycbc1?1VJYfSwJTephIZ3btQ6RJTBIzBf0QfLQkUwK4QBZaJtC0GkpNuk4YFVvI5thiwzu

Saskatchewan Surgical Care Network. (n.d.). Retrieved April 15, 2009, from Government of Saskatchewan: http://www.sasksurgery.ca/

Seeman, N. (2008). Inside the Health Blogosphere: Quality, Governance and the New Innovation Leaders. *ElectronicHealthcare, 7*(3), 101–108.

Shaw, A. (2009, March). *Telus Purchases MyChart from Sunnybrook.* Retrieved April 21, 2009, from Canadian Healthcare Technology: www.canhealth.com/mar09.html#09marstory1

Tan, H., & Ng, J. (2006). Googling for a Diagnosis - Use of Google as a Diagnostic Aid: Internet Based Study. *British Medical Journal,* 1143–1145.

Tapscott, D., & Williams, A. (2006). *Wikinomics: How Mass Collaboration Changes Everything.* Toronto: Penguin Group.

U.S. National Library of Medicine. (n.d.). *National Center for Biotechnology Information.* Retrieved April 12, 2008, from PubMed: www.pubmed.gov

Wikipedia. (2009, April 06). *Application Programming Interface.* Retrieved May 15, 2009, from Wikipedia: http://en.wikipedia.org/wiki/Application_programming_interface#cite_note-0

ADDITIONAL READING

Anderson, G. F., Bianca, K., Frogner, B. K., Johns, R. A., & Reinhardt, U. E. (2006). Health Care Spending and Use of Information Technology in OECD Countries. *Health Affairs, 25*(3), 819–831. doi:10.1377/hlthaff.25.3.819

Babin, G., Kropf, P., & Weiss, M. (2009). *E-Technologies: Innovation in an Open World,* Proceedings, 4th International Conference, MCETCH 2009, Ottawa, Canada, May 4 – 6, 2009.

Bodenheimer, T., & Wagner, E, H., & Grumbach, K. (2002). Improving Primary Care for Patients with Chronic Illness. *Journal of the American Medical Association, 288*(14), 1775–1779. doi:10.1001/jama.288.14.1775

Canada Health Infoway. EHR 2015: *Advancing Canada's Next Generation of Healthcare.* Canada Health Infoway, <www.infoway-inforoute.ca> Toronto.

Canada Health Infoway & Health Council of Canada. (2006). *Beyond Good Intentions: Accelerating the Electronic Health Record in Canada.* A policy conference. June 11–13, 2006, Montebello, QC <http://www.healthcouncilcanada.ca>

Cheung, K. H., Yip, K. Y., Townsend, J. P., & Scotch, M. (2008). HCLS 2.0/3.0: Health Care and Life Sciences Data Mashup Using Web 2.0.3.0. *Journal of Biomedical Informatics, 41,* 694–705. doi:10.1016/j.jbi.2008.04.001

Diamond, C. C., & Shirky, C. (2008). Health Information Technology: A Few Years of Magical Thinking. *Health Affairs, 27*(5), 383–390. doi:10.1377/hlthaff.27.5.w383

Ferguson, T. & the e-Patient Scholars Working Group. (2007). e-*Patients: How They Can Help Us Heal Health Care.* <http://e-patients.net/e-Patients_White_Paper.pdf>

Fyrat, F. A., & Vicdan, H. (2008). A New World of Literacy, Information Technologies, and the Incorporeal Selves: Implications for Macromarketing Thought. *Journal of Macromarketing, 28*(4), 381–396. doi:10.1177/0276146708325385

Gagliardi, A., & Alejandro, R. J. (2002). Examination of Instruments Used to Rate Quality of Health Information on the Internet: Chronicle of a Voyage with an Unclear Destination. *British Medical Journal, 324*(9), 569–573. doi:10.1136/bmj.324.7337.569

Gagnon, M. P., Legare, F., Labrecque, M., Fremont, P., Pluye, P., Gagnon, J., et al. Turcot. L., & Gravel, K. (2009*). Interventions for Promoting Information and Communication Technologies Adoption in Health Care Professionals* (Review) The Cochrane Collaboration. <http://www.thecochranelibrary.com>

Halamka, J. D. (2009). *Life as a Healthcare CIO.* Retrieved May 17, 2009 from http://geekdoctor. blogspot.com

Juzwishin, D. W. (2005). *Educating Publics and Policy Makers: Epistemic Committees and the Politics of Evidence-Based Health Reform in Alberta and Saskatchewan.* Dissertation. Edmonton, Alberta, Canada: University of Alberta

Juzwishin, D. W. (2009). *Political, Policy and Social Barriers to System Interoperability.* 4th International MCETECH Conference on eTechnologies. Ottawa: MCETECH 2009

Kushniruk, A. W., & Borycki, E. M. (2008). *Human, Social and Organizational Aspects of Health Information Systems.* Hershey, PA: IGI Global.

Lau, F. (2003). *A Pan-Canadian Health Informatics Education Strategy* (pp. 386–390). Proceedings American Medical Informatics Association.

Macmillan, P., Medd, A., & Hughes, P. (2009). *Change Your World or the World will Change You: The Future of Collaborative Government and Web 2.0.* Deloitte.

Martin, S., Kelly, G., Kernohan, W. G., McCreight, B., & Nugent, C. (2009). *Smart Home Technologies for Health and Social Care Support* (Review). The Cochrane Collaboration, http://www.thecochranelibrary.com

McDaniel, A. M., Schutte, D., & Keller, L. O. (2008). Consumer Health Informatics: From Genomics to Population Health. *Nursing Outlook, 56,* 216–223. doi:10.1016/j.outlook.2008.06.006

McDaniel, J. G. (2009). Advances in Information Technology and Communication in Health. In *Proceedings Information Technology in Community Health.* Victoria, Canada: ITCH.

McGee, J. B., & Begg, M. (2008). What Medical Educators Need to Know About "Web 2.0.". *Medical Teacher, 30*(2), 164–169. doi:10.1080/01421590701881673

Potts, H., Skiba, D., Paton, C., & Oh, H. (2008). Health 2.0 and Medicine 2.0: Tensions and Controversies in the Field. *Journal of Medical Internet Research, 10*(3), e23. doi:10.2196/jmir.1056

Protti, D. (1986). The Synergism of Health Information Science/Health Informatics. *Critical Reviews in Medical Informatics, 1*(2), 149–163.

Protti, D. (2008). e-Health in Canada: Lessons for European Health Systems. *Eurohealth, 14*(3), 30–32.

Tang, P. C., & Lee, T. H. (2009). Your Doctor's Office or the Internet? Two Paths to Personal Health Records. *The New England Journal of Medicine, 360*(13), 1276–1278. doi:10.1056/NEJMp0810264

Underhill, C., & McKeown, L. (2008). Getting a Second Opinion: Health Information and the Internet. Statistics Canada, Catalogue no. 82-003-X Health Reports, Ottawa.

Urowitz, S., Wiljer, D., Apatu, E., Eysenbach, G., DeLenardo, C., Harth, T., et al. (2008). Is Canada Ready for Patient Accessible Electronic Health Records? A National Scan. *Biomed Central, Medical Informatics and Decision Making, 8*(33). 24 July 2008 http://www.biomedcentral.com/1472-6947/8/33

Wiljer, D., Urowitz, S., Apatu, E., DeLenardo, C., Eysenbach, G., & Harth, T. (2008). Canadian Committee for Patient Accessible Health Records (CCPAEHR). Patient Accessible Electronic Health Records: Exploring Recommendations for Successful Implementation Strategies. *Journal of Medical Internet Research, 10*(4), e34. doi:10.2196/jmir.1061

Zeng, X., & Bell, P. (2008). Web 2.0 What the Health Care Manager Needs to Know. *The Health Care Manager, 27*(1), 58–70.

Compilation of References

@neWorld (2008). A Virtual Community for Kids with Cancer Retrieved October 15, 2008, from http://1worldonline.org/

Abdalla, J. A. (2006). A communication model for structural design objects: Performatives and protocols. *Advances in Engineering Software, 37*(6), 393–405. doi:10.1016/j.advengsoft.2005.09.001

Abdul-Kareem, S. (1998). A preliminary study of security in healthcare systems on the information superhighway: the Malaysian perspective. *Health Informatics Journal, 4*(3-4), 223–226. doi:10.1177/146045829800400314

Aboulnaga, A., & El Gebaly, K. (2007). µBE: automatic source selection and schema mediation for Internet scale data integration. In *Proceedings of IEEE International Conference on Data Engineering* (pp.186-195). Istanbul, Turkey: IEEE.

Adatia, F. A., & Bedard, P. L. (2002). Palm reading: 1. Handheld hardware and operating systems. *Canadian Medical Association Journal, 167*, 775–780.

Adatia, F., & Bedard, P. L. (2003). Palm reading: 2. Handheld software for physicians. *Canadian Medical Association Journal, 168*, 727–734.

Adragna, L. (1998). Implementing the enterprise master patient index. *Journal of American Health Information Management Association, 69*(9), 46–52.

Aetna, Inc. (2006, October 3). *Aetna introduces powerful, interactive personal health record.* Press release. Retrieved December 11, 2008, from http://www.aetna.com/news/2006/pr_20061003.htm.

Afework, A., Beynon, M. D., Bustamante, F., Cho, S., Demarzo, A., Ferreira, R., et al. (1998). Digital dynamic telepathology--the Virtual Microscope. In *Proceedings of the AMIA Symposium*, 912-916. Retrieved February 13, 2009, from http://www.pubmedcentral.nih.gov/articlerender.fcgi?artid=2232135

Aggarwal, P., Sardana, H. K., & Jindal, G. (2009). Content Based Medical Image Retrieval: Theory, Gaps and Future Directions. *ICGST-GVIP Journal, 9*(2), 27–37.

Aglets Workbench, I. B. M. (2001). IBM Japan Research Group. http://aglets.trl.ibm.co.jp

Agrawal, D., & Aggarwal, C. (2001). On the design and quantification of privacy preserving data mining algorithms. In *Proceedings of the Twentieth ACM SIGACT-SIGMOD-SIGART Symposium on Principles of Database Systems* (pp. 247–255). Santa Barbara, California, USA: ACM.

Ahmad, B., Omar, W., & Taleb-Bendiab, A. (2006). *Intelligent Monitoring Model For Sensing Financial Application Behaviour Based On Grid Computing Overlay.* Paper presented at the Submitted to 2006 IEEE International Conference on Services Computing (SCC 2006), USA.

AIIM. (2006, October 20). *Industry leaders join forces to advance portable healthcare document practices; new Best Practices Guide addresses exchange of healthcare information.* Press release. Retrieved November 8, 2008, from http://www.aiim.org/article-pr.asp?ID=32097.

AIIM. (n.d.). *PDF Healthcare Committee Web site.* Retrieved December 5, 2008, from http://www.aiim.org/standards.asp?ID=31832.

Aiken, L. H., Clarke, S. P., Sloane, D. M., Sochalski, J., & Silber, J. H. (2002). Hospital Nurse Staffing and Patient Mortality, Nurse Burnout, and Job Dissatisfaction. *Journal of the American Medical Association, 288*(16), 1987–1993. doi:10.1001/jama.288.16.1987

Alaoui, A., Collmann, J., Nguyen, D., Lindisch, D., Subbiah, R. T. N., Green, A., et al. (2003). *Implementing a secure Teleradiology system using the internet* Paper presented at the Computer Assisted Radiology and Surgery CARS 2003.

Copyright © 2010, IGI Global, distributing in print or electronic forms without written permission of IGI Global is prohibited.

Alcaniz, M., Botella, C., Banos, R., Perpina, C., Rey, B., & Lozano, J. A. (2003). Internet-based telehealth system for the treatment of agoraphobia. *Cyberpsychology & Behavior, 6*(4), 355–358. doi:10.1089/109493103322278727

Alexander, B. (2006). Web 2.0. A new wave of innovation for teaching and learning? *EDUCAUSE Review, 41*(2), 32–44.

Ali Shaikh, A., & Omer, R. (2005). *Formalising trust for online communities.* Paper presented at the Fourth international joint conference on Autonomous agents and multiagent systems, The Netherlands.

Aljareh, S., & Rossiter, N. (2002). Towards security in multi-agency clinical information services. *Health Informatics Journal, 8*(2), 95–103. doi:10.1177/146045820200800207

Allison, S. E., Wahlde, L., Shockley, T., & Gabbard, G. O. (2006). The Development of the Self in the Era of the Internet and Role-Playing Fantasy Games. *The American Journal of Psychiatry, 163*, 381–385. doi:10.1176/appi.ajp.163.3.381

Altman, G. (2004). *Delmar's fundamental and advanced nursing skills* (2nd ed.). Toronto: Thompson Delmar Learning.

Amabile, T., Patterson, C., Mueller, J., Wokocik, T., Odomirok, P. W., Marsh, M., & Kramer, S. (2001). Academic-practitioner collaboration in management research: A case of cross-profession collaboration. *Academy of Management Journal, 44*(2), 418–432. doi:10.2307/3069464

Amalberti, R., & Leape, L. L. (2002). *How Hazardous is Healthcare.* Paper presented at the 5th Joint Quality in Health Care Symposium.

America's Health Insurance Plans. (2006, December 13). *Industry leaders announce personal health record model; collaborate with consumers to speed adoption.* Press release. Retrieved December 14, 2008, from http://www.ahip.org/content/pressrelease.aspx?docid=18328.

America's Health Insurance Plans. (2006, June 20). *Health plans participate in CMS PHR pilot to help Medicare beneficiaries better manage their health.* Press release. June 20, 2006. Retrieved December 11, 2008, from http://www.ahip.org/content/pressrelease.aspx?docid=20043.

American Academy of Family Physicians. (n.d.). *ASTM Continuity of Care Record (CCR) Web site.* Retrieved November 8, 2008, from http://www.centerforhit.org/x201.xml.

American College of Radiology. (2003). American College of Radiology (ACR) Breast Imaging Reporting and Data System Atlas (BI-RADS® Atlas). Reston, VA.

American Health Information Management Association. (2007, June 19). *AHIMA calls on Congress to expand and standardize personal health information privacy protections.* Press release. Retrieved February 7, 2009, from http://www.ahima.org/press/press_releases/07.0619.asp.

American Health Information Management Association. (n.d.). *myPHR Web site.* Retrieved October 13, 2008, from http://www.myphr.com.

American Psychological Association. (1997). Services by telephone, teleconferencing, and Internet [Electronic Version], from http://www.apa.org/ethics/stmnt.01html

Ammenwerth, E., Schnell-Inderst, P., Machan, C., & Siebert, U. (2008). The effect of electronic prescribing on medication errors and adverse drug events: A systematic review. *Journal of the American Medical Informatics Association, 15*(5), 585–600. doi:10.1197/jamia.M2667

Anderson, G., & Knickman, J. (2001). Changing the chronic care system to meet people's needs. *Health Affairs, 20*(6), 146–160. doi:10.1377/hlthaff.20.6.146

Anderson, J. G., & Aydin, C. E. (2005). *Evaluating the organizational impact of healthcare information systems.* New York: Springer Verlag. doi:10.1007/0-387-30329-4

Anderson, P., Rothbaum, B., & Hodges, L. (2000). Virtual Reality: Using the virtual world to improve quality of life in the real world. *Menninger Winter Psychiatry Conference, 65*(1), 78-91.

Angelmar, R. (2007). Patient empowerment and efficient health outcomes. *Financing sustainable healthcare in Europe: New approaches for better outcomes,* 141. Retrieved February 28, 2009 from http://www.sustain-healthcare.org/cox.php

Ankolekar, A., Krötzsch, M., Tran, T., & Vrandecic, D. (2008). The two cultures: Mashing up Web 2.0 and the Semantic Web. *Web Semantics: Science. Services and Agents on the World Wide Web, 6*(1), 70–75.

Antani, S., Lee, D. J., Long, L. R., & Thoma, G. R. (2004). Evaluation of shape similarity measurement methods for spine X-ray images. *Journal of Visual Communication and Image Representation, 15*(3), 285–302. doi:10.1016/j.jvcir.2004.04.005

Antani, S., Long, L. R., & Thoma, G. R. (2004). Content-based image retrieval for large biomedical image archives.

Studies in Health Technology and Informatics, 107(Pt 2), 829–833.

Antoniou, G., & Harmelen, F. (2004). *A semantic web primer*. The MIT Press.

Antoniou, G., & Van Harmelen, F. (2004). Web ontology language: Owl. *Handbook on ontologies, 2*, 45-60.

Antoniou, P., Delidou, E., Aggeioplasti, K., & Kaldoudi, E. (2008) Astronomy Education for the Public via Web 2.0 technologies. In *Proceeding of ICERI2008 – International Conference of Education, Research and Innovation*, Madrid, Spain.

Anvari, M. (2007). Impact of Information Technology on Human Resources in Healthcare. *Healthcare Quarterly, 10*, 84-88. Retrieved November 9, 2008 from http://www.longwoods.com/product.php?productid=19320&cat=513&page=1

Araki, K., Ohashi, K., Yamazaki, S., Hirose, Y., Yamashita, Y., & Yamamoto, R. (2000). Medical markup language (MML) for XML-based hospital information interchange. *Journal of Medical Systems, 24*(3), 195–211. doi:10.1023/A:1005595727426

Archer, N. (2009). System Interoperability and Adoption in eHealth: Perspectives for the Canadian Healthcare System. *MCETECH 4th International Conference on eTechnologies*. Ottawa: MECTECH 2009.

Archer, P. (2005). *Quatro – a metadata platform for trustmarks*. Paper presented at the International Conference on Dublin Core and Metadata Applications: Vocabularies in Practice, Madrid, Spain.

Argawal, V. (2007). Podcasts for psychiatrists: a new way of learning. *Psychiatric Bulletin*, col 31, 270-271.

Arnaert, A., & Delesie, L. (2001). Telenursing for the elderly: The case for care via video-telephony. *Journal of Telemedicine and Telecare, 7*, 311–316. doi:10.1258/1357633011936912

Arnold, Y., Daum, M., & Krcmar, H. (2004). *Virtual Communities in Health Care: Roles, Requirements and Restrictions*. Paper presented at the Multikonferenz Wirtschaftsinformatik (MKWI) 2004.

Arnold, Y., Leimeister, J. M., & Krcmar, H. (2003). *CoPEP: A Development Process Model for Community Platforms for Cancer Patients*. Paper presented at the The XIth European Conference on Information Systems (ECIS).

Arora, M. (2009). CVS joins Google Health Rx network: millions can access medication records online. *Official blog from the Product Manager, Google Health*. Retrieved March 6, 2009, from http://www.socresonline.org.uk/12/5/17.html

Ash, J. S., & Bates, D. W. (2005). Factors and forces affecting EHR system adoption: report of a 2004 ACMI discussion. *Journal of the American Medical Informatics Association, 12*, 8–12. doi:10.1197/jamia.M1684

Ash, J. S., Berg, M., & Coiera, E. (2004). Some unintended consequences of information technology in health care: The nature of patient care information system related errors. *Journal of the American Medical Informatics Association, 11*(2), 121–124.

ASTM International. (2005). Designation [*Standard specification for continuity of care record][CCR]. E (Norwalk, Conn.)*, 2369–05.

Atack, L., Luke, R., & Chien, E. (2008). Evaluation of Patient Satisfaction With Tailored Online Patient Education Information. *Computers, Informatics, Nursing, 26*(5), 258–264. doi:10.1097/01.NCN.0000304838.52207.90

Athan, A., & Duchamp, D. (1993). *Agent-Mediated Message Passing for Constrained Environments*. In *Proceedings USENIX Symposium on Mobile and Location-Independent Computing* (pp. 103-1070). Cambridge, MA.

Atienza, A., Hesse, B., Baker, T., Abrams, D., Rimer, B., Croyle, R., & Volckmann, L. (2007). Critical issues in eHealth research. *American Journal of Preventive Medicine, 32*(5Suppl), S71–S74. doi:10.1016/j.amepre.2007.02.013

Atkinson, N. L., & Gold, R. S. (2002). The promise and challenge of eHealth interventions. *American Journal of Health Behavior, 26*, 494–503.

Aubrecht, P., Matousek, K., & Lhotská, L. (2008). On Designing an EHCR Repository. In L. Azevedo & A. R. Londral (Eds.), *Proc. of the International Conference on Health Informatics (HEALTHINF 08)* (pp. 280-285). Funchal, Madeira, Portugal.

Augar, N., Raitman, R., & Zhou, W. (2004). Teaching and learning online with wikis. In R. Atkinson, C. McBeath, D. Jonas-Dwyer & R. Phillips (Eds.), *Beyond the comfort zone: Proceedings of the 21st ASCILITE Conference* (pp. 95-104). Perth.

Awofeso, N., Dalhatu, A., & Schelokova, I. (2008). Training of Front-line Health Workers for Tuberculosis Control: Lessons from Nigeria and Kyrgyzstan. *Human Resources for Health, 6*(20). Retrieved October 28, 2008 from http://www.human-resources-health.com/content/6/1/20

Axup, J., Viller, S., & Bidwell, N. J. (2005, 15-20 May). *Usability of a mobile, group communication prototype while rendezvousing.* Paper presented at the The 2005 International Symposium on Collaborative Technologies and Systems, Queensland Univ., Qld., Australia.

Aziz, O., Lo, B., Pansiot, J., Atallah, L., Yang, G. Z., & Darzi, A. (2008). From computers to ubiquitous computing by 2010: health care. *Philos.Transact.A Math. Phys. Eng Sci., 366,* 3805–3811.

Bader, J., & Strickman-Stein, N. (2003). Evaluation of new multimedia formats for cancer communications. *Journal of Medical Internet Research, 5*(5).

Badrinath, B. R., Bakre, A., Imielinski, T., & Marantz, R. (1993). Handling Mobile Clients: A Case for Indirect Interaction. In *Proceedings of the 4th Workshop on Workstation Operating Systems, Aigen, Austria, October.*

Baeza-Yates, R., & Ribeiro-Neto, B. (1999). *Modern Information Retrieval.* New York: Addison Wesley.

Bagherzadeh, J., & Arun-Kumar, S. (2006). Flexible Communication of Agents based on FIPA-ACL. *Electronic Notes in Theoretical Computer Science, 159,* 23–39. doi:10.1016/j.entcs.2005.12.060

Bai, Q., & Zhang, M. (2006). Coordinating Agent Interactions Under Open Environments. In Fulcher, J. (Ed.), *Advances in applied artificial intelligence.* IGI.

Bai, X. (2005). Tabu Search Enhanced Markov Blanket Classifier for High Dimensional Data Sets. In *The Next Wave in Computing* (Vol. 29, pp. 337–354). Optimization, and Decision Technologies.

Bakken, S., Campbell, K. E., Cimino, J. J., Huff, S. M., & Hammond, W. E. (2000). Toward Vocabulary Domain Specifications for Health Level 7 – Coded Data Elements. *Journal of the American Medical Informatics Association, 7,* 333–342.

Baldwin, L., Clarke, M., Eldabi, T., & Jones, R. (2002). Telemedicine and its role in improving communication in healthcare. *Logistics Information Management, 15*(4), 309–319. doi:10.1108/09576050210436147

Ball, M. J., Costin, M. Y., & Lehmann, C. (2008). The personal health record: consumers banking on their health. *Studies in Health Technology and Informatics, 134,* 35–46.

Ball, M. J., Smith, C., & Bakalar, R. S. (2007). Personal health records: empowering consumers. *Journal of Healthcare Information Management, 21*(1), 76–86.

Bamidis, P. D., Constantinidis, S., Kaldoudi, E., Maglaveras, N., & Pappas, C. (2008). The use of Web 2.0 in teaching Medical Informatics to postgraduate medical students: first experiences. Published as Multimedia Appendix in G. Eysenbach (Ed.). Medicine 2.0: Social Networking, Collaboration, Participation, Apomediation, and Openness. *Journal of Medical Internet Research, 10*(3), e22. Retrieved from http://www.jmir.org/2008/3/e22/ doi:10.2196/jmir.1022-23

Bard, S. R. (1991). Virtual reality: an extension of perception. Noetic Sciences Review(Autumn), 7-16.

Barfield, W., & Weghorst, S. (1993). The sense of presence within virtual environments: A conceptual framework. In Salvendy, G., & Smith, M. (Eds.), *Human-computer interaction: Applications and case studies* (pp. 699–704). Amsterdam: Elsevier.

Baron, S., Spiliopoulou, M., & Günther, O. (2003). *Efficient monitoring of patterns in data mining environments. Advances in Databases and Information Systems* (pp. 253–265). Berlin, Heidelberg: Springer.

Bartle, R. (1999). *Early MUD History.* Retrieved February 28, 2009 from http://www.mud.co.uk/richard/mudhist.htm

Bashshur, R. L., Reardon, T. G., & Shannon, G. W. (2000). Telemedicine: A New Health Care Delivery System. *Annual Review of Public Health, 21,* 613–637. doi:10.1146/annurev.publhealth.21.1.613

Bates, D. W., Cohen, M., Leape, L. L., Overhage, J. M., Shabot, M. M., & Sheridan, T. (2001). Reducing the frequency of errors in medicine using information technology. *Journal of the American Medical Informatics Association, 8*(4), 299–308.

Bates, D. W., Teich, J. M., Lee, J., Seger, D., & Kuperman, G. J., Ma'Luf, N., Boyle, D., Leape, L. (1999). The impact of computerized physician order entry on medication error prevention. *Journal of the American Medical Informatics Association, 6*(4), 313–321.

Batet, M., Gibert, K., & Valls, A. (2007). The Data Abstraction Layer as Knowledge Provider for a Medical Multi-Agent System. In Riaño, D., & Campana, F. (Eds.), *Proc. of the From Knowledge to Global Care AIME 2007 Workshop K4CARE 2007* (pp. 87–100). Amsterdam, The Netherlands.

Batet, M., Gibert, K., & Valls, A. (2008). Tailoring of the Actor Profile Ontology in the K4Care Project. In D. Riaño (Ed.), *Proc. of the ECAI 2008 Workshop Knowledge Management for Health Care Procedures, K4HelP 2008* (pp. 104-122). Patras, Greece.

Battle, R., & Benson, E. (2008). Bridging the semantic Web and Web 2.0 with Representational State Transfer (REST). *Web Semantics: Science. Services and Agents on the World Wide Web, 6*(1), 61–69. doi:10.1016/j.websem.2007.11.002

Bauer, K.A. (2002). Using the Internet to Empower Patients and to Develop Partnerships with Clinicians. *World Hospital Health Services, 38*(2), 2-10 9.

Bazzocchi, M., Mazzarella, F., Del Frate, C., Girometti, F., & Zuiani, C. (2007). CAD systems for mammography: a real opportunity? A review of the literature. *La Radiologia Medica, 112*(3), 329–353. doi:10.1007/s11547-007-0145-5

Beach, R. D., Kuster, F. V., & Moussy, F. (1999). Subminiature implantable potentiostat and modified commercial telemetry device for remote glucose monitoring. *Instrumentation and measurement. IEEE Transactions on, 48*(6), 1239–1245.

Beardwood, J. P., & Kerr, J. A. (2005). Coming soon to a health sector near you: an advance look at the new Ontario Personal Health Information Protection Act (PHIPA): part II. *Healthcare Quarterly (Toronto, Ont.), 8*(1), 76–83.

Beck, A. T., Ward, C. H., Mendelson, M., Mock, J., & Erbaugh, J. (1961). An inventory for measuring depression. *Archives of General Psychiatry, 4*, 561–571.

Becker, S. A. (2004). A study of web usability for older adults seeking online health resources. [TOCHI]. *ACM Transactions on Computer-Human Interaction, 11*(4), 387–406. doi:10.1145/1035575.1035578

Beckwith, R. (2003). Designing for Ubiquity: The Perception of Privacy. *IEEE Pervasive Computing / IEEE Computer Society [and] IEEE Communications Society, 2*(2), 40–46. doi:10.1109/MPRV.2003.1203752

Beer, D., & Burrows, R. (2007). Sociology and, of and in Web 2.0: Some Initial Considerations. *Sociological Research Online, 12*(5). Retrieved March 6, 2009, from http://www.socresonline.org.uk/12/5/17.html

Belanger, Y. (2005). *Duke University iPod first year experience final evaluation report.* Durham, NC: Duke University. Retrieved November 14, 2008, from http://www.duke.edu/ddi/ipodfye.html

Bell, M. (2007, August). *By the Numbers: Quantitative Research Methods in Second Life.* Paper presented at the meeting of the Second Life Educator's Communities Conference, Chicago, IL.

Bellamy, M., & Connelly, C. (2009). *NHS Connecting for Health.* Retrieved 11/02/09, from http://www.connectingforhealth.nhs.uk/.

Bellifemine, F., Caire, G., & Greenwood, D. (2007). *Developing multi-agent systems with JADE.* Chichester, England: John Wiley and Sons. doi:10.1002/9780470058411

Bennett, K., Kabir, Z., Barry, M., Tilson, L., Fidan, D., & Shelley, E. (2008). *Cost-Effectiveness of Treatments Reducing Coronary Heart Disease Mortality in Ireland, 2000 to 2010.* Value.Health.

Bente, G., Rüggenberg, S., & Krämer, N. C. (2004). *Social presence and interpersonal trust in avatar-based, collaborative net-communications.* Paper presented at the 7th Annual International Workshop Presence 2004, Valencia.

Bente, G., Rüggenberg, S., & Krämer, N. C. (2005). *Virtual encounters. Creating social presence in net-based collaborations.* Paper presented at the 8th International Workshop on Presence.

Berenguer, V. J., Ruiz, D., & Soriano, A. (2008). *Application of Hidden Markov Models to Melanoma Diagnosis.* Paper presented at the International Symposium on Distributed Computing and Artificial Intelligence (DCAI 2008).

Berg, M. (1999). Patient care information systems and health care work: A sociotechnical approach. *International Journal of Medical Informatics, 55*(2), 87–101. doi:10.1016/S1386-5056(99)00011-8

Berler, A., Pavlopoulos, S., & Koutsouris, D. (2004). Design of an interoperability framework in a regional healthcare system. *Conference Proceedings. Annual International Conference of the IEEE Engineering in Medicine and Biology Society. IEEE Engineering in Medicine and Biology Society. Conference, 4*, 3093–3096.

Berliner, D., & Calfee, R. (Eds.). (1996). *Handbook of educational psychology.* New York: Macmillan.

Berners-Lee, T. (1997). *Axioms of Web Architecture: Metadata.* Retrieved June 5, 2009, from http://www.w3.org/DesignIssues/Metadata

Berners-Lee, T. (1998). *Semantic Web Road Map.* Retrieved June 5, 2009, from http://www.w3.org/DesignIssues/Semantic

Berners-Lee, T., Hendler, J., & Lassila, O. (2001). The semantic web. *Scientific American, 184*(5), 34–43. doi:10.1038/scientificamerican0501-34

Beth, D. S. (2008). Folksonomy and Health Information Access: How can Social Bookmarking Assist Seekers of Online Medical Information? *Journal of Hospital Librarianship*, *8*(1), 119–126. doi:10.1080/15323260801943570

Betts, G. H. (1909). *The distribution and function of mental imagery*. New York: Teachers College.

Bhanu, B., Peng, J., & Qing, S. (1998). Learning feature relevance and similarity metrics in image database. *IEEE Workshop Proceedings on Content-Based Access of Image and Video Libraries*, 14-18.

Bicer, V., Laleci, G. B., Dogac, A., & Kabak, Y. (2005, September). Artemis Message Exchange Framework: Semantic Interoperability of Exchanged Messages in the Healthcare Domain. *SIGMOD Record*, *34*(3), 71–76. doi:10.1145/1084805.1084819

Biocca, F. (1995). *Communication in the Age of Virtual Reality*. Lawrence Erlbaum Associates.

Biocca, F., Harms, C., & Burgoon, J. (2003). Toward a More Robust Theory and Measure of Social Presence: Review and Suggested Criteria. *Presence (Cambridge, Mass.)*, *12*(5), 456–480. doi:10.1162/105474603322761270

Bird, K. T. (1971). Telemedicine; a new health information exchange system. In *Annual Report no. 5*. Washingon: Veterans administration.

BIRN. (n.d.). http://www.nbirn.net/

Blechner, B., & Butera, A. (2002). Health Insurance Portability and Accountability Act of 1996 (HIPAA): a provider's overview of new privacy regulations. *Connecticut Medicine*, *66*(2), 91–95.

Blobel, B. G., Engel, K., & Pharow, P. (2006). Semantic interoperability--HL7 Version 3 compared to advanced architecture standards. *Methods of Information in Medicine*, *45*, 343–353.

Bloom, B. S. (2002). Crossing the Quality Chasm: A New Health System for the 21st Century. *JAMA: The Journal of the American Medical Association*, *287*, 646–64a. doi:10.1001/jama.287.5.646-a

Bock, B. C., Graham, A. L., Whiteley, J. A., & Stoddard, J. L. (2008). A review of web-assisted tobacco interventions (WATIs). *Journal of Medical Internet Research*, *10*, e39. doi:10.2196/jmir.989

Bodenheimer, T. (2005). High and Rising Health Care Costs. Part 1: Seeking an Explanation. *Annals of Internal Medicine*, *142*, 847–854.

Bodenheimer, T. (2005). High and Rising Health Care Costs. Part 2: Technologic Innovation. *Annals of Internal Medicine*, *142*, 932–937.

Bodenheimer, T. (2005). High and Rising Health Care Costs. Part 3: The Role of Health Care Providers. *Annals of Internal Medicine*, *142*, 996–1002.

Boehm, B. W. (1976). Software engineering. *IEEE Transactions on Computers*, •••, C-25.

Bojarczuk, C. C., Lopes, H. S., & Freitas, A. A. (2000). Genetic programming for knowledge discovery in chest pain diagnosis. *IEEE Engineering in Medicine and Biology Magazine*, *19*(4), 38–44. doi:10.1109/51.853480

Bojars, U., Breslin, J. G., Finn, A., & Decker, S. (2008). Using the Semantic Web for linking and reusing data across Web 2.0 communities. *Web Semantics: Science. Services and Agents on the World Wide Web*, *6*(1), 21–28. doi:10.1016/j.websem.2007.11.010

Bonetti, D., Eccles, M., Johnston, M., Steen, N., Grimshaw, J., & Baker, R. (2005). Guiding the design and selection of interventions to influence the implementation of evidence-based practice: an experimental simulation of a complex intervention trial. *Social Science & Medicine*, *60*(9), 2135–2147. doi:10.1016/j.socscimed.2004.08.072

Borg, I., & Groenen, P. J. F. (1997). *Modern multidimensional scaling: theory and applications*. New York: Springer.

Borycki, E. M., & Kushniruk, A. W. (2006). Identifying and preventing technology-induced error using simulations: Application of usability engineering techniques. *Healthcare Quarterly (Toronto, Ont.)*, *8*, 99–105.

Borycki, E. M., & Kushniruk, A. W. (2008). Where do technology induced errors come from? Towards a model for conceptualizing and diagnosing errors caused by technology. In Kushniruk, A. W., & Borycki, E. M. (Eds.), *Human and Social Aspects of Health Information Systems* (pp. 148–166). Hershey, PA: IGI Global.

Borycki, E. M., & Lemieux-Charles, L. (2008). Does a hybrid electronic-paper environment impact on health professional information seeking. *Studies in Health Technology and Informatics*, *136*, 505–510.

Borycki, E. M., Kushniruk, A. W., Kuwata, S., & Kannry, J. (2006). Use of simulation in the study of clinician workflow. *AMIA Annual Symposium Proceedings* (pp. 61-5).

Borycki, E. M., Kushniruk, A. W., Kuwata, S., & Watanabe, H. (2008). Using low-cost simulation approaches for assessing the impact of a medication administration system on workflow. *Studies in Health Technology and Informatics, 136*, 567–572.

Borycki, E. M., Kushniruk, A. W., Kuwata, S., & Watanabe, H. (2009). Simulations to assess medication administration systems. In Staudinger, B., Hob, V., & Ostermann, H. (Eds.), *Nursing and Clinical Informatics* (pp. 144–159). Hershey, PA: IGI Global.

Borycki, E. M., Lemieux-Charles, L., Nagle, L., & Eysenbach, G. (2009). Evaluating the impact of hybrid electronic-paper environments upon novice nurse information seeking. *Methods of Information in Medicine, 2*, 1–7.

Boulos, M. N. K. (2004). A first look at HealthCyberMap medical semantic subject search engine. *Technology and Health Care, 12*(1), 33.

Boulos, M. N. K., & Burden, D. (2007). Web GIS in practice V: 3-D interactive and real-time mapping in Second Life. *International Journal of Health Geographics, 27*(6), 51. doi:10.1186/1476-072X-6-51

Boulos, M. N. K., & Wheeler, S. (2007). The emerging Web 2.0 social software: an enabling suite of sociable technologies in health and health care education. *Health Information and Libraries Journal, 24*, 2–23. doi:10.1111/j.1471-1842.2007.00701.x

Boulos, M. N. K., Hetherington, L., & Wheeler, S. (2007). Second Life: and overview of the potential of 3-D virtual worlds in medical and health education. *Health Information and Libraries Journal, 24*(4), 233–245. doi:10.1111/j.1471-1842.2007.00733.x

Boulos, M. N., Marimba, I., & Wheeler, S. (2006). Wikis, blogs and podcasts: a new generation of Web-based tools for virtual collaborative clinical practice and education. *BMC Medical Education, 6*, 41–49. doi:10.1186/1472-6920-6-41

Boulos, M. N., Roudsari, A. V., & Carson, E. R. (2002). Towards a semantic medical Web: HealthCyberMap's tool for building an RDF metadata base of health information resources based on the Qualified Dublin Core Metadata Set. *Medical Science Monitor, 8*(7), MT124–MT136.

Bowers, K. W., Ragas, M. W., & Neely, J. C. (2009). Assessing the Value of Virtual Worlds for Post- Secondary Instructors: A Survey of Innovators, Early Adopters and the Early Majority in Second Life. *Intl. Journal of Humanities and Social Sciences, 3*(1), 40–51.

BPEL. (2007). *Business Process Execution Language for Web Services*. Retrieved April 22, 2009, from, http://www.ibm.com/developerworks/library/specification/ws-bpel/

BPMN. (2009). *Business Process Modeling Notation (BPMN)*. Retrieved April 22, 2009, from http://www.bpmn.org/

Branko, C., Lovell, N., & Basilakis, J. (2003). Using information technology to improve the management of chronic disease. *The Medical Journal of Australia, 179*(5), 242–246.

Bratsas, C., Bamidis, P. D., Kaimakamis, E., & Maglaveras, N. (2008). Usage of Semantic Web Technologies (Web-3.0) Aiming to Facilitate the Utilisation of Computerized Algorithmic Medicine in Clinical Practice. Published as Multimedia Appendix in G. Eysenbach (Ed.), Medicine 2.0: Social Networking, Collaboration, Participation, Apomediation, and Openness. *J Med Internet Res, 10*(3), e22. Retrieved from http://www.jmir.org/2008/3/e22/ doi:10.2196/jmir.pp1038-39

Breiman, L., Friedman, J. H., Olshen, R. A., & Stone, C. J. (1984). *Classification and Regression Trees*. Belmont, CA: Wadsworth.

Brendel, R., & Krawczyk, H. (2008). *Detection of Roles of Actors in Social Networks Using the Properties of Actors' Neighborhood Structure*. Paper presented at the Dependability of Computer Systems, 2008. DepCos-RELCOMEX '08. Third International Conference on.

Brennan, P. (1992). Computer Networks Promote Caregiving Collaboration: the ComputerLink Project. *Procedings Annual Symposium Computer Application Medical Care* (pp. 156-160). Baltimore: American Medical Informatics Association.

Breton, V. (2005). *From Grid to Healthgrid: Prospects and Requirements*. Paper presented at the Healthgrid 2005. caBIG. (n.d.). https://cabig.nci.nih.gov/

Brewlow, L. A., & Aha, D. W. (1997). Simplifying decision trees: a survey. *The Knowledge Engineering Review, 12*(1), 1–40. doi:10.1017/S0269888997000015

Brickley D., & Guha, R.V. (2004, February). *RDF Vocabulary Description Language 1.0: RDF Schema*. W3C Recommendation.

Brodie, M., Flournoy, R., Altman, D., Blendon, R., Benson, J., & Rosenbaum, M. (2000). Health information, the Internet, and the digital divide. *Health Affairs, 19*(6), 255–265. doi:10.1377/hlthaff.19.6.255

Brown, B., Chalmers, M., Bell, M., Hall, I. M. M., & Rudman, P. (2005). *Sharing the square: collaborative leisure in the city streets*. Paper presented at the 9th European Conference on Computer-Supported Cooperative Work(ECSCW'05).

Brown, J. S., & Adler, R. P. (2008). Minds on Fire: Open Education, the Long Tail, and Learning 2.0. *EDUCAUSE Review, 43*(1), 16–32.

Brown, S. H., Elkin, P. L., Rosenbloom, S. T., Husser, C., Bauer, B. A., & Lincoln, M. J. (2004). VA National Drug File Reference Terminology: A Cross-Institutional Content Coverage Study. *Medinfo, 2004*, 477–481.

Brox, G. A. (2005). MPEG-21 as an access control tool for the National Health Service Care Records Service. *Journal of Telemedicine and Telecare, 11*, 23–25. doi:10.1258/1357633054461868

Brunett, G., & Buerkle, H. (2006). Information Exchange in Virtual Communities: A Comparative Study. *Journal of Computer-Mediated Communication, 9*(2).

Burstein, M., Bussler, C., Finin, T., Huhns, M. N., Paolucci, M., & Sheth, A. P. (2005). A semantic Web services architecture. *Internet Computing, IEEE, 9*(5), 72. doi:10.1109/MIC.2005.96

Bustos, B., Keim, D., Saupe, D., & Schreck, T. (2007). Content-based 3D object retrieval. *IEEE Computer Graphics and Applications, 27*(4), 22–27. doi:10.1109/MCG.2007.80

Cabrera, M., Burgelman, J.C., Boden, M., da Costa, O., & Rodriguez, C. (2004*). eHealth in 2010: Realizing a Knowledge-based Approach to Healthcare in the EU – Challenges for the Ambient Care System*. (Report on eHealth related activities by IPTS). European Commission, Directorate-General, Joint Research Centre.

Cafazzo, J. A. K.J, L., Easty, A., Rossos, P. G., & Chan, C. T. (2008). *Bridging the Self-Care Deficit Gap: Remote Patient Monitoring and the Hospital-at-Home*. Paper presented at the eHealth 2008.

Cahill, C., Canales, C., Le Van Gong, H., Madsen, P., Maler, E., & Whitehead, G. (2008). Liberty Alliance Web Services Framework: A Technical Overview. Liberty Alliance Project, New Jersey. Retrieved May 1, 2009, from http://www.projectliberty.org/liberty/resource_center/papers

Cai, W., Feng, D. D., & Fulton, R. (2000). Content-based retrieval of dynamic PET functional images. *IEEE Transactions on Information Technology in Biomedicine, 4*(2), 152–158. doi:10.1109/4233.845208

Caldwell, L., Davies, S., Stewart, F., Thain, A., & Wales, A. (2008). Scottish toolkit for knowledge management. *Health Information and Libraries Journal, 25*(2), 125–134. doi:10.1111/j.1471-1842.2007.00747.x

Camara, E. (1993). Virtual reality: applications in medicine and psychiatry. *Hawaii Medical Journal, 52*(12), 332–333.

Camarinha-Matos, L., & Afsarmanesh, H. (2001). Virtual Communities and Elderly Support. In *Advances in Automation, Multimedia and Video Systems, and Modern Computer Science* (pp. 279–284). WSES.

Campana, F., Moreno, A., Riaño, D., & Varga, L. (2008). K4Care: Knowledge-Based Homecare e-Services for an Ageing Europe. In Annicchiarico, R., Cortés, U., & Urdiales, C. (Eds.), *Agent Technology and e-Health* (pp. 95–115). Basel, Switzerland: Birkhäuser Basel. doi:10.1007/978-3-7643-8547-7_6

Campbell Collaboration. (n.d.). *What Helps? What Hurts? Based on What Evidence?* Retrieved May 15, 2009, from The Campbell Collaboration (C2): http://www.campbellcollaboration.org

Campbell, H., Hotchkiss, R., Bradshaw, N., & Porteous, M. (1998). Integrated care pathways. *BMJ (Clinical Research Ed.), 316*, 133–137.

Canada Health Infoway. (2006). *Benefits Evaluation Indicators, Technical Report*. (Version 1.0. September 2006). Retrieved March 6, 2009, from http://www2.infoway-inforoute.ca/Documents/BE%20Techical%20Report%20(EN).pdf

Canadian Cochrane Centre. (n.d.). *The Cochrane Library*. Retrieved April 30, 2009, from Canadian Cochrane Centre: www.ccnc.cochrane.org

Canadian Institute for Health Information. (2007). *Health Care in Canada*. Ottawa, Ontario: Canadian Institute for Health Information.

Canadian Public Health Association. (2008). *Health Literacy Portal*. Retrieved January 23, 2009, from Canadian Public Health Association: http://www.cpha.ca/en/portals/h-l.aspx

CapMed and Staywell Health Managment Offer PHR/Wellness Program Presentations at AHIP 2008. (2008). Retrieved March 10, 2009, from http://www.bioimaging.com/assets/pdf/press_release/2008/2008-CapMed-Staywell-Collaborate.pdf

Carter, M. (1998). From security to trust. *Health Informatics Journal, 4*(3-4), 167–173. doi:10.1177/146045829800400306

Casals, J., Gibert, K., & Valls, A. (2007). Enlarging a medical actor profile ontology with new care units. In Riaño, D. (Ed.), *Proc. of the From Knowledge to Global Care AIME 2007 Workshop K4CARE 2007* (pp. 101–116). Amsterdam, The Netherlands.

Casanueva, J. S., & Blake, E. H. (2001). *The Effects of Avatars on Co-presence in a Collaborative Virtual Environment*. South Africa: Department of Computer Science, University of Cape Towno.

Cashen, M. S., Dykes, P., & Gerber, B. (2004). eHealth technology and Internet resources: barriers for vulnerable populations. *The Journal of Cardiovascular Nursing, 19*(3), 209–214.

Cattuto, C., Benz, D., Hotho, A., & Stumme, G. (2008). Semantic Grounding of Tag Relatedness in Social Bookmarking Systems. In A.P. Sheth, S. Staab, M. Dean, M. Paolucci, D. Maynard, T. Finin, K. Thirunarayan (Eds), *International Semantic Web Conference (ISWC 2008)* (LNCS 5319, pp. 615-631). Springer Verlag.

Cauwenberghs, G., & Poggio, T. (2000). *Incremental and Decremental Support Vector Machine Learning.* Paper presented at the NIPS.

Cavoukian, A. (2004). *A Guide to the Personal Health Information Act.*

CCITT (1987), *Draft Recommendation on Message Handling Systems, X 400, Version 5,* November.

CEN 13606. (2006). HealthInformatics – Electronic Health Record communication, Part1: Reference Model. European Standard. Retrieved May 1, 2009, from http://www.chime.ucl.ac.uk/resources/CEN/EN13606-1/N06-02_prEN13606-1_20060209.pdf

Cervantes, L., Lee, Y.-S., Yang, H., Ko, S.-h., & Lee, J. (2007). Agent-Based Intelligent Decision Support for the Home Healthcare Environment (LNCS 4413, pp. 414-424).

Chan, H. P., Sahiner, B., Kam, K. L., Petrick, N., Helvie, M. A., Goodsitt, M. M., & Adler, D. D. (1998). Computerized analysis of mammographic microcalcifications in morphological and texture feature spaces. *Medical Physics, 25,* 2007–2019. doi:10.1118/1.598389

Chan, H.-P., Lam, K., Petrick, N., Helvie, M., Goodsitt, M., & Adler, D. (1998). Computerized analysis of mammographic microcalcifications in morphological and texture feature space. *Medical Physics, 25,* 2007–2019. doi:10.1118/1.598389

Charif, Y., & Sabouret, N. (2006). An Overview of Semantic Web Services Composition Approaches. *Electronic Notes in Theoretical Computer Science, 146*(1), 33. doi:10.1016/j.entcs.2005.11.005

Charles, C., Gafni, A., & Whelan, T. (1997). Shared decision-making in the medical encounter: what does it mean? (or it takes at least two to tango). *Social Science & Medicine, 44*(5), 681–692. doi:10.1016/S0277-9536(96)00221-3

Chasteen, J. E., Murphy, G., Forrey, A., & Heid, D. (2003). The Health Insurance Portability and Accountability Act: practice of dentistry in the United States: privacy and confidentiality. [Electronic Resource]. *The Journal of Contemporary Dental Practice, 4*(1), 59–70.

Chau, R., & Yeh, C. H. (2005). *Enabling a Semantic Smart WWW: A Soft Computing Framework for Automatic Ontology Development.*

Chau, R., Smith-Miles, K., & Yeh, C. (2006). *Ontology Learning from Text: A Soft Computing Paradigm. LNCS, 4234,* 295.

Chaudhry, B., Wang, J., Wu, S., Maglione, M., Mojica, W., & Roth, E. (2006). Systematic review: impact of health information technology on quality, efficiency, and costs of medical care. *Annals of Internal Medicine, 144,* 742–752.

Chen, E. S., Mendonca, E. A., McKnight, L. K., Stetson, P. S., Lei, J., & Cimino, J. J. (2004). PalmCIS: A wireless handheld application for satisfying clinician information needs. *Journal of the American Medical Informatics Association, 11*(1), 19–28. doi:10.1197/jamia.M1387

Chen, Y., Wang, J. Z., & Krovetz, R. (2005). CLUE: cluster-based retrieval of images by unsupervised learning. *IEEE Transactions on Image Processing, 14*(8), 1187–1201. doi:10.1109/TIP.2005.849770

Cheng, E. Y., & Arthur, D. (2002). *Constructing A Virtual Behavior Change Support System: A Mobile Internet Healthcare Solution For Problem Drinkers.* Paper presented at the European Conference on Information Systems.

Chess, D., Grosof, B., Harrison, C., Levine, D., Parris, C., & Tsudik, G. (1995). Itinerant Agents for Mobile Computing. *Journal IEEE Personal Communications, 2*(5).

Cheung, K.-H., Yip, K. Y., Townsend, J. P., & Scotch, M. (2008). HCLS 2.0/3.0: Health care and life sciences data mashup using Web 2.0/3.0. *Journal of Biomedical Informatics, 41*(5), 694–705. doi:10.1016/j.jbi.2008.04.001

Chhetri, M. B., Price, R., Krishnaswamy, S., & Seng, W. L. (2006). *Ontology-Based Agent Mobility Modelling.* Paper presented at the 39th Annual Hawaii International Conference on System Sciences (HICSS '06).

Chinn, S. (2002). E-health engineering economics. *International Journal of Healthcare Technology and Management, 4,* 451–455. doi:10.1504/IJHTM.2002.002423

Chorbev, I., & Mihajlov, M. (2008). Wireless Telemedicine Services as part of an Integrated System for E-Medicine. In *MELECON08, The 14th IEEE Mediterranean Electrotechnical Conference* (pp. 264-269), Ajaccio, France: IEEE

Chorbev, I., Mihajlov, D., & Jolevski, I. (2009). Web Based Medical Expert System with a Self Training Heuristic Rule Induction Algorithm. In *DBKDA 2009, The First International Conference on Advances in Databases, Knowledge, and Data Applications,* Cancun, Mexico: IEEE

Chung, E., et al. (2004). Development and Evaluation of Emerging Design Patterns for Ubiquitous Computing. *Patterns C1-C15, DIS2004.* Clarke, R. (n.d.). *Identification, Anonymity and Pseudonymity in Consumer Transactions: A Vital System Design and Public Policy Issue.* Retrieved from http://www.anu.edu.au/people/Roger.Clarke/DV/AnonPsPol.html

Ciccarese, P., Caffi, E., Boiocchi, L., Quaglini, S., & Stefanelli, M. (2004). A Guideline Management System. In M. Fieschi, E. Coiera & J. X. Li (Eds.), *Proc. of the 11th World Congress on Medical Informatics, MEDINFO 2004* (pp. 28-32). San Francisco, USA.

Cimino, J. J. (1998). Desiderata for Controlled Medical Vocabularies in the Twenty-First Century. *Methods of Information in Medicine, 37,* 394–403.

Cioffi, J., & Markham, R. (1997). Clinical decision making by midwives: Managing case complexity. *Journal of Advanced Nursing, 23,* 265–272. doi:10.1046/j.1365-2648.1997.1997025265.x

Clancy, H. (2008, May). 7 Security Questions to Ask Your SaaS Provider. *Information Security Magazine.* Retrieved January 25, 2009, from http://searchsecurity.techtarget.com/magazineFeature/0,296894,sid14_gci1313252,00.html

Clark, H. (1998). *Formal Knowledge Networks: A Study of Canadian Experiences Helping Knowledge Networks Work.* Winnipeg: International Institute for Sustainable Development.

Clark, P., & Boswell, R. (1991). Rule Induction with CN2: Some Recent Improvements. In Y. Kodratoff (Ed.), *Fifth European Conference on Machine Learning* (pp. 151-163). Berlin, Springer-Verlag.

Clark, R. A., Inglis, S. C., McAlister, F. A., Cleland, J. G., & Stewart, S. (2007). Telemonitoring or structured telephone support programmes for patients with chronic heart failure: systematic review and meta-analysis. *BMJ (Clinical Research Ed.), 334,* 942. doi:10.1136/bmj.39156.536968.55

Cleland, J. G. F. (2006). The Trans-European Network - Home-Care Management System (TEN-HMS) Study: An Investigation of the Effect of Telemedicine on Outcomes in Europe. *Disease Management & Health Outcomes, 14*(1), 23–28. doi:10.2165/00115677-200614001-00007

Cleland, J. G. F., Louis, A. A., Rigby, A. S., Janssens, U., & Balk, A. H. M. M. (2005). Noninvasive Home Telemonitoring for Patients With Heart Failure at High Risk of Recurrent Admission and Death. *Journal of the American College of Cardiology, 45*(10). doi:10.1016/j.jacc.2005.01.050

Clements, A. (2008). It's Good to Get a Second Opinion. *Human Resources, 66.* Retrieved November 9, 2008 from http://proquest.umi.com/pqdweb?did=1582613671&sid=7&Fmt=3&clientId=77774&RQT=309&VName=PQD

Coates, W. C., Ankel, F., Birnbaum, A., Kosiak, D., Broderick, K. B., & Thomas, S. (2004). The virtual advisor program: linking students to mentors via the world wide web. *Academic Emergency Medicine, 11,* 253–255. doi:10.1111/j.1553-2712.2004.tb02205.x

Cobus, L. (2009). Using blogs and wikis in a graduate public health course. *Medical Reference Services Quarterly, 28*(1), 22–32. doi:10.1080/02763860802615922

Coenen, A., Marin, H. F., Park, A., & Bakken, S. (2001). Collaborative Efforts for Representing Nursing Concepts in Computer-based Systems: International Perspectives. *Journal of the American Medical Informatics Association, 8,* 202–211.

Coffield, R. L., & DeLoss, G. E. (2008). The Rise of the Personal Health Record: Panacea or Pitfall for Health Information. *American Health Lawyers Association - Health Lawyers News, 12*(10). Retrieved May 1, 2009, from http://www.fsbwv.com/pdf/The_Rise_of_the_PHR_AHLA.pdf

Cohen, J. (1992). A power primer. *Psychological Bulletin, 112,* 155–159. doi:10.1037/0033-2909.112.1.155

Coiera, E. (2004). Four Rules for the Reinvention of Health Care. *British Medical Journal, 328,* 1197–1199. doi:10.1136/bmj.328.7449.1197

Collins, C., & Jennings, N. (2006, August). *Emerging Best Practices for Campus Builds in Second Life.* Paper presented at the meeting of the Second Life Educator's Communities Conference, San Fransisco, CA.

Collins, M. J., Hoffmeister, J., & Worrell, S. W. (2006). Computer-aided detection and diagnosis of breast cancer. *Seminars in Ultrasound, CT, and MR, 27*(4), 351–355. doi:10.1053/j.sult.2006.05.009

Collins, T. (2009). Minutes of Blair meeting which sparked £13bn NHS IT scheme. Retrieved March 7, 2009, from http://www.computerweekly.com/Articles/2009/02/11/234758/minutes-of-blair-meeting-which-sparked-13bn-nhs-it.html

Coma del Corral, M. J., Luquín, P. A., Guevara, J. C., Movilla, A. O., Torres, G. T., & Garcia, J. L. (2005). Utility of a thematic network in primary health care: a controlled interventional study in a rural area. *Human Resource for Health, 3,* 4-11. Retrieved November 9, 2008 from http://www.human-resources-health.com/content/3/1/4

Commission of the European Communities. (2004). e-Health - making health care better for European citizens: An action plan for a European e-Health Area. (COM 356). Communication from the Commission to the Council, the European Parliament, the European Economic and Social Committee and the Committee of the Regions, Brussels.

Conner, N. (2008). Google Apps: The Missing Manual. Sebastopol, CA: O'Reilly/Pogue Press.

Consolvo, S., Smith, I. E., Matthews, T., LaMarca, A., Tabert, J., & Powledge, P. (2005). *Location disclosure to social relations: why, when, & what people want to share.* Paper presented at the SIGCHI conference on Human factors in computing systems, Portland, Oregon, USA.

Cook, D. A. (2009). The failure of e-learning research to inform educational practice, and what we can do about it. *Medical Teacher, 31*(2), 158–162. doi:10.1080/01421590802691393

Cook, D., Levinson, A., Garside, S., Dupras, D., Erwin, P., & Montori, V. (2008). Internet-based Learning on the Health Professions: A Meta-analysis. *American Medical Association Journal, 300*(10), 1181–1196. doi:10.1001/jama.300.10.1181

Cornelia, M. R., Thomas, W., Marguerite, S., Gilbert, F., & Samir, M. K. (2003). Effects of a computerized system to support shared decision making in symptom management of cancer patients: Preliminary results. *Journal of the American Medical Informatics Association, 10*(6), 573. doi:10.1197/jamia.M1365

Cornoldi, C., De Beni, R., Giusberti, F., Marucci, F., Massironi, M., & G., M. (1991). The study of vividness of images. In R. H. Logie & M. Denis (Eds.), *Mental images in human cognition.* Amsterdam: North Holland.

Cortés, U., Annicchiarico, R., & Urdiales, C. (2008). Agents and Healthcare: Usability and Acceptance. In B. Basel (Ed.), Agent Technology and e-Health. Springer.

Cowan, D. F. (Ed.). (2005). *Informatics for the Clinical Laboratory. A practical guide for the pathologist.* New York: Springer. doi:10.1007/b99090

Cox, I. J., Miller, M. L., Minka, T. P., Papathomas, T. V., & Yianilos, P. N. (2000). The Bayesian image retrieval system, PicHunter: theory, implementation, and psychophysical experiments. *IEEE Transactions on Image Processing, 9*(1), 20–37. doi:10.1109/83.817596

Cresci, M., Morrell, R., & Echt, K. (2004). The Convergence of Health Promotion and the Internet. In Nelson, R., & Ball, M. (Eds.), *Consumer Informatics: Applications and Strategies in Cyber Health Care.* New York: Springer.

CRISP-DM. (2009). Cross Industry Standard Process for Data Mining. Retrieved May 1, 2009, from http://www.crisp-dm.org/Process/index.htm

Croll, P. R., & Croll, J. (2007). Investigating Risk Exposure in e-Health Systems. *International Journal of Medical Informatics, 76,* 460–465. doi:10.1016/j.ijmedinf.2006.09.013

Cronje, J. C. (2001). Metaphors and models in internet-based learning. *Computers & Education, 37*(3-4), 241–256. doi:10.1016/S0360-1315(01)00049-5

Cross, S. S., Dennis, T., & Start, R. D. (2002). Telepathology: current status and future prospects in diagnostic histopathology. *Histopathology, 41*(2), 91–109. doi:10.1046/j.1365-2559.2002.01423.x

Crosson, F. J., & Madvig, P. (2004). Does Population Management Of Chronic Disease Lead To Lower Costs Of Care? *Health Affairs, 23,* 76–78. doi:10.1377/hlthaff.23.6.76

Crounse, W. (2009, 2009/01/27). *The View on Mobile Solutions in Health.* Retrieved 11/2/09, from http://blogs.

msdn.com/healthblog/archive/2009/01/27/the-view-on-mobile-solutions-in-health.aspx.

Crowther, R., Gask, L., Ives, R., & Jakenfelds, J. (2001). A program designed to monitor the course and management of depressive illness across the primary/secondary interface. *Medinfo, 10,* 719–723.

Csikszentmihalyi, M. (1975). *Beyond Boredom and Anxiety.* San Francisco: Jossey-Bass.

Csikszentmihalyi, M. (1990). *Flow: The psychology of optimal experience.* New York: Harper Collins.

Cummings, E., & Turner, P. (2009). Patient self-management and chronic illness: evaluating outcomes and impacts of information technology. *Studies in Health Technology and Informatics, 143,* 229–234.

Curran, V. R. (2006). Tele-education. *Journal of Telemedicine and Telecare, 12,* 57–63. doi:10.1258/135763306776084400

Curry, S. J. (2007). eHealth research and healthcare delivery beyond intervention effectiveness. *American Journal of Preventive Medicine, 32*(5Suppl), S127–S130. doi:10.1016/j.amepre.2007.01.026

D'Amour, D., Ferrada-Videla, M., San Martin, R. L., & Beaulieu, M. D. (2005). The conceptual basis for interprofessional collaboration: core concepts and theoretical frameworks. *Journal of Interprofessional Care, 19*(Suppl 1), 116–131. doi:10.1080/13561820500082529

da Silva, P. P., McGuinness, D. L., & Fikes, R. (2006). A proof markup language for Semantic Web services. *Information Systems, 31*(4-5), 381. doi:10.1016/j.is.2005.02.003

Daconta, M., Obrst, L., & Smith, K. (2003). *The semantic web.* Indianapolis: John Wiley & Sons.

Dambisya, Y. A. (2007). Review of Non-financial Incentives for Health Care Worker Retention in East and Southern Africa. *Regional Network for Equity in Health in East and Southern Africa,* 1-72. Retrieved October 30, 2008 from http://www.equinetafrica.org/bibl/docs/DIS44HRdambisya.pdf

Daniel, C., Buemi, A., Ouagne, D., Mazuel, L., & Charlet, J. (2009, August). *Functional requirements of terminology services for coupling interface terminologies to reference terminologies.* Paper presented at MIE 2009: The XXII International Conference of the European Federation for Medical Informatics, Sarajevo, Bosnia and Herzegovina.

Daniel, C., Garcia-Rojo, M., Bourquard, K., Henin, D., Schrader, T., Della Mea, V., et al. (2009). Standards to Support Information Systems Integration in Anatomic Pathology. *Archives of Pathology & Laboratory Medicine, 133*(11), 1841-1849. Retrieved February 24, 2010 from http://www.archivesofpathology.org/doi/full/10.1043/1543-2165-133.11.1841

Darmoni, S. J., Leroy, J. P., Baudic, F., Douyere, M., Piot, J., & Thirion, B. (2000). CISMeF: a structured health resource guide. *Methods of Information in Medicine, 39*(1), 30–35.

Davenport, T. H., & Prusak, L. (2000). *Working Knowledge: How Organizations Manage What They Know.* Boston, MA: Harvard Business School Press.

Davies, J., Duke, A., & Sure, Y. (2003). *OntoShare: a knowledge management environment for virtual communities of practice.* Paper presented at the Proceedings of the 2nd international conference on Knowledge capture.

Davies, J., Fensel, D., & Harmelen, F. (2002). *Towards the semantic web: ontology driven knowledge management.* John Wiley & Sons.

Davis, K., Doty, M. M., Shea, K., & Stremikis, K. (2009). Health Information Technology and Physician Perceptions of Quality of Care and Satisfaction. *Health Policy (Amsterdam),* 239–246. doi:10.1016/j.healthpol.2008.10.002

Dawes, M., & Sampson, U. (2003). Knowledge management in clinical practice: a systematic review of information seeking behavior in physicians. *International Journal of Medical Informatics, 71*(1), 9–15. doi:10.1016/S1386-5056(03)00023-6

de Graaf, L. E., Gerhards, S. A., Evers, S. M., Arntz, A., Riper, H., & Severens, J. L. (2008). Clinical and cost-effectiveness of computerised cognitive behavioural therapy for depression in primary care: design of a randomised trial. *BMC Public Health, 8,* 224. doi:10.1186/1471-2458-8-224

de Keizer, N. (2008). The quality of evidence in health informatics: How did the quality of healthcare IT evaluation publications develop from 1982 to 2005? *International Journal of Medical Informatics, 77*(1), 41–49. doi:10.1016/j.ijmedinf.2006.11.009

de Keizer, N. F., Abu-Hanna, A., & Zwetsloot-Schonk, J. H. M. (2000). Understanding Terminological Systems I: Terminology and Typology. *Methods of Information in Medicine, 39,* 16–21.

De Lucia, A., Francese, R., Passero, I., & Tortora, G. (2009). Development and evaluation of a virtual campus on Second Life: The case of SecondDMI. *Computers & Education, 52*(1), 220–233. doi:10.1016/j.compedu.2008.08.001

Dean, J. C., & Ilvento, C. C. (2006). Improved cancer detection using computer-aided detection with diagnostic and screening mammography: prospective study of 104 cancers. *AJR. American Journal of Roentgenology, 187*(1), 20–28. doi:10.2214/AJR.05.0111

Dean, M., & Schreiber, G. (2004). *OWL Web Ontology Language Reference.* W3C Recommendation.

Deber, R. B., Kraetschmer, N., Urowitz, S., & Sharpe, N. (2005). Patient, consumer, client, or customer: what do people want to be called? *Health Expectations, 8*(4), 345–351. doi:10.1111/j.1369-7625.2005.00352.x

Deber, R. B., Kraetschmer, N., Urowitz, S., & Sharpe, N. (2007). Do people want to be autonomous patients? Preferred roles in treatment decision-making in several patient populations. *Health Expectations, 10*(3), 248–258. doi:10.1111/j.1369-7625.2007.00441.x

Dee, F. R., Donnelly, A., Radio, S., Leaven, T., Zaleski, M. S., & Kreiter, C. (2007). Utility of 2-D and 3-D virtual microscopy in cervical cytology education and testing. *Acta Cytologica, 51*, 523–529.

Del Bimbo, A. (1999). *Visual information retrieval.* San Francisco, CA: Morgan Kaufmann Publishers.

Demiris, G. (2005). Virtual Communities in Health Care. In B. Silverman, A. Jain, I. A. & L. Jain (Eds.), Intelligent Paradigms for Healthcare Enterprises (Vol. 184, pp. 121-137). Springer.

Demiris, G., Parker Oliver, D. R., Porock, D., & Courtney, K. L. (2004). The Missouri telehospice project: background and next steps. *Home Health Care Technology Report, 1*(4), 55–57.

Denis, A. (2002). The Internet and Health Communication. *Nurse Researcher, 9*(3), 89–91.

Dertouzos, M. (1997). *What will be* (pp. 175–189). London, UK: Judy Piatkus Ltd.

Deshpande, A., & Jadad, A. (2006). Web 2.0: Could it help move the health system into the 21st century? *Journal of Men's Health & Gender, 3*(4), 332–336. doi:10.1016/j.jmhg.2006.09.004

Dewey, J. (1944). *Democracy and Education.* New York: Free Press.

DICOM Working Group 26 Pathology (2008). *Digital Imaging and Communications in Medicine (DICOM) Supplement 122: Specimen Module and Revised Pathology SOP Classes.* Rosslyn, Virginia: DICOM Standards Committee. Retrieved February 16, 2009, from ftp://medical.nema.org/medical/dicom/final/sup122_ft2.pdf

DICOM Working Group 4. (2006). *Digital Imaging and Communications in Medicine (DICOM) Supplement 106: JPEG 2000 Interactive Protocol.* Rosslyn, Virginia: DICOM Standards Committee. Retrieved February 17, 2009, from ftp://medical.nema.org/medical/dicom/final/sup106_ft.pdf

Dieng-Kuntz, R., Minier, D., Ruzicka, M., Corby, F., Corby, O., & Alamarguy, L. (2006). Building and using a medical ontology for knowledge management and co-operative work in a health care network. *Computers in Biology and Medicine, 36*(7-8), 871–892. doi:10.1016/j.compbiomed.2005.04.015

Dieterle, E., & Clarke, J. (in press). Multi-user virtual environments for teaching and learning. In Pagani, M. (Ed.), *Encyclopedia of multimedia technology and networking* (2nd ed.). Hershey, PA: Idea Group, Inc.

Dieterle, E., & Clarke, J. (in press). Multi-user virtual environments for teaching and learning. In Pagani, M. (Ed.), *Encyclopedia of multimedia technology and networking* (2nd ed.). Hershey, PA: Idea Group, Inc.

Dietzel, G. T. (2002). Challenges of telematics and telemedicine for health care: from e-Europe 2002 to the electronic health passport. *International Journal of Computerized Dentistry, 5*(2-3), 107–114.

Dimech, M., & Beer, T. (2008). *Report of dermatopathology module results SM08-1.* Burwood, Australia: RCPA Quality Assurance Programs Pty Limited. Retrieved February 13, 2009, from http://www.rcpaqapa.netcore.com.au/notices/SM08-1_results.pdf

Dimech, M., & Davies, D. J. (2006). *Report of virtual microscopy pilot survey results 2005.* Burwood, Australia: RCPA Quality Assurance Programs Pty Limited. Retrieved February 13, 2009, from http://www.rcpaqapa.netcore.com.au/notices/VM_pilot_survey_results_VM05-1.pdf

Dolin, R. H., Alschuler, L., Boyer, S., & Beebe, C. (2000). *An update on HL7's XML-based document representation standards.* Paper presented at the AMIA Symposium.

Donnelly, K. (2008). Multilingual documentation and classification. *Studies in Health Technology and Informatics, 134*, 235–243.

Dorileo, E. A. G., Frade, M. A. C., Roselino, A. M. F., Rangayyan, R. M., & Azevedo-Marques, P. M. (2008). *Color image processing and content-based image retrieval techniques for the analysis of dermatological lesions.* Paper presented at the Engineering in Medicine and Biology Society, 2008. EMBS 2008. 30th Annual International Conference of the IEEE.

Dorsch, J. L. (2000). Information needs of rural health professionals: a review of the literature. *Bull Med Libr Assoc, 88*(4): 346-354. Retrieved November 9, 2008 from http://www.pubmedcentral.nih.gov/articlerender.fcgi?tool=pubmed&pubmedid=11055302

Dreyer, K. J. (2006). *PACS: a guide to the digital revolution* (2nd ed.). New York: Springer.

Dublin Core. (2009). The Dublin Core Metadata Initiative. Retrieved April 22, 2009, from, http://dublincore.org/

Duckett, S. (2009). *News and Views from the President/CEO.* Retrieved May 20, 2009, from Alberta Health Services Internal Blog: http://iblogs.albertahealthservices.ca/ceo/

Duda, R. O., & Hart, P. E. (1973). *Pattern classification and scene analysis.* New York: Wiley.

Duffy, M., Wimbush, E., Reece, J., & Eadie, D. (2003). Net profits? Web site development and health improvement. *Health Education, 103*(5), 278–285. doi:10.1108/09654280310499055

Dumontier, M., & Villanueva-Rosales, N. (2009). Towards pharmacogenomics knowledge discovery with the semantic web. *Briefings in Bioinformatics, 10*(2), 153–163. doi:10.1093/bib/bbn056

Dunbrack, L. A. (2007, April). The PHR maturity model: the road to interoperability. *Health Industry Insights.* #HI206237.

Dussault, G., & Franceschini, M. C. (2006). Not Enough There, Too Many Here: Understanding Geographical Imbalances in the Distribution of the Health Workforce. *Human Resources for Health*, 4, 12-28. Retrieved November 18, 2008 from http://www.human-resources-health.com/content/4/1/12

Dutta, M., Bodie, G., & Basu, A. (2008). Health Disparity and the Racial Divide among the Nation's Youth: Internet as a Site for Change? In Everett, A. (Ed.), *Learning Race and Ethnicity: Youth and Digital Media. The John D. and Catherine T. MacArthur. Foundation Series on Digital Media and Learning* (pp. 175–198). Cambridge, MA: The MIT Press.

Duval, E., & Hodgins, W. (2009). International LOM Survey: Report. Retrieved April 22, 2009, from, http://dlist.sir.arizona.edu/403/

Dy, J. G., Brodley, C. E., Kak, A., Broderick, L. S., & Aisen, A. M. (2003). Unsupervised Feature Selection Applied to Content-based Retrieval of Lung Images. *IEEE Transactions on Pattern Analysis and Machine Intelligence, 25*(3), 373–378. doi:10.1109/TPAMI.2003.1182100

Ebner, M., Holzinger, A., & Maurer, H. (2007). Web 2.0 Technology: Future Interfaces for Technology Enhanced Learning. In C. Stephanidis (Ed.), Universal Access in HCI, Part III, HCII 2007 (LNCS 4556, pp. 559-568). Berlin, Germany: Springer-Verlag.

Ebner, W., Leimeister, J. M., & Krcmar, H. (2004). *Trust in Virtual Healthcare Communities: Design and Implementation of Trust-Enabling Functionalities.* Paper presented at the Proceedings of the Proceedings of the 37th Annual Hawaii International Conference on System Sciences (HICSS'04) - Track 7 - Volume 7.

Echarte, F., & Astrain, J. J. Córdoba, & A., Villadangos, J. (2008). Pattern Matching Techniques to Identify Syntactic Variations of Tags in Folksonomies. In M.D. Lytras (Ed.), *First World Summit on the Knowledge Society: Emerging Technologies and Information Systems for the Knowledge Society* (WSKS 2008) (LNAI 5288, pp. 557–564). Springer Verlag.

Echarte, F., Astrain, J. J., Córdoba, A., & Villadangos, J. (2007). Ontology of Folksonomy: A New Modeling Method. In S. Handschuh, N. Collier, T. Groza, R. Dieng-Kuntz, M. Sintek, A. de Waard (Eds.), Semantic Authoring, Annotation and Knowledge Markup Workshop (SAAKM2007), CEUR-WS Vol. 289. SITE Central Europe: RWTH Aachen University.

Echarte, F., Astrain, J. J., Córdoba, A., & Villadangos, J. (2008). Self-adaptation of Ontologies to Folksonomies in Semantic Web. In *Proceedings of World Academy of Science* (*Vol. 33*). Engineering and Technology.

Echarte, F., Astrain, J. J., Córdoba, A., & Villadangos, J. (2009). Improving Folksonomies Quality by Syntactic Tag Variations Grouping. In S.Y. Shin, S. Ossowski (Eds.), *24th Annual ACM Symposium on Applied Computing* (pp. 1226-1230). New York: ACM.

Economist. (2009, April 16). A Special Report on Health Care and Technology. *The Economist.* London, Britain, UK: The Economist.

Eder, J., & Koncilia, C. (2002). *Incorporating ICD-9 and ICD-10 Data in a Warehouse.* Paper presented at the 15th IEEE Symposium on Computer-Based Medical Systems (CBMS'02).

Efron, B., & Tibshirani, R. (1993). *An introduction to the bootstrap*. New York: Chapman & Hall.

Ehlers, U. (2007). The new pathway for e-learning: From distribution to collaboration and competence in e-learning. *Association for the Advancement of Computing in Education Journal, 16*(2), 187–20.

El Emam, K., Jabbouri, S., Sams, S., Drouet, Y., & Power, M. (2006). Evaluating common de-identification heuristics for personal health information. *Journal of Medical Internet Research, 8*(4), e28. doi:10.2196/jmir.8.4.e28

El Maliki, T., & Seigneur, J. M. (2007). *A Survey of User-centric Identity Management Technologies.* Paper presented at IEEE SECUREWARE 2007, Int. Conf. on Emerging Security Information, Systems and Technologies.

El Morr, C. (2007). *Mobile Virtual Communities in Healthcare: Managed Self Care on the move.* Paper presented at the International Association of Science and Technology for Development (IASTED) - Telehealth (2007), Montreal, Canada.

El Morr, C., Subercaze, J., Maret, P., & Rioux, M. (2008). *A Virtual Knowledge Community for Human Rights Monitoring for People with Disabilities.* Paper presented at the IADIS International Conference on Web Based Communities.

El Naqa, I. (2002). Content-based image retrieval by similarity learning for digital mammography illinois Institute of Technology, Chicago, IL.

El Naqa, I., Wernick, M., Yang, Y., & Galatsanos, N. (2000). *Image retrieval based on similarity learning.* Paper presented at the *I*EEE Inter. Conf. on Image Processing, Vancouver, CA.

El Naqa, I., Wernick, M., Yang, Y., & Galatsanos, N. (2002). *Content-based image retrieval for digital mammography.* Paper presented at the IEEE Inter. Conf. on Image Processing, Rochester, NY.

El Naqa, I., Yang, Y., Galatsanos, N. P., & Wernick, M. N. (2003). *Relevance feedback based on incremental learning for mammogram retrieval.* Paper presented at the 2003 International Conference on Image Processing, 2003. ICIP 2003.

El Naqa, I., Yang, Y., Galatsanos, N. P., & Wernick, M. N. (2004). *Mammogram retrieval based on incremental learning.* Paper presented at the IEEE International Symposium on Biomedical Imaging: Nano to Macro, 2004.

El Naqa, I., Yang, Y., Galatsanos, N. P., Nishikawa, R. M., & Wernick, M. N. (2004). A similarity learning approach to content-based image retrieval: application to digital mammography. *IEEE Transactions on Medical Imaging, 23*(10), 1233–1244. doi:10.1109/TMI.2004.834601

Eldon, E. (2009, April). *Single sign-on service OpenID getting more usage.* Retrieved January 25, 2009, from http://venturebeat.com/2009/04/14/single-sign-on-service-openid-getting-more-usage/

Elmes, D. G., Kantowicz, B. H., & Roediger, H. L. (1981). *Research methods in psychology* (2nd ed.). St. Paul: West Publishing Company.

Elmore, J. G., Barton, M. B., Moceri, V. M., Polk, S., Arena, P. J., & Fletcher, S. W. (1998). Ten-Year Risk of False Positive Screening Mammograms and Clinical Breast Examinations. *The New England Journal of Medicine, 338*(16), 1089–1096. doi:10.1056/NEJM199804163381601

Elson, S. (2009). Regionalization of Health Care from a Political and Structural Perspective. *Healthcare Management Forum*, 6–11.

Ely, J. W., Burch, R. J., & Vinson, D. C. (1992). The information needs of family physicians: case-specific clinical questions. *The Journal of Family Practice, 35*(3), 265–269.

Ely, J. W., Osheroff, J. A., Ebell, M. H., Bergus, G. R., Levy, B. T., Chambliss, M. L., & Evans, E. R. (1999). Analysis of questions asked by family doctors regarding patient care. *BMJ (Clinical Research Ed.), 319*, 358–361.

Emanuel, E. (1975). A half-life of 5 years. *Canadian Medical Association Journal, 112*(5), 572.

Endsley, S., Kibbe, D. C., Linares, A., & Coloafi, K. (2006). An introduction to personal health records. *Family Practice Management, 13*(5), 57–62.

Eng, T. (2006). Healia, a search engine for finding high quality and personalized health information. *Journal of Men's Health & Gender, 3*(4), 418–419. doi:10.1016/j.jmhg.2006.09.005

Eng, T. R. (2001). *The eHealth Landscape: A Terrain Map of Emerging Information and Communication Technologies in Health and Health Care.* Princeton, NJ: The Robert Wood Johnson Foundation.

Ericsson, KA, Simon, HA. *Protocol analysis: Verbal reports as data* (2nd ed.). Cambridge, Massachusetts: MIT Press.

Eslami, S., Abu-Hanna, A., & deKeizer, N. F. (2007). Evaluation of outpatient computerized physician medication order entry systems: A systematic review. *Journal of the American Medical Informatics Association, 14*(4), 400–406. doi:10.1197/jamia.M2238

Eslami, S., deKeizer, N. F., & Abu-Hanna, A. (2008). The impact of computerized physician medication order entry in hospitalized patients: A systematic review. *International Journal of Medical Informatics, 77,* 365–376. doi:10.1016/j.ijmedinf.2007.10.001

Esquivel, A., Meric-Bernstam, F., & Bernstam, E.V. (2006). Accuracy and self correction of information received from an internet breast cancer list: content analysis. *British Medical Journal, 22;332*(7547), 939-942.

European commission. DG INFSO (2008). *Sources of financing and policy recommendations to Member States and the European Commission on boosting eHealth investment.* Brussels. Retrieved March 7, 2009, from http://www.financing-eHealth.eu/downloads/documents/FeH_D5_3_final_study_report.pdf

European Commission. i2010 (2009). *Benchmarking.* Brussels. Retrieved March 7, 2009, from http://ec.europa.eu/information_society/eeurope/i2010/benchmarking/index_en.htm

European Council. (2008). Presidency Conclusions of the Brussels European Council, 13/14 March 2008. Retrieved January 28, 2009, from http://www.consilium.europa.eu/ueDocs/cms_Data/docs/pressData/en/ec/99410.pdf

Evfimievski, A., Srikant, R., Agrawal, R., & Gehrke, J. (2002, July). Privacy preserving mining of association rules. In *Proceedings of The Eighth ACM SIGKDD International Conference on Knowledge Discovery and Data Mining* (pp. 217–228). Edmonton, Alberta, Canada.

Eysenbach, G. (2001). What is e-health? *Journal of Medical Internet Research, 3*(2), e20. Retrieved March 6, 2009, from http://www.jmir.org/2001/2/e20/

Eysenbach, G. (2005). The law of attrition. *Journal of Medical Internet Research, 7,* e11. doi:10.2196/jmir.7.1.e11

Eysenbach, G. (2007). From intermediation to disintermediation and apomediation: new models for consumers to access and assess the credibility of health information in the age of Web2.0. *Studies in Health Technology and Informatics, 129*(Pt 1), 162–166.

Eysenbach, G. (2008). Credibility of health information and digital media: new perspectives and implications for youth. In Metzger, M. J., & Flanagin, A. J. (Eds.), *Digital Media, Youth, and Credibility. The John D and Catherine T MacArthur Foundation Series on Digital Media and Learning.* Cambridge, MA: MIT Press.

Eysenbach, G. (2008). Medicine 2.0: Social Networking, Collaboration, Participation, Apomediation, and Openness. *Journal of Medical Internet Research, 10*(3), 1–14. doi:10.2196/jmir.1030

Eysenbach, G. (2009). Infodemiology and infoveillance: framework for an emerging set of public health informatics methods to analyze search, communication and publication behavior on the Internet. *Journal of Medical Internet Research, 11,* e11. doi:10.2196/jmir.1157

Eysenbach, G., & Jadad, A. (2001, June). Evidence-based Patient Choice and Consumer Health Informatics in the Internet Age. *Journal of Medical Internet Research,* 1–14.

Eysenbach, G., Kohler, C., Yihune, G., Lampe, K., Cross, P., & Brickley, D. (2001). A metadata vocabulary for self- and third-party labeling of health web-sites: Health Information Disclosure, Description and Evaluation Language (HIDDEL). In *Proc AMIA Symp* (pp. 169-173).

Eysenbach, G., Powell, J., Englesakis, M., Rizo, C., & Stern, A. (2004). Health related virtual communities and electronic support groups: systematic review of the effects of online peer to peer interactions. *BMJ (Clinical Research Ed.), 328*(7449), 1166. doi:10.1136/bmj.328.7449.1166

Eysenbach, G., Powell, J., Kuss, O., & Sa, E. (2002). Empirical Studies Assessing the Quality of Health Information for Consumers on the World Wide Web: a Systematic Review. *Journal of the American Medical Association,* 2691–2700. doi:10.1001/jama.287.20.2691

Fabri, M., Moore, D. J., & Hobbs, D. J. (1999). The Emotional Avatar: Nonverbal Communication between Inhabitants of Collaborative Virtual Environments. In Braffort (Ed.), Gesture-Based Communication in Human-Computer Interaction (LNCS 1739, pp. 245-248).

Facebook. (2008). Facebook Expands Power of Platform Across the Web and Around the World. Retrieved March 7, 2009, from http://www.facebook.com/press/releases.php?p=48242

Facey, K., Topfer, L., & Chan, L. (2009). *Glossary.* Retrieved February 14, 2009, from INAHTA Health Technology Assessment Glossary: http://www.inahta.org/GO-DIRECT-TO/Members/

Fayyad, U. M., Piatetsky-Shapiro, G., & Smyth, P. (1996). From data mining to knowledge discovery: an overview.

In Fayyad, U. M., Piatetsky-Shapiro, G., Smyth, P., & Uthurusamy, R. (Eds.), *Advances in Knowledge Discovery & Data Mining* (pp. 1–34). Menlo Park, CA, US: American Association for Artificial Intelligence.

Fellenstein, G. (2005). *On Demand Computing: Technologies and Strategies.* IBM Press.

Fenn, J. (2009, 2009/02/04). *Hype cycle - Wikipedia, the free encyclopedia.* Retrieved 11/02/09, from http://en.wikipedia.org/w/index.php?title=Hype_cycle&oldid=268502613.

Fensel, D., van Harmelen, F., Horrocks, I., McGuinness, D. L., & Patel-Schneider, P. F. (2001). OIL: an ontology infrastructure for the Semantic Web. *Intelligent Systems, IEEE, 16*(2), 38. doi:10.1109/5254.920598

Fenton, J. J., Taplin, S. H., Carney, P. A., Abraham, L., Sickles, E. A., & D'Orsi, C. (2007). Influence of computer-aided detection on performance of screening mammography. *The New England Journal of Medicine, 356*(14), 1399–1409. doi:10.1056/NEJMoa066099

Ferber, J. (1999). *Multi-Agent Systems. An Introduction to Distributed Artificial Intelligence.* Addison-Wesley.

Ferguson, T. (2007). ePatients white paper. www.e-patients.net. Retrieved March 6, 2009, from http://www.e-patients.net/e-Patients_White_Paper.pdf on 22/1/08

Ferreira, L., Berstis, V., Armstrong, J., Kendzierski, M., Neukoetter, A., & Takagi, M. (2003). *Introduction to Grid Computing with Globus.* IBM.

Ferreira, R., Moon, B., Humphries, J., Sussman, A., Saltz, J., Miller, R., & Demarzo, A. (1997). The Virtual Microscope. *Proceedings of the AMIA Annual Fall Symposium,* 449-453. Retrieved February 13, 2009, from http://www.pubmedcentral.nih.gov/articlerender.fcgi?tool=pubmed&pubmedid=9357666

Field, M. J., & Grigsby, J. (2002). Telemedicine and remote patient monitoring. *Journal of the American Medical Association, 288*(4), 423–425. doi:10.1001/jama.288.4.423

Fildes, J. (2007). Virtual treatment for US troops. Retrieved from http://news.bbc.co.uk/2/hi/science/nature/6375097.stm

Finegold, A. R. D., & Cooke, L. (2006). Exploring the Attitudes, Experiences and Dynamics of Interaction in Online Groups. *The Internet and Higher Education, 9,* 201–215. doi:10.1016/j.iheduc.2006.06.003

Finin, T., & Labrou, Y. (1997). KQML as an agent communication language. In Bradshaw, J. M. (Ed.), *Software Agents* (pp. 291–316). MIT Press.

FIPA. (2002). FIPA Interaction Protocol Library Specification (Specification No. DC00025F). Geneva, Switzerland: Foundation for Intelligent and Physical Agents (FIPA).

FIPA. (2009). FIPA Agent Communication specifications. Retrieved May 5, 2009, from www.fipa.org

FIPA. (n.d.). *Foundation of Intelligent Physical Agent.* Retrieved from http://ww.fipa.org/

Fireman, B., Bartlett, J., & Selby, J. (2004). Can Disease Management Reduce Health Care Costs By Improving Quality? *Health Affairs, 23,* 63–75. doi:10.1377/hlthaff.23.6.63

Fogel, K. (2005). *Producing open source software: how to run a successful free software project.* Retrieved January 7, 2009, from http://producingoss.com

Fontelo, P., DiNino, E., Johansen, K., Khan, A., & Ackerman, M. (2005). Virtual Microscopy: Potential Applications in Medical Education and Telemedicine in Countries with Developing Economies. *38th Hawaii International Conference on System Sciences.*

Fox, A., Gribble, S. D., Brewer, E. A., & Amir, E. (1996). *Adapting* to Network and Client Variability via On-Demand Dynamic Distillation. In *Proceedings of the ASPLOS-VII, Cambridge, MA, October.*

Fox, J., & Das, S. (2000). *Safe and Sound.* Menlo Park, CA, USA: AAAI and MIT Press.

Fox, J., Beveridge, M., & Glasspool, D. (2003). Understanding intelligent agents: analysis and synthesis. *AI Communications, 16*(3), 139–152.

Fox, S. (2006). Online health search 2006. Pew Internet and American Life Project 2005. Retrieved March 6, 2009, from www.pewinternet.org/PPF/r/190/report_display.asp.

France, F. H., & Gaunt, P. N. (1994). The need for security-a clinical view. *International Journal of Bio-Medical Computing, 35,* 189–194.

Fraser, H. S. F., Jazayeri, D., Nevil, P., Karacaoglu, Y., Farmer, P. E., Lyon, E., et al. (2004) An information system and medical record to support HIV treatment in rural Haiti. *BMJ, 329,* 1142-1146. Retrieved October 30, 2008 from http://www.bmj.com/cgi/content/full/329/7475/1142.

Freitas, A. A., & Lavington, S. H. (1998). *Mining Very Large Databases with Parallel Processing.* London, UK: Kluwer.

Freudenheim, M. (2007, April 16). AOL Founder hopes to build new giant among a bevy of health care Web sites. *New York Times*.

Frey, J. G. (2009). *The value of the Semantic Web in the laboratory*. Drug Discovery Today.

Friedman, C. P., & Wyatt, J. C. (2006). *Evaluation methods in biomedical informatics*. New York: Springer.

Frost, J., & Massagli, M. P. (2008). Social uses of personal health information within PatientsLikeMe, an online patient community: what can happen when patients have access to one another's data. *Journal of Medical Internet Research*, *10*(2), e15. doi:10.2196/jmir.1053

Furnell, S. M., Davey, J., Gaunt, P. N., Louwerse, C. P., Mavroudakis, K., & Treacher, A. H. (1998). The ISHTAR guidelines for healthcare security. *Health Informatics Journal*, *4*(3-4), 179–183. doi:10.1177/146045829800400308

Furness, P. (2007). A randomized controlled trial of the diagnostic accuracy of internet-based telepathology compared with conventional microscopy. *Histopathology*, *50*(2), 266–273. doi:10.1111/j.1365-2559.2006.02581.x

Furst, I. (2009). *Wait Time & Delayed Care*. Retrieved February 14, 2009, from Wait Time & Delayed Care: http://waittimes.blogspot.com

Fyrenious, A. (2005). Lectures in problem-based learning—Why, when and how? An example of interactive lecturing that stimulates meaningful learning. *Medical Teacher*, *27*(1), 61–65. doi:10.1080/01421590400016365

Gale, M. E., & Gale, D. R. (2000). DICOM modality worklist: an essential component in a PACS environment. *Journal of Digital Imaging*, *13*(3), 101–108. doi:10.1007/BF03168381

Garcia-Lizana, F., & Sarria-Santamera, A. (2007). New technologies for chronic disease management and control: a systematic review. *Journal of Telemedicine and Telecare*, *13*, 62–68. doi:10.1258/135763307780096140

Garshol, L. (2002). *What Are Topic Maps?* Graauw, M. (2002). *Business Maps: Topic Maps Go B2B*.

Gaudinat, A., Ruch, P., Joubert, M., Uziel, P., Strauss, A., & Thonnet, M. (2006). Health search engine with e-document analysis for reliable search results. *International Journal of Medical Informatics*, *75*(1), 73–85. doi:10.1016/j.ijmedinf.2005.11.002

Genes, N., & Parekh, S. (2009). Bringing journal club to the bedside in the form of a critical appraisal blog. [article in press, epub ahead of print]. *The Journal of Emergency Medicine*, (Jan): 24.

Georgiadis, P., Daskalakis, A., Nikiforidis, G., Cavouras, D., Sifaki, K., Malamas, M., et al. (2007). *PDA-based system with teleradiology and image analysis capabilities*. Paper presented at the Engineering in Medicine and Biology Society, 2007. EMBS 2007. 29th Annual International Conference of the IEEE.

Georgiadis, T. D. (2002). *Dynamic Creation of Collaborating System and Database Management, Using Mobile Agents*. Master thesis supervised by George Samaras, Computer Science Department, University of Cyprus, June.

Georgian-Smith, D., Moore, R. H., Halpern, E., Yeh, E. D., Rafferty, E. A., & D'Alessandro, H. A. (2007). Blinded comparison of computer-aided detection with human second reading in screening mammography. *AJR. American Journal of Roentgenology*, *189*(5), 1135–1141. doi:10.2214/AJR.07.2393

Geyman, J. P. (2007). Disease management: panacea, another false hope, or something in between? *Annals of Family Medicine*, *5*, 257–260. doi:10.1370/afm.649

Ghenniwa H., & Kamel M. (2000). Interaction Devices for Coordinating Cooperative Distributed Systems. *Journal of Intelligent Automation and Soft Computing*.

Ghenniwa, H., & Huhns, M. (2004). Intelligent Enterprise Integration: eMarketplace Model. In Gupta, J., & Sharma, S. (Eds.), *Creating Knowledge Based Organizations* (pp. 46–79). Hershey, PA: Idea Group Publishing.

Gialelis, J., Foundas, P., Kalogeras, A., Georgoudakis, M., Kinalis, A., & Koubias, S. (2008). Wireless Wearable Body Area Network Supporting Person Centric Health Monitoring. In *Proceedings of the 7th IEEE International Workshop on Factory Communication Systems (WFCS 2008), May 20-23, 2008*.

Giger, M., Huo, Z., Vyborny, C., Lan, L., Bonta, I., & Horsch, K. (2002). *Intelligent CAD workstation for breast imaging using similarity to known lesions and multiple visual prompt aids*. Paper presented at the SPIE.

Gilbertson, J. R., Ho, J., Anthony, L., Jukic, D. M., Yagi, Y., & Parwani, A. V. (2006). Primary histologic diagnosis using automated whole slide imaging: a validation study. *BMC Clinical Pathology*, *6*(4). Retrieved February 18, 2009, from http://www.biomedcentral.com/1472-6890/6/4

Gilbody, S., Bower, P., Fletcher, J., Richards, D., & Sutton, A. J. (2006). Collaborative care for depression: a cumulative meta-analysis and review of longer-term outcomes. *Archives of Internal Medicine*, *166*, 2314–2321. doi:10.1001/archinte.166.21.2314

Gilder, G. (1993, 2008/10/30). *Metcalfe's law - Wikipedia, the free encyclopedia.* Retrieved 11/02/09, from http://en.wikipedia.org/wiki/Metcalfe%http://en.wikipedia.org/w/index.php?title=Metcalfe%27s_law&oldid=248687837.

Gilfor, J. (2004). *Report on Electromagnetic Interference in Hospitals,* from http://www.pdacortex.com/EMI.htm.

Gilmour, J. A. (2007). Reducing disparities in the access and use of Internet health information. a discussion paper. *International Journal of Nursing Studies, 44,* 1270–1278. doi:10.1016/j.ijnurstu.2006.05.007

Giustini, D. (2006). How Web 2.0 is changing medicine. *British Medical Journal, 23;333*(7582), 1283-1284.

Giustini, D. (2006). Scrooge and intellectual property rights. *British Medical Journal, 333,* 179–1284.

Giustini, D. (2006, December 23-30). How Web 2.0 is Changing Medicine. *British Medical Journal,* –1284. doi:10.1136/bmj.39062.555405.80

Giustini, D. (2007, December 22-29). Web 3.0 and Medicine. *British Medical Journal, 335,* 1273–1274. doi:10.1136/bmj.39428.494236.BE

Glasgow, R. E. (2002). Evaluation of theory-based interventions: the RE-AIM model. Glanz, K., Lewis, F.M., & Rimer, B.K. (Ed.), Health behavior and health education (3rd ed., pp. 531-544). San Francisco CA: John Wiley & Sons.

Glasgow, R. E. (2007). eHealth evaluation and dissemination research. *American Journal of Preventive Medicine, 32,* S119–S126. doi:10.1016/j.amepre.2007.01.023

Glasgow, R. E., McKay, H. G., Piette, J. D., & Reynolds, K. D. (2001). The RE-AIM framework for evaluating interventions: what can it tell us about approaches to chronic illness management? *Patient Education and Counseling, 44,* 119–127. doi:10.1016/S0738-3991(00)00186-5

Glasgow, R. E., Vogt, T. M., & Boles, S. M. (1999). Evaluating the public health impact of health promotion interventions: the RE-AIM framework. *American Journal of Public Health, 89,* 1322–1327. doi:10.2105/AJPH.89.9.1322

Glissmann, S., Smolnik, S., Schierholz, R., Kolbe, L., & Brenner, W. (2005). *Proposition of an m-business procedure model for the development of mobile user interfaces.*

Global Kids Inc. (2008, August). Summer 2008 RezEd Report. *Global Kids, 1*(1). Retrieved February 28, 2009 from http://www.rezed.org/.

Gloth, M., Coleman, E., Philips, S., & Zorowitz, R. (2005). Using Electronic Health Records to Improved Care: Will "Hight Tech" Allow a Return to "High Touch" Medicine? *Journal of the American Medical Directors Association,* ▪▪▪, 270–275. doi:10.1016/j.jamda.2005.05.003

Glover, F. (1989). Tabu search - Part I. *ORSA Journal on Computing, 1*(3), 190-206.

Glueckauf, R. L., Pickett, T. C., Ketterson, T. U., Loomis, J. S., & Rozensky, R. H. (2003). Preparation for the Delivery of Telehealth Services: a Self-Study Framework for Expansion of Practice. *Professional Psychology, Research and Practice, 34*(2), 159–163. doi:10.1037/0735-7028.34.2.159

Goh, S. H. (2006). The internet as a health education tool: sieving the wheat from the chaff. *Singapore Medical Journal, 47*(1), 3–5.

Golbreich, C., Zhang, S., & Bodenreider, O. (2006). The foundational model of anatomy in OWL: Experience and perspectives. *Web Semantics: Science. Services and Agents on the World Wide Web, 4*(3), 181–195. doi:10.1016/j.websem.2006.05.007

Golder, S. A., & Huberman, B. A. (2005). The Structure of Collaborative Tagging Systems. *Journal of Information Science, 32*(2), 198–208. doi:10.1177/0165551506062337

Goldfield, G. S., & Boachie, A. (2003). Delivery of family therapy in the treatment of anorexia nervosa using telehealth. *Telemedicine Journal and e-Health, 9*(1), 111–114. doi:10.1089/153056203763317729

Goldschmidt, P. G. (2005). HIT and MIS: Implications of Health Information Technology and Medical Information Systems. *Communications of the ACM, 48*(10), 69–74.

Goldsmith, H., Manderscheid, W., & Merwin, E. (1995). Human Resource Issues in Rural Mental health Services. *Community Mental Health Journal, 31,* 525-537. Retrieved October 28, 2008 from http://www.springerlink.com/content/p68r402563qp0755/fulltext.pdf

Goldstein, D., Groen, P. J., Ponkshe, S., & Wine, M. (2007). *Medical Informatics 20/20: Quality and Electronic Health Records Through Collaboration, Open Solutions, and Innovation.* Sudbury, MA: Jones & Bartlett Publishers.

Gómez-Pérez, A., Fernández-López, M., & Corcho, O. (2004). *Ontological Engineering with examples from the areas of Knowledge Management, e-Commerce and the Semantic Web* (2nd ed.). Berlin, Germany: Springer Verlag.

Goode, A., & Satyanarayanan, M. A. (2008). *Vendor-neutral library and viewer for whole-slide images* (Opendiamond, report). Pittsburgh, PA: Carnegie Mellon University. Retrieved February 13, 2009, from http://diamond.cs.cmu.edu/papers/CMU-CS-08-136.pdf

Google Health. (2009). *Google Health.* Retrieved May 1, 2009, from https://www.google.com/health

Gopalan, J., Alhajj, R., & Barker, K. (2006). Discovering Accurate and Interesting Classification Rules Using Genetic Algorithm. In *International Conference on Data Mining, DMIN 2006* (pp. 389-395). Las Vegas, Nevada: CSREA Press

Gordon, M. S., Issenberg, S. B., Mayer, J. W., & Felner, J. N. (1999). Developments in the use of simulators and multimedia computer systems in medical education. *Medical Teacher, 21*, 32–36. doi:10.1080/01421599980002

Gorini, A., Gaggioli, A., & Riva, G. (2007). Virtual worlds, real healing. *Science, 318*(5856), 1549. doi:10.1126/science.318.5856.1549b

Gorini, A., Gaggioli, A., Vigna, C., & Riva, G. (2008). A second life for ehealth: Prospects for the use of 3-d virtual worlds in clinical psychology. *Journal of Medical Internet Research, 10*(3). doi:10.2196/jmir.1029

Gorman, P. J., Meier, A. H., Rawn, C., & Krummel, T. M. (2000). The future of medical education is no longer blood and guts, it is bits and bytes. *American Journal of Surgery, 180*, 353–356. doi:10.1016/S0002-9610(00)00514-6

Graham K., & Jeremy J.C. (2004, February). *Resource Description Framework (RDF): Concepts and Abstract Syntax.* W3C Recommendation.

Graham, P. (2005). Web 2.0. Retrieved from http://www.paulgraham.com/web20.html

Granlien, M. F., Herzum, M., & Gudmundsen, J. (2008). The gap between actual and mandated use of an electronic medication record three years after deployment. *Studies in Health Technology and Informatics, 136*, 419–424.

Gray, J., & Reuter, A. (1993). *Transaction Processing: Concepts and Techniques.* Morgan Kaufman Publishers, Inc.

Greaves, M., & Mika, P. (2008). Semantic Web and Web 2.0. *Web Semantics: Science Services and Agents on the World Wide Web, 6*(1), 1–3. doi:10.1016/j.websem.2007.12.002

Greenes, R. A. (Ed.). (2007). *Clinical Decision Support. The Road Ahead.* Elsevier.

Grid Services Provisioning. *Journal of Computer Sciences, 6*(2), 521-527.

Griffiths, F., Lindenmeyer, A., Powell, J., Lowe, P., & Thorogood, M. (2006). Why are health care interventions delivered over the internet? A systematic review of the published literature. *Journal of Medical Internet Research, 8*, e10. doi:10.2196/jmir.8.2.e10

Gritzalis, S. (2004). Enhancing Privacy and Data Protection in Electronic Medical Environments. *Journal of Medical Systems, 28*(6). doi:10.1023/B:JOMS.0000044956.55209.75

Grone, O., & Garcia-Barbero, M. (2001). Integrated care: a position paper of the WHO European Office for Integrated Health Care Services. *International Journal of Integrated Care, 1*, e21.

Grossman, D. A., & Frieder, O. (1998). *Information retrieval: algorithms and heuristics.* Boston: Kluwer.

Gruber, T. (1993). A Translation Approach to Portable Ontology Specifications. *Knowledge Acquisition, 5*(2), 199–220. doi:10.1006/knac.1993.1008

Gruber, T. R. (1993). Toward principles for the design of ontologies used for knowledge sharing. *Padua workshop on Formal Ontology.*

Guimond, A., & Subsol, G. (1997). Automatic MRI Database Exploration and Applications. *Pattern Recognition and Artificial Intelligence, 11*(8), 1345–1365. doi:10.1142/S0218001497000627

Guo, G. D., Jain, A. K., Ma, W. Y., & Zhang, H. J. (2002). Learning similarity measure for natural image retrieval with relevance feedback. *IEEE Transactions on Neural Networks, 13*(4), 811–820. doi:10.1109/TNN.2002.1021882

Guo, J., Takada, A., Tanaka, K., Sato, J., Suzuki, M., & Suzuki, T. (2004). The development of MML (Medical Markup Language) version 3.0 as a medical document exchange format for HL7 messages. *Journal of Medical Systems, 28*(6), 523–533. doi:10.1023/B:JOMS.0000044955.51844.c3

Gustafson, D. H., Hawkins, R. P., Boberg, E. W., McTavish, F., Owens, B., & Wise, M. (2002). CHESS: 10 years of research and development in consumer health informatics for broad populations, including the underserved. *International Journal of Medical Informatics, 65*(3), 169–177. doi:10.1016/S1386-5056(02)00048-5

Gustafson, D., Hawkins, R., Boberg, E., McTavish, F., Owens, B., & Wise, M. (2002). CHESS: 10 years of Research and Development in Consumer Health Informatics for Broad Populations Including the Underserved. *International Journal of Medical Informatics*, 167–177.

Guy, M., & Tonkin, E. (2006). Folksonomies - Tidying up Tags? *D-Lib Magazine*, *12*(1). doi:10.1045/january2006-guy

Guyon, I., & Elissee, A. (2003). An Introduction to Variable and Feature Selection. *Journal of Machine Learning Research*, *3*, 1157–1182. doi:10.1162/153244303322753616

Hadjiiski, L., Sahiner, B., Helvie, M. A., Chan, H. P., Roubidoux, M. A., & Paramagul, C. (2006). Breast masses: computer-aided diagnosis with serial mammograms. *Radiology*, *240*(2), 343–356. doi:10.1148/radiol.2401042099

Hafner, J., Sawhney, H. S., Equitz, W., Flickner, M., & Niblack, W. (1995). Efficient color histogram indexing for quadratic form distance functions. *IEEE Transactions on Pattern Analysis and Machine Intelligence*, *17*(7), 729–736. doi:10.1109/34.391417

Haimson, B. R., & Elfenbein, M. H. (1985). *Experimental methods in psychology*. Toronto: McGraw-Hill.

Häkkilä, J., & Chatfield, C. (2005). *'It's like if you opened someone else's letter': user perceived privacy and social practices with SMS communication.* Paper presented at the 7th international conference on Human computer interaction with mobile devices & services, Salzburg, Austria.

Halpert, B. J. (2005). *Authentication interface evaluation and design for mobile devices.* Paper presented at the 2nd annual conference on Information security curriculum development, Kennesaw, Georgia.

Hamlin, K. (2005). *Identity 2.0 Gathering: Getting to the Promised Land.* Retrieved January 25, 2009, from http://www.oreillynet.com/pub/a/policy/2005/10/07/identity-workshop.html

Han, J., & Kamber, M. (2006). *Data Mining: Concepts and Techniques* (2nd ed.). Morgan Kaufmann Publishers.

Hansen, M. A. (2008). User-controlled identity management: the key to the future of privacy? *International Journal of Intellectual Property Management*, *2*(4), 325–344.

Harden, R. M. (2000). Evolution or revolution and the future of medical education: replacing the oak tree. *Medical Teacher*, *22*, 435–442. doi:10.1080/01421590050110669

Harden, R. M., & Hart, I. R. (2002). An international virtual medical school (IVIMEDS): the future for medical education? *Medical Teacher*, *24*, 261–267. doi:10.1080/01421590220141008

Hardiker, N. R., Hoy, D., & Casey, A. (2000). Standards for Nursing Terminology. *Journal of the American Medical Informatics Association*, *7*, 523–538.

Hardy, B., Mur-Veemanu, I., Steenbergen, M., & Wistow, G. (1999). Inter-agency services in England and The Netherlands. A comparative study of integrated care development and delivery. *Health Policy (Amsterdam)*, *48*, 87–105. doi:10.1016/S0168-8510(99)00037-8

Harman, L. B. (2005). HIPAA: a few years later. *Online Journal of Issues in Nursing*, *10*(2), 31.

Harris, L. D. (1994). Psychodynamic effects of virtual reality. *The Arachnet Electronic Journal on Virtual Culture*, *2*(1).

Hassan-Montero, Y., & Herrero-Solana, V. (2006). Improving tag-clouds as visual information retrieval interfaces. In V.P. Guerrero-Bote (Ed.) *International Conference on Multidisciplinary Information Sciences and Technologies* (InSciT2006).

Hassol, A., Walker, J. M., Kidder, D., Rokita, K., Young, D., & Pierdon, S. (2004). Patient experiences and attitudes about access to a patient electronic health care record and linked web messaging. *Journal of the American Medical Informatics Association*, *11*(6), 505–513. doi:10.1197/jamia.M1593

Hastie, T., & Tibshirani, R. (1996). Discriminant Adaptive Nearest Neighbor Classification. *IEEE Transactions on Pattern Analysis and Machine Intelligence*, *18*(6), 10. doi:10.1109/34.506411

Health 2.0. (n.d.). *The Next Conference.* Retrieved April 29, 2009, from Health 2.0: http://health2con.com

Health Council of Canada. (2005). *Ten Steps to a Common Framework for Reporting on Wait Times.* Toronto: Health Council of Canada.

Health Council of Canada. (2008). *Rekindling Reform: Health Care Renewal in Canada 2003 - 2008.* Toronto: Health Council of Canada.

Health Council of Canada. (2008). *Sustainability in Public Health Care: What Does it Mean? A Panel Discussion Report.* Toronto: Health Council of Canada.

Health Insurance Portability and Accountability Act (HIPAA). Retrieved from http://www.intellimark-it.com/privacysecurity/hipaa.asp

Health Level Seven, Inc. (n.d.). *Personal Health Record System Functional Model.* Retrieved April 17, 2009, from http://www.hl7.org/ehr/.

Health Level Seven. (n.d.). HL7 Continuity of Care Document, a healthcare IT interoperability standard, is approved by balloting process and endorsed by healthcare IT standards panel. Press release. February 12, 2007. Retrieved December 11, 2008, from http://www.hl7.org/documentcenter/public/pressreleases/20070212.pdf.

Health Level Seven. (n.d.). *HL7 receives ANSI approval of three version 3 specifications including CDA, release 2.* Press release. May 5, 2005. Retrieved December 11, 2008, from http://www.hl7.org/documentcenter/public/pressreleases/20050505.pdf.

Health Level Seven. (n.d.). *The Clinical Document Architecture (CDA) Release 2.0.* Retrieved November 2, 2008, from http://www.hl7.org.

Health on the Net Foundation. (2009, March 9). *HONcode.* Retrieved May 15, 2009, from Health on the Net Foundation: http://www.hon.ch

Healthcare Information Management and Systems Society. (n.d.). *Personal Health Record Web site.* Retrieved July 3, 2008, from http://www.himss.org/ASP/topics_phr.asp.

HealthLinkBC. (2009). *HealthLink BC.* Retrieved May 15, 2009, from HealthLinkBC: www.healthlinkbc.ca

HealthVault. (2009). *Microsoft HealthVault.* Retrieved May 1, 2009, from http://www.healthvault.com

Heeks, R., Jang, S., Ko, K., & Lee, H. (2008). Analysing South Korea's ICT for Development Aid Programme *The Electronic Journal of Information Systems in Developing Countries, 35,* 1-15. Retrieved October 28, 2008 from http://www.ejisdc.org/ojs2/index.php/ejisdc/article/viewFile/496/252

Heflin, J., Hendler, J., & Luke, S. (1999). *SHOE: A Knowledge Representation Language for Internet Applications* (No. Technical Report CS-TR-4078): Department of Computer Science, University of Maryland.

Heiberg Engel, P. J. (2008). Tacit knowledge and visual expertise in medical diagnostic reasoning: implications for medical education. *Medical Teacher, 30*(7), e184–e188. doi:10.1080/01421590802144260

Henderson, L. N., & Tulloch, J. (2008). Incentives for Retaining and Motivating Health Workers in Pacific and Asian Countries. *Human Resources for Health, 6,* 18-37. Retrieved November 18, 2008 from http://www.human-resources-health.com/content/6/1/18

Hendrix, C., & Barfield, W. (1996). Presence within virtual environments as a function of visual display parameters. *Presence (Cambridge, Mass.), 5,* 274–289.

Henry, S. G., Zaner, R. M., & Dittus, R. S. (2007). Viewpoint: Moving beyond evidence-based medicine. *Academic Medicine, 82*(3), 292–297. doi:10.1097/ACM.0b013e3180307f6d

Hewitt, C. (2009). Perfect Disruption: The Paradigm Shift from Mental Agents to ORGs. *IEEE Internet Computing, 13*(1), 90–93. doi:10.1109/MIC.2009.15

Hewitt, M., & Ganz, P. (Eds.). (2006). *From Cancer Patient to Cancer Survivor: Lost in Transition.* Washington, DC: The National Academies Press.

Heymann, P., & García-Molina, H. H. (2006). *Collaborative Creation of Communal Hierarchical, Taxonomies in Social Tagging Systems* (Tech. Rep. No. 2006-10). Stanford InfoLab.

Hillestad, R., Bigelow, J., Bower, A., Girosi, R., Meili, R., Scoville, R., & Taylor, R. (2005). Can electronic medical record systems transform health care: potential health benefits, savings, and costs? *Health Affairs, 24,* 1103–1117. doi:10.1377/hlthaff.24.5.1103

Hillmann, D. (2005). Using Dublin Core Retrieved June 5, 2009, from http://dublincore.org/documents/usageguide/

Hinchcliffe, D. (2008). *What Is WOA? It's The Future of Service-Oriented Architecture (SOA).* Retrieved March 22, 2009, from http://hinchcliffe.org/archive/2008/02/27/16617.aspx

HIPAA. (1996). *Health Insurance Portability and Accountability Act.* United States Congress, United States. Retrieved May 1, 2009, from http://aspe.hhs.gov/admnsimp/pl104191.htm

HL7 CDA. (2009). *Clinical Document Architecture (CDA).* Retrieved May 1, 2009, from http://xml.coverpages.org/healthcare.html #cda

HL7. (2009). *Health Level Seven.* Retrieved May 1, 2009, from http://www.hl7.org

HL7. (2009). *Work Groups. Anatomic Pathology.* Ann Arbor, MI: Health Level Seven, Inc. Retrieved February 23, 2009, from http://www.hl7.org/Special/committees/anatomicpath/index.cfm

Ho, D. (2009, January). *Tutorial: OpenID authentication with SSO (PHP).* Retrieved April 3, 2009, from http://www.mti.epita.fr/blogs/serveur/2009/01/12/tutorial-authentification-sso-avec-openid-en-php/

Hoffmann, R. (2008). A wiki for the life sciences where authorship matters. *Nature Genetics, 40*(9), 1047–1051. doi:10.1038/ng.f.217

Holdener, A. T., III. (2008). Ajax: The Definitive Guide. Sebastopol, CA, US: O'Reilly Media, Inc.

Holi, M., & Hyvonen, E. (2004). *A method for modeling uncertainty in semantic web taxonomies*. Paper presented at the Proceedings of the 13th international World Wide Web conference on Alternate track papers & posters.

Holland, J. H. (1986). Escaping brittleness: the possibilities of general purpose algorithms applied to parallel rule-based systems. In Michalski, R. S., Carbonell, J. G., & Mitchell, T. M. (Eds.), *Machine Learning, an AI Approach* (*Vol. 2*, pp. 593–623). San Mateo, California: Morgan Kaufmann.

Holmes, G., & Cunningham, S. J. (1993). Using data mining to support the construction and maintenance of expert systems. In *Artificial Neural Networks and Expert Systems*. (pp. 156-159). First New Zealand International Two-Stream Conference.

Hongoro, C., & McPake, B. (2004). How to Bridge the Gap In Human Resources for Health. *Lancet, 364*, 1451–1456. doi:10.1016/S0140-6736(04)17229-2

Horrocks, I., Patel-Schneider, P. F., & van Harmelen, F. (2003). From SHIQ and RDF to OWL: the making of a Web Ontology Language. *Web Semantics: Science. Services and Agents on the World Wide Web, 1*(1), 7. doi:10.1016/j.websem.2003.07.001

Housel, B. C., Samaras, G., & Lindquist, D. B. (1996). *WebExpress: A Client/Intercept Based System for Optimizing Web Browsing in a Wireless Environment. Journal ACM/Baltzer Mobile Networking and Applications (MONET)*. Special Issue on Mobile Networking on the Internet.

Howe, N., & Strauss, W. (2000). *Millennials Rising: The Next Great Generation.*

Hu, J., & Peyton, L. (2009). Integrating Identity Management with Federated Healthcare Data Models. In *Proceedings of the 4th International MCeTech Conference on eTechnologies* (pp. 100-112). Ottawa, Canada. LNBIP 26, Springer.

Hu, J., Peyton, L., Turner, C., & Bishay, H. (2008). A Model of Trusted Data Collection for Knowledge Discovery in B2B Networks. In *Proceedings of the 3rd International MCETECH Conference on e-Technologies* (pp. 60-69). Montreal, Canada.

Hubert, R. (2006). Accessibility and usability guidelines for mobile devices in home health monitoring. *SIGACCESS Accessibility and Computing*(84), 26-29.

Huff, S. M., Rocha, R. A., McDonald, C. J., DeMoor, J. E., & Fiers, T. (1998). Development of the logical observation identifier names and codes (LOINC) vocabulary. *Journal of the American Medical Informatics Association, 5*, 276–292.

Hughes, B., & Wareham, J. (2008). Democratized Collaboration in Big Pharma. In G. Soloman (Ed.), *Proceedings of the Academy of Management Conference, 13th August 2008, Anaheim, CA.*

Hughes, B., Joshi, I., & Lemonde, H. (2008). To 2.0 or not to 2.0? Young doctors have already answered the question. In G. Eysenbach (Ed.), *Proceedings of the Medicine 2.0 congress, 4-5th September 2008, Toronto* (p. 39).

Hughes, B., Joshi, I., & Wareham, J. (2008). Medicine 2.0: Tensions and controversies in the field. *Journal of Medical Internet Research, 6;10*(3), e23. Retrieved March 7, 2009, from http://www.jmir.org/2008/3/e23/

Hughes, B., Joshi, I., Lemonde, H., & Wareham, J. (2009). Junior physician's use of Web 2.0 for information seeking and medical education: a qualitative study. *International Journal of Medical Informatics.*

Hunkeler, E. M., Katon, W., Tang, L., Williams, J. W. Jr, Kroenke, K., & Lin, E. H. (2006). Long term outcomes from the IMPACT randomised trial for depressed elderly patients in primary care. *BMJ (Clinical Research Ed.), 332*, 259–263. doi:10.1136/bmj.38683.710255.BE

Hussein, R., Engelmann, U., Schroeter, A., & Meinzer, H. P. (2004). *DICOM Structured Reporting Part 1. Overview and Characteristics 1* (*Vol. 24*, pp. 891–896). RSNA.

Hutchinson, C., Ward, J., & Castilon, K. (2009). Navigating the Next-Generation Application Architecture. *IT Professional, 11*(2), 18–22. doi:10.1109/MITP.2009.33

IBM. (2003). Autonomic Computing. May 2004, from http://www.research.ibm.com/autonomic

ICD-10. (n.d.). http://www.who.int/classifications/icd/en/index.html.

Initiative for Privacy Standardization in Europe (IPSE). Retrieved from http://www.hi-europe.info/files/2002/9963.htm

Institute of Aging-University of British Columbia. (2007). *The Future is AGING: Institute of Aging Strategic Plan 2007 – 2012.* Canadian Institutes of Health Research.

International Organization for Standardization. (n.d.). *ISO/TR 20514:2005Health informatics — Electronic health record — Definition, scope, and context*. Retrieved January 17, 2009, from http://www.iso.org/iso/iso_catalogue/catalogue_tc/catalogue_detail.htm?csnumber=39525.

International Study of Asthma and Allergies in Children (ISAAC) Steering Committee. (1998). Worldwide variations in the prevalence of asthma symptoms: The International Study of Asthma and Allergies in Children. *The European Respiratory Journal, 12*(2), 315–335. doi: 10.1183/09031936.98.12020315

International Telecommunication Union (ITU). (2009). *Measuring the Information Society: The ICT Development Index, 2009 Edition. Geneva, Switzerland*. Retrieved April 21, 2008 from http://www.itu.int/ITU-D/ict/publications/idi/2009/material/IDI2009_w5.pdf

International, I. H. E. (2008). *Anatomic Pathology Technical Framework. Volume 1 (PAT TF-1). Profiles. Revision 1.2 – Trial Implementation*. Retrieved February 17, 2009, from http://www.ihe.net/Technical_Framework/upload/ihe_anatomic-path_TF_rev1-2_TI_vol1_2008-11-24.pdf

International, I. H. E. (2008). *Anatomic Pathology Technical Framework. Volume 2 (PAT TF-2). Transactions. Revision 1.2 – Trial Implementation*. Retrieved February 17, 2009, from http://www.ihe.net/Technical_Framework/upload/ihe_anatomic-path_TF_rev1-2_TI_vol2_2008-11-24.pdf

Ipsos Reid. (2009). *Online Healthcare: Coming of Age*. Calgary: Ipsos Reid.

Isern, D., Millan, M., Moreno, A., Pedone, G., & Varga, L. Z. (2008). Home Care Individual Intervention Plans in the K4Care Platform. In S. Puuronen, M. Pechenizkiy, A. Tsymbal & D.-J. Lee (Eds.), *Proc. of the 21st IEEE International Symposium on Computer-Based Medical Systems, 2008 IEEE CBMS* (pp. 455-457). Jywaskyla, Finland.

Isern, D., Moreno, A., Sánchez, D., Hajnal, A., Pedone, G., & Varga, L. Z. (2010). Agent-based execution of personalised home care treatments. *Applied Intelligence*. doi:.doi:10.1007/s10489-009-0187-6

Isern, D., Sánchez, D., & Moreno, A. (2010). Agents Applied in Health Care: A Review. *International Journal of Medical Informatics, 75*(3), 145–166. doi:10.1016/j.ijmedinf.2010.01.003

Ishikawa, K., Konishi, N., Tsukuma, H., Tsuru, S., Kawamura, A., & Iwata, N. (2004). A clinical management system for patient participatory health care support. Assuring the patients' rights and confirming operation of clinical treatment and hospital administration. *International Journal of Medical Informatics, 73*(3), 243–249. doi:10.1016/j.ijmedinf.2003.11.021

Ishikawa, K., Ohmichi, H., Umeatso, Y., Terasaki, H., Tsukuma, H., & Iwata, N. (2007). The guideline of the personal haelth data structure to secure safety healthcare: The balance between use and protection to satisfy the patients' needs. *International Journal of Medical Informatics, 76*, 412–418. doi:10.1016/j.ijmedinf.2006.09.005

ISO. (2003). The Dublin Core metadata element set *ISO 15836:2003*. Retrieved June 5, 2009, from http://www.iso.org/iso/en/CatalogueDetailPage.CatalogueDetail?CSNUMBER=37629&scopelist=PROGRAMME

Issenberg, S. B., McGaghie, W. C., Hart, I. R., Mayer, J. W., Felner, J. M., & Petrusa, E. R. (1999). Simulation technology for health care professionals skills training and assessment. *Journal of the American Medical Association, 282*(9), 861–866. doi:10.1001/jama.282.9.861

Issenberg, S. B., McGaghie, W. C., Petrusa, E. R., Gordon, D. L., & Scalese, R. J. (2005). Features and uses of high-fidelity medical simulations that lead to effective learning: A BEME systematic review. *Medical Teacher, 27*(1), 10–28. doi:10.1080/01421590500046924

Ito, M. (2007). Limitations and diagnostic responsibility in telepathology. In T. Sawai (Ed.), Telepathology in Japan. Development and practice (pp. 60-65). Morioka, Iwate, Japan: Celc, Inc.

Jablin, F. M., & Putnam, L. L. (2001). *The new handbook of organizational communication: Advances in theory, research and methods*. New York: Sage.

Jackson, W., & Verberg, N. (2006). *Methods: Doing social research* (4th ed.). Toronto: Pearson Prentice Hall.

Jacobs, J., Caudell, T., Wilks, D., Keep, M. F., Mitchell, S., & Buchanan, H. (2003). Integration of advanced technologies to enhance problem-based learning over distance: Project TOUCH. *The Anatomical Record, 270B*, 16–22. doi:10.1002/ar.b.10003

JADE. (n.d.). Java Agent Development Framework: Jade. Retrieved from http://www.jade.cselt.it/

Jagannathan, V., Reddy, Y. V., Srinivas, K., Karinthi, R., Shank, R., Reddy, S., et al. (1995). *An overview of the CERC ARTEMIS project*. Paper presented at the Symposium on Computer Applications in Medical Care.

Jerome, L. W., DeLeon, P. H., James, L. C., Folen, R., Earles, J., & Gedney, J. J. (2000). The coming of age of telecommunications in psychological research and practice. *The American Psychologist*, *55*(4), 407–421. doi:10.1037/0003-066X.55.4.407

Jiang, G., Pathak, J., & Chute, C. G. (2009). Formalizing ICD coding rules using Formal Concept Analysis. *Journal of Biomedical Informatics*, *42*(3), 504–517. doi:10.1016/j.jbi.2009.02.005

Jing, F., Li, M., Zhang, H. J., & Zhang, B. (2004). An efficient and effective region-based image retrieval framework. *IEEE Transactions on Image Processing*, *13*(5), 699–709. doi:10.1109/TIP.2004.826125

Johnson, C. M., & Turley, J. P. (2006). The significance of cognitive modeling in building healthcare interfaces. *International Journal of Medical Informatics*, *75*, 163–172. doi:10.1016/j.ijmedinf.2005.06.003

Johnson, G., & Ambrose, G. (2006). Neo-Tribes: The Power and Potential of Online Communities in Health Care. *Communications of the ACM*, *49*(1), 107–113. doi:10.1145/1107458.1107463

Johnson, O., & Liu, J. (2006). A traveling salesman approach for predicting protein functions. *Source Code for Biology and Medicine*, *1*(3), 1–7.

Joinson, A. (1999). Social desirability, anonymity, and Internet-based questionnaires. *Behavior Research Methods, Instruments, & Computers*, *31*(3), 433–438.

Joinson, A. (2001). Self-disclosure in computer-mediated communication: the role of self awareness and visual anonimity. *European Journal of Social Psychology*, *31*(2), 177–192. doi:10.1002/ejsp.36

Joint Commission for Health Care Quality. (2008). Safely implementing health information and converging technologies. Retrieved April 14, 2009 from http://www.jointcommission.org/SentinelEventAlert/sea_42.htm

Jones, J., Wilson, A., Parker, H., Wynn, A., Jagger, C., Spiers, N., & Parker, G. (1999). Economic evaluation of hospital at home versus hospital care: cost minimisation analysis of data from randomised controlled trial. *British Medical Journal*, *319*(7224), 1547–1550.

Jones, M. T. (2008). Cloud computing with Linux Cloud computing platforms and applications. *IBM Research Journal*. Retrieved April 25, 2009, from http://www.ibm.com/developerworks/library/l-cloud-computing/index.html

Jones, R., Higgs, R., de Angelis, C., & Prideaux, D. (2001). Changing face of medical curricula. *Lancet*, *357*(9257), 699–703. doi:10.1016/S0140-6736(00)04134-9

Jones, T. M. (2003). Patient participation in EHR benefits. *Health Management Technology*, *24*(10).

Joseph, B. (2007, August). *Global Kids Inc.'s Best Practices in Using Virtual Worlds for Education*. Paper presented at the meeting of the Second Life Educator's Communities Conference, Chicago, IL.

Jovicic, A., Holroyd-Leduc, J. M., & Straus, S. E. (2006). Effects of self-management intervention on health outcomes of patients with heart failure: a systematic review of randomized controlled trials. *BMC Cardiovascular Disorders*, *6*, 43. doi:10.1186/1471-2261-6-43

Jun, J. B., Jacobson, S. H., & Swisher, J. R. (1999). Application of discrete-event simulation in health care clinics: A Survey. *The Journal of the Operational Research Society*, *50*(2), 109–123.

Jung, F. (2009). XML-based prescription drug database helps pharmacists advise their customers. Retrieved April 22, 2009, from, http://www.softwareag.com/xml/applications/sanacorp.htm

Jurgen, B., Felix, G., & Harald, V. (2004). Dependability Issues of Pervasive Computing in a Healthcare Environment". In *Security in Pervasive Computing 2003* (LNCS 2802). Retrieved from http://www.vs.inf.ethz.ch/res/papers/bohn_pervasivehospital_spc_2003_final.pdf

Kabene, S. M., Orchard, C., Howard, J. M., Soriano, M. A., & Leduc, R. (2006). The importance of human resources management in health care: a global context. *Human Resources for Health*, *4*, 20–36. doi:10.1186/1478-4491-4-20

Kaelber, D. C., Jha, A. K., Johnston, D., Middleton, B., & Bates, D. W. (2008). A research agenda for personal health records (PHRs). *Journal of the American Medical Informatics Association*, *15*(6), 729–736. doi:10.1197/jamia.M2547

Kahan, M. (2000). Integration of Psychodynamic and Cognitive–Behavioral Therapy in a Virtual Environment. *Cyberpsychology & Behavior*, *3*(2), 179–183. doi:10.1089/109493100316021

Kaldoudi, E., Bamidis, P. D., Papaioakeim, M., & Vargemezis, V. (2008). Problem-based learning via Web 2.0 technologies. In *Proceedings of CBMS2008: The 21th IEEE International Symposium on Computer-Based Medical Systems, Special Track: Technology Enhanced Learning in Medical Education*. (pp. 391-396). Jyväskylä, Finland: IEEE Computer Society.

Kaldoudi, E., Bamidis, P. M., & Pattichis, C. (2009). Multi-type content repurposing and sharing in medical education. In *Proceedings of INTED2009: International Technology, Education and Development Conference*, Valencia, Spain: International Association of Technology, Education and Development.

Kaldoudi, E., Papaioakeim, M., Bamidis, P. M., & Vargemezis, V. (2008b). Towards expert content sharing in medical education. In *Proceedings of INTED2008: International Technology, Education and Development Conference*, Valencia, Spain: International Association of Technology, Education and Development.

Kaliski, B. (2008, October). *Multi-tenant Cloud Computing: From Cruise Liners to Container Ships*. Paper presented at the Trusted Infrastructure Technologies Conference, APTC '08. Third Asia-Pacific, 4 – 4.

Kallergi, M. (2004). Computer-aided diagnosis of mammographic microcalcification clusters. *Medical Physics, 31*, 314–326. doi:10.1118/1.1637972

Kamel, B. M. N., & Wheeler, S. (2007). The emerging Web 2.0 social software: an enabling suite of sociable technologies in health and healthcare education. *Health Information and Libraries Journal, 24*(1), 2–23. doi:10.1111/j.1471-1842.2007.00701.x

Karin, S. C., Mary Kay, M., Tessa, K.-M., Timothy, M. B., Ronald, K., & Matthew, D. P. (2004). The impact of diabetic retinopathy: perspectives from patient focus groups. *Family Practice, 21*, 447–453. doi:10.1093/fampra/cmh417

Karkalis, G. I., & Koutsouris, D. D. (October 2006). *E-health and the Web 2.0*. Paper presented at The International Special Topic Conference on Information Technology in Biomedicine, Greece 2006.

Kavanagh, S., & Knapp, M. (2002). Costs and cognitive disability: modelling the underlying associations. *The British Journal of Psychiatry, 180*, 120–125. doi:10.1192/bjp.180.2.120

Kawash, J., El Morr, C., & Itani, M. (2007). A Novel Collaboration Model for Mobile Virtual Communities. *International Journal for Web Based Communities, 3*(1).

Kayser, K., Szymas, J., & Weinstein, R. S. (Eds.). (1999). *Telepathology. Telecommunication, electronic education and publication in Pathology*. Berlin: Springer.

Kelton, A. J. (2008). Virtual worlds. Outlook good. *EDUCAUSE Review, 43*(5), 5–22.

Kemp, J. (2006). Second Life Heart Murmur Sim video demonstration. Retrieved from http://it.youtube.com/watch?v=xJY2Iwbzop4

Kennedy, R., Lee, Y., Van Roy, B., Reed, C. D., & Lippman, R. P. (1998). *Solving data mining problems through pattern recognition*. Prentice Hall.

Kessler, R. C., Berglund, P., Demler, O., Jin, R., Koretz, D., & Merikangas, K. R. (2003). The epidemiology of major depressive disorder: results from the National Comorbidity Survey Replication (NCS-R). *Journal of the American Medical Association, 289*, 3095–3105. doi:10.1001/jama.289.23.3095

Ketchell, D. S., St Anna, L., Kauff, D., Gaster, B., & Timberlake, D. (2005). PrimeAnswers: A practical interface for answering primary care questions. *Journal of the American Medical Informatics Association, 12*(5), 537–545. doi:10.1197/jamia.M1601

Khazab, M., Tweedale, J., & Jain, L. C. (2009). Interoperable Intelligent Agents in a Dynamic Environment. In Nakamatsu, K., Phillips-Wren, G., & Jain, L. C. (Eds.), *New Advances in Intelligent Decision Technologies*. doi:10.1007/978-3-642-00909-9_18

Kim, H. L., Scerri, S., Breslin, J. G., Decker, S., & Kim, H. G. (2008). The state of the art in tag ontologies: a semantic model for tagging and folksonomies. In *Proceedings of the 2008 International Conference on Dublin Core and Metadata Applications, Berlin, Germany* (pp. 128-137).

Kim, H. N. (2008). The phenomenon of blogs and theoretical model of blog use in educational contexts. *Computers & Education, 51*(3), 1342–1352. doi:10.1016/j.compedu.2007.12.005

Kindig, D., & Stoddart, G. (2003). What is Population Health? *American Journal of Public Health*, 380–383. doi:10.2105/AJPH.93.3.380

Kinoshita, S. K., de Azevedo-Marques, P. M., Pereira, R. R. Jr, Rodrigues, J. A., & Rangayyan, R. M. (2007). Content-based retrieval of mammograms using visual features related to breast density patterns. *Journal of Digital Imaging, 20*(2), 172–190. doi:10.1007/s10278-007-9004-0

Kirkpatrick, D. (1998). *Evaluating Training Programs: The Four Levels*. San Francisco, CA: Berrett-Koehler.

Kirkpatrick, S., Gelatt, C. D. Jr, & Vecchi, M. P. (1983). Optimization by Simulated Annealing. *Science, 220*(4598), 671–680. doi:10.1126/science.220.4598.671

Kittler, A. F., Carlson, G. L., Harris, C., Lippincott, M., Pizziferri, L., & Volk, L. A. (2004). Primary care physician attitudes towards using a secure web-based portal designed to facilitate electronic communication with patients. *Informatics in Primary Care, 12*(3), 129–138. ·

Kluge, E. H. (1993). Advanced patient records: some ethical and legal considerations touching medical information space [see comment]. *Methods of Information in Medicine, 32*(2), 95–103.

Kneebone, R. (2005). Evaluating clinical simulation for learning procedural skills: A theory-based approach. *Academic Medicine, 80*(6), 549–553. doi:10.1097/00001888-200506000-00006

Kobb, R., Chumbler, N. R., Brennan, D. M., & Rabinowitz, T. (2008). Home telehealth: mainstreaming what we do well. *Telemed. J. E. Health, 14*, 977–981.

Koch, M., & Möslein, K. M. (2005). Identity Management for Ecommerce and Collaborative Applications. *International Journal of Electronic Commerce, 9*(3), 11–29.

Kokolakis, S., Gritzalis, D., & Katsikas, S. (1998). Generic security policies for healthcare information systems. *Health Informatics Journal, 4*(3-4), 184–195. doi:10.1177/146045829800400309

Kolb, T. M., Lichy, J., & Newhouse, J. H. (2002). Comparison of the Performance of Screening Mammography, Physical Examination, and Breast US and Evaluation of Factors that Influence Them: An Analysis of 27,825 Patient Evaluations. *Radiology, 225*(1), 165–175. doi:10.1148/radiol.2251011667

Koocher, G. P., & Morray, E. (2000). Regulation of Telepsychology: A survey of state attorneys general. *Professional Psychology, Research and Practice, 31*, 503–508. doi:10.1037/0735-7028.31.5.503

Kopans, D. B. (2007). *Breast imaging* (3rd ed.). Baltimore, MD: Lippincott Williams & Wilkins.

Koppel, R., & Kreda, D. (2009). Health care information technology vendors' "hold harmless" clause: Implications for clinicians. *Journal of the American Medical Association, 301*(12), 1276–1278. doi:10.1001/jama.2009.398

Koppel, R., Metlay, J. P., Cohen, A., Abaluck, B., Localio, R., Kimmel, S. E., & Strom, B. L. (2005). Role of computerized physician order entry systems in facilitating medication errors. *Journal of the American Medical Association, 293*(10), 1197–1203. doi:10.1001/jama.293.10.1197

Korhonen, I., Parkk, J., & Van Gils, M. (2003). Health Monitoring in the Home of the Future. *IEEE Engineering in Medicine and Biology Magazine, 22*(3), 66–73. doi:10.1109/MEMB.2003.1213628

Korp, P. (2006). Health on the Internet: implications for health promotion. *Health Education Research, 21*(1), 78–86. doi:10.1093/her/cyh043

Korthaus, A., & Hildenbrand, T. (2003). *Creating a Java- and CORBA-Based Enterprise Knowledge Grid Using Topic Maps.* Paper presented at the Workshop on Knowledge Grid and Grid Intelligence.

Krcmar, H., Arnold, Y., Daum, M., & Leimeister, J. M. (2002). Virtual communities in health care: the case of "krebsgemeinschaft.de". *SIGGROUP Bull., 23*(3), 18–23.

Krohn. M., Yip, A., Brodsky, M., Morris, R., & Walfish, M. (November 2007). *A world wide web without walls.* ACM Workshop on Hot Topics in Networks presentated at HotNets-VI, Atlanta, GA.

Krueger, M. W. (1991). *Artificial reality II.* New York: Addison-Wesley.

Kukafka, R. (2007). Guest Editorial: Public Health Informatics. *Journal of Biomedical Informatics, 40*, 365–369. doi:10.1016/j.jbi.2007.07.005

Kulma, M., & Springer, B. (2006). Easing the bottom-line impact of staffing shortages: A case study in shift bidding. *Healthcare Financial Management, 60*, 92–97.

Kumar, A., Quaglini, S., Stefanelli, M., Ciccarese, P., Caffi, E., & Boiocchi, L. (2002). A framework for representing and executing a clinical practice guideline for the management of high blood pressure in pregnancy. *Technology and Health Care, 10*(6), 517–519.

Kurtz, B., Fenwick, J., & Ellsworth, C. (2007). Using podcasts and tablet PCs in computer science. In *Proceedings of 45th ACM South East Conference* (pp. 484-489). Winston Salem, NC: ACM.

Kushniruk, A. W., & Borycki, E. M. (2006). Low-cost rapid usability engineering: Designing and customizing usable healthcare information systems. *Healthcare Quarterly (Toronto, Ont.), 9*(4), 98–100, 102.

Kushniruk, A. W., & Patel, V. L. (2004). Cognitive and usability engineering methods for the evaluation of clinical information systems. *Journal of Biomedical Informatics, 37*, 56–76. doi:10.1016/j.jbi.2004.01.003

Kushniruk, A. W., Borycki, E., Kuwata, S., & Kannry, J. (2006). Predicting changes in workflow resulting from healthcare information systems: Ensuring the safety of healthcare. *Healthcare Quarterly (Toronto, Ont.), 9*, 114–118.

Kushniruk, A. W., Kaufman, D. R., Patel, V. L., Levesque, Y., & Lottin, P. (1992). Assessment of a computerized patient record system: A cognitive approach to evaluating an emerging medical technology. *M.D. Computing, 13*(5), 406–415.

Kushniruk, A. W., Triola, M. M., Borycki, E. M., Stein, B., & Kannry, J. L. (2005). Technology induced error and usability: The relationship between usability problems and prescription errors when using a handheld application. *International Journal of Medical Informatics, 74,* 519–526. doi:10.1016/j.ijmedinf.2005.01.003

Kushniruk, A., & Patel, V. (2004). Cognitive and Usability Engineering Methods for the Evaluation of Clinical Information Systems. *Journal of Biomedical Informtics,* 56-76.

Kuwata, S., Kushniruk, A., Borycki, E., & Watanabe, H. (2006). Using simulation methods to analyze and predict changes in workflow and potential problems in the use of bar-coding medication order entry systems. *AMIA Annual Symposium Proceedings,* 994.

Kuziemsky, C. E., Borycki, E. M., Black, F., Boyle, M., Cloutier-Fisher, D., Fox, L., et al. (2007). A framework for interdisciplinary team communication and its implications for information systems design. wcmeb. *Eighth World Congress on the Management of eBusiness* (pp. 14).

Lacovara, J. E. (2008). When searching for the evidence, stop using Wikipedia! *Medsurg Nursing, 17*(3), 153.

Lam, T. P. (2005). *The origin of problem based learning. Medical Teacher, 27(5), 473.* Letter to the Editor.

Lamminaho, V. (2000). Metadata specification: Forms, Menus for Description of Courses and All Other Objects. CUBER project: Deliverable D3.1

Lammond, D., Crow, R., Chase, J., Doggen, K., & Sinkels, M. (1996). Information sources used in decision making: Considerations for simulation development. *International Journal of Nursing Studies, 33*(1), 47–57. doi:10.1016/0020-7489(95)00064-X

Lamson, R. J. (1997). *Virtual therapy.* Montreal, Canada: Polytechnic International Press.

Landau, S. (Ed.). (2003). Liberty ID-WSF and Privacy Overview, version 1.0, Liberty Alliance Project. Retrieved May 1, 2009, from http://www.projectliberty.org/liberty/resource_center/papers

Landi, F., Onder, G., Russo, A., Tabaccanti, S., Rollo, R., & Federici, S. (2001). A new model of integrated home care for the elderly: impact on hospital use. *Journal of*

Clinical Epidemiology, 54(9), 968–970. doi:10.1016/S0895-4356(01)00366-3

Langheinrich, M. (2001). Privacy by Design: Principles of Privacy-Aware Ubiquitous Systems. In *Ubicomp 2001.* Retrieved from http://www.vs.inf.ethz.ch/publ/papers/privacy-principles.pdf.

Langheinrich, M. (2002). A Privacy Awareness System for Ubiquitous Computing Environments. *Ubicomp (. LNCS, 2498,* 237–245.

Lapointe, L., & Rivard, S. (2005). Clinical information systems: Understanding and preventing their premature demise. *Healthcare Quarterly (Toronto, Ont.), 3*(4), 92–99.

Lapointe, L., & Rivard, S. (2006). Getting physicians to accept new information technology: Insights from case studies. *Canadian Medical Association Journal, 174*(11), 1573–1578. doi:10.1503/cmaj.050281

Lau, L. M., & Shakib, S. (2005). Towards Data Interoperability: Practical Issues in Terminology Implementation and Mappingof the HIC 2005. *Thirteenth National Health Informatics Conference* (pp. 208-213). Melbourne, Australia.

Laura, G. M. (2006, June). Social bookmarking, folksonomies, and Web 2.0 tools. *Searcher, 14*(6), 26-38. Retrieved March 22, 2009, from http://www.accessmylibrary.com/coms2/summary_0286-16124325_ITM

Le Bozec, C., Henin, D., Fabiani, B., Schrader, T., Garcia-Rojo, M., & Beckwith, B. (2007). Refining DICOM for pathology-progress from the IHE and DICOM pathology working groups. *Studies in Health Technology and Informatics, 129*(Pt 1), 434–438.

Ledbetter, C. S., & Morgan, M. W. (2001). Toward Best Practice: Leveraging the Electronic Patient Record as a Clinical Data Warehouse. *Journal of Healthcare Information Management, 15*(2). Retrieved May 1, 2009, from http://www.himss.org/content/files/jhim/15-2/him15205.pdf

Lee, K. M. (2004). Why Presence Occurs: Evolutionary Psychology, Media Equation, and Presence. *Presence (Cambridge, Mass.), 13*(4), 494–505. doi:10.1162/1054746041944830

Lee, Y., & Geller, J. (2006). Semantic enrichment for medical ontologies. *Journal of Biomedical Informatics, 39*(2), 209. doi:10.1016/j.jbi.2005.08.001

Lehmann, T., Güld, M., & Thies, C. (2003). *Content-based image retrieval in medical applications for picture archiving and communication systems.* Paper presented at the Medical Imaging.

Lehmann, T., Guld, M., Thies, C., Plodowski, B., Keysers, D., & Ott, B. (2004). *IRMA - Content-based image retrieval in medical applications.* Paper presented at the 14th World Congress on Medical Informatics.

Leif, R. C., & Leif, S. B. (1998). A DICOM Compatible Format for Analytical Cytology Data. In Farkas, D. L., Tromberg, B. J., & Leif, R. C. (Eds.), *Optical Diagnostics of Living Cells II, Advanced Techniques in Analytical Cytology. SPIE Proceedings Series* (*Vol. 3260*, pp. 282–289). A. Katzir Biomedical Optics Series.

Leijdekkers, P., Gay, V., & Lawrence, E. (2007). *Smart Homecare System for Health Tele-monitoring.* Paper presented at the Digital Society, 2007. ICDS '07. First International Conference on the.

Leimeister, J. M., Daum, M., & Krcmar, H. (2002). *Mobile Communication and Computing in Healthcare: Designing and Implementing Mobile Virtual Communities for Cancer Patients.* Paper presented at the Tokyo Mobile Business Roundtable.

Leimeister, J. M., Daum, M., & Krcmar, H. (2003). *Towards m-communities: the case of COSMOS healthcare.* Paper presented at the The 36th Annual Hawaii International Conference on System Sciences.

Leonard, K. (2009, January 30). *One Patient, One Record (OPOR).* Retrieved April 29, 2009, from Patient Destiny: http://patientdestiny.typepad.com

Leonard, K. J. W., D., & Casselman, M. (2008a). An Innovative Information Paradigm for Consumers with Chronic Conditions: The value proposition. The Journal on Information Technology in Healthcare.

Leonard, K. J., & Wiljer, D. (2007). Patients Are Destined to Manage Their Care. *Healthcare Quarterly (Toronto, Ont.), 10*(3), 76–78.

Leonard, K. J., Casselman, M., & Wiljer, D. (2008). Who will demand access to their personal health record? A focus on the users of health services and what they want. *Healthcare Quarterly (Toronto, Ont.), 11*(1), 92–96.

Leonard, K., Wiljer, D., & Urowitz, S. (2008). Yes Virginia, There Are System Benefits to be Gained from Providing Patients Access to Their Own Health Information. *Healthcare Quarterly (Toronto, Ont.), 11*(4), 66–70.

Lepine, J. P., Gastpar, M., Mendlewicz, J., & Tylee, A. (1997). Depression in the community: the first pan-European study DEPRES (Depression Research in European Society). *International Clinical Psychopharmacology, 12*, 19–29.

Levenson, N. (1995). *Safeware: System safety and computers.* Reading, Massachusetts: Addison-Wesley.

Levine, L. A. (2006). Introduction to RIS and PACS. In Dreyer, K. J., Hirschorn, D. S., Thrall, J. H., & Mehta, A. (Eds.), *PACS. A guide to the digital revolution* (2nd ed., pp. 27–44). New York: Springer.

Lhotská, L., Aubrecht, P., Valls, A., & Gibert, K. (2008). Security recommendations for implementation in distributed healthcare systems. In M. Klima (Ed.), *Proc. of the 42th IEEE Int. Carnahan Conference on Security Technology (IEEE ICCST 08)* (pp. 76-83). Prague, Czech Republic.

Li, J., & Shaw, M. (2004). Protection of Health Information in Data Mining. *International Journal of Healthcare Technology and Management, 6*(2), 210–222. doi:10.1504/IJHTM.2004.004977

Li, Q., Li, F., Shiraishi, J., Katsuragawa, S., Sone, S., & Doi, K. (2003). Investigation of new psychophysical measures for evaluation of similar images on thoracic CT for distinction between benign and malignant nodules. *Medical Physics, 30*, 2584–2593. doi:10.1118/1.1605351

Lin, E. H., Von, K. M., Katon, W., Bush, T., Simon, G. E., & Walker, E. (1995). The role of the primary care physician in patients' adherence to antidepressant therapy. *Medical Care, 33*, 67–74. doi:10.1097/00005650-199501000-00006

Lin, G., Dasmalchi, G., & Zhu, J. (2008, September). *Cloud Computing and IT as a Service: Opportunities and Challenges.* Paper presented at ICWS '08. IEEE International Conference on Web Services, 5 – 5.

Lin, H., Davis, J., & Zhou, Y. (2009). *An Integrated Approach to Extracting Ontological Structures from Folksonomies.* Presented at 6th Annual European Semantic Web Conference (ESWC2009)

Lin, J. C. (1999) Applying telecommunication technology to health-care delivery. *Engineering in Medicine and Biology Magazine, IEEE*, 28-31. Retrieved November 9, 2008 from http://ieeexplore.ieee.org/xpls/abs_all.jsp?arnumber=775486

Lindberg, D., Humphreys, B., & McCray, A. (1993). The Unified Medical Language System. *Methods of Information in Medicine, 34*, 281–291.

Linden Lab. (2008). *Second Life – Economy Stats 11/2008.* Retrieved February 28, 2009 from http://static.secondlife.com/economy/stats_200811.xls

Linden Lab. (2009). *Second Life Economic* Statistics. Retrieved February 28, 2009 from http://secondlife.com/statistics/economy-data.php

Linden Lab. (2009). *Second Life System Requirements.* Retrieved February 28, 2009 from http://secondlife.com/support/sysreqs.php

Linden Lab. (2009). *What is Second Life?* Retrieved February 28, 2009 from http://secondlife.com/whatis/

Lintonen, T. P., Konu, A. I., & Seedhouse, D. (2008). Information technology in health promotion. *Health Education Research, 23*(3), 560–566. doi:10.1093/her/cym001

Lipnack, J., & Stamps, J. (2000). *VIRTUAL TEAMS: People Working Across Boundaries with Technology* (2nd ed.). New York: John Wiley & Sons.

Lisac, M., Blum, K., & Schlette, S. (2008). Health Systems and Health Reform in Europe. *Inter Economics, 43*(4), 184–218. doi:10.1007/s10272-008-0253-z

Liu, C. (2006, August). *Second Life Learning Community: A Peer-Based Approach to Involving More Faculty Members in Second Life.* Paper presented at the meeting of the Second Life Educator's Communities Conference, San Fransisco, CA.

Liu, X., Hui, Y., Sun, W., & Liang, H. (2007). Towards Service Composition Based on Mashup. *IEEE Congress on Services (SERVICES 2007).*

Liu, Y., Lazar, N., & Rothfus, W. (2002). *Semantic-based Biomedical Image Indexing and Retrieval.* Paper presented at the *Int'l Conf. on Diagnositc Imaging and Analysis.*

Live. (2006). *Introduction to Windows Live ID, Windows Live Development Center.* Retrieved May 1, 2009, from http://msdn.microsoft.com/en-us/library/bb288408.aspx

LOM. (2004). *Learning Object Metadata.* Retrieved April 22, 2009, from, http://ltsc.ieee.org/wg12/

Longo, F. (2007). Implementing managerial innovations in primary care: Can we rank change drivers in complex adaptive organizations? *Health Care Management Review, 32*(3), 213–225.

Lopes, H. S., Coutinho, M. S., & Lima, W. C. (1998). An evolutionary approach to simulate cognitive feedback learning in medical domain. In Sanchez, E., Shibata, T., & Zadeh, L. A. (Eds.), *Genetic Algorithms and Fuzzy Logic Systems: Soft Computing Perspectives* (pp. 193–207). Singapore: World Scientific.

Lopez Osornio, A., Luna, D., Gambarte, M. L., Gomez, A., Reynoso, G., & Gonzalez Bernaldo de Quiros, F. (2007). Creation of a Local Interface Terminology to SNOMED CT. In K.A. Kuhn, J.R. Warren, T.Y. Leong (Eds.), *Medinfo 2007: Proceedings of the 12th World Congress on Health (Medical) Informatics; Building Sustainable Health Systems* (pp. 765-769). Amsterdam: IOS Press.

Lopez, D. M., & Blobel, B. (2009). Enhanced semantic interoperability by profiling health informatics standards. *Methods of Information in Medicine, 48*, 170–177.

Lorig, K. R., Sobel, D. S., Ritter, P. L., Laurent, D., & Hobbs, M. (2001). Effect of a self-management program on patients with chronic disease. *Effective Clinical Practice, 4*(6), 256–262.

Lu, S., Dong, M., & Fotouhi, F. (2002). The Semantic Web: opportunities and challenges for next-generation Web applications. *Information Research, 7*(4), 7–4.

Ludwick, D. A., & Doucette, J. (2009). Primary Care Physicians' Experience with Electronic Medical Records: Barriers to Implementation in a Fee-for-Service Environment. *Int. J. Telemed. Appl., 2009*, 853524.

Ludwick, D. A., & Doucette, J. (2009). The implementation of operational processes for Alberta Electronic Health Record: Lessons for Electronic Medical Record Adoption in primary care. *Healthcare Quarterly (Toronto, Ont.), 7*(4), 103–107.

Luiz Olavo Bonino da Silva, S., Renata, S. S. G., & Marten van, S. (2005). *Agent-oriented context-aware platforms supporting communities of practice in health care.* Paper presented at the The fourth international joint conference on Autonomous agents and multiagent systems, The Netherlands.

Lukasiewicz, T., & Straccia, U. (2008). Managing uncertainty and vagueness in description logics for the Semantic Web. *Web Semantics: Science. Services and Agents on the World Wide Web, 6*(4), 291–308. doi:10.1016/j.websem.2008.04.001

Madden, M., & Fox, S. (2005). *Finding answers online in sickness and in health.* Washington, DC: Pew Internet and American Life Project.

Maheu, M. M., Whitten, P., & Allen, A. (2001). *E-Health, Telehealth, and Telemedicine.* John Wiley and Sons.

Malich, A., Fischer, D. R., & Bottcher, J. (2006). CAD for mammography: the technique, results, current role and further developments. *European Radiology, 16*(7), 1449–1460. doi:10.1007/s00330-005-0089-x

Malik, S. S., Qureshi, N. A., Ali, A., Ahmad, H. F., & Suguri, H. (2005). *Inter platform agent mobility in FIPA compliant multi-agent systems.* Paper presented at the 2005 International Conference on Active Media Technology (AMT 2005).

Maloney-Krichmar, D. (2002). *An ethnographic study of an online, mutual-aid health community: group dynamics, roles, and relationships.* Paper presented at the CHI '02 extended abstracts on Human factors in computing systems, Minneapolis, Minnesota, USA.

Maloney-Krichmar, D., & Preece, J. (2005). A multi-level analysis of sociability, usability, and community dynamics in an online health community. *ACM Transactions on Computer-Human Interaction, 12*(2), 201–232. doi:10.1145/1067860.1067864

Mamlin, B. W., Biondich, P. G., Wolfe, B. A., Fraser, H., Jazayeri, D., Allen, C., et al. (2006). Cooking up an open source EMR for developing countries: OpenMRS – a recipe for successful collaboration. *AMIA 2006 Symposium Proceedings* (pp. 529-533).

Manhattan Research Group. (2007). White Paper: Physicians and Web 2.0: 5 Things You Should Know about the Evolving Online Landscape for Physicians. Retrieved March 6, 2009, from http://www.manhattanresearch.com/TTPWhitePaper.aspx

Manhattan Research. (n.d.). *Cybercitizen Health v8.0.* Retrieved January 7, 2009, from http://www.manhattanresearch.com/products/Strategic_Advisory/CCH/default.aspx.

Manning, M., Aggarwal, A., Gao, K., & Tucker-Kellogg, G. (2009). Scaling the walls of discovery: using semantic metadata for integrative problem solving. *Briefings in Bioinformatics, 10*(2), 164–176. doi:10.1093/bib/bbp007

Mannino, D. M., Homa, D. M., Akinbami, L. J., Moorman, J. E., Gwynn, C., & Redd, S. C. (2002). Surveillance for asthma, United States, 1980-1999.

Maret, P., Hammoud, M., & Calmet, J. (2004). *Muti Agent Based Virtual Knowledge Communities for Distributed Knowledge Management.* Paper presented at the International Workshop on Engineering Societies in the Agents World (ESAW), Toulouse, France.

Markle Foundation. (2006, December). Americans see access to their medical information as a way to improve quality, reduce health care costs. News release. Retrieved October 13, 2008, from http://www.markle.org/downloadable_assets/news_release_120706.pdf.

Markle Foundation. (2006, December). *Connecting Americans to Their Health Care: A Common Framework for Networked Personal Health Information.* Retrieved November 8, 2008, from http://www.connectingforhealth.org/commonframework/docs/P9_NetworkedPHRs.pdf.

Markle Foundation. (2006, November). Survey finds Americans want electronic personal health information to improve own health care. News release. Retrieved July 3, 2008, from http://www.markle.org/downloadable_assets/research_doc_120706.pdf.

Markle. (2003). Connecting for Health: A Public-Private Collaborative. http://www.connectingforhealth.org/resources/final_phwg_report1.pdf. Accessed: 2008-09-22. (Archived by WebCite® at http://www.webcitation.org/5b24kHscL).

Marks, E. A. (2006). *Service-oriented architecture: a planning and implementation guide for business and technology / Eric A. Marks, Michael Bell.* Hoboken, NJ: Wiley.

Marks, J. S. (2008). *Targeting Arthritis: Improving Quality of Life for More Than 46 Million Americans. Centers for Disease Control and Prevention.* CDC.

Marmor, T., Oberlander, J., & White, J. (2009). The Obama Administration's Options for Health Care Cost Control: Hope Versus Reality. *Annals of Internal Medicine, 150*, 485–489.

Martin Moreno, J., Ruiz Fernandez, D., Soriano Paya, A., & Berenguer Miralles, V. J. (2008). *Monitoring 3D movements for the rehabilitation of joints in physiotherapy.* Paper presented at the 30th Annual International Conference of the IEEE Engineering in Medicine and Biology Society.

Martin, D., Burstein, M., Hobbs, J., Lassila, O., McDermott, D., McIlraith, S., et al. (2004). Semantic Markup for Web Services. *OWL-S.* Retrieved June 5, 2009, from http://www.w3.org/Submission/OWL-S/

Marton, F., Dahlgren, L.-O., Svensson, L., & Saljo, R. (1977). Inlarning och omvarldsuppfattning. Stockholm, Sweden: Almqvist och Wiksell forlag AB.

Mason, H., & Moutahir, M. (2006, August). *Multidisciplinary Experiential Education in Second Life: A Global Approach.* Paper presented at the meeting of the Second Life Educator's Communities Conference, San Francisco, CA.

Mathews, S. (1998). Protection of personal data--the European view. *Journal of American Health Information Management Association, 69*(3), 42–44.

Mattocks, E. (2009) Managing Medical Ontologies using OWL and an e-business Registry / Repository. Retrieved April 22, 2009, from, http://www.gca.org/xmlusa/2004/slides/mattocks&dogac/Mattocks%20-%20Managing%20Medical%20Ontologies%20using%20OWL%20and%20an%20e-business%20Registry%20%20Repository.ppt

Mayer, M. A., Karkaletsis, V., Stamatakis, K., Leis, A., Villarroel, D., & Thomeczek, C. (2006). MedIEQ–Quality Labelling of Medical Web Content Using Multilingual Information Extraction. *Press Medical and Care Compunetics, 3*, 183–190.

McAfee, A. (2006). Enterprise 2.0: The dawn of emergent collaboration. *MIT Sloan Management Review, 47*(3), 21–28.

McArthur, V. (2008). Real ethics in a virtual world. *Conference on Human Factors in Computing (CHI) Proceedings* (pp. 3315-3320).

McDaniel, A., Schutte, D., & Keller, L. (2008). Consumer Health Informatics: from Genomics to Population Health. *Nursing Outlook*, 216–223. doi:10.1016/j.outlook.2008.06.006

McDonald, C. J., Huff, S. M., Suico, J. G., Hill, G., Leavelle, D., & Aller, R. (2003). LOINC, a Universal Standard for Identifying Laboratory Observations: A 5-Year Update. *Clinical Chemistry, 49*(4), 624–633. doi:10.1373/49.4.624

McDonald, C. J., Schadow, G., Barnes, M., Dexter, P., Overhage, J. M., Mamlin, B., & McCoy, J. M. (2003). Open source software in medical informatics – why, how and what. *International Journal of Medical Informatics, 69*, 175–184. doi:10.1016/S1386-5056(02)00104-1

McGee, J. B., & Begg, M. (2008). What medical educators need to know about "Web 2.0". *Medical Teacher, 30*(2), 164–169. doi:10.1080/01421590701881673

McGee, M. K. (2006, December 13). Insurers push patients toward e-health records. *InformationWeek*. Retrieved December 19, 2008, from http://www.informationweek.com/story/showArticle.jhtml?articleID=196603941.

McGinty, K. L., Saeed, S. A., Simmons, S. C., & Yildirim, Y. (2006). Telepsychiatry and e-Mental Health Services: Potential for Improving Access to Mental Health Care. *The Psychiatric Quarterly, 77*(4), 335–342. doi:10.1007/s11126-006-9019-6

McGraw, D., Dempsey, J. X., Harris, L., & Goldman, J. (2009). Privacy As An Enabler, Not An Impediment: Building Trust Into Health Information Exchange. *Health Affairs, 28*, 416–427. doi:10.1377/hlthaff.28.2.416

McGuinness, D. L., Fikes, R., Hendler, J., & Stein, L. A. (2002). DAML+OIL: an ontology language for the Semantic Web. *Intelligent Systems, IEEE, 17*(5), 72. doi:10.1109/MIS.2002.1039835

McIlraith, S. A., Son, T. C., & Honglei, Z. (2001). Semantic Web services. *Intelligent Systems, IEEE, 16*(2), 46. doi:10.1109/5254.920599

McLaughlin, C. P., & Kaluzny, A. D. (2006). *Continuous quality improvement in healthcare: Theory, implementations and applications* (3rd ed.). Toronto: Jones and Bartlett.

McLean, R., Richards, B. H., & Wardman, J. I. (2007). The effect of Web 2.0 on the future of medical practice and education: Darwikinian evolution or folksonomic revolution? *The Medical Journal of Australia, 187*(3), 174–177.

Medicine 2.0. (2009). *Medicine 2.0*. Retrieved April 29, 2009, from Medicine 2.0 2009: http://www.medicine-20congress.com

Meersman, D., Scheunders, P., & Van Dyck, D. (1998). *Classification of microcalcifications using texture-based features*. Paper presented at the 4th International Workshop on Digital Mammography.

Meglič, M. (2007, September). *Care management using BPM: case of depression*. Paper presented at EFMI Special Topic Conference on Open Source in Health care, London, United Kingdom.

Menezes, A. M. B., Perez-Padilla, R., Jardim, J. R. B., Muino, A., Lopez, M. V., Valdivia, G., et al. (2005). Chronic obstructive pulmonary disease in five Latin American cities (the PLATINO study): a prevalence study. *The Lancet, 366*(9500), 1875(1877).

Merali, Y., & Davies, J. (2001). *Knowledge capture and utilization in virtual communities*. Paper presented at the Proceedings of the 1st international conference on Knowledge capture.

MetaMap. (2009). *Meta Map Portal*. Retrieved April 22, 2009, from http://metamap.nlm.nih.gov/

Meuser, J., Bean, T., Goldman, J., & Reeves, S. (2006). Family health teams: A new Canadian interprofessional initiative. *Journal of Interprofessional Care, 20*(4), 436–428. doi:10.1080/13561820600874726

Michael, J. (2006). Where's the evidence that active learning works? *Advances in Physiology Education, 30*(4), 159–167. doi:10.1152/advan.00053.2006

Michlmayr, E. (2005). A Case Study on Emergent Semantics in Communities. In *Workshop on Social Network Analysis, International Semantic Web Conference.*

Mika, P., & Tummarello, G. (2008). Web Semantics in the Clouds. *Intelligent Systems. IEEE, 23*(5), 82–87. doi:10.1109/MIS.2008.94

Miller, G. (2007). The promise of parallel universes. *Science, 317*(5843), 1341–1343. doi:10.1126/science.317.5843.1341

Miller, T. W., Kraus, R. F., Kaak, O., Sprang, R., & Burton, D. (2002). Telemedicine: a child psychiatry case report. *Telemedicine Journal and e-Health, 8*(1), 139–141. doi:10.1089/15305620252933482

Mingers, J. (1986). Expert Systems-Experiments with Rule Induction. *The Journal of the Operational Research Society, 37*(11), 1031–1037.

Ministry of Health and Long-Term Care. (n.d.). *Ontario Wait Times.* Retrieved April 12, 2009, from Government of Ontario: http://www.health.gov.on.ca/transformation/wait_times/wait_mn.html

Mitchell, P. (1998). France gets smart with health a la carte. *Lancet, 351*(9104), 7. doi:10.1016/S0140-6736(05)78518-4

Mitchell, R., Agle, B., & Wood, D. (1997). Towards a theory of stakeholder identification and salience. *Academy of Management Review, 22*(4), 853–887. doi:10.2307/259247

Mitra, S. K., Lee, T.-W., & Goldbaum, M. (2005). A Bayesian network based sequential inference for diagnosis of diseases from retinal images. *Pattern Recognition Letters, 26*(4), 459–470. doi:10.1016/j.patrec.2004.08.010

Mohan, C. (1997). *Recent Trends in Workflow Management Products, Standards and Research* (pp. 396–409). Workflow Management Systems and Interoperability.

Mohan, J. (1995). *A National Health Service?: The Restructuring of Health Care in Britain Since 1979.* St. Martin's Press.

Mohanty, S. K., Mistry, A. T., Amin, W., Parwani, A. V., Pople, A. K., Schmandt, L., et al. (2008). The development and deployment of Common Data Elements for tissue banks for translational research in cancer - an emerging standard based approach for the Mesothelioma Virtual Tissue Bank. *BMC Cancer, 8,* 91. Retrieved February 16, 2009, from http://www.biomedcentral.com/1471-2407/8/91

Moreno, A., & Garbay, C. (2003). Software agents in health care. *Artificial Intelligence in Medicine, 27*(3), 229–232. doi:10.1016/S0933-3657(03)00004-6

Moreno, A., & Isern, D. (2002). *A first step towards providing health-care agent-based services to mobile users.* Paper presented at the first international joint conference on Autonomous agents and multiagent systems: part 2, Bologna, Italy.

Moreno, A., & Nealon, J. L. (Eds.). (2003). *Applications of Software Agent Technology in the Health Care Domain.* Springer.

Mortensen, E. (1985). Trends in electronic Mail and its role in office automation. *Electronic Publishing Review, 5*(4), 257–268.

Müller, H., Michoux, N., Bandon, D., & Geissbuhler, A. (2004). A review of content-based image retrieval systems in medical applications-clinical benefits and future directions. *International Journal of Medical Informatics, 73*(1), 1–23. doi:10.1016/j.ijmedinf.2003.11.024

Mukherjee, A., & McGinnis, J. (2007). E-healthcare: an analysis of key themes in research. *International Journal of Pharmaceutical and Healthcare Marketing, 1*(4), 349–363. doi:10.1108/17506120710840170

Muller, H., Rosset, A., Garcia, A., Vallee, J. P., & Geissbuhler, A. (2005). Informatics in radiology (infoRAD): benefits of content-based visual data access in radiology. *Radiographics, 25*(3), 849–858. doi:10.1148/rg.253045071

Muller, H., Rosset, A., Vallee, J., & Geissbuhler, A. (2004). *Comparing features sets for content-based image retrieval in a medical-case database.* Paper presented at the *PACS and Imaging Informatics*

Muneera, S. U. (2006). *Graphic Design: Collaborative Processes = Understanding Self and Others, Art 325: Collaborative Processes.* Corvallis, Oregon: Fairbanks Hall, Oregon State University.

Muramatsu, C., Li, Q., Schmidt, R., Suzuki, K., Shiraishi, J., & Newstead, G. (2006). Experimental determination of subjective similarity for pairs of clustered microcalcifications on mammograms: observer study results. *Medical Physics, 33*(9), 3460–3468. doi:10.1118/1.2266280

Muramatsu, C., Li, Q., Suzuki, K., Schmidt, R. A., Shiraishi, J., & Newstead, G. M. (2005). Investigation of psychophysical measure for evaluation of similar images for mammographic masses: preliminary results. *Medical Physics, 32*(7), 2295–2304. doi:10.1118/1.1944913

Murch, R. (2004). *Autonomic Computing*. Prentice Hall.

Murray, C. J. L., & Frenk, J. (2000). A framework for assessing the performance of health systems. *Bulletin of the World Health Organization, 78*(6), 717–731.

Murray, C. J. L., Salomon, J. A., & Mathers, C. D. (2000). A critical examination of summary measures of population health. *Bulletin of the World Health Organization, 78*(8), 981–994.

Murray, E., Burns, J., Tai, S., Lai, R., & Nazareth, J. (2005). *Interactive Health Communication Applications for People with Chronic Disease*. Oxford: Cochrane Collboration.

Mushlin, A. I., Kouides, R. W., & Shapiro, D. E. (1998). Estimating the accuracy of screening mammography: a meta-analysis. *American Journal of Preventive Medicine, 14*(2), 143–153. doi:10.1016/S0749-3797(97)00019-6

Musser, J. (2006, Fall). *Web 2.0 Principles and Best Practices*. Retrieved April 24, 2009, from O'Reilly Radar: http://oreilly.com/catalog/web2report/chapter/web20_report_excerpt.pdf

Myerson, S. G., & Mitchell, A. R. (2003). Mobile phones in hospitals. *BMJ (Clinical Research Ed.), 326*(7387), 460–461. doi:10.1136/bmj.326.7387.460

Nagy, P. G. (2007). The future of PACS. *Medical Physics, 34*(7), 2676–2682. doi:10.1118/1.2743097

Najjar, J., Ternier, S., & Duval, E. (2003). The Actual Use of Metadata in ARIADNE: an Empirical Analysis. *3rd Annual Ariadne Conference*, K.U.Leuven, Leuven, Belgium.

Nakayama, R., Uchiyama, Y., Hatsukade, I., Yamamoto, K., Watanabe, R., & Namba, K. (1999). Discrimination of malignant and benign microcalcification clusters on mammograms. *J Comp Aid Diag Med Imag, 3*, 1–7.

Narayan, K. M. V., Boyle, J. P., Thompson, T. J., Sorensen, S. W., & Williamson, D. F. (2003). [JAMA]. *Lifetime Risk for Diabetes Mellitus in the United States The Journal of the American Medical Association, 290*, 1884–1890.

National Institute of Standards and Technology. (2001, November 26). *Federal Information Processing Standards (FIPS) Publication 197, Advanced Encryption Standard (AES)*.

National Library of Medicine Board of Regents. (2006, September). Charting a Course for the 21st Century: NLM's [from http://www.nlm.nih.gov/pubs/plan/lrp-docs.html.]. *Long Range Planning*, 2006–2016. Retrieved November 5, 2008.

National Library of Medicine. (n.d.). *Unified Medical Language System Web site*. Retrieved January 11, 2009, from http://www.nlm.nih.gov/research/umls/umlsmain.html.

National Research Council. (1999). *How people learn*. Washington, DC: National Academy Press.

Nealon, J. L., & Moreno, A. (2003). Agent-Based Applications in Health Care. In Nealon, J. L., & Moreno, A. (Eds.), *Applications of Software Agent Technology in the Health Care Domain* (pp. 3–18). Basel, Switzerland: Birkhäuser Verlag.

Neame, R. L., & Olson, M. (1996). Measures implemented to protect personal privacy for an on-line national patient index: a case study. *Topics in Health Information Management, 17*(2), 18–25.

Nelson, E. L., Barnard, M., & Cain, S. (2003). Treating childhood depression over videoconferencing. *Telemedicine Journal and e-Health, 9*(1), 49–55. doi:10.1089/153056203763317648

NetworkedPlanet. (2005). Topic Maps in Web-site Architecture.

Neuhauser, L., & Kreps, G. L. (2003). Rethinking communication in the e-health era. *Journal of Health Psychology, 8*(1), 7–22. doi:10.1177/1359105303008001426

Neumeyer-Gromen, A., Lampert, T., Stark, K., & Kallischnigg, G. (2004). Disease management programs for depression: a systematic review and meta-analysis of randomized controlled trials. *Medical Care, 42*, 1211–1221. doi:10.1097/00005650-200412000-00008

New Media Consortium. (2008, May). *Spring 2007 Survey Educators in Second Life*. [Online].

Newcomb, S., & Durusau, P. (August 2005). *Multiple Subject Map Patterns for Relationships and TMDM Information Items*. Paper presented at the Extreme Markup Languages 2005, Montréal, Canada.

Newsroom, F. A. O. (2004). Retrieved March 10, 2009, from http://www.fao.org/english/newsroom/news/2003/26919-en.html

Niblack, W., Barber, R., Equitz, W., Flickner, M., Glasman, E., & Petkovic, D. (1993). The QBIC project: Querying images by content using color, texture, and shape. *SPIE Proc. on Storage and Retrieval for Image and Video Databases, 1908*, 137–146.

NISO. (2004). Understanding Metadata Retrieved June 5, 2009, from http://www.niso.org/standards/resources/UnderstandingMetadata.pdf

No Surrender. (n.d.). Retrieved April 12, 2009, from No Surrender Charitable Trust: http://www.no-surrender. org

Norman, G. J., Zabinski, M. F., Adams, M. A., Rosenberg, D. E., Yaroch, A. L., & Atienza, A. A. (2007). A review of eHealth interventions for physical activity and dietary behavior change. *American Journal of Preventive Medicine, 33*, 336–345. doi:10.1016/j.amepre.2007.05.007

Novak, P., & Dix, J. (2006). *Modular BDI architecture.* Paper presented at the 5th International Conference on Autonomous Agents.

Nugent, C. D., Wang, H., Black, N. D., Finlay, D. D., & Owens, F. J. (2006). ECG Telecare: Past, present and future. In Istepanian, R. S. H., Laxminarayan, S., & Pattichis, C. S. (Eds.), *M-Health. Emerging Mobile Health Systems* (pp. 375–388). Springer.

O'Connor, A., Stacey, D., Entwistle, V., Llewellyn-Thomas, H., Rovner, D., Holmes-Rovner, M., et al. (2002). Decision aids for people facing health treatment or screening decisions. (Publication no. 10.1002/14651858. CD001431).

O'Connor, M. (2006). A review of factors affecting individual performance in team environments. *Library Management, 27*(3), 135–143. doi:10.1108/01435120610652888

O'Grady, L., Witteman, H., Bender, J. L., Urowitz, S., Wiljer, D., & Jadad, A. R. (2009). Measuring the Impact of a Moving Target: Towards a Dynamic Framework for Evaluating Collaborative Adaptive Interactive Technologies. *Journal of Medical Internet Research, 11*(2), e20. doi:10.2196/jmir.1058

O'Malley, D. P. (2008). Practical Applications of Telepathology Using Morphology-Based Anatomic Pathology. *Archives of Pathology & Laboratory Medicine, 132*(5), 743–744.

O'Reilly, T. (2005). *What is Web 2.0: Design patterns and business models for the next generation of software.* Retrieved February 1, 2008, from http://www.oreillynet. com/pub/a/oreilly/tim/news/2005/09/30/what-is-web-20. html

O'Sullivan, T., & Studdert, R. (2005). *Agent technology and reconfigurable computing for mobile devices.* Paper presented at the 2005 ACM symposium on Applied computing, Santa Fe, New Mexico.

Odlyzko, A., & Tilly, B. (2005). *A refutation of Metcalfe's Law and a better estimate for the value of networks and network interconnections.* Minneapolis, Minnesota, USA: University of Minnesota.

Oh, H., Rizo, C., Enkin, M., & Jadad, A. (2005). What Is eHealth (3): A Systematic Review of Published Definitions. *Journal of Medical Internet Research, 7*(1), e1. Retrieved March 7, 2009, from http://www.jmir. org/2005/1/e1/

Ohler, J. (2008). The semantic web in education. *EDUCAUSE Quarterly, 31*(4), 7–9.

Olariu, S., Maly, K., Foudriat, E. C., & Yamany, S. M. (2004). Wireless support for telemedicine in disaster management. *Tenth International Conference on Parallel and Distributed Systems* (pp. 649-656).

Omar, W., & Taleb-Bendiab, A. (2006). E-Health Support Services Based On Service Oriented Architecture. *IEEE IT Professional, 8*(2), 35–41. doi:10.1109/ MITP.2006.32

Omar, W., Ahmad, B., & Karam, Y. (2006). Autonomic Middleware Services for Just-In-Time

Omar, W., Ahmad, B., & Taleb-Bendiab, A. (2006). *Grid Overlay for Remote E-Health Monitoring.* Paper presented at the The 4th ACS/IEEE International Conference on Computer Systems and Applications (AICCSA-06).

Omar, W., Ahmad, B., Taleb-Bendiab, A., & Karam, Y. (2005, 24-28, May). *A Software Framework for Open Standard Self-Managing Sensor Overlay For Web Services.* Paper presented at the 7th International Conference on Enterprise Information Systems (ICEIS2005), MIAMI BEACH- FLORIDA-USA.

Omar, W., Taleb-Bendiab, A., & Karam, Y. (2005, 19-21, September). *PlanetLab Overlay: Experimenting With Sensing and Actuation Support For Situated Autonomic Computing Services For The Planetary- Scale System.* Paper presented at the iiWAS, Malaysia.

Omar, W., Taleb-Bendiab, A., & Karam, Y. (2005, 27-28, June). *PlanetLab Overlay: Experimenting with Sensing and Actuation Support for Situated Autonomic Computing Services.* Paper presented at the 6th PG net2005 conference, Liverpool, UK.

Omar, W., Taleb-Bendiab, A., & Karam, Y. (2006). Autonomic Middleware Services for Just-In-Time Grid Services Provisioning. *Journal of Computer Sciences, 6*(2), 521–527.

Omnimedix Institute. (2008, December 11). *Major U.S. employers join to provide lifelong personal health records for employees; independent system will give individuals access to complete medical information whenever and wherever they need it.* Press release. December 6,

2006. Retrieved December 11, 2008, from http://www.omnimedix.org/pr_2006.12.06.html.

OpenEHR. (2009). *The openEHR Foundation.* Retrieved May 1, 2009, from http://www.openehr.org/shared-resources/getting_started/openehr_primer.html

OpenSSO. (2009). *Sun OpenSSO.* Retrieved May 1, 2009, from http://www.sun.com/software/products/opensso_enterprise/index.xml

Oracle (1997). *Oracle Mobile Agents Technical Product Summary.* Retrieved from www.oracle.com/products/networking/mobile/agents/html

Orchard, M., Green, E., Sullivan, T., Greenberg, A., & Mai, V. (2008). Chronic disease prevention and management: implications for health human resources in 2020. *Healthcare Quarterly (Toronto, Ont.), 11*(1), 38–43.

Orlikowski, W. J. (1992). The duality of technology: Rethinking the concept of technology in organizations. *Organization Science, 3*(3), 398–427. doi:10.1287/orsc.3.3.398

OSCAR. (n.d.). *Welcome to OSCAR Canada Users Society.* Retrieved May 17, 2009, from OSCAR: http://www.oscarcanada.org/

Ossowski, S. (2008). *Coordination and Agreement in Multi-Agent Systems.* Paper presented at the Cooperative Information Agents,12th International Workshop.

Otero, F. E. B., Silva, M. M. S., Freitas, A. A., & Nievola, J. C. (2003). Genetic Programming for Attribute Construction in Data Mining. In *Genetic Programming* (pp. 384–393). Berlin, Heidelberg: Springer. doi:10.1007/3-540-36599-0_36

Øvretveit, J. (1998). *Evaluating health interventions.* London: Open University Press.

OWL. (2003). *WEB Ontology Language.* Retrieved April 22, 2009, from http://www.w3.org/TR/owl-ref/

Ozbolt, J. (2000). Terminology Standards for Nursing: Collaboration at the Summit. *Journal of the American Medical Informatics Association, 7*(6), 517–522.

Padgham, L., & Lambrix, P. (2005). Formalisations of Capabilities for BDI-Agents. *Autonomous Agetns and Multi-agent Systems, 10*(3), 249–271. doi:10.1007/s10458-004-4345-2

Page, J., Zaslavsky, A., & Indrawan, M. (2004). *A buddy model of security for mobile agent communities operating in pervasive scenarios.* Paper presented at the second workshop on Australasian information security, Data Mining and Web Intelligence, and Software Internationalisation - Volume 32, Dunedin, New Zealand.

Paindaveine, S. N. a. Y. (2002). *HealthGrid Terms of Reference.*

Pallapa, G., & Das, S. (2007). *Resource Discovery in Ubiquitous Health Care.* Paper presented at the Advanced Information Networking and Applications Workshops

Pampallona, S., Bollini, P., Tibaldi, G., Kupelnick, B., & Munizza, C. (2002). Patient adherence in the treatment of depression. *The British Journal of Psychiatry, 180,* 104–109. doi:10.1192/bjp.180.2.104

Panteli, N. (2003). *DITIS: An eHealth Mobile Application in Cyprus. A user's Perspective.* May, Internal DITIS report. Retrieved from http://www.ditis.ucy.ac.cy/publications/internalreports.htm

Panteli, N., & Dibben, M. R. (2001). Reflections on Mobile communication systems. *Futures, 33*(5), 379–391. doi:10.1016/S0016-3287(00)00081-1

Panteli, N., Pitsillides, B., Pitsillides, A., & Samaras, G. (2006). An E-healthcare Mobile application: A Stakeholders' analysis. In Al-Hakim, L. (Ed.), *Web Mobile-Based Applications for Healthcare Management.* Hershey, PA: IGI Global.

Papaioakeim, M., Kaldoudi, E., Vargemezis, V., & Simopoulos, K. (2006). Confronting the problem of ever expanding core knowledge and the necessity of handling overspecialized disciplines in medical education. In *Proceedings of ITAB 2006: IEEE International Special Topic Conference on Information Technology in Biomedicine.* Ioannina, Greece: IEEE.

Parepinelli, R. S., Lopes, H. S., & Freitas, A. (2002). An Ant Colony Algorithm for Classification Rule Discovery. In Abbass, H. A., Sarker, R. A., & Newton, C. S. (Eds.), *Data Mining: Heuristic Approach* (pp. 191–208). Hershey, PA: Idea Group Publishing.

Parker, K. R., & Chao, J. T. (2007). Wiki as a teaching tool. *Interdisciplinary Journal of Knowledge and Learning Objects, 3,* 57–72.

Parsons, T. D., & Rizzo, A. A. (2008). Affective outcomes of virtual reality exposure therapy for anxiety and specific phobias: a meta-analysis. *Journal of Behavior Therapy and Experimental Psychiatry, 39*(3), 250–261. doi:10.1016/j.jbtep.2007.07.007

Partners, G. T. (2002). *The Autonomic Computing Report – Characteristics of Self Managing IT Systems.*

Passant, A. (2007). Using Ontologies to Strengthen Folksonomies and Enrich Information Retrieval in Weblogs: Theoretical background and corporate use-case. In *International Conference on Weblogs and Social Media* (ICWSM 2007).

Patel, V. L., & Groen, G. J.The general and specific nature of medical expertise: A critical look. In Ericsson, K. A., & Smith, J. (Eds.), *Toward a general theory of expertise prospects and limits. New York* (pp. 93–125). Cambridge.

Patel, V. L., Kushniruk, A. W., Yang, S., & Yale, J.-F. (2000). Impact of a computer-based patient record system on data collection, knowledge organization, and reasoning. *Journal of the American Medical Informatics Association, 7*(6), 569–585.

Paterson, B. L. (2001). The shifting perspectives model of chronic illness. *Journal of Nursing Scholarship, 33*(1), 21–26. doi:10.1111/j.1547-5069.2001.00021.x

Patients First Review. (2009, January). Retrieved April 10, 2009, from Government of Saskatchewan: http://www.patientfirstreview.ca/

PatientsLikeMe. (n.d.). *PatientsLikeMe: Patients Helping Patients Live Better Every Day*. Retrieved April 10, 2009, from www.Patientslikeme.com

Patrick, J., Wang, Y., & Budd, P. (2007). An automated system for conversion of clinical notes into snomed clinical terminology. In *Proceedings of the fifth Australasian symposium on ACSW frontiers* (pp. 219–226). Darlinghurst, Australia: Australian Computer Society, Inc.

Patterson, E. S., Cook, R. I., & Render, M. L. (2002). Improving patient safety by identifying side effects from introducing bar coding in medication administration. *Journal of the American Medical Informatics Association, 9*(5), 540–553. doi:10.1197/jamia.M1061

Patterson, V. (2005). Teleneurology. *Journal of Telemedicine and Telecare, 11*(2), 55–59. doi:10.1258/1357633053499840

Pautasso, C., Zimmermann, O., & Leymann, F. (2008). RESTful Web Services vs. "Big" Web Services: Making the Right Architectural Decision. WWW 2008 / Refereed Track: Web Engineering - Web Service Deployment Beijing, China

Peleg, M., & Tu, S. W. (2006). Decision Support, Knowledge Representation and Management in Medicine. In Haux, R., & Kulikowski, C. (Eds.), *International Medical Informatics Association (IMIA) Yearbook of Medical Informatics 2006. Schattauer GmbH*. Germany: International Medical Informatics Association.

Peleg, M., Tu, S. W., Bury, J., Ciccarese, P., Fox, J., & Greenes, R. A. (2003). Comparing Computer-Interpretable Guideline Models: A Case-Study Approach. *Journal of the American Medical Informatics Association, 10*(1), 52–68. doi:10.1197/jamia.M1135

Pender, M. P., Lasserre, K., Kruesi, L., Del Mar, C., & Anuradha, S. (2008). Putting Wikipedia to the test: a case study. In *Proceedings of the Special Libraries Association Annual Conference*. Seattle, Washington.

Peng, J., Bhanu, B., & Qing, S. (1999). Probabilistic feature relevance learning for content-based image retrieval. *Computer Vision and Image Understanding, 75*(1-2), 150–164. doi:10.1006/cviu.1999.0770

Pepper, S. (2002). The TAO of Topic Maps.

Percia, L., & Motta, E. (2007). Integrating folksonomies with the Semantic Web. In Lecture Notes in Computer Science, vol. 4519, The Semantic Web: Research and Applications (pp. 624-639). Berlin/Heidelberg: Springer.

Petushi, S., Marker, J., Zhang, J., Zhu, W., Breen, D., & Chen, C. (2008). A visual analytics system for breast tumor evaluation. *Analytical and Quantitative Cytology and Histology, 30*(5), 279–290.

Peyton, L., & Hu, J. (2007). Knowledge Discovery in a Circle of Trust. In Zanasi, A., Brebbia, C., & Ebecken, N. (Eds.), *Data Mining VIII: Data, Text and Web Mining and their Business Applications* (pp. 235–244). Billerica, MA, USA: WIT Press.

Peyton, L., Hu, J., Doshi, C., & Seguin, P. (2007). Addressing privacy in a federated identity management network for e-health. In *Proceedings* of *Eighth World Congress on the Management of eBusiness,* Toronto.

PHIPA. (2004). *Personal Health Information Protection Act*. Government of Ontario, Canada. Retrieved May 1, 2009, from http://www.e-laws.gov.on.ca/html/statutes/english/elaws_statutes_04p03_e.htm

Pickard, B. (2007, June 19). *Hearing on protecting patient privacy in healthcare information systems*. U.S. House of Representatives Committee on Oversight and Government Reform, Subcommittee on Information Policy, Census and National Archives (Testimony of the President of the American Health Information Management Association (AHIMA)). Retrieved November 8, 2008, from http://ahima.org/dc/CommentsTestimony.asp.

PIPEDA. (2000). *The Personal Information Protection and Electronic Documents Act*. Department of Justice, Canada. Retrieved May 1, 2009, from http://laws.justice.gc.ca/en/P-8.6/text.html

Pitsillides, A., Pitsillides, B., Samaras, G., Dikaiakos, M., Christodoulou, E., & Andreou, P. (2004). DITIS: A collaborative virtual medical team for home healthcare of cancer patients. In Istepanian, R. H., Laxminarayan, S., & Pattichis, C. S. (Eds.), *M-Health: Emerging Mobile Health Systems* (pp. 247–266). Springer.

Pitsillides, A., Samaras, G., Dikaiakos, M., & Christodoulou, E. (1999), *DITIS: Collaborative Virtual Medical team for home healthcare of cancer patients*. Conference on the Information Society and Telematics Applications, Catania, Italy, 16-18 April.

Plant, R. T., Murrell, S., & Moreno, H. R. (1994). Prototype decision support system for a differential diagnosis of psychotic, mood, and organic mental disorders: Part II. *Medical Decision Making, 14*, 273–288. doi:10.1177/0272989X9401400310

Podgorelec, V., Kokol, P., Molan Stiglic, M., Heričko, M., & Rozman, I. (2005). Knowledge Discovery with Classification Rules in a Cardiovascular Database. *Computer Methods and Programs in Biomedicine, 80*, S39–S49. doi:10.1016/S0169-2607(05)80005-7

Pokahr, A., Braubach, L., & Lamersdorf, W. (2005). *A BDI architecture for goal deliberation*. Paper presented at the 4th International Conference on Autonomous Agents.

Polanyi, M. (1958, 1998). Personal knowledge. Towards a post critical philosophy. London: Routledge.

Porter, M. E., & Teisberg, E. O. (2006). *Redefining health care*. Boston: Harvard Business School Press.

Porter, R. (Ed.). (2006). *The Cambridge History of Medicine* (1st ed.). Cambridge University Press.

Potts, H. W. (2006). Is e-health progressing faster than e-health researchers? *Journal of Medical Internet Research, 8*(3), e23. Retrieved March 7, 2009, from http://www.jmir.org/2006/3/e23/

Powell, G. (2006). *Beginning XML Databases*. Wrox.

Powers, M. B., & Emmelkamp, P. M. (2008). Virtual reality exposure therapy for anxiety disorders: A meta-analysis. *Journal of Anxiety Disorders, 22*(3), 561–569. doi:10.1016/j.janxdis.2007.04.006

Preece, J. (2000). *Online Communities: Designing Usability, Supporting Sociability*. Chichester, England: Wiley & Sons Ltd.

Pritchard, L. (2003). Great Scots! *Medical Education, 37*, 493–494. doi:10.1046/j.1365-2923.2003.01529.x

Public Health Agency of Canada. (1999). Measuring Up: A Health Surveillance Update on Canadian Children and Youth (No. 0-662-27888-7): Ottawa: Minister of Public Works and Government Services Canada.

Public Health Agency of Canada. (2002). Canadian Paediatric Society, College of Family Physicians and Canadian Teachers' Federation Call for Urgent Action to Boost Physical Activity Levels in Children and Youth Retrieved June 10, 2008, from http://www.phac-aspc.gc.ca/pau-uap/paguide/child_youth/media/realease.html

Puech, P., Chazard, E., Lemaitre, L., & Beuscart, R. (2007). *DicomWorks Teleradiology: Secure transmission of medical images over the Internet at low cost*. Paper presented at the Engineering in Medicine and Biology Society, 2007. EMBS 2007. 29th Annual International Conference of the IEEE.

Puustjärvi, J. (2004). Integrating e-Learning Systems. *Proc. of the International Conference on Web-Based Education* (pp. 417-421).

Puustjärvi, J., & Pöyry, P. (2003). Searching learning objects from virtual universities. In *Proc. of the International Workshop on Multimedia Technologies in e-Learning and Collaboration (WOMTEC)*.

Puustjärvi, J., & Puustjärvi, L. (2006). The challenges of electronic prescription systems based on semantic web technologies. In *Proc. of the 1st European Conference on eHealth* (pp. 251-261).

Pyper, C., Amery, J., Watson, M., & Crook, C. (2004). Patients' experiences when accessing their on-line electronic patient records in primary care. *The British Journal of General Practice, 54*(498), 38–43.

Pyper, C., Amery, J., Watson, M., Crook, C., & Thomas, B. (2002). Patients' access to their online electronic health records. *Journal of Telemedicine and Telecare, 2*, 103–105. doi:10.1258/135763302320302244

Qayami, A. K., & Qayami, T. (1999). Computer-assisted learning: cyperPatient™ - A step in the future of surgical education. *Journal of Investigative Surgery, 12*, 307–317. doi:10.1080/089419399272296

Qi, H., & Snyder, W. E. (1999). Content-based image retrieval in picture archiving and communications systems. *Journal of Digital Imaging, 12*(2Suppl 1), 81–83. doi:10.1007/BF03168763

Quinlan, J. R. (1986). Induction of deciscion trees. *Machine Learning, 1*(1), 81–106. doi:10.1007/BF00116251

Quinlan, J. R. (1987). Generating production rules from decision trees. In *International Joint Conference on Artificial Intelligence: Vol. 1. Knowledge Representation* (pp. 304-307). San Francisco: CA: Morgan Kaufmann.

Quinlan, J. R. (1993). *C4.5: Programs for Machine Learning*. San Francisco, CA: Morgan Kaufmann.

Quinlan, K. M., & Ã…kerlind, G. S. (2000). Factors affecting departmental peer collaboration for faculty development: Two cases in context. *Higher Education, 40*(1), 23–52. doi:10.1023/A:1004096306094

Quteishat, A., Peng Lim, C., Tweedale, J., & Jain, L. C. (2009). A neural network-based multi-agent classifier system. *Neurocomputing, 72*(7-9), 1639–1647. doi:10.1016/j.neucom.2008.08.012

Rabinowitz, E. (1999). Is there a doctor in the house? *Managed Care (Langhorne, Pa.), 8*(9), 42–44.

Rakotomamonjy, A. (2003). Variable Selection Using SVM-based Criteria. *Journal of Machine Learning Research, 3*(7/8).

Ralston, J. D., Carrell, D., Reid, R., Anderson, M., Moran, M., & Hereford, J. (2007). Patient Web Services Integrated with a Shared Medical Record: Patient Use and Satisfaction. *Journal of the American Medical Informatics Association, 14*(6), 798–806. doi:10.1197/jamia.M2302

Rath, H. (2003). *The Topic Maps Handbook: empolis GmbH*. Germany: Gutersloh.

Raymond, E. (1999). *The Cathedral and the Bazaar*. Sebastapol, CA: O'Reilly Media.

RDFS. (2000). *Resource Description Framework (RDF) Schema Specification 1.0*. Retrieved April 22, 2009, from http://www.w3.org/TR/2000/CR-rdf-schema-20000327/

Recordon, D., & Reed, D. (2006), OpenID 2.0: a platform for user-centric identity management. In *Proceedings of the Second ACM Workshop on Digital Identity Management* (pp. 11-16). Alexandria, Virginia, USA. DIM '06. ACM, New York, NY, 11-16.

Reddy, K. S., Shah, B., Varghese, C., & Ramadoss, A. (2005). Responding to the threat of chronic diseases in India.(Author abstract)(Report). *The Lancet, 366*(9498), 1744(1746).

Reddy, R., Jagannathan, V., Srinivas, K., Karinthi, R., Reddy, S. M., Gollapudy, C., & Friedman, S. (1993). *ARTEMIS: a collaborative framework for health care*. Paper presented at the Annual Symposium on Computer Application [sic] in Medical Care.

Reed, D. (2009, 2009/01/27). *Reed's law - Wikipedia, the free encyclopedia*. Retrieved 11/02/09, from http://en.wikipedia.org/w/index.php?title=Reed%27s_law&oldid=266758174.

Reese, S. (2007, June 1). The value of PHRs depends on the quality of data inputs. *Managed Healthcare Executive*. Retrieved December 14, 2008, from http://www.managedhealthcareexecutive.com.

Rehank, D. R., Dodds, P., & Lannom, L. (2005). A model and infrastructure for federated learning content repositories. In *Proceedings of the 14th International World Wide Web Conference, Chiba, Japan: W3C et al.*

Reid, R. J., & Wagner, E. H. (2008). Strengthening primary care with better transfer of information. *Canadian Medical Association Journal, 179*(10), 987–988. doi:10.1503/cmaj.081483

Reif, G., et al. (2001). A Web-based peer-to-peer architecture for collaborative nomadic working. *10th IEEE Workshops on Enabling Technologies: Infrastructures for Collaborative Enterprises (WETICE 2001), Boston, MA, USA* (pp. 334-339).

Reiher, P., Popek, J., Gunter, M., Salomone, J., & Ratner, D. (1996). Peer-to-Peer Reconciliation Based Replication for Mobile Computers. In *Proceedings of the European Conference on Object Oriented Programming 2nd Workshop on Mobility and Replication, June*.

Reiner, B. I., & Siegel, E. L. (2006). Introduction to RIS and PACS. In Dreyer, K. J., Hirschorn, D. S., Thrall, J. H., & Mehta, A. (Eds.), *PACS. A guide to the digital revolution* (2nd ed., pp. 27–44). New York: Springer.

Renahy, E., Parizot, I., & Chauvin, P. (2008). Health information seeking on the Internet: a double divide? Results from a representative survey in the Paris metropolitan area, France, 2005-2006. *BMC Public Health, Feb 21, 8*(1), 69.

Reponen, J., Niinimäki, J., Kumpulainen, T., Ilkko, E., Karttunen, A., & Jartti, P. (2005). *Mobile teleradiology with smartphone terminals as a part of a multimedia electronic patient record*. Paper presented at the CARS 2005: Computer Assisted Radiology and Surgery.

Retrieved May 1, 2009, from http://doi.ieeecomputersociety.org/10.1109/MCETECH.2008.22

Rhee, M. Y. (2003). *Internet Security: Cryptographic Principles, Algorithms and Protocols*. Wiley.

Rheingold, H. (1993). *The virtual community: Homesteading on the electronic frontier*. Reading, MA: Addison-Wesley.

Rheingold, H. (2001, July). Face-to-Face with Virtual Communities. *Campus Technology, 14*, 8–12.

Riaño, D. (2007). The SDA* Model: A Set Theory Approach In P. Kokol, V. Podgorelec, M. Dušanka, M. Zorman & M. Verlic (Eds.), *Proc. of the 20th IEEE International Symposium on Computer-Based Medical Systems, IEEE CBMS 2007* (pp. 563-568). Maribor, Slovenia.

Riaño, D., Real, F., Campana, F., Ercolani, S., & Annicchiarico, R. (2009). An Ontology for the Care of the Elder at Home In C. Combi, Y. Shahar & A. Abu-Hanna (Eds.), *Proc. of the 12th Conference on Artificial Intelligence in Medicine, AIME 2009* (pp. 235-239). Verona, Italy.

Richman, W. L., Kiesler, S., Weisband, S., & Drasgow, F. (1999). A meta-analytic study of social desirability distortion in computer-administered questionnaires, and interviews. *The Journal of Applied Psychology, 84*, 754–775. doi:10.1037/0021-9010.84.5.754

Richter, J., Anderson-Inman, L., & Frisbee, M. (August, 2007). *Critical engagement of teachers in second life: Progress in the SaLamander project.* Paper presented at the meeting of the Second Life Educator's Communities Conference, Chicago, IL.

Riva, G. (2000). From telehealth to e-health: Internet and distributed virtual reality in health care. *Cyberpsychology & Behavior, 3*, 989–998. doi:10.1089/109493100452255

Riva, G. (2004). Immersive Virtual Telepresence: virtual reality meets eHealth. *Studies in Health Technology and Informatics, 99*, 255–262.

Riva, G. (2005). Virtual reality in psychotherapy [review]. *Cyberpsychology & Behavior, 8*(3), 220–230, discussion 231–240. doi:10.1089/cpb.2005.8.220

Riva, G. (2007). Virtual reality and telepresence. *Science, 318*(5854), 1240–1242. doi:10.1126/science.318.5854.1240d

Riva, G. (2009). Interreality: A new paradigm for E-health. *Studies in Health Technology and Informatics,* 144.

Riva, G., & Davide, F. (Eds.). (2003). *Being there: concepts, effects and measurements of user presence in synthetic environments.* Amsterdam, The Netherlands: IOS Press.

Riva, G., Anguera, M. T., Wiederhold, B. K., & Mantovani, F. (Eds.). (2006). *From Communication to Presence: Cognition, Emotions and Culture towards the Ultimate Communicative Experience.* Amsterdam: IOS Press.

Riva, G., Mantovani, F., Capideville, C. S., Preziosa, A., Morganti, F., & Villani, D. (2007). Affective interactions using virtual reality: the link between presence and emotions. *Cyberpsychology & Behavior, 10*(1), 45–56. doi:10.1089/cpb.2006.9993

Robbins, S. (2006, August). *"Image Slippage": Navigating the Dichotomies of an Academic Identity in a Non-academic Virtual World.* Paper presented at the meeting of the Second Life Educator's Communities Conference, San Fransisco, CA.

Robbins, S. (2007). *A Futurist's View of Second Life Education: A Developing Taxonomy of Digital Spaces.* Paper presented at the meeting of the Second Life Educator's Communities Conference, Chicago, IL.

Robert, M.E., Lamps, L., & Lauwers, G.Y., & Association of Directors of Anatomic and Surgical Pathology. (2008). Recommendations for the reporting of gastric carcinoma. *Human Pathology, 39*(1), 9–14. doi:10.1016/j.humpath.2007.05.024

Robertson, L., Smith, M., & Tannenbaum, D. (2005). Case management and adherence to an online disease management system. *Journal of Telemedicine and Telecare, 11*(Suppl 2), S73–S75. doi:10.1258/135763305775124885

Robertson, L., Smith, M., Castle, D., & Tannenbaum, D. (2006). Using the Internet to enhance the treatment of depression. *Australasian Psychiatry, 14*, 413–417.

Robinson, K. S. (2003). Online Bidding Fills Nursing Jobs. HRMagazine. Alexandria, 44.

Rodden, T. (1991). A Survey of CSCW Systems. *Interacting with Computers, 3*(3), 319–353. doi:10.1016/0953-5438(91)90020-3

Rogers, E. M. (2003). *Diffusion of innovations* (5th ed.). New York: Free Press.

Rogova, G., Stomper, P., & Ke, C.-C. (1999). *Microcalcification texture analysis in a hybrid system for computer-aided mammography.* Paper presented at the Medical Imaging: Image Processing.

Rojo, M. G. (2009). *Standards in digital pathology and telepathology. IHE-Pathology.* Retrieved February 18, 2009, from http://www.conganat.org/digital/index.htm#ihe

Rojo, M. G., Gallardo, A. J., González, L., Peces, C., Murillo, C., González, J., & Sacristán, J. (2008). Reading virtual slide using web viewers: results of subjective experience with three different solutions. *Diagnostic Pathology, 3*(Suppl 1), S23. doi:10.1186/1746-1596-3-S1-S23

Rojo, M. G., Garcia, G. B., Mateos, C. P., Garcia, J. G., & Vicente, M. C. (2006). Critical comparison of 31 commercially available digital slide systems in pathology. *International Journal of Surgical Pathology, 14*(4), 285–305. doi:10.1177/1066896906292274

Romanosky, S., et al. (2005). *Privacy Patterns for Online Interactions*. Paper presented at Plop 2005, Monticello, Illinois, Sept. 7-10, 2005.

Romm, C., Pliskin, N., & Clarke, R. (1997). Virtual Communities and Society: Toward an Integrative Three Phase Model. *International Journal of Information Management, 17*(4), 261–270. doi:10.1016/S0268-4012(97)00004-2

Rosenbloom, S. T., Brown, S. H., Froehling, D., Bauer, B. A., Wahner-Roedler, D. L., Gregg, W. M., & Elkin, P. L. (2009). Using SNOMED CT to represent two interface terminologies. *Journal of the American Medical Informatics Association, 16*(1), 81–88. doi:10.1197/jamia.M2694

Rosenbloom, S. T., Miller, R. A., & Johnson, K. B. (2006). Interface terminologies: facilitating direct entry of clinical data into electronic health record systems. *Journal of the American Medical Informatics Association, 13*(3), 277–288. doi:10.1197/jamia.M1957

Rossille, D., Laurentc, J.-F., & Burguna, A. (2005). Modelling a decision-support system for oncology using rule-based and case-based reasoning methodologies. *International Journal of Medical Informatics, 74*(2), 299–306. doi:10.1016/j.ijmedinf.2004.06.005

Rotheram-Borus, M. J., & Flannery, N. D. (2004). Interventions that are CURRES: costeffective, useful, realistic, robust, evolving, and sustainable. In Rehmschmidt, H., Belfer, M., & Goodyer, I. M. (Eds.), *Facilitating pathways: care, treatment, and prevention in child and adolescent health*. New York: Springer.

Rothwell, D., & Côté, R. (1996). Managing Information with SNOMED: Understanding the Model. *SCAMC*, 80-83.

Rourke, J. T. B. (2002). Building the new Northern Ontario Rural Medical School. *The Australian Journal of Rural Health, 10*, 112–116.

Rubner, Y., Tomasi, C., & Guibas, L. J. (1998). *A metric for distributions with applications to image databases*. Paper presented at the Sixth International Conference on Computer Vision, 1998.

Rui, Y., & Huang, T. S. (1998). Relevance feedback: A power tool for interactive content-based image retrieval.

IEEE Transactions on Circuits and Systems for Video Technology, 8(5).

Ruiz Fernandez, D., & Soriano Paya, A. (2009). A Distributed Approach of a Clinical Decision Support System Based on Cooperation. In Olla, P., & Tan, J. (Eds.), *Mobile Health Solutions for Biomedical Applications* (pp. 92–110). Hershey, PA: IGI Global.

Ruiz, D., Soriano, A., Montejo, C. A., & Bueno, A. (2006). *Ubiquitous diagnosis: assurance through distribution and collaboration*. Paper presented at the Pervasive Health Conference 2006.

Russell, S. J., & Norvig, P. (2003). *Artificial Intelligence: A Modern Approach* (2nd ed.). Prentice Hall.

Russell, T. L. (2001). *The no significant difference phenomenon*. Montgomery, USA: IDECC.

Rutten, L., Arorab, N., Bakosc, A., Azizb, N., & Rowland, J. (2005). Information needs and sources of information among cancer patients: a systematic review of research (1980-2003). *Patient Education and Counseling, 57*(3), 250–261. doi:10.1016/j.pec.2004.06.006

Ruttenberg, A., Clark, T., Bug, W., Samwald, M., Bodenreider, O., & Chen, H. (2007). Advancing translational research with the Semantic Web. *BMC Bioinformatics, 8*(Suppl 3), S2. doi:10.1186/1471-2105-8-S3-S2

Saba, V. K. (1989). *Nursing Information Systems. Classification systems for describing nursing practice: working papers* (pp. 55–61). American Nurses Association.

Sait. S. M., & Youssef, H. (1999). *General Iterative Algorithms for Combinatorial Optimization*. Los Alamitos, California, USA: IEEE Computer Society.

Samaras, G., & Pitsillides, A. (1997). Client/Intercept: a Computational Model for Wireless Environments. In *Proceedings of the 4th International Conference on Telecommunications (ICT'97), Melbourne, Australia, April*.

Sampat, M. P., Markey, M. K., & Bovik, A. C. (2005). Computer-aided detection and diagnosis in mammography. In Bovik, A. C. (Ed.), *Handbook of Image and Video Processing* (2nd ed., pp. 1195–1217). Elsevier. doi:10.1016/B978-012119792-6/50130-3

San Martin-Rodriguez, L., Beaulieu, M. D., D'Amour, D., & Ferrada-Videla, M. (2005). The determinants of successful collaboration: a review of theoretical and empirical studies. *J Interprof Care, 19*(Suppl 1)\, 132-147.

Sandars, J., & Haythornthwaite, C. (2007). New horizons for e-learning in medical education: ecological and

Web 2.0 perspectives. *Medical Teacher, 29*(4), 307–310. doi:10.1080/01421590601176406

Sandars, J., & Schroter, S. (2007). Web 2.0 technologies for undergraduate and postgraduate medical education: an online survey. *Postgraduate Medical Journal, 83*, 759–762. doi:10.1136/pgmj.2007.063123

Sandars, J., Homer, M., Pell, G., & Croker, T. (2008). Web 2.0 and social software: the medical student way of e-learning. *Medical Teacher, 83*(986), 759–762.

Sandelowski, M. (1991). Combining qualitative and quantitative sampling, data collection and analysis techniques in mixed-method studies. *Research in Nursing & Health, 23*, 2046–2255.

Santos, L. O. B. S., Guizzardi, R. S. S., & Sinderen, M. v. (2005). *Agent-oriented context-aware platforms supporting communities of practice in health care.* Paper presented at the Proceedings of the fourth international joint conference on Autonomous agents and multiagent systems, The Netherlands.

Sarasohn-Kahn, J. (2008). *The Wisdom of Patients. California Healthcare Foundation.* Oakland: California Healthcare Foundation.

Sarma, A., Dong, X., & Halevy, A. (2008, June). Bootstrapping pay-as-you-go data integration systems. In *Proceedings of ACM SIGMOD International Conference on Management of Data.*

Saskatchewan Health Quality Council. (2007). *Finding the Time to Shorten the Wait Time for Patients.* Retrieved January 23, 2009, from Health Quality Council: https://www.hqc.sk.ca/portal.jsp;jsessionid=uyam4ycbc1?1VJ YfSwJTephIZ3btQ6RJTBIzBf0QfLQkUwK4QBZaJt C0GkpNuk4YFVvI5thiwzu

Saskatchewan Surgical Care Network. (n.d.). Retrieved April 15, 2009, from Government of Saskatchewan: http://www.sasksurgery.ca/

Sato, K. (2007). Mobile communications in Japan. In T. Sawai (Ed.), Telepathology in Japan. Development and practice (pp. 232-234). Morioka, Iwate, Japan: Celc, Inc.

Sattar, K. (2007). A Sustainable Model for Use of ICTs in Rural Pakistan. *International Journal of Education and Development using Information and Communication Technology, 3*, 89-97. Retrieved October 30, 2008 from http://proquest.umi.com/pqdweb?did=1409299671&Fmt =4&clientId=11263&RQT=309&VName=PQD

Sawai, T. (2007). A survey of telepathology in the public hospitals of Iwate prefecture. In T. Sawai (Ed.), Telepathology in Japan. Development and practice (pp. 105-109). Morioka, Iwate, Japan: Celc, Inc.

Sawai, T. (2007). The state of telepathology in Japan. In T. Sawai (Ed.), Telepathology in Japan. Development and practice (pp. 3-9). Morioka, Iwate, Japan: Celc, Inc.

Schaffert, S., Bischof, D., Buerger, T., Gruber, A., Hilzensauer, W., & Schaffert, S. (2006). Learning with semantic wikis. In *Proceedings of the First Workshop on Semantic Wikis – From Wiki To Semantics (SemWiki2006)* (pp.109-123). Budva, Montenegro.

Schiffbauer, J., O'Brien, J. B., Timmons, B. K., & Kiarie, W. N. (2008). The Role of Leadership in HRH Development in Challenging Public Health Settings. *Human Resources for Health, 6*, 23. Retrieved October 30, 2008 from http://www.human-resources-health.com/content/pdf/1478-4491-6-23.pdf

Schmidt, H. G., Vermeulen, L., & van der Molen, H. T. (2006). Longterm effects of problem-based learning: a comparison of competencies acquired by graduates of a problem-based and a conventional medical school. *Medical Education, 40*(6), 562–567. doi:10.1111/j.1365-2929.2006.02483.x

Schmidt, K., & Bannon, L. (1992). Taking CSCW seriously. [CSCW]. *Computer Supported Cooperative Work, 1*(1). doi:10.1007/BF00752449

Schoenburg, R. (2005). Security of Healthcare Information Systems. In D. Lewis, G. Eysenbach, R. Kukafka, P. Z. Stavri & H. Jimison (Eds.), Consumer Health Informatics. New York: Springer Science+Business Media Inc.

Schott, G., & Hodgetts, D. (2006). Health and digital gaming: the benefits of a community of practice. *Journal of Health Psychology, 11*, 309–316. doi:10.1177/1359105306061189

Schroeder, R. (2002). *The Social Life of Avatars.* New York: Springer.

Schuable, L., & Glaser, R. (Eds.). (1996). Innovations in learning. New Jersey: Mahwah.

Schubert, P., & Hampe, J. F. (2005). *Business Models for Mobile Communities.* Paper presented at the 38th Annual Hawaii International Conference on System Sciences(HICSS '05).

Schumacher, M. (2002). *Security Patterns and Security Standards - With Selected Security Patterns for Anonymity and Privacy.* Paper presented at European Conference on Pattern Languages of Programs, (EuroPLoP), 2002

Scott, R. E., & Saeed, A. (2008). Global eHealth–Measuring Outcomes: Why, What, and How. Report commissioned by WHO's Global Observatory for eHealth. Retrieved March 6, 2009, from http://www.eHealth-connection.org/files/conf-materials/Global%20eHealth%20-%20Measuring%20Outcomes_0.pdf

Scoville, S. A., & Buskirk, T. D. (2007). Traditional and virtual microscopy compared experimentally in a classroom setting. *Clinical Anatomy (New York, N.Y.)*, *20*(5), 565–570. doi:10.1002/ca.20440

Scuvee-Moreau, J., Kurz, X., & Dresse, A. (2002). National dementia economic study group. The economic impact of dementia in Belgium: results of the National Dementia Economic Study (NADES). *Acta Neurologica Belgica*, *102*(3), 104–113.

Secretariat of the Commission for Environmental Cooperation (CEC). (2006). *Toxic Chemicals and Children's Health in North America*. Montreal: Commission for Environmental Cooperation.

Seeman, N. (2008). Inside the Health Blogosphere: Quality, Governance and the New Innovation Leaders. *ElectronicHealthcare*, *7*(3), 101–108.

Setness, P. (2003). When privacy and the public good collide. Does the collection of health data for research harm individual patients? *Postgraduate Medicine*, *113*(5), 15. doi:10.3810/pgm.2003.05.1418

Shachak, A., Hadas-dayagi, M., Ziv, A., & Reis, S. (2009). Primary care physicians' use of an electronic medical record system: A cognitive task analysis. *Journal of General Internal Medicine*, *24*(3), 341–348. doi:10.1007/s11606-008-0892-6

Shadish, W. R., Cook, T. D., & Campbell, D. T. (2002). *Experimental and quasiexperimental design for generalized causal inference*. Boston, MA: Houghton Mifflin.

Shahar, Y., Young, O., Shalom, E., Galperin, M., Mayaffit, A., Moskovitch, R., & Hessing, A. (2004). A Framework for a Distributed, Hybrid, Multiple-Ontology Clinical-Guideline Library and Automated Guideline-Support Tools. *Journal of Biomedical Informatics*, *37*(5), 325–344. doi:10.1016/j.jbi.2004.07.001

Shamian, J. (1988). The effect of the teaching of decision analysis on student nurses' clinical intervention decision making. Unpublished doctorial dissertation. Case Western Reserve University, Clevland, Ohio.

Shapiro, J. S., Kannry, J., Lipton, M., Goldberg, E., Conocenti, P., & Stuard, S. (2006, October). Approaches to Patient Health Information Exchange and Their Impact on Emergency Medicine. *Annals of Emergency Medicine*, *48*(4), 426–432. doi:10.1016/j.annemergmed.2006.03.032

Shaw, A. (2009, March). *Telus Purchases MyChart from Sunnybrook*. Retrieved April 21, 2009, from Canadian Healthcare Technology: www.canhealth.com/mar09.html#09marstory1

Shaw, N. T. (2002, May). 'CHEATS': a generic information communication technology (ICT) evaluation framework. [PMID: 11922936]. *Computers in Biology and Medicine*, *32*(3), 209–220. doi:10.1016/S0010-4825(02)00016-1

Shearer, C. (2000). The CRISP-DM model: the new blueprint for data mining. *Journal of Data Warehousing*, *5*(4), 13–22.

Sheehan, P. W. (1967). A shortened form of Bett's questionnaire upon mental imagery. *Journal of Clinical Psychology*, *23*, 386–389. doi:10.1002/1097-4679(196707)23:3<386::AID-JCLP2270230328>3.0.CO;2-S

Shepitsen, A., Gemmel, J., Mobasher, B., & Burke, R. (2008). Personalized Recommendation in Social Tagging Systems Using Hierarchical Clustering. In J.A. Konstan (Ed.), *2nd ACM Conference on Recommender Systems* (pp. 259–266). New York: ACM.

Sheppard, L., & Mackintosh, S. (1998). Technology in education: what is appropriate for rural and remote allied health professionals? *Aust J Rural Health*, *6*, 189-193. Retrieved November 9, 2008 from http://www3.interscience.wiley.com/journal/119830096/abstract

Shi, J., & Malik, J. (2000). REGULAR PAPERS - Perceptual Grouping - Normalized Cuts and Image Segmentation. *IEEE Transactions on Pattern Analysis and Machine Intelligence*, *22*(8), 18.

Shoham, Y., & Leyton-Brown, K. (2009). *Multiagent Systems. Algorithmic, Game-Theoretic, and Logical Foundations*. Cambridge University Press.

Shortell, S. M., & Kaluzny, A. D. (2006). *Health care management: Organization design and behaviour* (5th ed.). Canada: Thompson Delmar Learning.

Shortliffe, E. H., & Cimino, J. J. (2008). *Biomedical Informatics: Computer Applications in Healthcare and Biomedicine*. New York: Springer.

Shulman, R., Singer, M., Goldstone, J., & Bellingan, G. (2005). Medication errors: A prospective cohort study of hand-written and computerized physician order entry in the intensive care unit. *Critical Care (London, England)*, *9*(8), 516–521. doi:10.1186/cc3793

Shyu, C. R., Brodley, C. E., Kak, A. C., Kosaka, A., Aisen, A., & Broderick, L. S. (1999). ASSERT: A Physician-in-the-loop Content-based Retrieval System for HRCT Image Database. *Computer Vision and Image Understanding*, *75*(1-2), 111–132. doi:10.1006/cviu.1999.0768

Siau, K., & Shen, Z. (2006). Mobile healthcare informatics. *Informatics for Health & Social Care*, *31*(2), 89–99. doi:10.1080/14639230500095651

Siegel, E. L., Reiner, B. I., & Knight, N. (2006). Introduction to RIS and PACS. In Dreyer, K. J., Hirschorn, D. S., Thrall, J. H., & Mehta, A. (Eds.), *PACS. A guide to the digital revolution* (2nd ed., pp. 27–44). New York: Springer.

Silver, B. G., Andonyadis, C., & Morales, A. (1998). Web-based healthcare agents; the case of reminders and to-dos. *Artificial Intelligence in Medicine*, *14*(3), 295–316. doi:10.1016/S0933-3657(98)00039-6

Simpson, J. A., & Weiner, E. S. C. (1989). *Collaboration. Oxford English Dictionary* (2nd ed.). Oxford University Press.

Siriwardena, A. N., Lawson, S., Vahl, M., Middleton, H., & de Zeeuv, G. (2008). Emerging technologies for developing and improving patients' health experience. *Quality in Primary Care*, *16*, 1–5.

Sixsmith, A., & Johnson, N. (2004). A Smart Sensor to Detect the Falls of the Elderly. *IEEE Pervasive Computing / IEEE Computer Society [and] IEEE Communications Society*, *3*(2), 42–47. doi:10.1109/MPRV.2004.1316817

Skiba, D. J. (2006). Web 2.0: next great thing or just marketing hype? *Nursing Education Perspectives*, *27*(4), 212–214.

Sklansky, J., Tao, E. Y., Bazargan, M., Ornes, C. J., Murchison, R. C., & Teklehaimanot, S. (2000). Computer-aided, case-based diagnosis of mammographic regions of interest containing microcalcifications. *Academic Radiology*, *7*(6), 395–405. doi:10.1016/S1076-6332(00)80379-7

Smedley, B. D., Stith, A. Y., & Nelson, A. R. (2003). *Unequal Treatment; Confronting Racial and Ethnic Disparities in Healthcare*. Washington, DC: National Academies Press.

Smeulders, A. W. M., & Worring, M. (2000). Content-Based Image Retrieval at the End of the Early Years. *IEEE Transactions on Pattern Analysis and Machine Intelligence*, *22*(12). doi:10.1109/34.895972

Smith, A. (2007). Telepaediatrics. *Journal of Telemedicine and Telecare*, *13*(4), 163–166. doi:10.1258/135763307780908021

Smith, B., & Ceusters, W. (2006). HL7 RIM: An incoherent standard. *Studies in Health Technology and Informatics*, *124*, 133.

Smith, G. (2006). Introduction to RIS and PACS. In Dreyer, K. J., Hirschorn, D. S., Thrall, J. H., & Mehta, A. (Eds.), *PACS. A guide to the digital revolution* (2nd ed., pp. 9–25). New York: Springer.

Smith, M.K., Welty, C., & McGuinness, D.L. (2004, February). *OWL Web Ontology Language Guide*. W3C Recommendation.

Smith, R. (1996). What clinical information do doctors need? *BMJ (Clinical Research Ed.)*, *313*, 1062–1068.

Smith, T., Orleans, C., & Jenkins, C. (2004). Prevention and Health Promotion: Decades of Progress, New Challenges, and an Emerging Agenda. *Health Psychology*, *23*(2), 126–131. doi:10.1037/0278-6133.23.2.126

SNOMED-CT. (n.d.). http://www.nlm.nih.gov/research/umls/Snomed/snomed_main.html.

Soenksen, D. G. (2005). A fully integrated virtual microscopy system for analysis and discovery. In J. Gu, R.W. Ogilvie, R.W. (Eds.), Virtual microscopy and virtual slides in teaching, diagnosis, and research. Series Advances in Pathology, Microscopy & Molecular Morphology. (pp. 35-47). Boca Ratón, FL: Taylor & Francis.

Sollazzo, T., Handschuh, S., Staab, S., & Frank, M. (2002). *Semantic Web Service Architecture -- Evolving Web Service Standards toward the Semantic Web*. Paper presented at the the15th International FLAIRS Conference, Pensacola, Florida.

Solomonides, T. (Eds.). (2005). *From Grid to Healthgrid: Prospects and Requirements*. IOS Press.

Somol, P., Pudil, P., & Kittler, J. (2004). Fast Branch & Bound Algorithms for Optimal Feature Selection. *IEEE Transactions on Pattern Analysis and Machine Intelligence*, *26*(7). doi:10.1109/TPAMI.2004.28

Spackman, K., & Campbell, K. (1998). Compositional concept using SNOMED: towards further convergence of clinical terminologies. *J Am Med Inform Assoc Annual Symposium*; 740-744.

SPARQL. (2008). *SPARQL Query Language for RDF*. Retrieved April 22, 2009, from http://www.w3.org/TR/rdf-sparql-query/

Spaulding, W. B. (1969). The undergraduate medical curriculum (1969 model): McMaster University. *Canadian Medical Association Journal, 100*(14), 659–664.

Specia, L., & Motta, E. (2007) Integrating Folksonomies with the Semantic Web. In *European Semantic Web Conference* (ESWC 2007), *The Semantic Web: Research and Applications* (LNCS 4519, pp. 624-639). Springer Verlag.

Spitzer, R. L., Kroenke, K., Linzer, M., Hahn, S. R., Williams, J. B., & deGruy, F. V. III (1995). Health-related quality of life in primary care patients with mental disorders. Results from the PRIME-MD 1000 Study. *JAMA: The Journal of the American Medical Association, 274*, 1511–1517. doi:10.1001/jama.274.19.1511

Spyglass Consulting (2006). *Spyglass Studies the Current State of Mobile Communications Adoption by Clinicians.* Marietta, GA: Spyglass Consulting Group.

Spyrou, C., Samaras, G., Pitoura, E., & Evripidou, P. (2004). Mobile agents for wireless computing: the convergence of wireless computational models with mobile-agent technologies. *Mobile Networks and Applications, 9*(5), 517–528. doi:10.1023/B:MONE.0000034705.10830.b7

Staab, S., Schnurr, H., Studer, R., & Sure, Y. (2001). Knowledge process and ontologies. *IEEE Intelligent Systems, 16*(1), 26–34. doi:10.1109/5254.912382

Starfield, B. (2007). Pathways of influence on equity in health. *Social Science & Medicine, 64*(7), 1355–1362. doi:10.1016/j.socscimed.2006.11.027

Steuer, J. S. (1992). Defining virtual reality: dimensions determining telepresence. *The Journal of Communication, 42*(4), 73–93. doi:10.1111/j.1460-2466.1992.tb00812.x

Stevens, V. J., Funk, K. L., Brantley, P. J., Erlinger, T. P., Myers, V. H., & Champagne, C. M. (2008). Design and implementation of an interactive website to support long-term maintenance of weight loss. *Journal of Medical Internet Research, 10*, e1. doi:10.2196/jmir.931

Strickland, R. N., & Hee II, H. (1996). Wavelet transforms for detecting microcalcifications in mammograms. *Medical Imaging. IEEE Transactions on, 15*(2), 218–229.

Studer, R., Benjamins, V. R., & Fensel, D. (1998). Knowledge Engineering: Principles and Methods. *IEEE Transactions on Knowledge and Data Engineering, 25*(1-2), 161–197.

Stumme, G., Hotho, A., & Berendt, B. (2006). Semantic Web Mining: State of the art and future directions. *Web Semantics: Science. Services and Agents on the World Wide Web, 4*(2), 124. doi:10.1016/j.websem.2006.02.001

Sturmberg, J. P., & Martin, C. M. (2008). Knowing--in medicine. *Journal of Evaluation in Clinical Practice, 14*(5), 767–770.

Su, Z., Zhang, H., Li, S., & Ma, S. (2003). Relevance feedback in content-based image retrieval: Bayesian framework, feature subspaces, and progressive learning. *IEEE Transactions on Image Processing, 12*(8), 924–937. doi:10.1109/TIP.2003.815254

Sulaiman, R., Sharma, D., Ma, W., & Tran, D. (2007). A Multi-agent Security Framwork for e-Health Services. In *Knowledge-Based Intelligent Information and Engineering Systems* (Vol. 4693). Springer. doi:10.1007/978-3-540-74827-4_69

Sung, M., Marci, C., & Pentland, A. (2005). Wearable feedback systems for rehabilitation. *Journal of Neuroengineering and Rehabilitation, 2*, 17. doi:10.1186/1743-0003-2-17

Sutton, D. R., & Fox, J. (2003). The syntax and semantics of the PROforma guideline modeling language. *Journal of the American Medical Informatics Association, 10*(5), 433–443. doi:10.1197/jamia.M1264

Swett, H. A., & Miller, P. I. (1987). ICON: a computer-based approach to differential diagnosis in radiology. *Radiology, 163*, 555–558.

Swett, H. A., Fisher, P. R., Cohn, A. I., Miller, P. I., & Mutalik, P. G. (1989). Expert system controlled image display. *Radiology, 172*, 487–493.

Swett, H. A., Mutalik, P. G., Neklesa, V. P., Horvath, L., Lee, C., & Richter, J. (1998). Voice-activated retrieval of mammography reference images. *Journal of Digital Imaging, 11*(2), 65–73. doi:10.1007/BF03168728

Tagare, H. D., Jaffe, C. C., & Duncan, J. (1997). Medical image databases: a content-based retrieval approach. *Journal of the American Medical Informatics Association, 4*(3), 184–198.

Tahir, M. A., Bouridane, A., Kurugollu, F., & Amira, A. (2005). A Novel Prostate Cancer Classification Technique Using Intermediate Memory Tabu Search. *EURASIP Journal on Applied Signal Processing*, (14): 2241–2249. doi:10.1155/ASP.2005.2241

Talmon, J., Ammenwerth, E., Brender, J., de Keizer, N., Nykänen, P., & Rigby, M. (2008). STARE-HI—Statement on reporting of evaluation studies in Health Informatics. *International Journal of Medical Informatics, 78*(1), 1. doi:10.1016/j.ijmedinf.2008.09.002

Tan, A., Freeman, D. H. Jr, Goodwin, J. S., & Freeman, J. L. (2006). Variation in false-positive rates of mammography reading among 1067 radiologists: a population-based assessment. *Breast Cancer Research and Treatment, 100*(3), 309–318. doi:10.1007/s10549-006-9252-6

Tan, H., & Ng, J. (2006). Googling for a Diagnosis - Use of Google as a Diagnostic Aid: Internet Based Study. *British Medical Journal*, 1143–1145.

Tan, J. (2005). *The Next Health Care Frontier*. San Francisco: Jossey-Bass.

Tan, J. (Ed.). (2005). *E-health care information systems: an introduction for students and professionals* (1st ed.). San Francisco, USA: Jossey-Bass.

Tan, L. T. (1995). National patient master index in Singapore. *International Journal of Bio-Medical Computing, 40*(2), 89–93. doi:10.1016/0020-7101(95)01130-7

Tang, H., & Ng, J.H.K. (2006). Googling for a diagnosis – use of Google as a diagnostic aid: internet based study. *British Medical Journal, 2;333*(7579), 1143-1145.

Tang, P. C., Ash, J. S., Bates, D. W., Overhage, J. M., & Sands, D. Z. (2006). Personal health records: definitions, benefits, and strategies for overcoming barriers to adoption. *Journal of the American Medical Informatics Association, 13*(2), 121–126. doi:10.1197/jamia.M2025

Tanne, J. (2007). Google launches free Electronic Health Records service for patients. *British Medical Journal, 336*, 1207. doi:10.1136/bmj.a208

Tapscott, D., & Williams, A. (2006). *Wikinomics: How Mass Collaboration Changes Everything*. Toronto: Penguin Group.

Tara, M. (2007). Development and evaluation of a knowledge requirements engineering model to support design of a quality knowledge-intensive eHealth application. Canada, Victoria.

Tatemura, J., Sawires, A., Po, O., Chen, S., Candun, K., Agrawal, D., & Goveas, M. (2007). Mashup feeds: continuous queries over Web services. In *Proceedings of ACM SIGMOD International Conference on the Management of Data* (pp. 1128-1130). Beijing, China.

Taylor, P., Fox, J., & Pokropek, A. (1999). The development and evaluation of CADMIUM: a prototype system to assist in the interpretation of mammograms. *Medical Image Analysis, 3*, 321–337. doi:10.1016/S1361-8415(99)80027-9

Taylor, Y., Eliasson, A., Andrada, T., Kristo, D., & Howard, R. (2006). The role of telemedicine in CPAP compliance for patients with obstructive sleep apnea syndrome. *Sleep and Breathing, 10*(3), 132–138. doi:10.1007/s11325-006-0059-9

te Brake, G. M., Karssemeijer, N., & Hendriks, J. H. (2000). An automatic method to discriminate malignant masses from normal tissue in digital mammograms. *Physics in Medicine and Biology, 45*(10), 2843–2857. doi:10.1088/0031-9155/45/10/308

Telus Health. (2009). Telus Health Solutions. Retrieved May 1, 2009, http://telushealth.com

Temesgen, Z., Knappe-Langworthy, J. E., Marie, M. M. S., Smith, B. A., & Dierkhising, R. A. (2006). Comprehensive Health Enhancement Support System (CHESS) for People with HIV Infection. *AIDS and Behavior, 10*(1), 35–40. doi:10.1007/s10461-005-9026-x

Tennenhouse, D. L., Smith, J. M., Sincoskie, W. D., & Minden, G. J. (1996). A Survey of Active Network Research. *Journal IEEE Communication Magazine, 35*(1), 80–86. doi:10.1109/35.568214

The Association of American Physicians and Surgeons. (n.d.). Doctors Lie to Protect Patient Privacy–Poll Survey. Retrieved from http://www.aapsonline.org/press/nrnewpoll.html

The Center for Health Enhancement Systems Studies. (2008). Comprehensive Health Enhancement Support System. Retrieved October 15, 2008, from https://chess.wisc.edu/chess/home/home.aspx

The Center for Information Technology Leadership. (n.d.). *The Value of Personal Health Record*s. Retrieved January 7, 2009, from http://www.citl.org/_pdf/CITL_PHR_Report.pdf

The Gene Ontology Consortium. (2000). Gene Ontology: tool for the unification of biology. *Nature Genetics, 25*, 25–29. doi:10.1038/75556

The National Committee on Vital and Health Statistics. (n.d.). *A Strategy for Building the National Health Information Infrastructure (NHII)*. Retrieved January 21, 2009, from http://aspe.hhs.gov/sp/NHII/Documents/NHIIReport2001/default.htm.

Thirion, B., Loosli, G., Douyere, M., & Darmoni, S. J. (2003). Metadata element set in a quality-controlled subject gateway: a step to a health semantic Web. *Studies in Health Technology and Informatics, 95*, 707–712.

Thomsen, E. (2002). *OLAP Solutions: Building Multidimensional Information Systems.* New York: John Wiley & Sons, Inc.

Tiwana, A. (2000). From Intuition to Institution: Supporting Collaborative Diagnoses in Telemedicine Teams. In *Proceedings of the 33rd Hawaii International Conference on System Sciences.*

Tobias, J., Chilukuri, R., Komatsoulis, G. A., Mohanty, S., Sioutos, N., & Warzel, D. B. (2006). The CAP cancer protocols-a case study of caCORE based data standards implementation to integrate with the Cancer Biomedical Informatics Grid. *BMC Medical Informatics and Decision Making, 6*(25).

Tobin, K. W., Abramoff, M. D., Chaum, E., Giancardo, L., Govindasamy, V. P., Karnowski, T. P., et al. (2008). *Using a patient image archive to diagnose retinopathy.* Paper presented at the Engineering in Medicine and Biology Society, 2008. EMBS 2008. 30th Annual International Conference of the IEEE.

Tofukuji, I. (2007). Current implementations of telepathology. In T. Sawai (Ed.), Telepathology in Japan. Development and practice (pp. 39-42). Morioka, Iwate, Japan: Celc, Inc.

Tofukuji, I. (2007). Electronic medical records and the Integrating the Healthcare Enterprise initiative. In T. Sawai (Ed.), Telepathology in Japan. Development and practice (pp. 235-238). Morioka, Iwate, Japan: Celc, Inc.

Tofukuji, I. (2007). Virtual slides and telepathology. In T. Sawai (Ed.), Telepathology in Japan. Development and practice (pp. 223-226). Morioka, Iwate, Japan: Celc, Inc.

Tompa, E. (2002). The Impact of Health on Productivity: Empirical Evidence and Policy Implications. In Banting, K., Sharpe, A., & St-Hilaire, F. (Eds.), *Review of Economic Performance and Social Progress* (*Vol. 2,* pp. 181–202). Centre for the Study of Living Standards and the Institute for Research on Public Policy.

Tonkin, E. (2005). Making the case for a wiki. *Ariadne,* 42. Retrieved November 14, 2008, from http://www.ariadne.ac.uk/issue42/tonkin/

TopicMaps.Org. (n.d.). XML Topic Maps (XTM) 1.0.

Topps, D. (2005). *Implementing an EMR across multiple academic family medicine teaching sites.* Calgary: University of Calgary.

Topps, D., Evans, R., Khan, L., & Hays, R. B. (2004). *Personal Digital Assistants in Vocational Training (Adobe PDF).* Townsville, Queensland: James Cook University.

Topps, D., Thomas, R., & Crutcher, R. (2003). Introducing personal digital assistants to family physician teachers. *Family Medicine, 35*(1), 55–59.

Toro-Troconis, M., Mellström, U., Partridge, M., Meeran, K., Barrett, M., & Higham, J. (2008, July). Designing game-based learning activities for virtual patients in Second Life. *Journal of CyberTherapy & Rehabilitation, 1*(3), 227–239. Retrieved February 28, 2009 from http://www.elearningimperial.com/SL/J-CyberTherapy-Rehab_Toro-Troconis_V04.pdf

Toro-Troconis, M., Partridge, M., Barrett, M., & Mellström, U. (2008, July). Game-based learning for the delivery of virtual patients in Second Life. *The Academy Subject Centre for Medicine, Dentistry and Veterinary Medicine Newsletter, 1*(17). Retrieved February 28, 2009 from http://www.medev.ac.uk/external_files/pdfs/01_newsletter/0117_lo_res.pdf

Toro-Troconis, M., Partridge, M., Mellström, U., Meeran, K., & Higham, J. (2008, July). Technical infrastructure and initial findings in the design and delivery of game-based learning for virtual patients in Second Life. In *Proceedings of Researching Learning in Virtual Environments.* Milton Keynes: The Open University. Retrieved February 28, 2009 from http://www.elearningimperial.com/SL/ReLIVE_paper_Maria_Toro_Troconis_V03.pdf

Tot, T. (2005). Correlating the ground truth of mammographic histology with the success or failure of imaging. *Technology in Cancer Research & Treatment, 4*(1), 23–28.

Tourassi, G. D., Harrawood, B., Singh, S., Lo, J. Y., & Floyd, C. E. (2007). Evaluation of information-theoretic similarity measures for content-based retrieval and detection of masses in mammograms. *Medical Physics, 34*(1), 140–150. doi:10.1118/1.2401667

Tourassi, G. D., Ike, R. III, Singh, S., & Harrawood, B. (2008). Evaluating the effect of image preprocessing on an information-theoretic CAD system in mammography. *Academic Radiology, 15*(5), 626–634. doi:10.1016/j.acra.2007.12.013

Tourassi, G. D., Vargas-Voracek, R., Catarious, D. M. Jr, & Floyd, C. E. Jr. (2003). Computer-assisted detection of mammographic masses: a template matching scheme based on mutual information. *Medical Physics, 30*(8), 2123–2130. doi:10.1118/1.1589494

Trentin, G. (2009). Using a wiki to evaluate individual contribution to a collaborative learning project. *Journal of Computer Assisted Learning, 25*(1), 43–55. doi:10.1111/j.1365-2729.2008.00276.x

Trivedi, M. H., Daly, E. J., Kern, J. K., Grannemann, B. D., Sunderajan, P., & Claassen, C. A. (2009). Barriers to implementation of a computerized decision support system for depression: an observational report on lessons learned in "real world" clinical settings. *BMC Medical Informatics and Decision Making, 9,* 6. doi:10.1186/1472-6947-9-6

Trivedi, M. H., Kern, J. K., Grannemann, B. D., Altshuler, K. Z., & Sunderajan, P. (2004). A computerized clinical decision support system as a means of implementing depression guidelines. *Psychiatric Services (Washington, D.C.), 55,* 879–885. doi:10.1176/appi.ps.55.8.879

TriZetto. (n.d.). http://integratedhealth.trizetto.com/main/pages/TriZetto/IHMX/ShowCollateral.aspx?oid =26955&ssid=0&hid=0&sid=0&cp=1950.

Tsuchihashi, Y., Takamatsu, T., Hashimoto, Y., Takashima, T., Nakano, K., & Fujita, S. (2008). Use of virtual slide system for quick frozen intra-operative telepathology diagnosis in Kyoto, Japan. *Diagnostic Pathology, 3*(Suppl 1), S6. doi:10.1186/1746-1596-3-S1-S6

Tuchinda, R., Szekely, P., & Knoblock, C. A. (2008). *Building Mashups by example.* Paper presented at the 13th international conference on Intelligent user interfaces, Gran Canaria, Spain.

Tufano, J. T., & Karras, B. T. (2005). Mobile eHealth interventions for obesity: a timely opportunity to leverage convergence trends. *Journal of Medical Internet Research, 7,* e58. doi:10.2196/jmir.7.5.e58

Tulu, B., & Chatterjee, S. (2005). A Taxonomy of Telemedicine Efforts with respect to Applications, Infrastructure, Delivery Tools, Type of Setting and Purpose. *38th Hawaii International Conference on System Sciences* (pp. 147.2).

Tuominen, V. J., & Isola, J. (2009). Linking whole-slide microscope images with DICOM by using JPEG2000 Interactive Protocol. [Epub ahead of print]. *Journal of Digital Imaging,* (May): 5.

Tweedale, J., Ichalkaranje, N., Sioutis, C., Jarvis, B., Consoli, A., & Phillips-Wren, G. (2007). Innovations in multi-agent systems. *Journal of Network and Computer Applications, 30*(3), 1089–1115. doi:10.1016/j.jnca.2006.04.005

U.S. Department of Health and Human Services. (2006, February). Personal Health Records and Personal Health Record Systems: A Report and Recommendations from the National Committee on Vital and Health Statistics. *National Cancer Institute, National Institutes of Health, and National Center for Health Statistics, Centers for Disease Control and Prevention.* Retrieved July 3, 2008, from http://www.ncvhs.hhs.gov/0602nhiirpt.pdf.

U.S. National Library of Medicine. (2009). Unified Medical Language System, Bethesda, MD: National Institutes of Health. Retrieved February 20, 2009, from http://www.nlm.nih.gov/research/umls/

U.S. National Library of Medicine. (n.d.). *National Center for Biotechnology Information.* Retrieved April 12, 2008, from PubMed: www.pubmed.gov

Uauy, R., Albala, C., & Kain, J. (2001). Obesity Trends in Latin America: Transiting from Under- to Overweight. *The Journal of Nutrition, 131*(3), 893S–899.

Ullman, J., & Widom, J. (1998). *Principles of Database Systems.* Prentice Hall.

United Nations. (2005). *Information Economy Report.* Paper presented at the United Nations Conference on trade and Development.

Unutzer, J., Choi, Y., Cook, I. A., & Oishi, S. (2002). A web-based data management system to improve care for depression in a multicenter clinical trial. *Psychiatric Services (Washington, D.C.), 53,* 671–673, 678. doi:10.1176/appi.ps.53.6.671

Urbain, J. L. (2005). Breast cancer screening, diagnostic accuracy and health care policies. *Canadian Medical Association Journal, 172*(2), 210–211. doi:10.1503/cmaj.1041498

Urowitz, S., & Deber, D. (2008). How Consumerist Do People Want to Be? Preferred Role in Decision-Making of Individuals with HIV/AIDS. *Health Policy (Amsterdam), 3*(3).

Urowitz, S., Wiljer, D., Apatu, E., Eysenbach, G., DeLenardo, C., Harth, T., et al. (2008). Is Canada ready for patient accessible electronic health records? A national scan. *Journal, 8.* Retrieved from http://www.pubmedcentral.nih.gov/articlerender.fcgi?tool=pubmed&pubmedid=18652695

Ustinova, A. (2008). Developers compete at Facebook conference. San Francisco Chronicle. Retrieved March 7, 2009, from http://www.sfgate.com/cgi-bin/article.cgi?f=/c/a/2008/07/23/BU7C11TAES.DTL

Vafaie, H., & Imam, I. (1994). *Feature selection methods: Genetic algorithms vs. greedy-like search.* Paper presented at the International Conference on Fuzzy and Intelligent Control Systems.

Vaidya, J., & Clifton, C. (2004). *Privacy-preserving data mining: why, how, and what for?* IEEE Security & Privacy.

van Bemmel, J. H., & Musen, M. A. (Eds.). (1997). *Handbook of Medical Informatics* (1st ed.). Houten, the Netherlands: Springer-Verlag.

van der Bijl, N. (1998). Security of information in trusts. *Health Informatics Journal*, 4(3-4), 210–215. doi:10.1177/146045829800400312

Van Rensburg, D., Steyn, F., Schneider, H., & Loffstadt, L. (2008). Human Resource Development and Antiretroviral Treatment in Free State Province, South Africa. *Human Resources for Health*, 6, 15. Retrieved October 28, 2008 from http://www.human-resources-health.com/content/6/1/15

Vander Wal, T. (2007). *Folksonomy*. Retrieved February 2, 2007, from http://vanderwal.net/folksonomy.html.

Vandervalk, B. P., McCarthy, E. L., & Wilkinson, M. D. (2009). Moby and Moby 2: Creatures of the Deep (Web). *Briefings in Bioinformatics*, 10(2), 114–128. doi:10.1093/bib/bbn051

Vannier, M. W., & Summers, R. M. (2003). Sharing images. *Radiology*, 228(1), 23–25. doi:10.1148/radiol.2281021654

Vapnik, V. (1998). *Statistical Learning Theory*. New York: Wiley.

Venkatasubramanian, K., & Gupta, S. (2007). Security Solutions for Pervasive Healthcare. In Security in Distributed, Grid, Mobile, and Pervasive Computing (pp.349-366).

Venkatesh, V., Morris, M. G., Davis, G. B., & Davis, F. D. (2003). User Acceptance of Information Technology: Toward a Unified View. *Management Information Systems Quarterly*, 27(3), 425–478.

Verdicchio, M., & Colombetti, M. (2009). Communication languages for multiagent systems. *Computational Intelligence*, 25(2), 136–159. doi:10.1111/j.1467-8640.2009.00333.x

Verizon Communications, Inc. (2007, May 9). *Verizon CEO announces implementation of new online personal health records program for company employees*. Press release. May 9, 2007. Retrieved December 19, 2008, from http://newscenter.verizon.com/press-releases/verizon/2007/verizon-ceo-announces.html.

Versel, N. (2008). Health 2.0. Will its promise be realized? *Managed Care (Langhorne, Pa.)*, 17(3), 49–52.

Vian, T., Richards, S. C., McCoy, K., Connelly, P., & Feeley, F. (2007). Public-Private Partnerships to Build Human Capacity in Low Income Countries: Findings from the Pfizer Program. *Human Resources for Health*, 5, 8-19. Retrieved November 18, 2008 from http://www.human-resources-health.com/content/5/1/8

Vicente, K. (2004). *The Human Factor*. Toronto: Vintage Canada.

Vilamovska, A. M., & Hatziandreu, E. Schindler, H.R., van Oranje-Nassau, C., de Vries, H., & Krapels, J. (2009). Study on the requirements and options for RFID application in healthcare: Identifying areas for Radio Frequency Identification deployment in healthcare delivery: A review of relevant literature. Rand Europe, European Commission. Retrieved May 4, 2009 from http://www.rand.org/pubs/technical_reports/TR608/

Vimarlund, V., & Olve, N. G. (2005). Economic analyses for ICT in elderly healthcare: questions and challenges. *Health Informatics Journal*, 11(4), 309–321. doi:10.1177/1460458205058758

Vitacca, M., Mazzù, M., & Scalvini, S. (2009). Sociotechnical and organizational challenges to wider e-Health implementation. *Chronic Respiratory Disease*, 6, 91–97. doi:10.1177/1479972309102805

Voelker, R. (2003). Virtual patients help medical students link basic science with clinical care. *Journal of the American Medical Association*, 290, 1700–1701. doi:10.1001/jama.290.13.1700

Vogel, L. H., & Perreault, L. E. (2006). Management of Information in Healthcare Organizations. In Edward, H., & Cimino, J. J. (Eds.), *Biomedical Informatics; Computer Applications in Health Care and Biomedicine* (pp. 476–510). Berlin, Heidelberg: Springer.

Vogt, W. P. (1999). *Dictionary of statistics and methodology* (2nd ed.). Thousand Oaks: Sage.

Vygotsky, L. S. (1978). *Mind Society: the Development of Higher Mental Processes*. Cambridge, MA: Harvard University Press.

W3C (2004). Concepts and Abstract Syntax. *Resource Description Framework (RDF)*. Retrieved June 5, 2009, from http://www.w3.org/TR/rdf-concepts/

W3C (2004). OWL Web Ontology Language. Retrieved from http://www.w3.org/tr/owl-features

Wagner, C.S. & Leydesdorff, L. (2005). *The diffusion of international collaboration and the formation of a core group. Globalisation in the network of science in 2005*.

Walker, A. (1999). South Australia: best practice guidelines for patient master index maintenance. *Health Information Management*, 29(1), 43–45.

Walker, J., Pan, E., Johnston, D., Adler-Milstein, J., Bates, D. W., & Middleton, B. (2005). *The value of health care information exchange and interoperability. Health Affairs* (pp. W5-10–W5-18). Millwood: Web Exclusives.

Wallerstein, N. (2006). *What is the evidence on effectiveness of empowerment to improve health?* Albuquerque: Europe's Health Evidence Network.

Wang, S. S., Green, M., & Malkawi, M. (2002). *Mobile positioning technologies and location services.*

Wangberg, S. C., Andreassen, H. K., Prokosch, H. U., Santana, S. M., Sørensen, T., & Chronaki, C. E. (2008). Relations between Internet use, socio-economic status (SES), social support and subjective health. *Health Promotion International, 23*(1), 70–77. doi:10.1093/heapro/dam039

Ward, J. P. T., Gordon, J., Field, M. J., & Lehmann, H. P. (2001). Communication and information technology in medical education. *Lancet, 357*, 792–796. doi:10.1016/S0140-6736(00)04173-8

Wei, C., Li, C., & Wilson, R. (2006). *A Content-based approach to medical image database retrieval Database Modeling for Industrial Data Management: Emerging Technologies and Applications* (pp. 258–291). Hershey, PA: Idea Group Publishing.

Wei, D., Chan, H. P., Helvie, M. A., Sahiner, B., Petrick, N., & Adler, D. D. (1995). Classification of mass and normal breast tissue on digital mammograms: multiresolution texture analysis. *Medical Physics, 22*(9), 1501–1513. doi:10.1118/1.597418

Wei, L., Yang, Y., Nishikawa, R. M., & Jiang, Y. (2005). A study on several machine-learning methods for classification of malignant and benign clustered microcalcifications. *IEEE Transactions on Medical Imaging, 24*(3), 371–380. doi:10.1109/TMI.2004.842457

Wei, L., Yang, Y., Nishikawa, R. M., Wernick, M. N., & Edwards, A. (2005). Relevance vector machine for automatic detection of clustered microcalcifications. *IEEE Transactions on Medical Imaging, 24*(10), 1278–1285. doi:10.1109/TMI.2005.855435

Wei, L., Yang, Y., Wernick, M. N., & Nishikawa, R. M. (2009). Learning of Perceptual Similarity From Expert Readers for Mammogram Retrieval. *Selected Topics in Signal Processing. IEEE Journal of, 3*(1), 53–61.

Weinstein, R. S., Descour, M. R., Liang, C., Richter, L., Russum, W. C., Goodall, J. F., et al. (2005). Reinvention of light microscopy. Array microscopy and ultrarapidly scanned virtual slides for diagnostic pathology and medical education. In J. Gu, R.W. Ogilvie, R.W. (Eds.), Virtual microscopy and virtual slides in teaching, diagnosis, and research. Series Advances in Pathology, Microscopy & Molecular Morphology. (pp. 10-34). Boca Ratón, FL: Taylor & Francis.

Weise, T., Achler, S., G"ob, M., Voigtmann, C., & Zapf, M. (2007). Evolving Classifiers – Evolutionary Algorithms in Data Mining. [KIS]. *Kasseler Informatikschriften, 2007*, 1–20.

Weiss, S. M., & Kulikowski, C. A. (1991). *Computer Systems that Learn.* San Francisco, CA: Morgan Kaufmann.

Wen, J., & Tan, J. (2005). Mapping e-health strategies: thinking outside the traditional healthcare box. *International Journal of Electronic Healthcare, 1*(3), 261–276. doi:10.1504/IJEH.2005.006474

Wenger, E. (2000). Communities of practice and social learning systems. *Organization, 7*(2), 225–246. doi:10.1177/135050840072002

Wenger, E. (2001). *Etienne Wenger's 2001 study of technology for communities of practice.* Retrieved 11/2/09, from http://www.ewenger.com/tech/.

Westberg, E. E., & Miller, R. A. (1998). The Basis for Using the Internet to Support the Information Needs of Primary Care. *Journal of the American Medical Informatics Association, 6*, 6–25.

Weyns, D., Helleboogh, A., Holvoet, T., & Schumacher, M. (2009). The agent environment in multi-agent systems: A middleware perspective. *Multiagent and Grid Systems -. International Journal (Toronto, Ont.), 5*, 93–108.

White, A. (2006). *Introduction to BPMN,* Retrieved April 22, 2009, from http://www.bpmn.org/Documents/Introduction%20to%20BPMN.pdf

White, J. E. (1996). *Mobile Agents* [General Magic White Paper]. Retrieved from http://www.genmagic.com/agents.

WHO. (2006). Basic Documents. Constitution of the World Health Organization. 45. from http://www.who.int/governance/eb/who_constitution_en.pdf

WHO. (2006, May). *WHO eHealth: standardized terminology.* EXECUTIVE BOARD EB118/8, 118th Session 25, Provisional agenda item 8.4. Retrieved January 13, 2009, from http://apps.who.int/gb/ebwha/pdf_files/EB118/B118_8-en.pdf

Wibulpolprasert, S., & Pengpaibon, P. (2003). Integrated Strategies to Tackle the Inequitable Distribution of doctors in Thailand: Four Decades of Experience. *Human*

Resources for Health, 1, 12. Retrieved November 18, 2008 from http://www.human-resources-health.com/content/1/1/12

Wickramasinghe, N. S., & Fadlalla, A. M. A. (2005). A framework for assessing e-health preparedness. *International Journal of Electronic Healthcare*, *1*(3), 316–334. doi:10.1504/IJEH.2005.006478

Wiecha, J., & Pollard, T. (2004). The Interdisciplinary eHealth Team: Chronic Care for the Future. *Journal of Medical Internet Research*, *6*(3). doi:10.2196/jmir.6.3.e22

Wiederhold, B. K., & Wiederhold, M. D. (2004). *Virtual Reality Therapy for Anxiety Disorders*. American Psychological Association Press.

Wikipedia. (2009, April 06). *Application Programming Interface*. Retrieved May 15, 2009, from Wikipedia: http://en.wikipedia.org/wiki/Application_programming_interface#cite_note-0

Wiklund, H., & Lindh, J. (2005). Development Without Strategy – the case of web-based health care services in Swedish city councils. *International Journal of Public Information Systems*, *1*, 71–80.

Wiljer, D., Bogomilsky, S., Catton, P., Murray, C., Stewart, J., & Minden, M. (2006). Getting results for hematology patients through access to the electronic health record. *Canadian Oncology Nursing Journal*, *16*(3), 154–164.

Wilkinson, R. G. (2007). Comment on: The changing relation between mortality and income. *International Journal of Epidemiology*, *36*(3), 484–490. doi:10.1093/ije/dym077

Wilkinson, R.G. (1997). Socioeconomic determinants of health. Health inequalities: relative or absolute material standards? *British Medical Journal*, *22;314*(7080), 591-5.

Willard, T. (2001). *Helping Knowledge Networks Work*. Winnipeg: International Institute for Sustainable Development.

Williams, P. A. H. (2008). When trust defies common security sense. *Health Informatics Journal*, *14*(3), 211–221. doi:10.1177/1081180X08092831

Williamson, K. B., Kang, Y. P., Steele, J. L., & Gunderman, R. B. (2002). The Art of Asking: Teaching Through Questioning. *Academic Radiology*, *9*(12), 1419–1422. doi:10.1016/S1076-6332(03)80669-4

Wilson, G. (2006) 'No show' hospital patients cost NHS £700m, *Telegraph.co.uk*, retrieved February 23, 2009 from http://www.telegraph.co.uk/news/uknews/1517730/%27No-show%27-hospital-patients-cost-NHS-andpound700m.html

Wilson, P., Bunn, F., & Morgan, J. (2009). A mapping of the evidence on integrated long term condition services. *British Journal of Community Nursing*, *14*, 202–206.

Wilson, P., Petticrew, M., & Booth, A. (2009). After the gold rush? A systematic and critical review of general medical podcasts. *Journal of the Royal Society of Medicine*, *102*(2), 69–74. doi:10.1258/jrsm.2008.080245

Winkelman, W. J., & Choo, C. W. (2003). Provider-Sponsored Virtual Communities for Chronic Patients: Improving Health Outcomes through Organizational Patient-Centred Knowledge Management. *Health Expectations*, *6*(4), 352–259. doi:10.1046/j.1369-7625.2003.00237.x

Women's Health Matters Network. (2008). Retrieved October 15, 2008, from http://www.womenshealthmatters.ca/

WONCA International Classification Committee. (1998). *ICPC-2, International Classification of Primary Care* (2nd ed.). Oxford University Press.

Wong, J., & Hong, J. I. (2007). *Making mashups with marmite: towards end-user programming for the web.* Paper presented at the Human Factors in Computing Systems, San Jose, California, USA

Wooldridge, M. (2000). Intelligent Agents. In Weiss, G. (Ed.), *Multiagent Systems: A Modern Approach to Distributed Artificial Intelligence*. The MIT Press.

Wooldridge, M. (2002). *An Introduction to multiagent systems*. West Sussex, England: John Wiley and Sons, Ltd.

Wootton, R., Craig, J., & Patterson, V. (Eds.). (2006). *Introduction to Telemedicine* (2nd ed.). Rittenhouse Book Distributors.

World Factbook. (2009, March 5, 2009). Retrieved March 10, 2009, from https://www.cia.gov/library/publications/the-world-factbook/print/xx.html

World Health Organization (WHO). (2006) *Building Foundations for eHealth: Progress of Member States: Report of the Global Observatory for eHealth*. Geneva, Switzerland; WHO. Retrieved November 9, 2008 from http://www.who.int/ehealth/resources/bf_full.pdf

World Health Organization. (2003). The World Health Report 2003—Shaping the Future. Geneva, Switzerland: World Health Organization (WHO).

World Health Organization. (2005). Preventing Chronic Disease: A Vital Investment. Geneva, Switzerland: World Health Organization (WHO).

WorldVistA Web site. (n.d.). Retrieved December 11, 2008, from http://www.worldvista.org

Wuerdeman, L., Volk, L., Pizziferri, L., Ruslana, T., Harris, C., Feygin, R., et al. (2005). *How Accurate is Information that Patients Contribute to their Electronic Health Record?* Paper presented at the AMIA 2005.

Wyatt, J. C., & Liu, J. L. Y. (2002). Basic concepts in medical informatics. *Journal of Epidemiology and Community Health, 56*(11), 808–812. doi:10.1136/jech.56.11.808

Wyatt, J., & Sullivan, F. (2005). eHealth and the future: promise or peril? *Journal*. Retrieved from http://www.bmj.com/cgi/content/full/331/7529/1391

Xiao, L., Vicente, J., Saez, C., Gibb, A., Lewis, P., Dasmahapatra, S., et al. (2008). *A Security Model and its Application to a Distributed Decision Support System for Healthcare.* Paper presented at the Third International Conference on Availability, Reliability and Security.

Xiao, Y., & Chen, H. (Eds.). (2008). *Mobile telemedicine: a computing and networking perspective*. Boca Raton: CRC Press.

Xu, Z., Fu, Y., Mao, J., & Su, D. (2006). Towards the Semantic Web: Collaborative Tag Suggestions. In *Workshop on Collaborative Web tagging* (WWW2006).

Xue, Z., Antani, S., Long, L. R., Jeronimo, J., & Thoma, G. R. (2007). Investigating CBIR techniques for cervicographic images. *AMIA... Annual Symposium Proceedings / AMIA Symposium. AMIA Symposium*, 826–830.

Yach, D., Hawkes, C., Gould, C. L., & Hofman, K. J. (2004). The Global Burden of Chronic Diseases: Overcoming Impediments to Prevention and Control. *Journal of the American Medical Association, 291*(21), 2616–2622. doi:10.1001/jama.291.21.2616

Yagi, Y. (2007). *Critical comparison of digital pathology systems*. Retrieved February 16, 2009, from http://www.bioimagene.com/pdfs/Study%20Yagi%20et%20al%20070501.pdf

Yan, H., Jiang, Y., Zheng, J., Peng, C., & Li, Q. (2005). A multilayer perceptron-based medical decision support system for heart disease diagnosis. *Expert Systems with Applications, 30*(2), 272–281. doi:10.1016/j.eswa.2005.07.022

Yang, S. K., Moon, W. K., Cho, N., Park, J. S., Cha, J. H., & Kim, S. M. (2007). Screening mammography-detected cancers: sensitivity of a computer-aided detection system applied to full-field digital mammograms. *Radiology, 244*(1), 104–111. doi:10.1148/radiol.2441060756

Yang, Y. F., Lohmann, P., & Heipke, C. (2008). Genetic algorithms for multi-spectral image classification. In Schiewe, J., & Michel, U. (Eds.), *Geoinformatics paves the Highway to Digital Earth:Festschrift zum 60* (pp. 153–161). Geburtstag von Prof. M. Ehlers.

Yee, G., Korba, L., & Song, R. (2006). Ensuring Privacy for E-Health Service. In *Proceedings of the First International Conference on Availability, Reliability and Security (ARES 2006)*. Vienna, Austria. April, 2006

Yee, N., & Bailenson, J. N. (2007). The Proteus effect: Self transformations in virtual reality.

Yellowlees, P. M., & Cook, J. N. (2006). Education about hallucinations using an internet virtual reality system: a qualitative survey. *Academic Psychiatry, 30*(6), 534–539. doi:10.1176/appi.ap.30.6.534

Young, O., & Shahar, Y. (2005). The Spock System: Developing a Runtime Application Engine for Hybrid-Asbru Guidelines. In S. Miksch, J. Hunter & E. Keravnou (Eds.), *Proc. of the 10th Conference on Artificial Intelligence in Medicine, AIME 2005* (pp. 166-170). Aberdeen, Scotland. Key Terms Medical Informatics, Ubiquitous Health care, Web 2.0 approaches for clinical practice, design and development of ICT methodologies for health care.

Youseff, L., Butrico, M., & Da Silva, D. (2008, Nov. 12-16). Toward a Unified Ontology of Cloud Computing. *Grid Computing Environments Workshop, 2008. GCE, 08*, 1–10.

Yu, S., & Guan, L. (2000). A CAD system for the automatic detection of clustered microcalcifications in digitized mammogram films. *IEEE Transactions on Medical Imaging, 19*(2), 115–126. doi:10.1109/42.836371

Yusuf, S., Reddy, S., Ounpuu, S., & Anand, S. (2001). Global Burden of Cardiovascular Diseases: Part I: General Considerations, the Epidemiologic Transition, Risk Factors, and Impact of Urbanization. *Circulation, 104*(22), 2746–2753. doi:10.1161/hc4601.099487

Zarocostas, J. (2008). World Medical Association scales up training for multidrug resistant tuberculosis to fight epidemic. *BMJ (Clinical Research Ed.), 336*, 1155. doi:10.1136/bmj.39584.662130.DB

Zeineh, J. (2005). Reinvention of light microscopy. (2005). The Trestle Digital Backbone. In J. Gu, R.W. Ogilvie, R.W. (Eds.), *Virtual microscopy and virtual slides in* teaching, diagnosis, and research. Series Advances in Pathology, Microscopy & Molecular Morphology. (pp. 77-96). Boca Ratón, FL: Taylor & Francis.

Zenel, B., & Duchamp, D. (1997). General Purpose Proxies: Solved and Unsolved Problems. In *Proceedings of the Hot-OS VI*.

Zeng, Q. T., & Tse, T. (2006). Exploring and developing consumer health vocabularies. *Journal of the American Medical Informatics Association, 13*(1), 24–29. doi:10.1197/jamia.M1761

Zerhouni, E. (2003). The NIH roadmap. *Science, 302*(5642), 63–72. doi:10.1126/science.1091867

Zhang, C., Xi, J., & Yang, X. (2008). *An architecture for intelligent collaborative systems based on multiagent.* Paper presented at the Computer Supported Cooperative Work in Design. CSCWD 2008.

Zhang, H., & Sun, G. (2002). Feature selection using tabu search method. *Pattern Recognition, 35*(3), 701–711. doi:10.1016/S0031-3203(01)00046-2

Zhao, D. (1993). *Rule-based morphological feature extraction of microcalcifications in mammograms.* Paper presented at the Medical Imaging: Image Processing.

Zheng, B., Lu, A., Hardesty, L. A., Sumkin, J. H., Hakim, C. M., & Ganott, M. A. (2006). A method to improve visual similarity of breast masses for an interactive computer-aided diagnosis environment. *Medical Physics, 33*(1), 111–117. doi:10.1118/1.2143139

Zheng, B., Mello-Thoms, C., Wang, X., & Gur, D. (2007). *Improvement of visual similarity of similar breast masses selected by computer-aided diagnosis schemes.* Paper presented at the 4th IEEE International Symposium on Biomedical Imaging: From Nano to Macro.

Zheng, L., Wetzel, A. W., Gilbertson, J., & Becich, M. J. (2003). Design and analysis of a content-based pathology image retrieval system. *IEEE Transactions on Information Technology in Biomedicine, 7*(4), 249–255. doi:10.1109/TITB.2003.822952

Zhou, M., Bao, S., Wu, X., & Yu, Y. (2007). An Unsupervised Model for Exploring Hierarchical Semantics from Social Annotations. In K. Aberer, K.S. Choi, N. Noy, D. Allemang, K.I. Lee, L.J.B. Nixon, J. Golbeck, P. Mika, D. Maynard, G. Schreiber, & P. Cudré-Mauroux (Eds.) *International Semantic Web Conference* (ISWC 2007) (LNCS 4825, pp. 673-686). Springer Verlag.

Zielinski, K., Duplaga, M., & Ingram, D. (2006). *Information Technology Solutions for Health Care, Health Informatics Series.* Berlin: Springer-Verlag.

About the Contributors

Dr. Sabah Mohammed graduated in 1977 and joined Sony as a maintenance Engineer. In 1979 he joined Glasgow University for his graduate studies where he obtained his Post-Graduate Diploma and Masters in Computing Science. After that he continued his PhD graduate studies in Computer Science at Brunel University, London, UK where his PhD thesis was about developing an intelligent system for designing adaptive computer architectures. After his PhD graduation, Dr. Mohammed joined several academic institutions as Assistant/Associate Professor of Computer Science including (BU, Amman University, Philadelphia University, Applied Science University and HCT). During this period (1986-2001), Dr. Mohammed chaired several Computer Science and Information Systems departments including (Philadelphia University, Applied Science University, HCT). Since late 2001, Dr. Mohammed is full Professor of Computer Science with tenure at Lakehead University, Ontario, Canada. Dr. Mohammed also served as a Visiting Professor at the Laurentian University, Department of Math and Computer Science during winter 2007. Currently Dr. Mohammed is serving also as an Adjunct Research Professor at the University of Western Ontario (2009-2012). Dr. Mohammed has co-authored four text books in Compilers, Artificial Intelligence, Java Programming and Applied Image Processing. Dr. published over 90 refereed publications and was the MSc advisor for 17 students and 1 PhD student. Dr. Mohammed has received research support from a variety of governmental and industrial organizations. Dr. Mohammed organized two international conferences as well as chairing several conference sessions besides being as an IPC member of several notable conferences. Dr. Mohammed is the coordinator of Northern Ontario Web Intelligence research group that was established during 2003. Dr. Mohammed's research interests include Web Intelligence, Ubiquitous Computing, Web-Oriented Architectures, Ambient and Mobile Computing, Image Processing for Ubiquitous Images and Medical Informatics. Dr. Mohammed is the Editor-in-Chief of the Journal of Emerging Technologies in Web Intelligence-Academy Publisher-Finland. Dr. Mohammed is also on the editorial boards of several other journals (e.g. Computer Aided Engineering and Technology- Inderscience, Journal of Universal Computing-Springer, International Journal of Computing and Information Sciences-IJCIS Publishers, International Journal of Network Security- IJNS Publisher, International Journal of Pattern Recognition and Machine Intelligence- International Scientific Publishers and Journal of Computer Science-Academy Publisher). Dr. Mohammed is a member of the British Computer Society, Professional Software Engineer of Ontario, Professional member of the ACM, CIPS and IEEE.

Jinan Fiaidhi is a Tenure Full Professor and Graduate Coordinator at the Department of Computer Science - Lakehead University. She is also Adjunct Research Professor with the University of Western Ontario. She received a Ph.D. degree in Computer Science from Brunel University in 1986, a Post-graduate Diploma in Microprocessors Programming from Essex University in 1983 and a Diploma in

Copyright © 2010, IGI Global, distributing in print or electronic forms without written permission of IGI Global is prohibited.

Engineering Management from the University of Technology in 1978. Her research interest involves Personal Learning Environment, Collaborative Learning, Telemedical Education, Virtual Multimedia Learning Objects, Mobile Learning, Collaborative Learning at the Enterprise Level and at the Web, Applications of Mashups, Widgets and Rich Internet Applications in Learning, Developing Learning Infrastructures (e.g. P2P, Mobile, Wireless, Grid, Web 2.0), Learning Ontologies and Folksonomies, and Learning Reasoners. Dr. Fiaidhi have a long research and teaching experience as she held various academic positions including being a chairperson of the Department of Computer Science-University of Technology. Dr. Fiaidhi research is fully supported by NSERC and CFI research grants. Dr. Fiaidhi authored four books, five chapters in books and over than 100 refereed articles in highly reputed journals and conferences. Dr. Fiaidhi have several notable research achievements which include Virtual SceneBeans, DICOM Based Mobile Infrastructure for Telemedical Learning, Biomedical Semantic Blog, and Ontology Extracting Agent for Telemedical Blogging. Dr. Fiaidhi is a Professional Engineer of Ontario (PEng), a Senior Member of IEEE and member of CIPS, ACM and the BCS.

* * *

Norm Archer, Ph.D. is a Professor Emeritus in the DeGroote School of Business, McMaster University, Canada, and a Special Advisor to the McMaster eBusiness Research Centre. Norm and his graduate students and colleagues are intensively involved in studies of the adoption and use of electronic health records in Canada, identity theft and fraud, and a range of eBusiness issues.

Dr. José Javier Astrain has taught courses including programming, operating systems, ambient intelligence and wireless sensor networks, pattern recognition, database systems and computer networks at Universidad Pública de Navarra. Dr. Astrain holds an M.S. in Telecommunications Engineering from the Universidad Pública de Navarra in 1999 and a Ph.D. in Computer Science from the same university in 2004. He is currently an Assistant Professor of computer science. His current research interests include pattern recognition, semantic web and folksonomies.

Panagiotis D. Bamidis is an Assistant Professor of Medical Education Informatics at the Medical School of Aristotle University of Thessaloniki, Greece. He is a permanent member of the International Committee of the iSHIMR conferences, Editorial Board member of the Health Informatics Journal and the Hippokratia Journal, and a reviewer of the IEEE Transactions on Information Technology in BioMedicine, Computer Methods and Programs in BioMedicine, Personal and Ubiquitous Computing and others. His research interests are within Affective and Physiological Computing and HCI, affective and assistive technologies for the disabled and the elderly, technology enhanced learning in medical education, collaborative learning and content sharing and social educational networks, areas in which he has published over 80 papers in various journals and conference proceedings. He has been the Scientific Co-ordinator of 8 national and international grants, while he is currently the project director for the CIP-PSP Long Lasting Memories/LLM project and the eContentPlus2008 project mEducator.

Dr. Elizabeth Borycki is an Assistant Professor in the School of Health Information Science at the University of Victoria, British Columbia, Canada. Professor Borycki has worked in numerous roles among them Consultant, Disease Management Specialist, Clinical Informatics Specialist, and Researcher. Elizabeth teaches organizational behaviour and change management, systems evaluation, quality improvement, research methods and biomedical fundamentals in the undergraduate and graduate programs at the School of Health Information Science. Her research interests include clinical informatics, change management, health information system implementations, patient safety, project management and information seeking involving health information systems. Elizabeth has co-authored many papers evaluating the effects of health information systems upon information seeking and patient safety. More recently, she has edited a book on the Human, Social and Organizational Aspects of Health Information Systems.

Professor Dr. Andrej Brodnik BSc received his PhD in Computer Science from the University of Waterloo, Ontario, Canada. His main research interests are succinct data structures and efficient algorithms. He is an author of over 100 scientific papers and several international patents. Dr. Brodnik holds a position of Professor at the University of Primorska, and University of Ljubljana, Slovenia, and had a position of Adjoint Professor at the University of Technology, Lulea, Sweden. Before joining University of Primorska he was CTO at ActiveTools, Slovenia. At University of Primorska he served as a vice-rector. He is currently director of Primorska Institute of Natural Sciences and Technology at the University of Primorska. Dr. Brodnik is winner of, among others, "Boris Kidric Foundation" Award (Slovenian national scientific award), Fullbright Scholarship, ITRC/ICR Fellowship, Innovation Cup and IBM Faculty Award. He is member of IEEE and ACM.

Ivan Chorbev was born in Ohrid in the Republic of Macedonia, on April 27, 1980. He received his bachelor degree in computer science, automation and electrical engineering in 2004 and the M.Sci degree in computer science in 2006 from the Faculty of Electrical Engineering and Information Technology, University "St. Cyril and Methodius" in Skopje, R. of Macedonia. He received his PhD in the area of e-medicine and telemedicine at the same university in 2009. His employment experience includes Macedonian Telecommunications - T-Home. Now he teaches C/C++ programming, Computer Graphics, Computer Animation and Web Design at the Faculty of Electrical Engineering and Information Technology in Skopje. His fields of interest include combinatorial optimization, constraint programming, machine learning, web programming technologies, the application of computers in medicine and medical information systems. He is a member of the IEEE.

Eleni Christodoulou is currently a senior researcher in the Computer Science Department of the University of Cyprus carrying out research in the areas eServices (eHealth, eGovernment), collaborative working environments and mobile wireless computing, She gained a Ph.D. in Medical Informatics and she has an over 20 years working experience in the Information Technology business and academia sector both in Germany and Cyprus especially in the provision of consultancy and implementations in the eHealth sector. She has been participating, as an expert and as a project coordinator in over 15 internationally and nationally funded projects and studies, including different IST and eTen projects related to eGovernment and eHealth like: Mpower, HealthService24, LinkCare, MEMO, eUser. She has been the coordinator of the IPE funded DITIS project, which was ranked seventh among over eighty products at the World Summit Award (WSA) Competition in 2003 and among the finalists in the eHealth Ministerial conference 2003.

Dr. Alberto Córdoba has taught courses including software engineering, Web 2.0 and Semantic Web at Universidad Pública de Navarra and Universidad Nacional de Educación a Distancia. His research focus is on object design, Web 2.0, Semantic Web and folksonomies. Dr. Córdoba received the MS degree in physics from the Universidad del País Vasco in 1982 and the PhD degree in physics from the same university in 1991. He is currently an Associate Professor in the Department of Mathematics Engineering and Computer Science. He is member of the ACM.

Christel Daniel (MD, PhD, MCU-PH) is a computer science senior researcher at the department of information systems of the Hospital Europeen Georges Pompidou in Paris, France, and at the French National Institute for Health and Medical Research (INSERM). Dr. Daniel is the editor of the IHE Anatomic Pathology Technical Framework, vol. 1 & 2. She has published multiple papers on the use of virtual slides in pathology, the role of terminologies and ontologies in electronic health records, and the use of medical standards in pathology.

Ivica Dimitrovski was born in Kratovo in the Republic of Macedonia, on December 18, 1981. He received his bachelor and master degrees in computer science, automation and electrical engineering in 2005 and 2008, respectively, from the Faculty of Electrical Engineering and Information Technology, University „St. Cyril and Methodius" in Skopje, R. of Macedonia. Now he is working on his PhD thesis in the area of content-based image retrieval. At present he is a teaching and research assistant at the Faculty of Electrical Engineering and Information Technology in Skopje. His fields of interest include image processing, medical images, machine learning, content-based retrieval of multimedia data and web programming technologies.

D. Francisco Echarte received his MS degree in computer science from the Universidad del País Vasco in 1999. He is currently a PhD student in computer science at the Universidad Pública de Navarra. He is also working as IT specialist at the Healthcare Service of Navarra Government. His current research interests include semantic web, folksonomies and social webs.

Prof. Christo El Morr (PhD Biomedical Engineering, Compiègne University of Technology-France, 1997). He served in computer science and MIS in Lebanon and UAE. He is currently an Assistant Professor of Health Informatics at York University, Canada. His research projects cover healthcare, computer science engineering and social sciences. His research interests are multidisciplinary, they include mainly e-Health, e-Collaboration, Virtual Communities, Software Accessibility for people with Visual Disability, PACS and Health Information Systems integration. He consulted for international organization and served as an Expert Reviewer for the Ministry of Research and Innovation — Ontario, Canada (Ontario Research Fund).

Daniel Ruiz Fernández received his Bachelors degree in Computer Science from the University of Alicante (Spain) in 1998 and his Ph degree in Computer Science from the same university in 2003. Between 1999 and 2004 he worked as a lecturer at the University of Alicante. Since 2004, he has been an Associate Professor in the Department of Computer Technology and Information at the University of Alicante. Additionally, he is a founding member of the IBIS research group of the University of Alicante, and a member of IEEE and Computer Society. He has been a leader of several national projects related to medical informatics and he is also a member of several conferences committees and editorial board member of international publications. His research interests are focused in medical informatics, computer architectures, distributed computing and computer networks.

Andrea Gaggioli is Research Professor of General Psychology and Senior Researcher of the Interactive Communication and Ergonomics of New Technologies — ICE-NET - Lab at the Università Cattolica del Sacro Cuore, and Deputy Head Researcher at the Applied Technology for Neuro-Psychology Laboratory — ATNP-Lab — at the Istituto Auxologico Italiano in Milan, Italy. Gaggioli obtained his M.S. degree in Psychology from University of Bologna and a Ph.D. in Psychobiology from the Faculty of Medicine of the University of Milan. In the past, he collaborated with the Competence Center for Virtual Reality at the Fraunhofer Institute for Industrial Engineering in Stuttgart, Germany. His research goal is to investigate how new technologies can be used to enhance people well-being and promote positive social change.

Marcial García-Rojo (MD, PhD) is the coordinator of information systems of the Hospital General de Ciudad Real, Spain. He is member of the Council of the Spanish Society of Health Informatics (SEIS) and the Spanish Society of Pathology-Spanish Division of the International Academy of Pathology (SEAP-DEAIP), and editor of the Spanish Journal of Pathology (Revista Española de Patología). Main research areas are medical informatics, immunohistochemistry and molecular pathology. He is chair of the European project EURO-TELEPATH, Anatomic Telepathology Network, Action IC0604 of the European Cooperation in the field of Scientific and Technical Research (COST).

Dimosthenis Georgiadis is currently a PhD candidate in the Computer Science of the University of Cyprus. Due to the last years he worked in numerous projects evolved in the eHealth domain. Such projects are DITIS, Linkcare, HS24, mPower and MELCO. During these projects he advanced in user requirements collection, building intelligent web interfaces, carried out surveys, collect and analyze data and conduct interviews and trainings with healthcare professionals. Within the next months he's planning to complete his PhD thesis that is focused in wireless collaboration that is focused in the eHealth domain.

Panagiotis Germanakos is Assistant Professor in the Depart-ment of Management and MIS, University of Nicosia (since 2008). He obtained his PhD from the University of Athens (2008) and his MSc in International Marketing Management from the Leeds University Business School (1999). His B.Sc. was in Computer Science (1998) and also holds a HND Diploma of Technician Engineer in the field of Computer Studies (1996). He is also a Research Scientist, in the Semantic and Cognitive Research Adaptivity Technologies (SCRAT) research group of the Department of Computer Science, University of Cyprus (since 2003) and in the Faculty of Communication & Media Studies, University of Athens (since 2004). His research interest is in Web Adaptation and Personalization Environments and Systems based on user profiling encompassing amongst others visual, cognitive and emotional processes, implemented on desktop and mobile / wireless platforms. He has several publications, including co-edited books, chapters, articles in journals, and conference contributions, including a best student paper award (Adaptive Hypermedia 2008 conference).

Dr. Hamada Ghenniwa is Associate Professor at the University of Western Ontario, and is the head of Cooperative Distributed Systems Engineering Group. Dr. Ghenniwa internationally renowned for his expertise in computational intelligence for coordination and cooperation in distributed "systems" environments. It includes theoretical and engineering foundation of agent-oriented, service-oriented, and Grid computing to improve the "quality" of cooperative distributed systems. Application areas include enterprise integration, electronic business, collaborative manufacturing and complex real-time systems. He published the findings of his research in more than 150 publications in world-class journals, books and conference proceedings. Dr. Ghenniwa's research activities also include industrial R&D in collaboration with industrial partners and government institutes to develop sophisticated system architectures, tools and prototypes that range from mobile physical robots, to integration and collaborative tools, to intelligent manufacturing and business solutions. All of these activities are conducted in three specialized Labs: Distributed Intelligent Systems Lab focuses on complex real-time systems and intelligent manufacturing; Software Engineering Lab focuses on cooperative distributed systems architecture and technologies; EK3 Innovation Lab focuses on information technology & knowledge engineering.

Dr. Candace J. Gibson is an associate professor in the Department of Pathology at the Schulich School of Medicine and Dentistry, the University of Western Ontario, in London, ON. She has been involved in medical research, teaching to undergraduate baccalaureate, medical, nursing and dental students, and administration in the department's graduate and undergraduate degree programs. Over the past decade she has been actively engaged in the introduction of teaching in health informatics as a medical school elective and in the health information management program in the Faculty of Health Sciences. In the latter program she teaches courses in pathology, health informatics and health information management. Her current interests include the development of effective e-learning tools, HI and HIM curriculum development, and the introduction and use of the electronic health record.

Alessandra Gorini was born in 1976 in Milan, Italy, where she obtained her degree in experimental psychology at the Università Vita e Salute San Raffaele. Successively she obtained a master degree in Clinical Neuropsychology at the University of Padova, Italy, and a Master in Affective Neuroscience at the Maastricht University, The Netherlands, where she is actually completing her Ph.D. in Affective Neuroscience. After some years of clinical activities and research on anxiety disorders, now she works at the Applied Technology for Neuro-Psychology Laboratory – ATNP-Lab – at the Istituto Auxologico Italiano in Milan, Italy studying the clinical applications of virtual reality and new technologies for the treatment of anxiety disorders.

W. Ed Hammond is Professor-emeritus, Department of Community and Family Medicine and Professor-emeritus, Department of Biomedical Engineering, Duke University and Adjunct Professor in the Fuqua School of Business at Duke University. He is a Past President of the American Medical Informatics Association (AMIA). He is in his third term as Chair of Health Level 7; he is Co-chair of the Advisory Council; and co-chair of the Clinical Interoperability Council. He was Chair of the Data Standards Working Group of the Connecting for Health Public-Private Consortium. Dr. Hammond was a member of the IOM Committee on Patient Safety Data Standards and a member of the Panel for the evaluation of ONC. He served as President of the American College of Medical Informatics and as Chair of the Computer-based Patient Record Institute. He served as the Convenor of ISO Technical Committee 215, Working Group 2 for 6 years and is currently ISO TC 215's Ambassador to Developing Countries. He is chair of the ISO/CEN/HL7/CDISC/IHTSDO Joint Initiative Council. He is a founding fellow of ACMI and a founding fellow of AIMBE. He was a member of the National Library of Medicine's Long Range Planning Committee (2006) and a member of the Healthcare Information Technology Advisory Panel of the Joint Commission on Accreditation of Healthcare Organizations (2006). He was an advisor to the American Hospital Association Information Technology Standards Initiative Strategy Committee and a member of the Tolven Institute Governing Board. Dr. Hammond was awarded the Paul Ellwood Lifetime Achievement Award in 2003 and the ACMI Morris F. Collen Award of Excellence in November 2003. He has published over 350 technical articles.

Ben Hughes is a researcher at ESADE Business School, examining diverse topics such as open innovation in pharmaceutical companies, knowledge management in consulting companies, or the use of the internet to promote healthcare. He has published related materials in journals such as the Journal Medical Internet Research, the International Journal for Medical Informatics, or R&D management, and has worked as a consultant with McKinsey & Company advising clients in the health care sector on issues around the use of the internet. He holds a Master in Research in Social Science from ESADE Business School, an MBA from HEC Business School, a M.Sci. in Physics from University College London, and is currently completing his PhD at ESADE.

Jun Hu is a systems analyst at Health Canada and a Ph.D. candidate in Computer Science at the University of Ottawa. Her research interests are in application architecture, distributed data mining and privacy. She has a M.Sc. (2006) and B.Sc. (2004) in Computer Science from the University of Ottawa.

David Isern is a researcher of the University Rovira i Virgili's Department of Computer Science and Mathematics. He is also associate professor of the Open University of Catalonia. He received his PhD in Artificial Intelligence (2009) and an MSc (2005) from the Technical University of Catalonia. His research interests are intelligent software agents, distributed systems, user's preferences management, and ontologies, especially applied in healthcare and information retrieval systems. He has been involved in several research projects (National and European), and published several papers and conference contributions.

Boban Joksimoski was born February 3rd 1986 in Skopje, Republic of Macedonia. In 2008 he received his bachelor degree in Information Science, Informatics and Computer Engineering at the Faculty of Electrical Engineering and Information Technology, University "St. Cyril and Methodius" in Skopje, R. of Macedonia. Currently he is continuing his education for his Master Degree at the same faculty. His interests include Computer Graphics, Visualization, Computer Animation, Geographical Information Systems and application of Information Sciences in medicine. Currently he is teaching and research assistant at the Faculty of Informatics, European University – Republic of Macedonia. Other significant work experience includes freelance 2D and 3D graphical artist. He is a member of IEEE.

Erin Jones completed both her undergraduate degree in Psychology, and her Master of Information Studies at the University of Toronto. The early part of her career was spent in research and development of Internet Communication Technologies (ICTs), Knowledge Management, and eLearning solutions at Princess Margaret Hospital – a part of the University Health Network and Canada's premier cancer-treatment facility. At Princess Margaret Hospital, Erin's work focused on human-centred design, needs investigation, and usability testing research, with an eye to encouraging patient empowerment and a client-focused approach to care. Erin is currently with the department of Research and Innovation at George Brown College in Canada, where she specializes in innovations in health technology.

Donald Juzwishin Ph.D. is principal of Juzwishin Consulting Inc. and adjunct associate professor in the Health Information Science program at the University of Victoria. His firm specializes in helping organizations with health reform initiatives and information needs to improve internal processes and serve patients more effectively. Formerly, as the CEO of the Health Council of Canada and as Director of Health Technology Assessment at the Alberta Heritage Foundation for Medical Research, Dr. Juzwishin pioneered methods and tools that help bridge knowledge creation to decision making. He has 30 years of experience in health care working as an administrator, policy maker, researcher and advisor and has served on the Board of the Canadian Agency for Drugs and Technology in Health and the Partners in Health Advisory Board of the Canadian Society for International Health. Dr. Juzwishin has published in the fields of health services administration, policy making, health care politics, accountability and health technology assessment.

Dr. Stefane M. Kabene is a faculty member in the Aubrey Dan Management and Organizational Studies Program with a cross appointment in the Faculty of Health Science at the University of Western Ontario, London, Ontario, Canada. His primary interests are in healthcare, information and communication technology and human resources for health. His focus is in Interprofessional collaborative practice, knowledge transfer, quality of care and patient involvement in clinical decision making. The future of health care lies in health professionals' capacity and willingness to develop new ways of working together for the benefit of the patient. Knowledge and power sharing, role valuing, use of information and communication technology and patients' participation in decision making are only a few of the variables we need to better understand. Dr. Kabene is involved in research projects with the Schulich School of Medicine and Dentistry, the School of Nursing, and the Faculty of Social Sciences.

Eleni Kaldoudi is an Assistant Professor of Physics of Medical Imaging and Telemedicine at the School of Medicine, Democritus University of Thrace, Greece. Her research interests are within medical informatics and telematics, with emphasis on technologies supporting medical education, home care telematics, medical image management, and magnetic resonance imaging, areas in which she has published one book and over 50 papers in various journals and conference proceedings. She is currently acting as an expert in the EU FP7 Programme "Capacities: Regions of Knowledge, Research Potential and Coherent Development of Policies", and has been an Associate Editor in the field of "eLearning" for the journal of IEEE Transactions on Information Technology in Biomedicine. She has been a reviewer in a number of scientific journals and a member of the scientific committee for a number of international conferences in the field of medical informatics and telematics, and a scientific/technical coordinator in 6 national and EU grants.

Lisa King recently completed her Honors BA in Psychology at the University of Western Ontario, London, Ontario, Canada. She hopes to continue her studies in the graduate program in Psychology at UWO. Her interests reside in health psychology and human factors. While completing her degree she was a research assistant in the field of human resources for health and technology working with Dr. Stefane Kabene. This is her first published contribution.

Stathis Konstantinidis has received a Bachelor Degree in Computer Science, University of Crete, Greece, and an MSc in Medical Informatics, Aristotle University of Thessaloniki, Greece. He is currently a PhD Candidate in Medical Education Informatics, Aristotle University of Thessaloniki, Greece, and he is also working as research associate at the Laboratory of Medical Informatics of Medical School of Aristotle University of Thessaloniki and teaching at Technological Educational Institute of West Macedonia, Kozani, Greece.

Dr. Andre Kushniruk is a Professor at the School of Health Information Science at the University of Victoria, British Columbia, Canada. Dr. Kushniruk conducts research in a number of areas including electronic health records, evaluation of the effects of technology, human-computer interaction in health care and other domains as well as cognitive science. His work is known internationally and he has published widely in the area of health informatics. He focuses on developing new methods for the evaluation of information technology and studying human-computer interaction in health care in studies of technology designed for healthcare providers and patients. Dr. Kushniruk has held academic positions at a number of Canadian universities and worked with a number of major hospitals in Canada, the United States and Europe. He holds undergraduate degrees in Psychology and Biology, as well as a M.Sc. in Computer Science and a Ph.D. in Cognitive Psychology.

Dr. Rebecca E. Lee serves as director of the Texas Obesity Research Center in the Department of Health and Human Performance at the University of Houston, and is an associate professor in the Department and holds a courtesy appointment at the University of Texas School of Public Health. She is an editorial board member of the International Journal of Women's Health and the American Journal of Health Promotion. She has authored and co-authored numerous studies in peer-reviewed publications, serves as a charter member on the Community Level Health Promotion Study Section for the Center for Scientific Review at the National Institute of Health, and has received many honors and awards, including the College of Education Research Excellence Award in 2005 and 2008, at the University of Houston, the Award for Outstanding Achievement from the Texas Council on Cardiovascular Disease (CVD) and Stroke, and is a Fellow of the Society of Behavioral Medicine. She is principal investigator for several federally and privately funded research grants including the International Health Challenge in Second Life, funded by the USC Annenberg School for Communication.

Dr. Simon Y. Liu is the Director of Information Systems at the National Library of Medicine, National Institutes of Health. Prior to that, he was the Deputy Director of Information Management and Security at the Department of Justice; the Information Technology Architect at the Treasury Department; and a program manager in the private sector. Dr. Liu has published over 60 book chapters, journal articles, and conference papers. He holds two doctoral degrees in Computer Science and Higher Education Administration; three master degrees in Government, Business Administration, and Computer Science; and a bachelor degree in Mathematics. He is the Associate Editor-in-Chief of the IT Professional magazine published by the Computer Society, the Institute of Electrical and Electronics Engineers.

Suzana Loskovska received the bachelor and master degrees in computer science and automation from the Faculty of Electrical Engineering and Information Technology, University „Ss. Cyril and Methodius", Skopje, R. of Macedonia, in 1989 and 1992, respectively, and the PhD from Technical University of Wien, Wien, Austria in 1995. At present, she is a professor at the Department of Computer Science and Engineering at the Faculty of Electrical Engineering and Information Technology, University „Ss. Cyril and Methodius" in Skopje, R. of Macedonia. Her research interests include programming, visualization, human-computer interaction, virtual reality, medical imaging, modeling and visualization of processes in medical praxis.

Dr. AbdulMutalib Masaud-Wahaishi is an Assistant Professor at the United Arab Emirates University, College of Information Technology Dr. AbdulMutalib received a B.Sc. degree (1986) in Computer Engineering from Al-Fateh University, Tripoli Libya; M. Eng. Sc. (2003) and Ph.D. (2007) degrees in Software Engineering from the University of Western Ontario , Department of Electric and Computer Engineering, London, Canada. His research expertise includes theoretical and engineering foundations of computational intelligence with a special focus on agent-orientation, coordination and cooperation in distributed "systems" environments; Engineering design of agent-oriented, service-oriented (SO), and Grid computing to improve the "quality" of cooperative distributed systems. Application areas include enterprise integration, electronic business and Information gathering. His research has resulted in several publications in world-class conference proceedings. Prior to joining the academia, Dr. AbdulMutalib had more than 14 years of industrial experience. Duties include technical supervision, support and design, and project management.

Assist. Matic Meglič, MD cum lauda is working as Slovene Research Agency Research Fellow at UP PINT, Slovenia, where he is currently finishing his PhD. His research field within eHealth covers novel web based and mobile health care services, patient empowerment and process support for integrated health care and public health. He is a regular presenter or co-author at international conferences (i.e. eHealth, WoHIT, Medicine2.0, EFMI), member of Programme Committee of eHealth2009 as well as editorial and organizational boards of several expert events and publications. He is intensively involved in Slovene national eHealth strategy implementation where he is currently head of Expert Group for National Health Care Portal and member of Health Care Informatics Standardization Board, Teleradiology Council (all at Ministry of Health of the Republic of Slovenia). He is also Cotrugli Business School E-MBA Fellow, CEO of a consulting not-for-profit company and founder of an award winning web2.0 start-up.

Antonio Moreno is a Lecturer at the University Rovira i Virgili's Computer Science and Mathematics Department. He is the founder and head of the ITAKA research group (Intelligent Techniques for Advanced Knowledge Acquisition). His main research interests are the application of agent technology to problems in diverse domains (health care, Tourism) and ontology learning from the Web. He was the coordinator of the Spanish network on agents and multi-agent technology. He has organised several workshops on agents applied in healthcare in the most prestigious international scientific conferences. He has acted as invited editor of special issues in AI Communications, Artificial Intelligence in Medicine and IEEE Intelligent Systems, and he has also edited several books.

Costas Mourlas is Assistant Professor in the National and Kapodistrian University of Athens (Greece), Department of Communication and Media Studies since 2002. He obtained his PhD from the Department of Informatics, University of Athens in 1995 and graduated from the University of Crete in 1988 with a Diploma in Computer Science. In 1998 was an ERCIM fellow for post-doctoral studies through research in STFC, UK. He was employed as Lecturer at the Univeristy of Cyprus, Department of Computer Science from 1999 till 2002. His previous research work focused on distributed multimedia systems with adaptive behaviour, Quality of Service issues, streaming media and the Internet. His current main research interest is in the design and the development of intelligent environments that provide adaptive and personalized context to the users according to their preferences, cognitive characteristics and emotional state. He has several publications including edited books, chapters, articles in journals and conference contributions. Dr. C. Mourlas has taught various undergraduate as well as postgraduate courses in the Dept. of Computer Science of the University of Cyprus and the Dept. of Communication and Media Studies of the University of Athens. Furthermore, he has coordinated and actively participated in numerous national and EU funded projects.

Issam El Naqa received his B.Sc. (1992) and M.Sc. (1995) in Electrical and Communication Engineering from the University of Jordan, Jordan, Ph.D. (2002) in Electrical Engineering from Illinois Institute of Technology, Chicago, IL, USA, and M.A. (2007) in Biology Science from Washington University in St. Louis, St. Louis, MO, USA. He is currently an assistant professor at the department of Radiation Oncology at Washington University School of medicine, St. Louis, MO, USA. He is a member of IEEE, AAPM, and ASTRO. His current research interests include image processing, pattern recognition, machine learning, biomarkers discovery, and treatment outcomes.

Dr. Wail M. Omar is the dean of the Faculty of Computing and Information Technology at Sohar University-Sultanate of Oman. Dr. Omar is the member from grand research committee in Research Council of Oman. Dr. Omar is reviewer for many journals and international conferences. Dr. Omar is member from the Global Digital Literacy Committee (GDLC) in the United State of America. His research interests are in the field of Grid Computing, Service Oriented Architecture, Web Services, Web X, E-Health, Large Scale Enterprise Applications, and monitoring system. Dr. Omar has a Ph.D. in Computing and Software Engineering from Liverpool John Moores University (Liverpool-UK), M.Sc. in Computer Engineering from Al Nahrain University (Baghdad-Iraq), and B.Sc. in Electronic and Communication Engineering from Al Nahrain University (Baghdad-Iraq).

Liam Peyton, Ph.D., P.Eng., is a principal investigator for the Intelligent Data Warehouse laboratory and Associate Professor at the University of Ottawa which he joined in 2002 after spending 10 years as an industry consultant and instructor specializing in business process automation, performance management, and software development methodologies. He has degrees from Aalborg University (Ph.D. 1996), Stanford University (M.Sc. 1989), and McGill University (B.Sc. 1984).

J. Puustjarvi obtained his B.Sc. and M.Sc degree in computer science in 1985 and 1990, respectively, and his PhD.degree in computer science in 1999, all from the University of Helsinki, Finland. Since 2004 he has been a professor of information society technologies. He is also an adjunct professor of eBussines technologies at the Technical University of Helsinki, and an adjunct professor of computer science at the University of Helsinki. His research interests include eLearning, eHealth, eBussines, knowledge management, semantic web and databases.

L. Puustjarvi obtained her M.Sc degree in pharmacy in 1981, and her professional development exam in community pharmacy in 2005, both from the University of Helsinki, Finland. She has worked in several pharmacies as well as in research groups focusing on medicinal information systems. Currently she is pharmacy owner in Kaivopuisto Pharmacy in Helsinki. In addition, she participates in many medicinal researches and advises thesis focusing on medicinal information systems. Her current research interest includes electronic prescriptions, medicinal ontologies and medicinal information systems.

Giuseppe Riva is Associate Professor of General Psychology and Communication Psychology and Director of the Interactive Communication and Ergonomics of New Technologies — ICE-NET - Lab at the Università Cattolica del Sacro Cuore, and Head Researcher of the Applied Technology for Neuro-Psychology Laboratory — ATNP-Lab — at the Istituto Auxologico Italiano in Milan, Italy. Riva conducted several researches and published many papers about methods and assessment tools in psychology and about the use of Virtual Reality in medicine and in training. Member of the New York Academy of Science and the American Psychological Association, Riva is also Associate Editor for the journal "CyberPsychology & Behavior" and Content Editor of the "International Journal of Virtual Reality".

Dr. Samaras is currently a Professor of Computer Science at the University of Cyprus. He was previously at IBM Research Triangle Park, USA and taught at the University of North Carolina at Chapel Hill (adjunct Assistant Professor, 1990-93). He served as the lead architect of IBM's distributed commit architecture (1990-94) and co-authored the final publication of the architecture (IBM Book, SC31-8134-00, September 1994). He was member of IBM's wireless division and participated in the design/architecture of IBM's WebExpress, a wireless Web browsing system. He co-authored a book on data management for mobile computing (Kluwer A.P, 1997). His work on utilizing mobile agents for Web database access has received the best paper award of the 1999 IEEE International Conference on Data Engineering (ICDE'99). He has been invited as a program committee member in most conferences and workshops on mobile databases, mobile commerce and mobile computing. He has a number of patents relating to intelligent user interfaces, transaction processing technology and numerous technical conference and journal publications. Prof. Samaras participates in a number of EU's IST projects related to mobile, wireless computing and tiny devices as the Scientific coordinator of the Cyprus participation.

David Sánchez is a Lecturer at the University Rovira i Virgili's Computer Science and Mathematics Department. He is a member of the ITAKA research group (Intelligent Techniques for Advanced Knowledge Acquisition). His research interests are intelligent agents and ontology learning from the Web. He received a PhD on Artificial Intelligence from UPC (Technical University of Catalonia) in 2008.

Sameer Siddiqi is a Research Assistant in the Texas Obesity Research Center in the Department of Health and Human Performance at the University of Houston and Mayoral Intern in the City of Houston Mayor's Office of Health and Environmental Policy. He has been actively involved in the International Health Challenge in Second Life since its inception, and has significantly contributed to and managed various aspects of its development and ongoing execution. He has co-authored a number of works on Second Life and health interventions in peer-reviewed publications, and has received many honors, including the Barbara Jordan Health Policy Scholars Program Award in 2009.

Daniel Slamanig is a research assistant in the Healthcare Information Technology and Information Security Group at the Carinthia University of Applied Sciences. He holds a MSc degree in Medical Informatics and is currently a PhD student in computer science in the field of cryptography with the System Security Group at the University of Klagenfurt, Austria. His main research interests are applied cryptography and network security and especially cryptographic primitives supporting anonymity and their application in eHealth. He has published numerous papers and articles at national and international conferences and journals. He is a member of the International Association for Cryptologic Research (IACR) and the Austrian Computer Society (OCG).

Albert Solé-Ribalta received the Computer Science Engineering degree and Master in Artificial Intelligence degree, from the Universitat Rovira i Virgili (URV), in 2007. From 2005 to 2008 he was employed at Universitat Rovira i Virgili as a collaborator professor. From 2006 to 2008, he worked on ITAKA research group where he researched in web based interfaces for multi-agent systems. On 2007, with collaboration of IRCV research group, he published some papers about path planning and robot exploration. On 2008, he received a pre-doctoral research grand from Universitat Rovira i Virgili. He is currently researching in structural and syntactical pattern recognition based on graphs, at "Sistemes Sensorials Aplicats a la Indústria" (SSAI) research group with collaboration with Univeristat Politècnica de Catalunya (UPC).

Christian Stingl is a Professor for Healthcare Information Technology and Information Security at the School of Medical Information Technology, Carinthia University of Applied Sciences, Austria. He received his MSc in Mathematics from the University of Klagenfurt, Austria. Subsequently he was a research associate at the University of Klagenfurt where he received his PhD in mathematics in the field of cryptography. After 10 years of international consulting in the field of information systems and being a part time lecturer at the Carinthia University of Applied Sciences he became a Professor at this institution. His research interests include health care information systems and especially information security in context of Electronic and Personal Health Records. Dr. Stingl has published numerous articles and papers in national and international journals and peer reviewed conferences in the aforementioned fields.

Mahmood Tara is a physician and a health informatician, graduating from the University of Victoria, Canada. Mahmood is a fan computer application in improving the quality of healthcare services and medical education. He has been involved in research, teaching and the provision of services in health/medical informatics area since 1993, serving in a wide range of positions from computer technical assistant in the School of Medicine (Mashad University of Medical Sciences-MUMS), co-founder and editor of the Journal of Computer in Medicine (MUMS), to team member of the national initiatives toward "the personal health record for all Canadian citizens" (e-Health group of the National Research Council (NRC) of Canada), and to the founder and director of the Biomedical Informatics Department (MUMS). Dr. Tara's main area of research includes quality health system/software design and electronic knowledge provision.

Dr David Topps is a family physician and currently the Director of Clinical Informatics at the Northern Ontario School of Medicine. He started at NOSM in 2005, along with the charter students, in the first new medical school in Canada in 35 years. He has been working in medical, educational and clinical informatics for over 20 years. Author of the first peer networked electronic medical record in Canada, with novel features such as automatic problem list generation, he has continued to innovate in clinical informatics, and point of care medicine and education. With a varied background in rural, academic and interprofessional care, he brings a breadth of experience to his teaching and research interests. He has presented widely on communication issues, mobile and ubiquitous computing. His current research includes virtual patients, medical simulation and collaborative care support systems.

Sara Urowitz, PhD is the Manager of Educational Informatics at the Princess Margaret Hospital/University Health Network. She is also Assistant Professor in the Department of Psychiatry in the Faculty of Medicine at the University of Toronto. Her portfolio includes leading a national social networking initiative for cancer survivors, www.CaringVoices.ca, which enables survivors to connect from across the country in real-time and through forums. In addition to providing a platform for peer-to-peer support, Caring Voices, provides barrier free access to health care professionals and community organizations. Dr. Urowitz is currently involved in research that explores providing people with access to elements of their electronic health record, coupled with tailored education information. Her interests are focused on understanding how this type of access can activate people to be participants in their own health and wellness, and its impact on the provider-patient relationship.

Laszlo Zsolt Varga is a senior scientific associate and head of the System Development Department at MTA SZTAKI. He was visiting researcher in CERN and in the Department of Electronic Engineering at Queen Mary & Westfield College, University of London where his research focused on basic and applied research into the development of multi-agent systems. His current research interests include agent, grid and web computing for semantic interoperability in scientific and business applications. He has Ph.D. in informatics from the Electronic Engineering and Informatics Faculty of the Technical University of Budapest. He is steering committee member of the Artificial Intelligence Special Interest Group of the John von Neumann Computing Society.

Dr. Jesús Villadangos holds an M.S. in Physics from the Universidad del País Vasco in 1991 and a Ph.D. in Computer Science from the Universidad Pública de Navarra in 1999. He is currently an Associate Professor of Computer Science at the same university. His research focus is on distributed algorithms, and the combination of semantic web and software quality. He is member of the ACM.

Liyang Wei received the B.S. and M.S. from Department of biomedical engineering, Xi'an Jiaotong University (Xi'an, China) in 1998 and 2001, respectively. She received her Ph.D. from Department of biomedical engineering, Illinois institute of technology (Chicago, US) in 2006. Her research interests include medical image analysis, machine learning, pattern recognition and computer-aided diagnosis.

Dr. David Wiljer is the Director of Knowledge Management and eHealth Innovation for Oncology Education and the Radiation Medicine Program at Princess Margaret Hospital/University Health Network. He is also an Assistant Professor and the Director of Continuing Education in the Department of Radiation Oncology in the Faculty of Medicine at the University of Toronto. David is the founding Chair of a national working group, the Canadian Committee for Patient Accessible Health Records (CCPAEHR), dedicated to involving patients in their EHR. He has led the research, development, implementation and assessment of complex informatics initiatives for cancer care. His work includes an online social networking software, Caring Voices, and Infowell, a portal providing patients access to elements of their health record. David received the Cancer Patient Education Network (CPEN) Gold Star Award for his contribution in the field of informatics for patient education.

Yongyi Yang received the B.S.E.E. and M.S.E.E. degrees from Northern Jiaotong University, Beijing, China, in 1985 and 1988, respectively. He received the M.S. degree in applied mathematics and the Ph.D. degree in electrical engineering from Illinois Institute of Technology (IIT), Chicago, in 1992 and 1994, respectively. Dr. Yang is currently on the faculty of the department of electrical and computer engineering at IIT, where he is a Professor. Prior to this position, He was a faculty member with the Institute of Information Science, Northern Jiaotong University. His research interests are in signal and image processing, medical imaging, machine learning, pattern recognition, and biomedical applications. He is a co-author of *Vector Space Projections: A Numerical Approach to Signal and Image Processing, Neural Nets, and Optics*, John Wiley & Sons, Inc., 1998. He is an Associate Editor for the *IEEE Transactions on Image Processing*.

Index

Symbols

3D modeling 423

3-D virtual worlds
532, 536, 538, 545, 547, 549

5th freedom 140

A

Academic Family Health Team 350, 355,
357, 358, 359, 360, 362, 363, 366

access control lists (ACLs) 287

action research model 350

active learning 127, 128, 130, 136, 137,
141, 142, 144, 147

actor agents 378, 381, 382, 385

actor profile ontology (APO)
374, 375, 379, 384, 385, 387

actuators 218

advanced encryption standard (AES) 279

agent-based 370, 373, 378

agent communication languages (ACLs)
217, 224

ameliorate 359

anatomic pathology 457, 458, 459, 460,
461, 463, 466, 467, 468, 470, 471,
472, 473, 474, 475, 479, 480

anonymizer 302, 312, 313, 323

anonymous authentication 285, 288, 291, 292

ant colony optimization (ACO) 114

Ant Miner 114, 118, 120

apomediation 132, 145

application programming interface (API)
132, 384, 437

a priori 227

arbitrator 302, 308, 309, 310, 322

artificial intelligence (AI) 248, 251

ASCII 3

automated image analysis 459, 460, 467

autonomous agent 372, 374

autostainers 459

availability awareness 432

avatars 413, 414, 419, 422, 423, 424, 426,
429, 430

B

beam search 114

Beck depression inventory 401, 402, 403

belief-desire-intention (BDI) 218, 230

benchmarking 342, 344

beta blockers 173

biobanks 459

biomedical knowledge 128

biopsy 487, 489, 490

black box 234

body area networks 393, 406

body sensor networks 406

bottom-up 9, 10

breast imaging reporting and data system (BI-
RADS) 489, 491

brokering agent 313, 317, 318, 319, 325

brokering session 317

business process definition metamodel (BPDM)
396

business process diagram (BPD)
161, 162, 163

business process execution language (BPEL)
161, 164, 396

business process management (BPM)
396, 400, 410

business process modeling notation (BPMN)
161, 164, 165, 396

Copyright © 2010, IGI Global, distributing in print or electronic forms without written permission of IGI Global is prohibited.